Current Vascular Surgery: 2012

Mark K. Eskandari, MD

James S.T. Yao, MD, PhD
Professor of Education in Vascular Surgery
Professor of Radiology and Cardiology
Chief, Division of Vascular Surgery
Department of Surgery
Northwestern University
Feinberg School of Medicine
Chicago, IL

William H. Pearce, MD

Violet R. And Charles A. Baldwin
Professor of Vascular Surgery
Division of Vascular Surgery
Department of Surgery
Northwestern University
Feinberg School of Medicine
Chicago, IL

James S.T. Yao, MD, PhD

Professor Emeritus
Division of Vascular Surgery
Department of Surgery
Northwestern University
Feinberg School of Medicine
Chicago, IL

People's Medical Publishing House-USA
2 Enterprise Drive, Suite 509
Shelton, CT 06484
Tel: 203-402-0646
Fax: 203-402-0854
E-mail: info@pmph-usa.com

PMPH-USA

13 14 15 16/QG/9 8 7 6 5 4 3 2 1

ISBN-13   978-1-60795-175-9
ISBN-10   1-60795-175-4
eISBN-13 978-1-60795-254-1

Printed in the United States by Quad Graphics
Editor: Jason Malley; Copyeditor/Typesetter: diacriTech; Cover designer: Mary McKeon

Library of Congress Cataloging-in-Publication Data

Current vascular surgery 2012 / [edited by] Mark K. Eskandari, William H. Pearce, James S.T. Yao.
    p. ; cm.
Compendium book to the Northwestern University Vascular Symposium.
Includes bibliographical references and index.
ISBN-13: 978-1-60795-175-9
ISBN-10: 1-60795-175-4
ISBN-13: 978-1-60795-254-1 (eISBN)
I. Eskandari, Mark K. II. Pearce, William H. III. Yao, James S. T. IV. Northwestern University Vascular Symposium.
[DNLM: 1. Vascular Surgical Procedures—methods. 2. Surgical Procedures, Minimally Invasive—methods. 3. Vascular Diseases—surgery. WG 170]
LC Classification not assigned

617.4'13—dc23

2012035155

Sales and Distribution

Canada
McGraw-Hill Ryerson Education
Customer Care
300 Water St
Whitby, Ontario L1N 9B6
Canada
Tel: 1-800-565-5758
Fax: 1-800-463-5885
www.mcgrawhill.ca

Foreign Rights
John Scott & Company
International Publisher's Agency
P.O. Box 878
Kimberton, PA 19442
USA
Tel: 610-827-1640
Fax: 610-827-1671

Japan
United Publishers Services Limited
1-32-5 Higashi-Shinagawa
Shinagawa-ku, Tokyo 140-0002
Japan
Tel: 03-5479-7251
Fax: 03-5479-7307
Email: kakimoto@ups.co.jp

United Kingdom, Europe, Middle East, Africa
McGraw Hill Education
Shoppenhangers Road
Maidenhead
Berkshire, SL6 2QL
England
Tel: 44-0-1628-502500
Fax: 44-0-1628-635895
www.mcgraw-hill.co.uk

Singapore, Thailand, Philippines, Indonesia
Vietnam, Pacific Rim, Korea
McGraw-Hill Education
60 Tuas Basin Link
Singapore 638775
Tel: 65-6863-1580
Fax: 65-6862-3354
www.mcgraw-hill.com.sg

Australia, New Zealand
Elsevier Australia
Locked Bag 7500
Chatswood DC NSW 2067
Australia
Tel: 161 (2) 9422-8500
Fax: 161 (2) 9422-8562
www.elsevier.com.au

Brazil
SuperPedido Tecmedd
Beatriz Alves, Foreign Trade
Department
R. Sansao Alves dos Santos, 102 | 7th floor
Brooklin Novo
Sao Paolo 04571-090
Brazil
Tel: 55-16-3512-5539
www.superpedidotecmedd.com.br

*India, Bangladesh, Pakistan, Sri Lanka,
Malaysia*
CBS Publishers
4819/X1 Prahlad Street 24
Ansari Road, Darya Ganj,
New Delhi-110002
India
Tel: 91-11-23266861/67
Fax: 91-11-23266818
Email:cbspubs@vsnl.com

People's Republic of China
People's Medical Publishing House
International Trade Department
No. 19, Pan Jia Yuan Nan Li
Chaoyang District
Beijing 100021
P.R. China
Tel: 8610-67653342
Fax: 8610-67691034
www.pmph.com/en/

Preface

Welcome to our 37th Annual Vascular Symposium sponsored by the Division of Vascular Surgery, Feinberg School of Medicine, Northwestern University. Originally developed by Drs. Bergan and Yao, who currently reside in Chicago, our annual symposium has hosted renowned leaders in vascular surgery who have provided thought provoking and spirited discussions centered on the evolution of vascular and endovascular surgery. Over the years, the program has morphed from a topic oriented program to a more comprehensive overview as developed by Dr. Pearce. This year we have brought together 50 national experts for our 2 ½ day annual meeting to address contemporary topics and controversies in vascular and endovascular surgery. As has been the tradition, presentations cover the full spectrum of vascular surgery including changes in management of extracranial cerebrovascular disease, new treatment options for lower extremity arterial occlusive disease, novel techniques for complex venous disease, as well as recent cutting-edge developments in aortic stent graft repair in the chest and abdomen. In conjunction with the presentations are corresponding chapters found in this hardcover book with more in depth details and "pearls" from the experts. Over the last 3 decades, our symposium has been held at iconic hotels in the heart of Chicago, including the Drake and Fairmont; this year we have again chosen the InterContinental Hotel as the venue for our December Symposium, given its prime location in the heart of Chicago along the Magnificent Mile. It is our sincere hope that you will find the contributions in this book valuable to your practice of vascular and endovascular surgery. We thank you for your interest and support of our annual meeting.

Acknowledgments

We thank our esteemed authors who have thoughtfully contributed to this year's book. Their willingness to share their personal expertise and knowledge is what makes our book a success to other practitioners. Special thanks to Sara Minton, administrative coordinator, for her hard work in assembling and proofing the chapters and for keeping us on track with the deadlines of the Symposium. Without her, the symposium and book would not have been possible. We would also like to thank W.L. Gore & Associates, Incorporated for their continued generous educational grant which helps support the Symposium and printing of the book.

Mark K. Eskandari, MD
William H. Pearce, MD
James S.T. Yao, MD, PhD

Contents

4 Early CEA After Stroke   29

Dhiraj M. Shah, MD, Philip S.K. Paty, MD, Sean P. Roddy, MD, Manish Mehta, MD, MPH, Kathleen J. Ozsvath, MD, and R. Clement Darling III, MD

5 Cognitive Changes After Carotid Endarterectomy and Carotid Artery Stenting   35

Brajesh K. Lal, MD

SECTION II Supra-aortic Trunk Disease   45

6 Current Management of Acute Spontaneous Carotid Dissections   47

Rudy J. Rahme, MD, Salah G. Aoun, MD, Tarek El Ahamdieh, MD, Yvonne Curran, MD, and Bernard R. Bendok, MD

12 Hybrid Approaches for Ilio-femoral Arterial Occlusive Disease   115

Michele Piazza, MD and Joseph J. Ricotta II, MD, MS

13 Sutureless Anastomosis in Femoral-Popliteal Bypass for Lower Extremity Revascularization   127

Syed M. Hussain, MD and Nabeel R. Rana, MD

14 Update on Clinical Trials Evaluating the Effect of Biologic Therapy in Patients with Critical Limb Ischemia   139

Richard J. Powell, MD

15 Liquid Cast Arterial Stents: Stents of the Future   145

Melina R. Kibbe, MD and Guillermo A. Ameer, ScD

SECTION IV Lower Extremity Venous Disease   155

16 Management of Venous Trauma: Civilian and Military Injuries   157

Xzabia A. Caliste, MD and Colonel (ret) David L. Gillespie, MD

17 Iatrogenic Venous Injuries   167

Charles L. Mesh, MD and Creighton B. Wright, MD, MBA

18 Common Femoral Endovenectomy for Postthrombotic Syndrome   185

Anthony J. Comerota, MD

23 EVAR Explants Definitive Remediation   245

Sean P. Lyden, MD

24 Perigraft Seromas Following Open Aortic Reconstruction   253

Joseph L. Karam, MD and Alexander D. Shepard, MD

25 Aortic Surgery and Interventions in Patients with Connective Tissue Disorders   265

James H. Black, III, MD

SECTION VI Visceral and Renal Artery Disease   283

26 Visceral Artery Reconstruction   285

Thomas D. Willson, MD and Heron E. Rodriguez, MD

27 *In Situ* Renal Artery Aneurysm Repair   297

William P. Robinson III, MD

28 Open Surgical Treatment of Mesenteric Occlusive Disease   317

Margaret C. Tracci, MD, JD and Kenneth J. Cherry, MD

29 Contemporary Management of Acute Type B Aortic Dissection   335

Colin P. Ryan, MS and Timur P. Sarac, MD

34 Management of Late TEVAR Failures   393

Mark K. Eskandari, MD and Courtney M. Daly, MD

SECTION VIII Thoracoabdominal Disease   407

35 Disease Progression After Surgery for Takayasu Arteritis   409

Sung Wan Ham, MD and Fred A. Weaver, MD, MMM

36 Hybrid Endovascular Repair of Thoracic and Thoracoabdominal Aortic Aneurysms   421

Gustavo S. Oderich, MD and Bernardo C. Mendes, MD

37 Chimney, Snorkel, Periscope Combined with EVAR/TEVAR 431

Chandu Vemuri, MD and Luis A. Sanchez, MD

38 Branched and Fenestrated TEVAR for Thoracoabdominal Disease 443

Mark A. Farber, MD and Raghuveer Vallabhaneni, MD

39 Spinal Cord Protection After Open Thoracoabdominal Aortic Aneurysm Repair 451

Ali Azizzadeh, MD, Maria Codreanu, MD, Anthony L. Estrera, MD, Kristofer Charlton-Ouw, MD, and Hazim J. Safi, MD

SECTION IX Complex Venous Problems 465

Contributors

Ali F. AbuRahma, MD
West Virginia University
Charleston, WV

Tarek El Ahamdieh, MD
Northwestern University
Feinberg School of Medicine
Chicago, IL

Guillermo A. Ameer, ScD
Northwestern University
Evanston, IL

Suman Annambhotla, MD
Northwestern University
Feinberg School of Medicine
Chicago, IL

Sameer A. Ansari, MD, PhD
Northwestern University
Feinberg School of Medicine
Chicago, iL

Salah G. Aoun, MD
Northwestern University
Feinberg School of Medicine
Chicago, IL

Shipra Arya, MD, SM
University of Michigan
Ann Arbor, MI

Efthymios D. Avgerinos, MD
University of Pittsburgh School of
    Medicine
Pittsburgh, PA

Ali Azizzadeh, MD
University of Texas Health Science Center
Houston Medical School
Houston, TX

Bernard Bendok, MD
Northwestern University
Feinberg School of Medicine
Chicago, IL

James H. Black III, MD
Johns Hopkins University School of
    Medicine
Baltimore, MD

Thomas C. Bower, MD
Mayo College of Medicine
Rochester, MN

Xzabia A. Caliste, MD
University of Rochester Medical Center
Rochester, NY

Rabih A. Chaer, MD
University of Pittsburgh School of
    Medicine
Pittsburgh, PA

Kristofer M. Charlton-Ouw, MD
University of Texas Medical School
Houston, TX

Kenneth J. Cherry, MD
University of Virginia
Charlottesville, VA

Anthony J. Comerota, MD
Jobst Vascular Institute
Toledo, OH

Maria E. Codreanu, MD
University of Texas Medical School
Houston, TX

Michael S. Conte, MD
University of California, San Francisco
San Francisco, CA

Joseph S. Coselli, MD
Baylor College of Medicine
Houston, TX

Enrique Criado, MD
University of Michigan School of Medicine
Ann Arbor, MI

Yvonne Curran, MD
Northwestern University
Feinberg School of Medicine
Chicago, IL

Courtney M. Daly, MD
Northwestern University
Feinberg School of Medicine
Chicago, IL

R. Clement Darling, III, MD
Albany Medical College
Albany, NY

Sapan S. Desai, MD, PhD
University of Texas Medical School
Houston, TX

Paul D. DiMusto, MD
University of Michigan
Ann Arbor, MI

Mark K. Eskandari, MD
Northwestern University
Feinberg School of Medicine
Chicago, IL

Anthony M. Esparaz, BA
Northwestern University
Feinberg School of Medicine
Chicago, IL

Anthony L. Estrera, MD
University of Texas Medical School
Houston, TX

Grant T. Fankhauser, MD
Mayo Clinic College of Medicine
Phoenix, AZ

Mark Farber, MD
University of North Carolina
Chapel Hill, NC

Julie Freischlag, MD
Johns Hopkins University
Baltimore, MD

Manuel Garcia-Toca, MD
Alpert Medical School
Brown University
Providence, RI

Nitin Garg, MBBS, MPH
Medical University of South Carolina
Charleston, SC

David L. Gillespie, MD
University of Rochester Medical Center
Rochester, NY

Peter Gloviczki, MD
Mayo Clinic
Rochester, MN

Roger Gregory, MD
Eastern Virginia Medical School (Retired)
Norfolk, VA

Sung Wan Ham, MD
University of Southern California
Keck School of Medicine
Los Angeles, CA

Peter Henke, MD
University of Michigan School of Medicine
Ann Arbor, MI

Benjamin J. Herdrich, MD
University of Pennsylvania
Philadelphia, PA

Andrew W. Hoel, MD
Northwestern University
Feinberg School of Medicine
Chicago, IL

Syed M. Hussain, MD
University of Illinois College of Medicine
Peoria, IL

Geetha Jeyabalan, MD
University of Pittsburgh School of Medicine
Pittsburgh, PA

Jill K. Johnstone, MD
Alpert Medical School
Brown University
Providence, RI

William D. Jordan, Jr., MD
University of Alabama @ Birmingham
Birmingham, AL

Joseph L. Karam, MD
Henry Ford Hospital
Detroit, MI

Melina R. Kibbe, MD
Northwestern University
Feinberg School of Medicine
Chicago, IL

Christopher Kwolek, MD
Harvard Medical School
Boston, MA

Brajesh K. Lal, MD
University of Maryland Medical School
Baltimore, MD

Jason T. Lee, MD
Stanford University School of Medicine
Stanford, CA

Marlon A. Lee, MD
Northwestern University
Feinberg School of Medicine
Chicago, IL

Scott A. LeMaire, MD
Baylor College of Medicine
Houston, TX

Sean P. Lyden, MD
Cleveland Clinic
Cleveland, OH

James F. McKinsey, MD
Columbia University
New York, NY

Bernardo C. Mendes, MD
Mayo Clinic
Rochester, MN

Charles L. Mesh MD
Jewish Hospital of Mercy Health
Cincinnati, OH

Samuel R. Money, MD, MBA
Mayo Clinic Arizona
Phoenix, AZ

Gustavo S. Oderich, MD
Mayo Clinic
Rochester, MN

Marc A. Passman, MD
University of Alabama @ Birmingham
Birmingham, AL

Biraj M. Patel, MD
Northwestern University
Feinberg School of Medicine
Chicago, IL

Shonak B. Patel, MD
University of Alabama @ Birmingham
Birmingham, AL

Virendra I. Patel, MD
Harvard Medical School
Boston, MA

Philip S.K. Paty, MD
Albany Medical College
Albany, NY

William H. Pearce, MD
Northwestern University
Feinberg School of Medicine
Chicago, IL

Michele Piazza, MD
Padova University School of Medicine
Padova, ITALY

Richard J. Powell, MD
Dartmouth-Hitchcock
Lebanon, NH

Brandon W. Propper, MD
Johns Hopkins Medical Center
Baltimore, MD

Rudy J. Rahme, MD
Northwestern University
Feinberg School of Medicine
Chicago, IL

Nabeel Rana, MD
OSF/HeartCare Midwest
Peoria, IL

Norman M. Rich, MD
Uniformed Services University of
    Health Sciences
Bethesda, MD

Joseph J. Ricotta II, MD, MS
Emory University School of Medicine
Atlanta, GA

William P. Robinson III, MD
University of Massachusetts School of
    Medicine
Worcester, MA

Heron E. Rodriguez, MD
Northwestern University
Feinberg School of Medicine
Chicago, IL

Robert Ryu, MD
Northwestern University
Feinberg School of Meidine
Chicago, IL

Colin P. Ryan, MS
Case Western Reserve University
Cleveland, OH

Hazim J. Safi, MD
University of Texas Medical School at
    Houston
Houston, TX

Luis A. Sanchez, MD
Washington University School of Medicine
St. Louis, MO

Timur Sarac, MD
Case Western Reserve University
Lerner School of Medicine
Cleveland, OH

Dhiraj M. Shah, MD
Albany Medical College
Albany, NY

Alexander D. Shepard, MD
Wayne State University School
    of Medicine
Detroit, MI

Jeffrey Slaiby, MD
Alpert Medical School
Brown University
Providence, RI

Taylor A. Smith MD
Ochsner Clinic Foundation
New Orleans, LA

W. Charles Sternbergh, III, MD
Ochsner Clinic Foundation
New Orleans, LA

William M. Stone, MD
Mayo Clinic Arizona
Phoenix, AZ

Nikolaos Tsilimparis, MD
Emory University School of Medicine
Atlanta, GA

Margaret C. Tracci, MD, JD
University of Virginia
Charlottesville, VA

Gilbert R. Upchurch, Jr., MD
University of Virginia Health System
Charlottesville, VA

Raghuveer Vallabhaneni, MD
University of North Carolina
Chapel Hill, NC

Chandu Vemuri, MD
Washington University School of Medicine
St. Louis, MO

Fred A. Weaver, MD, MMM
University of Southern California
Keck School of Medicine
Los Angeles, CA

Thomas D. Willson, MD
Saint Joseph Hospital
Chicago, IL

Edward Y. Woo, MD
University of Pennsylvania Health System
Philadelphia, PA

Creighton B. Wright, MD, MBA
University of Cincinnati
Cincinnati, OH

James S.T. Yao, MD, PhD
Emeritus
Northwestern University
Feinberg School of Medicine
Chicago, IL

Chin Chin Yeh, MD
Albany Medical College
Albany, NY

Interviews of Leaders and Contributors in Vascular Surgery

A New Initiative Sponsored by SVS

*James S. T. Yao, MD, PhD, Roger T. Gregory, MD, Norman M. Rich, MD, and the History Project Work Group of the Society for Vascular Surgery**

In our life, we can't escape from history. History is defined as the discovery, documentation, collection, organization, and presentation of information about past events, usually in written format. Jesse Thompson, past President of the Society for Vascular Surgery (SVS), often quoted the great historian Thomas Carlyle as saying, "History is the essence of innumerable biographies."[1] History is manmade and men and women make history. As Thompson said, "The basis for today's modern vascular surgery rests on achievements from the past."[1] In an effort to preserve the history of the Society for Vascular Surgery and vascular surgery as a distinct surgical specialty, the leadership of SVS launched a new initiative to collect the oral history of vascular surgery by conducting interviews of leaders and contributors in vascular surgery. This chapter attempts to familiarize vascular surgeons with this oral history and its importance in our surgical heritage.

In the history of vascular surgery, there are three eras. The First Era began with the repair of a brachial artery by Hallowell in 1761[2] and ended with the discovery of thromboendarterectomy for an occluded artery by dos Santos in 1946.[3] This was an era of indirect surgery on arteries and treatment was often by ligation or sympathectomy to increase blood flow.[3] The Second Era was one of direct surgery on arteries as dos Santo described. A breakthrough occurred in the decade of the 1950s when Kunlin[4] introduced the femoral-popliteal vein bypass graft for limb ischemia. Dubost used

---

* History Project Work Group: James S. T. Yao, M.D., Ph.D. (Chair), Norman M. Rich, M.D., Roger T. Gregory, M.D., Peter F. Lawrence, M.D., Mark K. Eskandari, M.D., Melina R. Kibbe, M.D., Walter J. McCarthy, M.D., William H. Baker, M.D., and Calvin B. Ernst, M.D. (Consultant)

1

homograft for replacement of abdominal aortic aneurysm[5] and carotid endarterectomy was first performed by DeBakey and later by Eastcott and Rob as a procedure to prevent stroke.[6,7] In this Era, the Society for Vascular Surgery was formed in 1946 and began to take a leadership role to develop vascular surgery. From the 1960s to the 1980s was the era of reconstructive surgery. Guided by selective catheter arteriogram, heparin, and Dacron graft, nearly every vascular bed in the body is correctable by surgery. The growth of operative surgery continued until 1989, when Juan Parodi successfully applied the endovascular graft technique for a patient with abdominal aortic aneurysm.[8] This heralded the Third Era, one of catheter-based endovascular techniques for vascular lesions. Endovascular procedures are minimally invasive and many patients who are poor surgical candidates can now undergo the procedure with eventual success. Balloon angioplasty with or without stent placement is now a common procedure for treatment of stenotic lesions of carotid, visceral, and infrainguinal arteries, and endovenous ablation and laser are common for treatment of varicose veins. As endovascular procedures proliferated, open procedures began to decline. Nearly 69% of vascular surgical procedures are now done with endovascular technique.[9] This era of endovascular explosion is technology driven and it is not far-fetched to foresee a complete replacement of open surgery by endovascular technique.

ORAL HISTORY OF SVS AND VASCULAR SURGERY

The Society for Vascular Surgery was founded in 1946. Several publications have documented the birth and the progress of the Society.[10,11] The history of vascular surgery is often mixed with that of general surgery[12,13] and there are few books devoted to vascular surgery alone. These include *CLIO Chirurgica: The Arteries* by Wiley Barker[14] and *A History of Vascular Surgery* by Steven Friedman.[2] There is only one oral history in vascular surgery—*Band of Brothers: Creators of Modern Vascular Surgery* by Andrew Dale.[15] The other major history book in vascular surgery is *The Classics of Vascular Surgery* in which the author, Charles Rob, selected 27 articles considered to be classics in the literature.[16] For the history of the Society for Vascular Surgery, the volume by Shumacker, *The Society for Vascular Surgery: A History 1945–1983*[10] and the special issue of *Journal of Vascular Surgery* edited by Calvin Ernst and James S.T. Yao, which was published in June 1996 on the 50th anniversary of SVS, provide a complete history of SVS in the first 5 decades.[11]

Oral history is the oldest type of historical inquiry as well as one of the most modern. It has been said that "oral history is history come alive." The modern concept of oral history was developed in 1940 by Allan Nevins of Columbia University, using the tape recorder, and has progressed to high definition digital videography (DVD).[17] Oral history collects memories and personal commentaries of historical significance through recorded interviews. The discipline came into its own in the 1960s and early 1970s when inexpensive tape recorders became available to document social movements such as civil rights, feminism, and the Vietnam War protest. Many writers have employed oral history in their books. One good example is the book on President Truman, *Plain Speaking: An Oral Biography of Harry S. Truman*.[18] The author talked in total frankness with Truman for hundreds of hours spanning many months in the early 1960s, recorded in tapes and notes. He also interviewed many of those close to Truman. In the book *Shadow: Five Presidents and the Legacy of Watergate*, Bob Woodward used hundreds of recorded interviews with first hand witnesses to reconstruct the story.[19]

An oral history interview generally consists of a well prepared interviewer questioning the subject and recording their exchange in audio and video format. Unlike audio recording alone, the addition of video makes the interview a dynamic experience. The reaction of the interviewee to questioning, facial expressions, and body language are clearly visible when videotaping is added. It is a powerful tool for documenting historical events. Oral history is now an accepted part of history collecting methods and there are many oral history associations. In addition, many universities have academic programs in oral history.

The first oral history book on vascular surgery was by Andrew Dale.[15] Dale interviewed 36 vascular surgeons and one owner and engineer of a prosthetic graft manufacturer for *Band of Brothers*. (Figure 1-1) Unfortunately, he died of leukemia on September 22, 1990, and the book was completed by his trusted friends, Drs. George Johnson and James DeWeese. Dale was interested in learning about the early training and experiences that led to the interviewees' lives in vascular surgery rather than their contributions, which are common knowledge. He called this group "Creators of Modern Vascular Surgery." Dale wrote the foreword in January 1989. At that time, most of the interviewees already had been president of either SVS or ISCVS-NA. Four of the exceptions were Malcolm Perry, James S. T. Yao, Thomas Fogarty, and Frank Veith, all of whom were elected to president in the years subsequent to the interviews. Of the 37 individuals interviewed, only 8 were not elected to the presidency of either SVS or ISCVS-NA. The book provides interesting reading about the times and life of these surgical leaders.

During the 50th anniversary celebration of SVS, the Society sponsored VHS tape interviews of the two sole survivors of the 31 founders: Michael DeBakey and Harris Shumacker, Jr. Part of the interview of DeBakey was transcribed and published in the *Journal of Vascular Surgery*.[20] Both interviews have been converted to DVD and are now accessible via the SVS website (http://www.vascularweb.org). The interview with DeBakey is more than one hour long and provides detailed stories on how he built the Department of Surgery at Baylor College of Medicine into a major cardiovascular center. The interview of Shumacker recalled the time that he collected the membership fees and luncheon expenses by passing the hat for collection from the few SVS members attending the meetings. Other VHS tapes recently acquired by SVS are: (1) Frank J. Veith, *The Origin of a Species & Future of a Specialty* (VHS); (2) Michael E. DeBakey, *Rudolph Matas: How I Remember Him* (VHS); (3) John L. Ochsner, *Giants in Vascular Surgery—Childhood Memories* (VHS). These three VHS tapes are interviews by Roger Gregory, who has generously donated them to the Society, and have been converted to DVD for internet release. The SVS received three additional DVDs of interviews with Charles Rob, Emerick Szilagyi, and Harris Shumacker, Jr. The interview by Norman Rich of Charles Rob is titled *Reflections of Charles G. Rob: Early Years and Vascular Years* and centers on his military experience. Charles Rob has again said that the greatest invention in vascular surgery since World War II is the Fogarty balloon catheter. Judging from what we have seen with current endovascular technology, he is absolutely correct in that statement—Fogarty deserves the credit for the current endovascular revolution in vascular surgery. In the DVD of Shumacker, Norman Rich conducts the interview, again in two parts—the early years and the vascular years. Both DVDs on Rob and Shumacker were given to SVS courtesy of Norman Rich. Both are in the Military Surgical Heritage Series produced by Uniformed Service University. The interview with Szilagyi was conducted at Henry Ford Hospital, focuses on the management of aortic aneurysm, and contains the first aneurysm surgery to be performed live

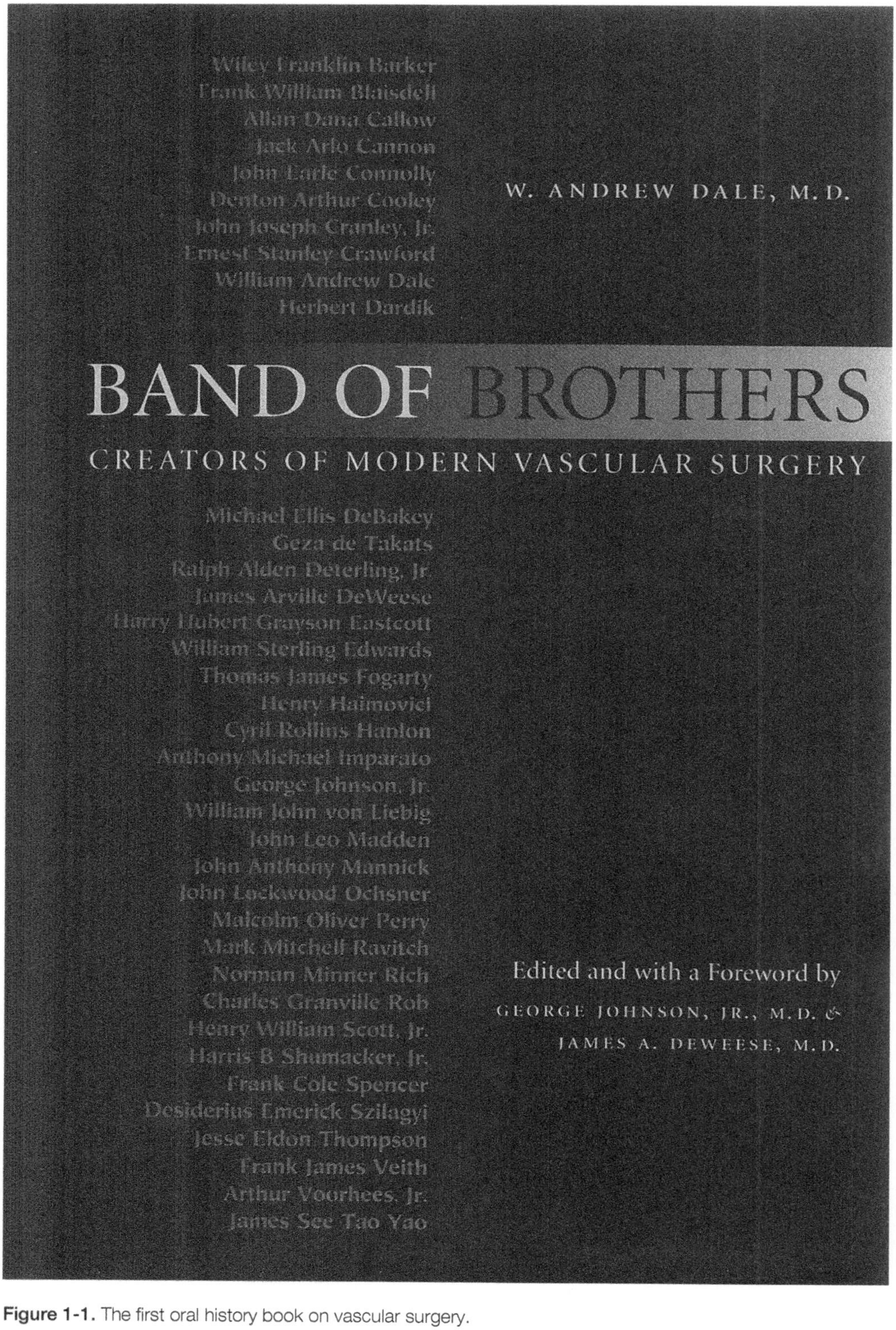

Figure 1-1. The first oral history book on vascular surgery.

on screen. The subtitle of the interview is what Szilagyi is known for: *The Conscience of Vascular Surgery*. We also received a DVD on the memorial service of Szilagyi and stories told by his former fellows. Both DVDs were given to SVS courtesy of Daniel Reddy.

DIGITAL VIDEOGRAPHY (DVD) INTERVIEWS WITH LEADERS IN VASCULAR SURGERY: A NEW INITIATIVE

Although the archive of oral history of the Society is somewhat small, the impact on history of the SVS is clearly shown. The SVS, under the current leadership of Richard Cambria and Peter Gloviczki, has decided to sponsor a series of audiovisual interviews to feature the outstanding leaders and contributors to the specialty of vascular surgery. It is hoped that, by the time we complete the planned interviews with leaders in vascular surgery, there will be sufficient materials to reconstruct the complete history of SVS.

A committee called the **History Project Work Group** was formed. The group is chaired by James S. T. Yao with Norman Rich and Roger Gregory as members and Calvin Ernst as consultant. After the first several interviews were conducted, the committee was enlarged to include younger members: Peter Lawrence, Mark Eskandari, Walter McCarthy, Melina Kibbe, and William Baker. The Work Group is charged (1) to develop a series of interviews with leaders in vascular surgery using standard definition videography (DVD) and (2) to acquire VHS interview tapes and convert the tapes to DVDs. All DVDs then will be uploaded to the SVS website (http://www.vascularweb.org) for internet access by members. The following are the steps taken by the Work Group:

Selection Criteria for Candidacy for Interview

The first task of the committee was to develop selection criteria for interview candidates. After a conference call, the following selection criteria were adopted:

1. Must be a member of Society for Vascular Surgery or International Society for Cardiovascular Surgery, North American Chapter;
   AND
2. Must have served as president of either Society for Vascular Surgery or International Society for Cardiovascular Surgery-North American Chapter or a regional vascular society nationally and internationally known as a contributor to the development of peripheral vascular surgery (local recognition, large number of cases, or newspaper fame were not counted);[†]
   OR
3. Be an inventor of an operative procedure or a medical device;
   OR
4. Have distinguished service to a vascular surgical society;
   OR
5. Be considered and universally acknowledged as an ultimate authority on a vascular disorder or surgical procedure.

While selection criteria are important, the Work Group will look at the total picture of the specialty to make sure all facets of vascular surgery are covered. As

---

[†] Adapted from Dale WA. Band of Brothers: Creators of Modern Vascular Surgery.[15]

stated previously, the development of vascular surgery involves multiple disciplines and we will strive to show this in our project. In the last several decades, we have witnessed the struggle of vascular surgery to be recognized as an independent surgical specialty. We will interview those who were involved in the process, including former officials from the American Board of Surgery and the American Board of Medical Specialties, to preserve an accurate history. Important events such as the change of the name of ISCVS-NA to American Association for Vascular Surgery (AAVS) and the eventual merger of SVS and ISCVS-NA (AAVS) and the impact of endovascular surgery on training and practice must be kept in our surgical heritage. In recent years, several leaders in vascular surgery have become deans of medical schools and a few have moved up to become CEOs of their own institutions. All these individuals may provide valuable information on how vascular surgeons should place themselves in the current tough economic situation. Finally, we have no desire to turn the interview project into a senior endeavor. The Work Group feels strongly that the younger generation of leaders must be part of the interviews to allow an accurate account of modern history of the Society and the specialty. America is led by young and vibrant leaders and such tradition must be kept when the history of the Society is being recorded.

Preparation for Interviews

The interviews take place in a quiet room with two comfortable chairs facing each other. Rooms close to heavy traffic by personnel should be avoided. A standard definition 4x3 video camera is used and, usually, we use the two camera technique to capture the interviewer and the interviewee. The interview, in general, takes about one hour to one hour and fifteen minutes. The interviewee is asked to submit (1) a current curriculum vitae (CV) and a short biosketch of less than 150 words, (2) a headshot, (3) a signed consent form approved by SVS legal counsel, and (4) no more than 10 photos of family, memorable events, prizes, and special occasions. These photos will be inserted in the recorded interview to highlight the events.

The interviewer must prepare for the interview. This consists of a review of the interviewee's CV, significant publications, usually the presidential address, and books edited or written by the interviewee. When necessary, inquiry to his or her colleagues may help to fashion the questioning. As pointed out recently in the Wall Street article by Funt, the best interviewers do their homework, put their own opinions aside, keep questions brief and listen closely for possible follow-ups.[21] The interview format utilized is somewhat fluid, allowing the interview to have considerable individual flexibility. Nonetheless, a basic review of the individual's early years, family background, and education is highlighted, with further attention to his/her surgical training, mentors, career highlights as well as low points, and his/her opinion of the reasons for his/her success. A final segment focuses on the interviewee's personal opinions of multiple topics.

The interviewer is advised to develop a master list of questions with important ones at the top. Members of the Work Group are encouraged to submit questions to the designated interviewer and the designated interviewer makes the final list of questions. The interviewer may show the questions to the interviewee prior to the interview. We believe an early acquaintance of the interviewer and interviewee adds value to the event.

After the completion of the interview and recording, editing of the tape is the final path to the product. Editing is often a tedious process. Judicious use of photos to highlight a memorable event or to illustrate an important occasion improves the visual value of the DVD. Once the editing is completed, the Work Group will select a subtitle for each of the DVDs. The DVD will be shown to the interviewee for his or her final approval before release to the public.

Lessons Learned from the Interviews

After experiencing many interviews with leaders in vascular surgery (DeBakey, Ochsner, Veith, Dietrich, Cooley, Imparato, Jacobson, Spencer, Villavicencio, Rich, Yao, Fogarty, Moore, Riles, Pearce) the author (RG) has the following impressions of these leaders. Interestingly, there were many common characteristics that all of these surgical giants shared:

1. All were intelligent. This is essentially a given in view of the rigors of medical school.
2. All worked hard. This is a consistent, common thread. Calvin Coolidge said, "...unrewarded genius is almost a proverb." Intelligence and talent is worthless without the added ingredient of hard work. Dr. Denton Cooley observes "The harder I worked, the luckier I got!"
3. All were opportunistic. Good fortune and "luck" probably played a role in all of their careers; however, when opportunity arose, it was recognized and utilized to the fullest.
4. All had mentors. These were teachers and role models who were interested in their success and offered sound advice and direction.
5. Most gravitated towards an academic career. This afforded maximum opportunity for teaching and research to complement a clinical practice that in all cases was vigorous.
6. Most were multi-dimensional, some more than others. This suggests an absence of "thought rigidity" and an ability to "think out of the box." Several were outstanding athletes, musicians, or artists.
7. Disappointment and failure, a constant in the human condition, only inspired determination and persistence.
8. All used deductive reasoning to recognize truth and reality. A blind alley was rarely pursued.
9. All had supportive families.
10. All were ambitious and most were not arrogant.
11. All were likeable and attractive leaders, despite occasional controversy.
12. All truly loved their patients and exhibited a passion for providing the best possible care for them.

SUMMARY

The purpose of the Society for Vascular Surgery is not just to hold an annual meeting but also to pursue social, financial, and political responsibilities. In addition, the Society leads in research, training, education, and practice (i.e., patient care). The current leadership of the SVS is dedicated to preserving the history of the Society. The History Project Work Group will execute the orders of the Society to develop a series of digital videography (DVD) recorded interviews with leaders in vascular surgery to be made available to our membership. Once the interviews are placed on the SVS website for internet access, they will become a permanent record. The information collected will form the basis for a second book—*Band of Brothers II* or perhaps *Band of Brothers and Sisters*—as part of the oral history of the Society for Vascular Surgery.

Acknowledgement

We thank Jan Goldstein for editorial preparation of the manuscript.

REFERENCES

1. Thompson JE. Vascular Surgical Techniques: Historical Perspective. In Bergan JJ, Yao JST, eds. *Techniques in Arterial Surgery*. Philadelphia: W.B. Saunders; 1990:3–13.
2. Friedman SG. *A History of Vascular Surgery*, 2nd Edition. Malden, MA: Blackwell-Futura; 2005.
3. dos Santos R, Lamas A, Pereira Caldas J. L'arteriographie dos members, de l'aorte et de ses branches abdominales. *Bull et Mem Soc Nat Chir*. 1929;55:587–601.
4. Kunlin J. Le traitement de l'ischeme arteritique par la greffe veineuse [Long vein transplantation in treatment of ischemia caused by arteritis]. *Rev Chir*. 1951;70:206–235.
5. Dubost C, Allary M, Oeconomos N. Resection of an aneurysm of the abdominal aorta: reestablishment of the continuity by a preserved human arterial graft, with result after five months. *AMA Arch Surg*. 1952;64:405–408.
6. DeBakey ME. Successful carotid endarterectomy for cerebrovascular insufficiency. Nineteen year follow-up. *JAMA*. 1975;233:1083–1085.
7. Eastcott HHG, Pickering GW, Rob CG. Reconstruction of internal carotid artery in a patient with intermittent attacks of hemiplegia. *Lancet*. 1954;267:994–996.
8. Parodi JC, Palmaz JC, Barone HD. Transfemoral intraluminal graft implantation for abdominal aortic aneurysms. *Ann Vasc Surg*. 1991;5:491–499.
9. Sambol EB, Kent KC. Operative Vascular Surgery in the Endovascular Era. In Pearce WH, Matsumura JS, Yao JST, eds. *Vascular Surgery in the Endovascular Era*. Evanston IL: Greenwood Academic Press; 2008:18–25.
10. Shumacker HB Jr. *The Society for Vascular Surgery—A History: 1945-1983*. Chicago: The Society for Vascular Surgery; 1984.
11. Ernst CB, Yao JST. Special issue: 50th anniversary, 1946-1996. *J Vasc Surg*. 1996;23:957–1160.
12. Wangensteen OH, Wagensteen SD. *The Rise of Surgery: From Empiric Craft to Scientific Discipline*. Minneapolis MN: University of Minnesota Press; 1978.
13. Rutkow IM. *American Surgery: An Illustrated History*. Philadelphia PA: Lippincott Williams & Wilkins; 1998.
14. Barker WF. *CLIO Chirurgica: The Arteries*. Austin TX: RG Landes Co.; 1992.
15. Dale WA. *Band of Brothers: Creators of Modern Vascular Surgery*. George Johnson and James DeWeese; 1996.
16. Rob CG. *The Classics of Vascular Surgery*. Medford, NJ: Apollo Press; 1982.
17. Oral History. Wikipedia, http://en.wikipedia.org/wiki/Oral_history, accessed 1/24/12.
18. Miller M. *Plain Speaking: An Oral Biography of Harry S. Truman*. New York: Berkley Publishing Corporation; 1973.
19. Woodward B. *Shadow: Five Presidents and the Legacy of Watergate*. New York: Simon & Schuster; 2000.
20. DeBakey ME, Blaisdell FW. The Society for Vascular Surgery: As I remember—An interview with Dr. Michael E. DeBakey. *J Vasc Surg*. 1996;23:1031–1034
21. Funt P. The lost art of the live interview. *Wall Street Journal*. April 9, 2012;A13.

SECTION I

Cerebrovascular Disease

2

Effects of Age on CAS Results: Data from CREST

Taylor A. Smith, MD and W. Charles Sternbergh, III, MD

INTRODUCTION

Carotid Endarterectomy (CEA) has been shown to be a safe and effective treatment for extra-cranial carotid artery atherosclerotic disease in both symptomatic and asymptomatic patients.[1,2] While CEA has remained the gold-standard treatment for carotid occlusive disease, carotid artery stenting (CAS) with distal embolic protection has been shown to be effective, with outcomes similar to endarterectomy, in certain high risk patient cohorts.[3,4]

The safety of CEA in octogenarians has been debated in statewide, multi-center, and Medicare population based analysis.[5–7] This debate led some to believe that patients over eighty years old should be considered high risk for CEA and were included as such in a randomized clinical trial[3] despite early evidence that the rate of stroke and death after CAS might actually be higher in octogenarians when compared to CEA.[8,9]

The Carotid Revascularization Endarterectomy versus Stenting (CREST) trial was designed as a multi-center, randomized, controlled trial to evaluate the safety and effectiveness of carotid stenting in patients who were not at high risk for CEA and included octogenarians. The CREST trial was originally designed to evaluate only symptomatic patients; however the inclusion criteria were expanded to include asymptomatic lesions in 2005. Physicians were allowed to participate in CREST if they possessed adequate catheter and wire skills and had acceptably low morbidity and mortality as determined by the CREST Interventional Management Committee. In order to credential the surgeons and interventionalists who would be performing CAS during the study, a lead-in phase was designed to ensure that all participants could safely perform CAS with distal embolic protection using the study devices (RX Acculink stent, RX Accunet anti-embolic device, Abbott Vascular, Santa Clara, CA, formerly Guidant). During this phase both asymptomatic and symptomatic patients were enrolled.

CREST LEAD-IN PHASE

An interim analysis of the lead-in phase to the CREST trial revealed a significantly higher risk of stroke and death after CAS among octogenarians when compared to non-octogenarians.[10] The outcomes of 740 of the 862 patients enrolled as of early 2004 were included in the interim analysis with ninety-nine of the 740 patients 80 years or older. The demographics between the octogenarians and non-octogenarians were similar with the exception of a higher incidence of diabetes, hyperlipidemia, and current smoking among the younger cohort.

When comparing these two groups, there was not a significant difference in 30-day mortality between octogenarians and non-octogenarians (2.02% vs 0.62%, $p = 0.1441$). However, there was a significant difference in the incidence of stroke within 30 days (12.12% vs 2.77%, $p < 0.0001$), giving a significant increase in the combined 30-day stroke and death rate (12.12% vs 3.23%, $p < 0.0001$). This statistically significant increased stroke risk held true when adjusting for symptomatic status, use of distal cerebral protection, percent stenosis, and gender. A statistically significant increase in the 30-day stroke and death rate among octogenarians was also found when comparing patients less than 60 years old, 60–69 years old, and 70–79 years old. (Figure 2-1)

Based on these findings, the investigators elected to stop enrolling octogenarians into the lead-in phase of the trial. However, octogenarians would be enrolled in the randomized portion of the CREST trial in order to asses if there was equivalent risk of CAS when compared to CEA. Given the significant effect of age on the peri-procedural stroke rate after CAS noted during the lead-in phase, a formal assessment of the impact of age on the efficacy of CEA and CAS was planned prior to the unblinding of randomized patient data.

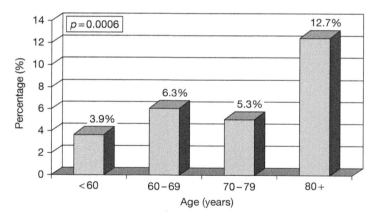

Figure 2-1. Incidence of 30-day stroke and death rate by patient age in CREST lead-in phase.

RESULTS FROM CREST

The results of the CREST trial were published in 2010 and failed to show a significant difference between CEA and CAS in the primary end-point defined as the combined peri-procedural incidence of heart attack, stroke and death and ipsilateral stroke up to four year follow-up.[11] In comparing the two groups, the incidence of the peri-procedural endpoints occurred in $5.2 \pm 0.6\%$ of CAS patients versus $4.5 \pm 0.6\%$ of CEA patients; a difference that did not reach statistical significance ($p = 0.38$). When examining the individual endpoints, there was no difference in the 30-day mortality rate between the CAS and CEA patients ($0.7 \pm 0.2\%$ vs. $0.3 \pm 0.2\%$, $p = 0.18$). There was a statistically significant higher incidence of stroke in the CAS group ($4.1 \pm 0.6\%$ vs. $2.3 \pm 0.4\%$, $p = 0.01$) and a statistically significant higher rate of myocardial infarction in the CEA group ($1.1 \pm 0.3\%$ vs. $2.3 \pm 0.4\%$, $p = 0.03$). The equivalence between the two groups was maintained at estimated four year follow-up (CEA 6.8%, CAS 7.2%, $p = 0.51$).

The pre-planned sub-analysis of the CREST trial was published in 2011.[12] This study included data from 2502 patients with a primary focus of determining the impact of age on the efficacy of CAS versus CEA as well as to evaluate the impact of age within each cohort of patients treated with either CEA or CAS. After adjusting for gender and symptomatic status, patient data were analyzed on an intention-to-treat basis using a proportional hazards model. Specific interaction points were added to the model to determine if an age-by-treatment effect exists for the primary outcome as a whole as well as for the individual components of peri-procedural stroke and heart attack. The frequency of death in the peri-procedural window was to low to allow for meaningful analysis of this individual end point. Prior to evaluating the data, $p < 0.10$ was considered suggestive of a treatment effect as determined by the study investigators. As an additional analysis, patients were divided into three groups based on age (less than 65, 65–74, 75 or older) to allow for assessment of events and efficacy of treatment within certain age ranges. Also examined were the impact of gender, symptomatic status, lesion characteristics, procedural details, and certain co-morbidities (hyperlipidemia, hypertension, and diabetes) as they relate to patient age and outcome.

In examining the cohort as a whole, the older patients tended to be caucasian, female, have lower incidence of diabetes, hypercholesterolemia, and smoking but have higher systolic blood pressures. None of these variables were significant across all age ranges for either the CAS or CEA treated patients.

The primary end point occurred in 7.2% of all patients treated with CAS. However, the incidence of the adverse outcomes was not uniform across the patient cohort. In those patients 75 years or older the incidence of heart attack, stroke, or death was 12.7%, compared with 6.3% for those 65–74 years old, and 3.9% for the youngest patients ($p < 0.0001$). No such age effect was seen in patients treated with CEA, however. Patients undergoing CEA had similar risk of in the three age categories (6.1% less than 64, 6.3% 65–74, 7.4% 75 years or older, $p = 0.5$). (Figures 2-2, 2-3) When comparing CEA and CAS, there was no difference in the incidence of the primary end point among patients in the two lower age strata. However, in patients 75 years or older the incidence was significantly higher (12.7% CAS vs. 7.4% CEA, $p = 0.05$) with a significant treatment by age interaction ($p = 0.02$). (Figure 2-4) The increased incidence of the primary end point in the CAS cohort is primarily driven by the increase in the rate of stroke as treatment age increases. This trend is not seen in patients treated with CEA.

When measuring age as a continuous variable, hazard ratios suggest the composite primary end point occurs with equal frequency between the two procedures at age 70, with CAS having more favorable outcomes in younger patients and CEA having better results in older patients. If comparing the incidence of stoke alone against advancing age, the hazard ratios suggest equivalence of the two procedures at 64 years old. (Figure 2-5) This implies that age has a larger magnitude of effect on the incidence of stroke than it does on the overall occurrence of the primary endpoint. The hazard

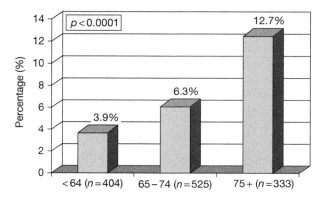

Figure 2-2. CAS outcome by age as reported in CREST.

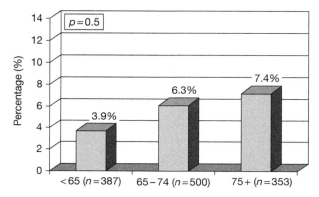

Figure 2-3. CEA outcome by age as reported in CREST.

ratios of CAS to CEA increase from 0.60 (95% CI, 0.31–1.18) in patients less than 65, to 1.08 (95% CI, 0.65–1.78) for those 65–74 years old, and 1.63 (95% CI, 0.99–2.69) for the oldest patients.

Patients treated with CAS have a 1.76 fold increased risk of the incidence of stroke (95% CI, 1.35–2.31) and an overall 1.77 fold increased risk of occurrence of the primary end point ($p < 0.0001$, 95% CI 1.38–2.28) with each 10 year increase in age. Those treated with CEA did not show an increased risk with increasing age for the composite end point (HR 1.16; 95% CI, 0.89–1.50; $p = 0.27$) or for stroke (HR 1.12; 95% CI, 0.82–1.54; $p = 0.45$).

Additional analysis showed no significant interaction between the treatment effect of age when compared to symptomatic status ($p = 0.96$), or gender ($p = 0.45$). The CAS cohort was also examined for the treatment effect of age as it relates to the incidence of diabetes, hypertension, hyperlipidemia, total procedure time, duration of fluoroscopy, and plaque characteristics. Of these, fluoroscopy time was the only variable found to be significant ($p = 0.046$) with only a minimal reduction in the hazard ratio (1.68 to 1.62) with each ten year advancement of age. The patients treated with CEA were not included in these sub-analyses as there was no variation in the incidence of the primary endpoints with increasing age.

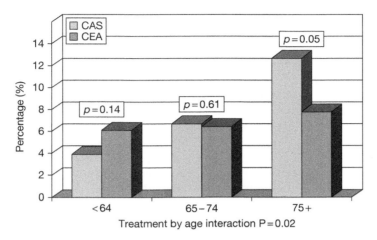

Figure 2-4. Comparison of the incidence of the Primary Endpoint between CAS and CEA. Patients subdivided by age.

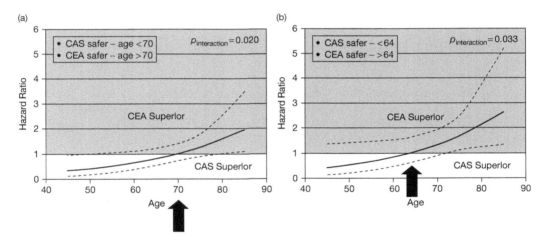

Figure 2-5. Hazard ratios comparing efficacy of CAS and CEA using age as a continuous variable. **A.** Comparison of the impact of age on the Primary Endpoint (MI, Death or Stroke). Equivalence (HR = 1.0) is reached at 70 years old with patients older than 70 years having superior outcomes after CEA. **B.** Comparison of the effect of age on the incidence of stroke or death. Equivalence between CAS and CEA is reached at 64 years old. Improved outcomes were seen in patients 64 years or older undergoing CEA. (From Age and Outcomes After Carotid Stenting and Endarterectomy: The Carotid Revascularization Endarterectomy Versus Stenting Trial, JH Voeks et al. Stroke 2011;42:3488. Copyright 2011 Wolters Kluwer Health. Reprinted with permission.)

DISCUSSION

The results of the CREST trial refute the notion that a less invasive procedure, CAS, would be more beneficial in older patients when compared to CEA. The increase in the rate of stroke with advancing age associated with CAS neutralizes the modest reduction in myocardial infarction when compared to CEA. Surprisingly, CAS was most beneficial in the youngest patient cohort; a group that may not have the same co-morbidities and risk factors needed to be considered high-risk for CEA.

Since the inception of the CREST trial, several reports have been published highlighting the increased risk of stroke in elderly patients.[9,13,14] A post-hoc analysis of the Stent-Protected Angioplasty versus Carotid Endarterectomy in Symptomatic Patients (SPACE) trial was published in 2008 to specifically define the clinical and angiographic risk factors leading to stroke or death.[15] The results of this subanalysis revealed that patients 68 years or older had an increased rate of adverse events (stroke or death within 30 days) following CAS than patients less than 68 (log-rank $p = 0.001$). This variation by age was not seen in patients treated with CEA. Patients 68 years or older also had an increased rate of adverse events when comparing CAS to CEA ($p = 0.026$). Also evaluated during this subanalysis were the effects of gender, qualifying event, side of intervention, degree of stenosis, and presence of high-grade contralateral stenosis. No significant interaction between these variables and the primary outcome measure were seen.

A preplanned meta-analysis of three previously published trials comparing CAS to CEA in symptomatic patients also revealed an increase in the risk of stroke and death in older patients.[16] Data from 3433 patients enrolled in the Endarterectomy versus Angioplasty in Patients with Symptomatic Severe Carotid Stenosis (EVA-3S), International Carotid Stenting Study (ICSS), and SPACE trials were pooled to determine the treatment effect of CAS verses CEA. Overall there was an increased risk of any stroke or death following CAS (7.7% vs. 4.4%, risk ratio 1.74; 95% CI 1.32–2.30, $p = 0.0001$). While the event rates between groups were equivalent in patients less than 70 years old (5.8% CAS vs. 5.7% CEA), patients 70 years or older had a two fold increase in the risk of stroke or death after treatment with CAS (12.0% vs. 5.9%, risk ratio 2.04; 95% CI 1.48–2.82, $p = 0.0053$).

Additionally, a recent review of the Nationwide Inpatient Sample from 2005 through 2008 analyzed the difference in outcomes for CAS and CEA based on patient age.[17] While several randomized trails have shown a difference between the two treatments with respect to age, the investigators wanted to evaluate their effect in a "real-world" general practice setting. Data from 495,331 patients were analyzed and divided based on patient age, less than 70 years or 70 years or greater, and treatment type, CAS or CEA. 88% of the patients underwent CEA while the remaining 12% underwent CAS. Approximately 96% and 93% percent of CEA and CAS patients were classified as asymptomatic and overall 59% of the procedures were performed in patients 70 years old or greater.

Data from this series showed that the incidence of stroke, cardiac complications, and mortality were higher within the older cohort regardless of the treatment used. Adjusted odds ratios of patients ≥70 years old, when compared to patients <70 years old, undergoing CAS was significantly higher for stroke (OR 1.7; 95% CI 1.2–2.5, $p = 0.0025$), while patients ≥70 years old undergoing CEA had a higher incidence of cardiac complications (OR 1.5; 95% CI 1.3–1.7, p<0.0001). The increased frequency of stroke and cardiac complications within the respective CAS and CEA cohorts also drove the incidence of stroke/cardiac complications and the composite end point to reach statistical significance.

When comparing the two treatment modalities in reference to patient age, CAS patients <70 years old had a significantly higher incidence of in-hospital mortality (0.76% vs. 0.29%, $p = 0.0008$) and cardiac complications (1.94% vs. 1.37%, $p = 0.0213$). The risk of stroke was not significantly different between CAS and CEA in patients <70 years old (1.35% vs. 1.02%, $p = 0.897$). In patients ≥70 years old the risk of postoperative stroke was significantly higher after CAS than after CEA (1.97% vs. 0.95%, $p < 0.0001$) with no significant difference in the incidence of cardiac complications (2.48% vs. 2.24%, $p = 0.3087$).

Several anatomic risk factors have been described that place elderly patients at higher risk for complications after CAS than younger patients. A single-center series of 133 patients treated with CAS demonstrated a significant increase in the risk of adverse outcome among patients ≥80 years old.[18] The patients within the older cohort had a statistically significant increase in the incidence of arch elongation, arch calcification, vessel origin stenosis, common carotid tortuosity, and severity of the target lesion stenosis when compared to patients less than 80 years old. These factors, when present, can increase the difficulty of successful wire and catheter manipulation leading to cerebral embolization of unstable plaque from either the arch, associated vessel or target lesion.

The impact of aortic arch calcification and elongation on the outcomes of CAS has been shown in several studies. In one series the aortic calcium content was calculated using a coronary calcium score from thoracic CT scans.[19] The results showed a correlation between increased aortic calcification and age 75 years or older. Older patients in this series were also more likely to have a type II arch. Another series showed an increase in the number of embolic lesions seen on post-CAS diffusion-weighted MRI among patients with severe aortic arch calcifications and ulceration of the target carotid lesion.[20] Octogenarians were found to have a significantly higher number of new embolic lesions than younger patients. This may be explained by the increased prevalence of arch calcifications and ulcerated carotid plaque among the older patients. A third study showed that aortic arch type was the only variable independently associated with adverse neurologic outcomes following CAS.[21]

In addition to unfavorable anatomic factors that occur in elderly patients, the cerebral reserve may also be decreased making them more susceptible to ischemic events after CAS. A review of 916 cerebral blood flow studies revealed an abnormal response to intra-cranial vasodilator administration indicating decreased cerebral vascular reserve in patients greater than 70 years old with significant carotid stenosis or peripheral vascular disease.[22] This would suggest that elderly patients are less tolerant to the cerebral embolization that occurs during CAS making them more likely to have a symptomatic ischemic event.

CONCLUSION

CAS has an increasingly higher risk of stroke with advancing age. Patients treated with CAS have a 1.76 fold increased risk of the incidence of stroke (95% CI, 1.35–2.31) with each 10 year increase in age. No such age effect is seen in patients treated with CEA. The cut point of equal outcome was 70 years of age in CREST[12] and 68 in SPACE[15]. Age is a critical variable in making informed choices regarding treatment of severe carotid artery stenosis.

REFERENCES

1. North American Symptomatic Endarterectomy Trial Collaborators. Beneficial effects of carotid endarterectomy in symptomatic patients with high grade stenosis. *N Engl J Med.* 1991;325:445–453.
2. Executive Committee for the Asymptomatic Carotid Atherosclerotic Study. Endarterectomy for asymptomatic carotid stenosis. *JAMA.* 1995;273:1421–1428.
3. Yadav JS, Wholey MH, Kuntz RE, et al. Protected Carotid-Artery Stenting versus Endarterectomy in High-Risk Patients. *N Engl J Med.* 2004;351:1493–1501.

4. The SPACE Collaborative Group. 30 day results from the SPACE trial of stent-protected angioplasty versus carotid endarterectomy in symptomatic patients: a randomized non-inferiority trial. *Lancet*. 2006;368:1239–1247.

5. Perler BA, Dardik A, Burleyson GP, et al. Influence of age and hospital volume on the results of carotid endarterectomy: a statewide analysis of 9918 cases. *J Vasc Surg*. 1998;27:25–33.

6. Fischer ES, Malenka DJ, Solomon NA, et al. Risk of carotid endarterectomy in the elderly. *Am J Public Health*. 1989;79:1617–1620.

7. Winslow CM, Solomon DH, Chassin MR, et al. The appropriateness of carotid endarterectomy. *N Engl J Med*. 1988;318:721–727.

8. Roubin GS, New G, Iyer SS, et al. Immediate and late clinical outcomes of carotid artery stenting in patients with symptomatic and asymptomatic carotid artery stenosis. *Circulation*. 2001;103:532–537.

9. Chastain HD II, Gomez CR, Iyer S, et al. for the UAB Neurovascular Angioplasty Team. Influence of age upon complications of carotid artery stenting. *J Endovasc Surg*. 1999;6:217–222.

10. Hobson RW II, Howard VJ, Roubin GS, et al. Carotid artery stenting is associated with increased complications in octogenarians: 30-day stroke and death rates in the CREST lead-in phase. *J Vasc Surg*. 2004;40:1106–1111.

11. Brott TG, Hobson RW II, Howard G, et al. Stenting versus endarterectomy for treatment of carotid-artery stenosis. *N Engl J Med*. 2010;363(1):11–23.

12. Voeks JH, Howard G, Roubin GS, et al. Age and outcomes after carotid stenting and end-arterectomy: the carotid revascularization endarterectomy versus stenting trial. *Stroke*. 2011;42:3484–3490.

13. International Carotid Stenting Study investigators. Carotid artery stenting compared with endarterectomy in patients with symptomatic carotid stenosis (International Carotid Stenting Study): an interim analysis of a randomised controlled trial. *Lancet*. 2010;375:985–997.

14. Kastrup A, Schulz JB, Raygrotzki S, et al. Comparison of angioplasty and stenting with cerebral protection versus endarterectomy for treatment of internal carotid artery stenosis in elderly patients. *J Vasc Surg*. 2004;40:945–951.

15. Stingele R, Berger J, Hans-Henning E, et al. Clinical and angiographic risk factors for stroke and death within 30 days after carotid endarterectomy and stent-protected angioplasty: a subanalysis of the SPACE study. *Lancet Neurol*. 2008;7:216–222.

16. Carotid Stenting Trialists' Collaboration. Short-term outcome after stenting versus endarterectomy for symptomatic carotid stenosis: a preplanned meta-analysis of individual patient data. *Lancet*. 2010;376:1062–1073.

17. Khatri R, Chaudrhy SA, Vazquez G, et al. Age differential between outcomes of carotid angioplasty and stent placement and carotid endarterectomy in general practice. *J Vasc Surg*. 2012;55:72–78.

18. Lam RC, Lin SC, DeRubertis B, et al. The impact of increasing age on anatomic factors affecting carotid angioplasty and stenting. *J Vasc Surg*. 2007;45:875–880.

19. Bazan HA, Pradhan S, Mojibian H, et al. Increased aortic arch calcification in patients older than 75 years: Implications for carotid artery stenting in elderly patients. *J Vasc Surg*. 2007;46:841–845.

20. Kastrup A, Gröschel K, Schnaudigel S, et al. Target lesion ulceration and arch calcification are associated with increased incidence of carotid stenting-associated ischemic lesions in octogenarians. *J Vasc Surg*. 2008;47:88–95.

21. Faggiolo GL, Ferri M, Freyrie A, et al. Aortic arch anomalies are associated with increased risk of neurologic events in carotid stent procedures. *Eur J Vasc Endovasc Surg*. 2007;33:436–441.

22. Chaer RA, Shen J, Rao A, et al. Cerebral reserve is decreased in elderly patients with carotid stenosis. *J Vasc Surg*. 2010;52:569–575.

3

Trans-cervical Carotid Stenting with Carotid Flow Reversal for Cerebral Protection

Enrique Criado, MD

RATIONALE FOR TRANS-CERVICAL CAROTID STENTING

During the last decade, carotid artery stenting (CAS) has become an accepted alternative treatment for carotid stenosis in selected patients with carotid artery disease. However, the major randomized clinical trials that compared CAS with carotid endarterectomy (CEA) have casted questions on the results of trans-femoral CAS with distal filter for cerebral protection, and have not produced a consensus on the equipoise between both therapeutic options. Most of the data accrued with CAS has been using the trans-femoral approach with distal filters for cerebral protection, while no major studies have compared transfemoral CAS with distal filter protection against other alternative carotid stenting techniques.

The embolic phenomena associated with CAS performed through a trans-femoral approach are directly related to the risk of stroke of the procedure. The intravascular instrumentation of the aortic arch, supra-aortic trunks and carotid lesion required for trans-femoral CAS have been shown to produce a very high rate of cerebral embolization as assessed with trans-cranial Doppler monitoring (TCD).[1-3] More recently, the detection of bilateral acute cerebral ischemic infarcts following trans-femoral CAS using MRI diffusion-perfusion imaging (DW-MRI) has raised great concern regarding the safety of trans-femoral CAS with distal filter protection.[4,5] The majority of the new ischemic hemispheric lesions following CAS are ipsilateral to the carotid intervention, which suggests that the manipulation of the ipsilateral carotid and stent delivery are related to the neurologic events.[6] However, between 19 and 32% of patients undergoing trans-femoral CAS sustain, in addition, contralateral hemisphere embolization, most likely secondary to the manipulation of the aortic arch and supra aortic trunks.[7]

It is obvious that the procedural steps that are particularly likely to produce emboli-zation during trans-femoral CAS are the introduction of guide-wires, catheters and sheaths into the aortic arch and supra-artic trunks, the advancement of these into the common carotid artery, crossing of the carotid lesion with the guide-wire and filter without protection, and balloon inflation and stent deployment.

Distal filter placement has become the most widely used and the only method approved by the USA regulatory bodies for cerebral protection during trans-femoral CAS. However, and paradoxically, the influence of access route and protection meth-odology on the results of CAS has not been addressed in any major trial, despite the clear fact that the results of carotid stenting are in great part determined by the access technique and the cerebral protection methods used in the procedure. Interestingly, the systematic use of distal filter protection for trans-femoral CAS was supported in a 2004 consensus document, published in the *Journal of Vascular Surgery*, without any comparative data to support such recommendation.

Several small, single center prospective trials comparing trans-femoral CAS with distal filter protection against carotid stenting without protection failed to show any reduction in the rate of micro embolic signals detected by trans-cranial Doppler (TCD) or in the number of new cerebral ischemic lesions in the ipsilateral hemisphere using DW-MRI.[8,9] In addition, the comparison of distal filter protection with other methods of cerebral protection has shown that distal filters increase the incidence of embolic signals detected in the middle cerebral artery by TCD.[10,11] These results, illustrate the limited cerebral protection provided by trans-femorally deployed distal filters.

It is important to consider that recent major trials evaluated the results of CAS based on a standard technique that uses the trans-femoral approach and distal filters for cerebral protection in most cases, and that these data are quickly becoming obso-lete as the technology and technique for CAS evolves. The two technical components of CAS, trans-femoral access and distal filter protection, are unrelated to stent per-formance, but are responsible for most neurological complications attributable to the procedure. Hence, it is quite plausible that the liabilities of trans-femoral CAS with distal filter protection could be eliminated by using an alternative access route and dif-ferent cerebral protection methodology. Therefore, it is hasty to pronounce a negative or a final evaluation of CAS based on recent large trial data, since the technique is still in its developmental stages and will likely improve. Based on the small differences in neurological complication rates between CAS and CEA found in randomized trials, it is very possible that a significant reduction in the embolic phenomena associated with CAS may produce neurological complication rates comparable, if not better, than those of CEA.

Over a decade ago, concerned with the intrinsic risks of trans-femoral carotid stenting with distal protection we developed an alternative technique that theo-retically could avoid those risks. We combined the ingenious concept of carotid flow reversal for cerebral protection developed by Juan Parodi with an alterna-tive access route that would avoid the embolic phenomena related to intravascular instrumentation. That was the original concept of our trans-cervical carotid artery stenting with carotid flow reversal for cerebral protection technique. The technique is simple and ideal for vascular surgeons familiar with carotid exposure. It consists in the creation of an arterio-venous fistula between the common carotid artery and the jugular or any other major vein using vascular sheaths and tubing connections. When common carotid artery flow is interrupted, the low resistance on the venous side reverses flow in the internal carotid artery towards the jugular vein through the arterio-venous connection, and the carotid stenting procedure can be conducted with uninterrupted reversal of flow in the internal carotid artery. Flow reversal throughout the procedure minimizes or eliminates the risk of cerebral embolization associated with CAS.

The transcervical approach for CAS eliminates the technical challenges and the inherent hazards related to the use of protection devices deployed through the transfemoral route.

Transcervical CAS with carotid flow reversal has several important advantages over other cerebral protection methods. It avoids crossing the carotid lesion without cerebral protection, and does not require negotiation of the aortic arch or aortic trunks that may be perilous in many cases and certainly always emboligenic. In addition, it is technically easier in patients with difficult arch anatomy, it requires minimal contrast volume, and with some experience it can be done faster that transfemoral CAS or carotid endarterectomy.

SURGICAL TECHNIQUE

Preoperative carotid ultrasound is the only imaging required in preparation for the procedure. A minimum of five centimeters from the clavicle to the carotid bifurcation, as is almost always the case, is required for the procedure because two or three centimeters of distance from the introducer sheath to the bifurcation are necessary to deploy the stent. Patients with significant stenosis or anterior calcific plaque in the mid common carotid should not be treated with transcervical CAS, but this has been rarely a problem in this author's experience. These anatomic restrictions should be assessed preoperatively with carotid ultrasonography.

Patients are treated preoperatively with aspirin and clopidogrel. Our technique for transcervical CAS was described in detail in our 2004 publication.[12] In summary, the technique consists in a 4 centimeter long, vertical incision starting above the superior edge of the clavicle between the heads of the sternocleidomastoid muscle. A two to three centimeter long segment of the common carotid artery and jugular vein are exposed, and the common carotid artery is controlled with an umbilical tape using a Rummel tourniquet. Using 4-French micropuncture kits for vascular access, an 8-French sheath is introduced in a cardiad direction in the jugular vein and another 8-F sheath antegradely in the common carotid artery. The sheaths are connected with intravenous line tubing and stopcocks to establish a common carotid to jugular vein fistula. (Figure 3-1) As the arterial sheath is placed, patients are anti-coagulated with 100 IU/kg of heparin to maintain an activated clotting time above 250 seconds. Using small volumes of hand injected contrast (5 mls), the carotid lesion is assessed and flow reversal in the carotid artery is ascertained by visualizing the lesion when contrast is injected antegradely into the common carotid, followed by contrast flowing retrogradely into the jugular vein from the carotid sheath after reopening the fistula at the end of the injection. The carotid lesion is crossed under flow reversal with a 0.014-inch guide-wire, and stenting is conducted under flow reversal in a standard fashion. (Figure 3-2) A completion carotid arteriogram is obtained to confirm satisfactory results. The post-dilation balloon is placed in the proximal internal carotid and inflated to allow re-establishment of antegrade flow initially into the ECA to flush particulate debris prior to re-establishing flow into the internal. In the presence of ECA

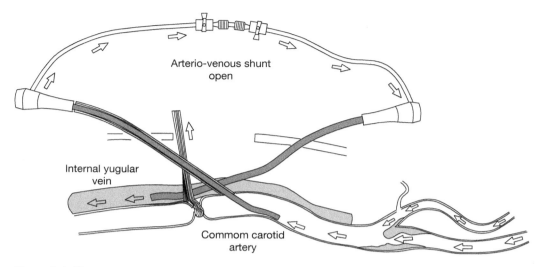

Figure 3-1. Through a small, low cervical incision the common carotid artery and internal jugular vein are exposed and cannulated with 8 French, 11 centimeter-long sheaths. The common carotid artery is controlled with a Rummel loop. The sheaths are connected with tubing using stopcocks to establish an arterio-venous communication between the common carotid and the jugular vein. When the common carotid artery is occluded, flow reverses in the internal carotid towards the jugular vein. The stopcocks allow contrast injection and control of the flow in the circuit. (Illustration courtesy of Juan Fontcuberta, MD)

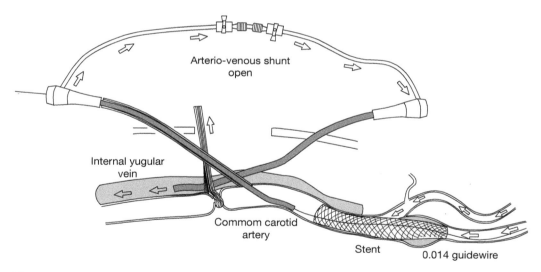

Figure 3-2. Through the 8 French common carotid sheath, the carotid lesion is crossed under flow reversal with a 0.014-inch guide-wire, and stenting is conducted under flow reversal in a standard fashion. (Illustration courtesy of Juan Fontcuberta, MD)

occlusion, blood is aspirated through the sheath with a 10 cc syringe to remove debris before antegrade carotid flow is restored. Upon completion, the sheaths are removed and the arteriotomy and venotomy are closed with polypropelene sutures. Before standard closure of the wound, meticulous hemostasis should be achieved to avoid neck hematomas. Daily aspirin and clopidogrel are given for one month after the procedure.

RESULTS OF TRANS-CERVICAL CAROTID ARTERY STENTING WITH CAROTID FLOW REVERSAL

During our early experience with trans-cervical CAS we demonstrated its' technical feasibility and that it could be safely done in awaked patients.[13] We showed that ipsilateral cerebral hemispheric oxygenation was not significantly reduced during flow reversal, and that carotid flow reversal was well tolerated in most awake patients without producing neurological impairment. In our initial experience with more than 100 patients, there were no deaths or major strokes, and we had a 2% incidence of minor stroke with full recovery. Tolerance to flow reversal occurred in 96% of our patients with a mean flow reversal time of 21 minutes. Two wound complications and one common carotid dissection related to access puncture occurred early in our experience, likely related to the learning curve.[14] In a recent prospective trial using preoperative and postoperative DW-MRI we investigated the difference in cerebral ischemic lesions between transcervical CAS with flow reversal and transfemoral CAS with distal filter protection, and found that after intervention, new post procedural DW-MRI ischemic infarcts occurred in 12.9% of transcervical cases while happened in 33.3% of patients undergoing trensfemoral CAS with distal filter. This almost three-fold difference in the incidence of brain infarction rates was statistically significant (p=0.03).[15]

The overall experience with trans-cervical CAS is limited and the technique in its infancy, but the results reported by several groups that have adopted this technique throughout the world have shown a remarkably low rate of major adverse events. The cumulative results with trans-cervical CAS are summarized in Table 3-1. A summary of the comparative incidence of major adverse events between trans-cervical CAS and those of trans-femoral CAS with distal filter protection and those of CEA drawn from major international trials is given in Table 3-2. From these data it is clear that the preliminary results with trans-cervical CAS with flow reversal can compare favorably with those of conventional CAS.

In regard to the effectiveness of cerebral protection during CAS, this is best assessed by data that incorporates DW-MRI imaging of the brain before and after intervention. Nothing could be more relevant than the incidence of cerebral

TABLE 3-1. CUMULATIVE RESULTS OF TRANS-CERVICAL CAROTID ARTERY STENTING WITH CAROTID FLOW REVERSAL

Author	# Of Patients	30 Day Death	Major Strokes	Minor Strokes	Freedom from Occlusion/ Re-stenosis
Pipinos[22]	17	0	0	0	100% at 24 months
Lin[23]	31	0	0	2	not reported (n/r)
Chang[24]	21	0	0	0	not reported
Alvarez[20]	219	1	3	0	92% at 36 months
Criado[14]	103	0	0	2	97% at 48 months
Faraglia[25]	52	0	1	1	100% at 6 months
Leal[7]	31	0	0	0	100% at 1 month
Pinter[26]	65	0	0	1	n/r
TOTAL	539	1 (0.18%)	4 (0.74%)	5 (0.92%)	

TABLE 3-2. COMPARISON OF DEATH AND MAJOR STROKE RATES BETWEEN TRANSFEMORAL CAS WITH DISTAL FILTER PROTECTION, CAROTID ENDARTERECTOMY (CEA) AND TRANS-CERVICAL CAROTID STENTING (METANALYSIS). BASED ON DATA REPORTED IN THE ICSS AND CREST TRIALS.

Study	Procedure	Embolic Protection	# Patients	% Death	% Major Stroke
ICSS[27]	Transfemoral CAS	Distal Filter	853	2.3%	1.7%
ICSS[27]	CEA	Clamp, backbleeding	857	0.8%	2.4%
CREST[16]	Transfemoral CAS	Distal Filter	1262	0.3%	1.5%
CREST[16]	CEA	Clamp, backbleeding	1240	0.7%	0.5%
Transcervical CAS	Transcervical CAS	Flow reversal	539	0%	0.7%

TABLE 3-3. COMPARISON OF BRAIN INFARCTION RATES (SILENT AND NOT SILENT) BETWEEN TRANSFEMORAL CAS, CAROTID ENDARTERECTOMY AND TRANS-CERVICAL CAS. BASED ON PROSPECTIVE DW-MRI PRE AND POST-OPERATIVE STUDIES FROM THE ICSS AND MO.MA. TRIALS

Study	Procedure	Embolic Protection	# Patients	% New DW-MRI Brain Lesions
ICSS[28]	Transfemoral CAS	Distal Filter	51	73%
Mo.Ma[29]	Transfemoral CAS	Proximal occlusion	127	30%
ICSS[28]	Carotid Endarterectomy	Clamp. backbleeding	107	17%
Leal et al.[7]	Transcervical CAS	Flow reversal	31	13%

embolization or of cerebral infarction in a carotid stenting trial. In this regard, it is disappointing, that all major sponsored trials conducted to establish the efficacy of transfemoral CAS in comparison with CEA have eluded the evaluation of cerebral embolization rates, while introducing the incidence of post-procedural troponin elevations, a parameter totally unrelated to the brain, as an endpoint in trial results. The comparative incidence of cerebral infarction rates between trans-cervical CAS, transfemoral CAS and CEA summarized in Table 3-3 speaks for itself and explains what many trials have deliberately eliminated from evaluation and analysis.

The clinical advantages of avoiding arch and supra-aortic trunk instrumentation are clearly seen in the differential results of carotid stenting in the elderly. The much higher prevalence of calcific atherosclerotic arch lesions and tortuous supra-aortic trunk anatomy in older patients are the reason for the higher neurological risk of CAS in this population. This risk has been well illustrated in the CREST trial[16] that reported a 12% stroke rate with trans-femoral CAS in octogenarians compared with a 3% rate in younger patients. Similarly, Lamb[17] reported an 11% stroke rate in octogenarian patients compared with a 1% stroke rate in the population under 80 years of age. Kastrup[18] also observed a significantly higher neurological complication rate in patients older than 75 years compared with the younger group. In a prospective study Roubin[19] found that age greater than 80 years was a strong predictor of major adverse events and late stroke. Strikingly, and in stark difference with the results of trans-femoral CAS, Alvarez et al[20] using trans-cervical carotid artery stenting with carotid flow reversal in 219 patients older than 70 years, reported a 2.2% combined incidence of stroke, death or myocardial infarction at 30 days, with no strokes occurring in patients who were asymptomatic (56% of total). These results in the elderly are clearly superior to those reported in any controlled trans-femoral CAS trial, and comparable, if not better, with historical results of CEA in the elderly.

The use of carotid flow reversal diminishes the incidence of embolic signals detected by TCD, which may actually be completely eliminated as Ribo[21] reported using this technique. Additionally, carotid flow reversal during CAS significantly reduces the number of new ischemic lesions detected by DW-MRI. This was seen in our comparative study of 31 patients who underwent trans-cervical CAS against a cohort undergoing trans-femoral CAS with distal filter protection. In our prospective, blinded comparison, trans-cervical CAS produced a remarkably lower incidence of DW-MRI detected brain infarcts than that with transfemoral, filter-protected CAS.[15]

In summary, carotid flow reversal using a trans-cervical approach for carotid artery stenting produces a significant reduction in the embolic signals and the development of new ischemic lesions in the brain. It is undeniable that a reduction in ischemic infarction following CAS is beneficial to the patient, most likely by reducing the short and long-term consequences of ischemic brain infarction. Trans-cervical carotid artery stenting avoids instrumentation of the arch and supra aortic trunks, thereby reducing the embolic phenomena from these arteries. More importantly, trans-cervical CAS crosses the carotid lesion after protection is in place. The need for a cervical incision could be considered a drawback of this technique, but is rather minimal, isexpeditious, safe and is well tolerated under local anesthesia. Trans-cervical CAS allows immediate ambulation following the procedure, making its performance on an ambulatory basis a realistic option. In addition, trans-cervical CAS eliminates the cost of transfemoral access devices and distal protection systems.

These important features make trans-cervical CAS an optimal alternative for high risk patients such as octogenarians, those with challenging arch anatomy or those in whom the transfemoral approach is impossible or contraindicated. Trans-cervical carotid stenting with carotid flow reversal is extremely safe and has the potential to be the best technique for CAS. An FDA sanctioned multicenter trial evaluating trans-cervical CAS is underway in the USA, and will shed light on the potential value of this technique. Based on our experience and that reported in the literature, in skilled hands, trans-cervical CAS with carotid flow reversal can yield lower neurological complication rates than those achieved with transfemoral distal filter protection, and potentially comparable if not better than those of CEA.

REFERENCES

1. Coggia M, Goeau-Brissonniere O, Duval JL, Leschi JP, Letort M, Nagel MD. Embolic risk of the different stages of carotid bifurcation balloon angioplasty: an experimental study. *J Vasc Surg*. 2000;31(3):550–557.
2. Rapp JH, Pan XM, Yu B, Swanson RA, Higashida RT, Simpson P, Saloner D. Cerebral ischemia and infarction from atheroemboli <100 microm in Size. *Stroke*. 2003;34(8):1976–1980.
3. Jordan WD, Jr., Voellinger DC, Doblar DD, Plyushcheva NP, Fisher WS, McDowell HA. Microemboli detected by transcranial Doppler monitoring in patients during carotid angioplasty versus carotid endarterectomy. *Cardiovasc Surg*. 1999;7(1):33–38.
4. Faraglia V, Palombo G, Stella N, Rizzo L, Taurino M, Bozzao A. Cerebral embolization during transcervical carotid stenting with flow reversal: a diffusion-weighted magnetic resonance study. *Ann Vasc Surg*. 2009;23(4):429–435.

5. Bonati LH, Jongen LM, Haller S, Zwenneke Flach H, et al. New ischaemic brain lesions on MRI after stenting or endarterectomy for symptomatic carotid stenosis: a substudy of the International Carotid Stenting Study (ICSS). *Lancet Neurol.* 2010;9:353–362.

6. Hammer FD, Lacroix V, Duprez T, Grandin C, Verhelst R, Peeters A, et al. Cerebral microembolization after protected carotid artery stenting in surgical high-risk patients: results of a 2-year prospective study. *J Vasc Surg.* 2005;42:847–53.

7. Leal JI, Orgaz A, Fontcuberta J, Flores A, Doblas M, Garcia-Benassi JM, Lane B, Loh C, Criado E. A prospective evaluation of cerebral infarction following transcervical carotid stenting with carotid flow reversal. *Eur J Vasc Endovasc Surg.* 2010;39:661–666.

8. Macdonald S, Evans DH, Griffiths PD et al: Filter-protected versus unprotected carotid artery stenting: a randomised trial. *Cerebrovasc Dis.* 2010;29:282–289.

9. Barbato JE, Dillavou E, Horowitz MB, Jovin TG, Kanal E, David S, Makaroun MS. A randomized trial of carotid artery stenting with and without cerebral protection. *J Vasc Surg.* 2008;47(4):760–765.

10. Rubartelli P, Brusa G, Arrigo A, Abbadessa F, Giachero C, Vischi M, Ricca MM, Ottonello GA. Transcranial Doppler monitoring during stenting of the carotid bifurcation: evaluation of two different distal protection devices in preventing embolization. *J Endovasc Ther.* 2006;13(4):436–442.

11. Crawley F, Stygall J, Lunn S, Harrison M, Brown MM., Newman S. Comparison of microembolism detected by transcranial Doppler and neuropsychological sequelae of carotid surgery and percutaneous transluminal angioplasty. *Stroke.* 2000;31:1329–1334.

12. Criado E, Doblas M, Fontcuberta J, Orgaz A, Flores A. Transcervical carotid artery angioplasty and stenting with carotid flow reversal: surgical technique. *Ann Vasc Surg.* 2004;18(2):257–261.

13. Criado E, Doblas M, Fontcuberta J, Orgaz A, Flores A, Lopez P, and Wall P. Carotid angioplasty with internal carotid artery flow reversal is well tolerated in the awake patient. *J Vasc Surg.* 2004;40:92–97.

14. Criado E, Fontcuberta J, Orgaz A, Flores A, Doblas M. Transcervical carotid stenting with carotid artery flow reversal: 3-year follow-up of 103 stents. *J Vasc Surg.* 2007;46(5):864–869.

15. Leal JI, Orgaz A, Flores A, Gil J, Rodriguez R, Peinado J, Criado E, Doblas M. A DW-MRI based study of transcervical carotid stenting with flow reversal versus transfemoral filter protected. *J Vasc Surg. 2012,* in press.

16. Brott TG, Hobson RW, Howard G, Roubin GA, Clark WM, et al. Stenting versus Endarterectomy for Treatment of Carotid-Artery Stenosis. *N Engl J Med.* 2010;363:11–23.

17. Lam RC, Lin SC, DeRubertis B, Hynecek R, Kent KC, Faries PL. The impact of increasing age on anatomic factors affecting carotid angioplasty and stenting. *J Vasc Surg.* 2007;45(5):875–880.

18. Kastrup A, Schulz JB, Raygrotzki S, Groschel K, Ernemann U. Comparison of angioplasty and stenting with cerebral protection versus endarterectomy for treatment of internal carotid artery stenosis in elderly patients. *J Vasc Surg.* 2004;40(5):945–951.

19. Roubin GS, New G, Iyer SS, Vitek JJ, Al-Mubarak N, Liu MW, Yadav J, Gomez C, Kuntz RE. Immediate and late clinical outcomes of carotid artery stenting in patients with symptomatic and asymptomatic carotid artery stenosis: a 5-year prospective analysis. *Circulation.* 2001;103(4):532–537.

20. Alvarez B, Matas M, Ribo M, Maeso J,Yugueros X, Alvarez-Sabin J. Transcervical carotid stenting with flow reversal is a safe technique for high risk patients older than 70 years. *J Vasc Surg.* 2012;55:978–984.

21. Ribo M, Molina CA, Alvarez B, Rubiera M, Alvarez-Sabin J, Matas M. Transcranial Doppler monitoring of transcervical carotid stenting with flow reversal protection: a novel carotid revascularization technique. *Stroke.* 2006;37(11):2846–2849.

22. Pipinos, II, Johanning JM, Pham CN, Soundararajan K, Lynch TG. Transcervical approach with protective flow reversal for carotid angioplasty and stenting. *J Endovasc Ther.* 2005;12(4):446–453.

23. Lin JC, Kolvenbach RR, Pinter L. Protected carotid artery stenting and angioplasty via transfemoral versus transcervical approaches. *Vasc Endovascular Surg.* 2005;39(6):499-503.

24. Chang DW, Schubart PJ, Veith FJ, Zarins CK. A new approach to carotid angioplasty and stenting with transcervical occlusion and protective shunting: why it may be a better carotid intervention. *J Vasc Surg.* 2004;39:994–1002.

25. Faraglia V, Palombo G, Stella N, Rizzo L, Taurino M, Bozzao A. Cerebral embolization during transcervical carotid stenting with flow reversal: a diffusion-weighted magnetic resonance study. *Ann Vasc Surg.* 2009;23(4):429–435.

26. Pinter L, Ribo M, Loh C, Lane B, Roberts T, Chou T, Kolvenbach RR. Safety and feasibility of a novel transcervical access neuroprotection system for carotid artery stentingin the PROOF study. *J Vasc Surg.* 2011;54:1317–23.

27. International Carotid Stenting Study Investigators. Carotid artery stenting compared with endarterectomy in patients with symptomatic carotid stenosis (International Carotid Stenting Study): an interim analysis of a randomized controlled study. *Lancet.* 2010; 375:985–997.

28. Bonati LH, Jongen LM, Haller S, Zwenneke Flach H, et al. New ischaemic brain lesions on MRI after stenting or endarterectomy for symptomatic carotid stenosis: a substudy of the International Carotid Stenting Study (ICSS). *Lancet Neurol.* 2010;9:353–362.

29. Biamino G. Deserve Study. Diffusion weighted MRI-based evaluation of the effectiveness of endovascular clamping during carotid artery stenting with the Mo.Ma. device. Presented at the 2011 EuroPCR Meeting, Paris, May 17-20, 2011.

4

Early CEA After Stroke

Dhiraj M. Shah, MD, Philip S.K. Paty, MD, Sean P. Roddy, MD, Manish Mehta, MD, MPH, Kathleen J. Ozsvath, MD, and R. Clement Darling III, MD

INTRODUCTION

Acute stroke is a prevalent disease in the United States. About 750,000 people suffer from acute stroke resulting in more than 140,000 deaths per year with a healthcare cost of approximately 20 billion dollars. A subset of these patients with acute stroke has significant extracranial carotid artery disease that may potentially benefit by undergoing carotid endarterectomy (CEA). However, there is controversy and continued debate about the timing of such intervention for the treatment of acute stroke.[1-8] Conventional wisdom suggests that carotid endarterectomy should be waived until six to eight weeks after the stroke for fear of extension of the stroke or converting an infarct into a hemorrhaging stroke.[8] On the other hand, there are studies that suggest that there is increased risk of recurrent stroke in the intervening period by waiting that long for surgery, therefore, the rationale for early CEA and debate continues as to the timing and size of the infarct for indication for carotid endarterectomy.[3] We have reviewed our data retrospectively from 1980 to 2007 for the purpose of gaining support from our experience for early CEA. All patients who had preoperative stroke within a month are included in this study.

METHODS

Records of all patients undergoing CEA at Albany Medical Center Hospital who had carotid endarterectomy within four weeks of their preoperative stroke were reviewed. We further subdivided those patients who had surgery within one week, one to two weeks, two to three weeks, and three to four weeks after the stroke and reported by us.[5] Excluded from this study are those patients who had symptomatic carotid disease but operated on more than a month after the stroke, acute hemorrhagic stroke, dense hemispheric paralysis or patients in a vegetative state, and also patients having acute MI or other medical conditions contraindicating surgery. Preoperatively, diagnosis of a stroke was made by clinical examination usually by a neurologist, by imaging studies—either a CT or magnetic resonance imaging enhanced with contrast, ultrasound of the carotid artery, and conventional contrast angiogram if needed.[9–11] The presence of 50% or greater stenosis of the ipsilateral carotid artery was considered for operative treatment. The procedure is usually done under regional cervical block anesthesia with the patient awake but a group of patients are operated on under general anesthesia according to surgeon's preference. The majority of patients underwent eversion carotid endarterectomy. Earlier in this series a small number of patients had longitudinal carotid endarterectomy with or without patch as needed. Shunts are usually used on demand in awake patients. Shunts are used in all patients undergoing general anesthesia. Preoperatively, the stroke size was measured in the brain and the location of the infarct was identified. Correlations are sought between the demographic presentations, extent of preoperative infarct, location, time between stroke and operation, as well as operative parameters and the risk factors. The majority of patients are seen by a neurologist, especially after 1999. Preoperative and postoperative National Institute of Health Stroke Scale score (NIHSS) are determined by the neurologist. The statistical analysis was done between the groups by using the analysis of variants, ANOVA, and chi square tests or Fischer Exact test.

The technique of eversion carotid endarterectomy has been described by us and others and its results in patients with extracranial carotid disease are well established.[12]

RESULTS

During this period, we have performed over 7,000 carotid endarterectomies at our center. The majority of these cases were done using the eversion technique in awake patients. Greater than 70% of these carotid endarerectomies were done in asymptomatic patients and 30% were done for symptomatic patients. Of this subset, there were 452 carotid endarterectomies done for acute stroke (i.e. within a month of ipsilateral hemispheric event). Although a small group of patients ultimately underwent bilateral carotid endarterectomy, in this analysis only the symptomatic unilateral CEA were included. The data was analyzed for patients' demographics in addition to onset of first symptom. Sixty-one percent of the patients were men, 39% women. The mean age was 70 years (range: 34–94 years). Associated risk factors included diabetes mellitus (27%), smoking (33%), hypertension (65%), and coronary artery disease (37%). None of these risk factors were significant for outcome. Twelve patients underwent emergency carotid endarterectomy when the stroke evolution was diagnosed (Table 4-1).

The rates of neurologic deficit after CEA were not statistically different from overall CEA in all comers. Preoperative brain imaging studies were available for over 75% of the patients. Lesions found on MRI or CT scans were utilized according to NASCET criteria. There was 37% cortical infarct, 17% borderline infarct and 14% deep infarcts in the perforators vascular territory.[13] Approximately one third of the patients did not show any infarct in prior imaging studies. The location and size of the infarct as well as the timing of surgery were not statistically significant factors for outcome in our earlier paper (Table 4-2). Interval between timing of the carotid endarterectomy and stroke rate was not different in larger database (Table 4-3). There was no statistical difference of stroke rates when surgery was done within a week, one to two weeks, two to three weeks, or three to four weeks after preoperative stroke. Therefore, we

TABLE 4-1. CEA FOR ACUTE STROKE

	Total		<1 week		1–4 weeks	P Value
Total Procedures	452		154		298	
Demographics						
male	275	60.84%	95	61.69%	180	
female	177	39.16%	59	38.31%	118	
diabetic	120	26.55%	40	25.97%	80	
smoker	150	33.19%	51	33.12%	99	
mean age	70		70		69	
age range	34–94		34–94		35–93	
Operative Parameters						
eversion	359	79.42%	137	88.96%	222	
elective shunt	63	13.94%	33	21.43%	30	
shunt on demand	30	6.64%	10	6.49%	20	
patch	7	1.55%	1	0.65%	6	
general anesthesia	52	11.50%	19	12.34%	33	
cervical block	399	88.27%	134	87.01%	265	
block -> general	1	0.22%	1	0.65%	0	
Operative Mortality	6	1.33%	1	0.65%	5	NS
cardiac	3	0.66%	0	0.00%	2	
stroke	3	0.66%	1	0.65%	2	
pulmonary	1	0.22%	0	0.00%	1	
Stroke/Mortality	16	3.54%	7	4.55%	9	NS
Non-fatal Complications						
TND	12	2.65%	5	3.25%	7	NS
PND	10	2.21%	6	3.90%	4	NS
hematoma	7	1.55%	4	2.60%	3	
arterial bleed	0	0.00%	0	0.00%	0	
immediate occlusion	5	1.11%	2	1.30%	3	
carotid bypass	3	0.66%	1	0.65%	2	
CEA thrombectomy	2	0.44%	1	0.65%	1	
wound infection	0	0.00%	0	0.00%	0	
Nerve injury	2	0.44%	1	0.65%	1	
intra-op TND w/o shunt	4	0.88%	1	0.65%	3	
intracerebral bleed	3	0.66%	1	0.65%	2	
cardiac	8	1.77%	1	0.65%	7	
seizures	1	0.22%	0	0.00%	1	
respiratory	2	0.44%	1	0.65%	1	
re-stenosis	4	0.88%	0	0.00%	4	
follow-up (months)						
mean	31		31		31	
range	1–246		1–148		1–246	

TABLE 4-2. LOCATION AND SIZE OF PREOPERATIVE INFARCT AND TIME INTERVAL FOR CEA

Interval between Stroke Onset and CEA (wk)	Cortical Infarct n (%)	Borderzone Infarct n (%)	Deep Infarct n (%)	No Infarct n (%)	Infarct Size (cm) (Mean± SD)	Patients with Data	Patients with No Data
0–1	21 (38%)	10 (17%)	7 (12%)	18 (33%)	1.4±1.6	56	13
1–2	14 (39%)	4 (11%)	6 (17%)	12 (33%)	1.3±1.3	36	21
2–3	4 (21%)	3 (16%)	3 (16%)	9 (47%)	0.7±0.9	19	9
3–4	18 (34%)	10 (19%)	5 (9%)	20 (38%)	1.0±1.4	53	21

TABLE 4-3. NIH STROKE SCALE SCORE

	Interval Between Stroke Onset and Surgery (wk)			
	0–1	1–2	2–3	3–4
Number of Patients	21	9	3	1
NIHSS Score (mean±SD) Preoperative	6.38±2.8*	3.67±1.7	0	1
Postoperative	5.9±3.2*	3.44+1.67	0	3
	Depth and Location of Infarct			
	Cortical	Borderzone	Deep	None
Number of Patients	19	8	2	3
NIHSS Score (mean±SD) Preoperative	5.4±3.2	5.0±3.0	4.0±1.4	4.3±3.8
Postoperative	5.3±3.5	3.6±2.0	4.0±1.4	4.3±3.8

*$p<0.05$

grouped the patients as 1 week and 1 to 4 weeks (Table 4-1). Overall stroke rate for this group was 3.1% including permanent and transient stroke and that was not statistically significant from our overall result of carotid endarterectomy where the stroke rate was 1.9% in 13,200 carotid endarterectomies performed to date. Eighty-eight percent of the operations were done under cervical block anesthesia without shunt. Others were done with general anesthesia and using shunt. Overall the utilization of shunt was about 15%. Shunt was used on demand in awake patients in 7%. There are no differences in the results when the patient was awake or under general anesthesia or the technique of endarterectomy (i.e. eversion vs. longitudinal), although the majority of patients underwent eversion carotid endarterectomy.[14] The operative mortality for the entire group was 1.3%. Therefore, the combined permanent stroke mortality rate was 3.2%. Postoperative stroke patients were further evaluated by imaging studies for extension of previous infarct, hemorrhage around it, or for any new infarct. Five of these patients had postoperative CEA thrombosis. All of these patients were taken back to the operating room due to development of progressive neurological deficit.[15] Emergent reconstruction was done in all the patients which included carotid artery bypass in four patients and rethrombectomy in one patient. Two patients who had permanent stroke had conversion of the previous infarct into hemorrhagic stroke. Transient neurologic deficits occurred in about 2% of the patients and symptoms resolved within 24 hours after the operation and did not have any infarct on imaging studies. No new neurologic deficits occurred in 12 patients who underwent carotid endarterectomy within 24 hours of the stroke in evolution. Other complications included hematoma, bleeding, cranial nerve injuries and non-fatal MI which is minor in 2% of patients (Table 4-2). Mean hospital stay varied between seven to nine days for those with previous neurologic deficit. NIHSS score compiled for 34 patients in our published series undergoing CEA within one week of stroke had significantly greater scores both preoperatively and postoperatively compared with patients who underwent CEA at any other interval (p<.05). There are no significant differences between distribution or location of infarcts in NIHSS score before and after CEA. There is however a significant relationship between perioperative infarct size and the NIHSS score. Preoperative infarct size greater than 3.5 cm±.85x correlated with postoperative stroke rate with the p-value<.01.

DISCUSSION

The rationale for performance of carotid endarterectomy for acute extracranial carotid disease in patients with stroke to prevent further stroke exacerbation is well documented in our experience. The goal of surgery is to prevent further stroke even if there is no improvement of prior neurological deficit. However, many published reports suggest this may possibly be obtained with significant perioperative complication and stroke rate. According to some series, the perioperative mortality of 21% and improvement of stroke status in only 47% of the patients dissuade these investigators from doing CEA in acute strokes. There are other reports which suggest that CEA in acute cases is worthwhile. The waiting period of four to six weeks after the stroke may result in a significant number of second strokes. Whittemore et al showed that CEA could be performed within one month after non disabling stroke with acceptable mortality and morbidity.[16] The review of our experience suggests that carotid endarterectomy can be done with optimal results within one to four weeks after the stroke. The stroke rate and mortality in our experience is acceptable and does not show any difference from our results of overall CEA.

Of course there is always selection bias in retrospective review because some of the patients that are excluded in our series might have been included in others. Selected patients as outlined in our series, who have reasonable neurological state, do not have infarct size greater than 5 cm, and have other acceptable perioperative risk factors, should enjoy an optimum result after early carotid endarterectomy following acute stroke.

Although the results of our retrospective review showed that larger infarct may increase the risk of peri or postoperative permanent neurological deficit, it remains unclear whether waiting longer than four weeks will reduce this risk. We limited our review of CEA only up to one month following the stroke and have not compared this further out because the stroke rate in our symptomatic patients did not differ from that of asymptomatic patients overall. With increasing acceptance of our eversion CEA technique, the carotid endarterectomy can be done expediently with an average of 10 minutes of cross-clamp time. We have experienced lower neurologic deficit in eversion endarterectomy compared to longitudinal endarterectomy. The use of shunt is controversial, although we have used more shunts later on in stroke patients to prevent even 10 minutes of surgical ischemia. This paradigm is instituted by most vascular surgeons in other studies. Prophylactic use of shunt may demonstrate a lower stroke rate, however, routine shunting was not our usual practice.

In conclusion, carotid endarterectomy can be done safely in patients who have stroke within one month prior to surgery for significant carotid artery disease when it is done expediently with an acceptable surgical technique that provides optimal results. Therefore, we suggest in patients with no hemorrhage, no dense paralysis, and small infarct size, urgent carotid endarterectomy should be recommended.

REFERENCES

1. Ballotta E, DaGiau G, Baracchini C, et al. Early versus delayed carotid endarterectomy after a nondisabling ischemic stroke: a prospective randomized study. *Surgery.* 2002;131:287–93.
2. Gasecki AP, Ferguson GG, Eliasziw M, et al. Early endarterectomy for severe carotid artery stenosis after a non-disabling stroke: results from the North American Symptomatic Carotid Endarterectomy Trial. *J Vasc Surg.* 1994;20:288–95.
3. Giordano JM, Trout HH III, Kozloff L, et al. Timing of carotid endarterectomy after stroke. *J Vasc Surg.* 1985;2:250–4.
4. Meyer FB, Piepgras DG, Sandok BA, et al. Emergency carotid endarterectomy for patients with acute carotid occlusion and profound neurologic deficits. *Ann Surg.* 1986;203:82–9.
5. Paty PSK, Darling RC III, Woratyla S, et al. Timing of carotid endarterectomy in patients with recent stroke. *Surgery.* 1997;122:850–5.
6. Piotrowski JJ, Bernhard VM, Rubin JR, et al. Timing of carotid endarterectomy after acute stroke. *J Vasc Surg.* 1990;11:45–52.
7. Ricco JB, Illuminati G, Bouin-Pineau MH, et al. Early carotid endarterectomy after a non-disabling stroke: a prospective study. *Ann Vasc Surg.* 2000;14:89–94.
8. Wylie EJ, Hein MF, Adams JE. Intracranial hemorrhage following surgical revascularization for treatment of actue stroke. *J Neurosurg.* 1964;21:212–5.
9. Damsio H. Computed tomographic guide to the identification of cerebral vascular territories. *Arch Neurol.* 1983;40:138–42.
10. Dosick SM, Whalen RC, Gale SS, et al. Carotid endarterectomy in the stroke patient: computerized axial tomography to determine timing. *J Vasc Surg.* 1985;2:214–9.
11. Ricotta JJ, Ouriel K, Green RM, et al. Use of computerized cerebral tomography in selection of patients for elective and urgent carotid endarterectomy. *Ann Surg.* 1985;202:783–87.
12. Shah DM, Darling RC III, Chang BB, et al. Carotid endarterectomy by eversion techniques. *Adv Surg.* 1999;33:459–76.
13. Ghika J. Bogousslavsk J. Regli F. Deep perforators from the carotid system: template of the vascular territories. *Arch Neurol.* 1990;47:1097–1100.
14. Corson JD, Chang BB, Shah DM, et al. The influence of anesthetic choice on carotid endarterectomy outcome. *Arch Surg.* 1987;122:807–12.
15. Rob C. Operation for acute completed stroke due to thrombosis of the internal carotid artery. *Surgery.* 1969;65:862–5.
16. Whittemore AD, Ruby ST, Couch NP, et al. Early carotid endarterectomy in patients with small, fixed neurologic deficits. *J Vasc Surg.* 1984;1:795–9.

5

Cognitive Changes After Carotid Endarterectomy and Carotid Artery Stenting

Brajesh K. Lal, MD

ABSTRACT

Cognitive function is an important outcome measure that affects patient well-being and functional status. However, it has not been evaluated systematically in the context of carotid revascularization. Clinical trials comparing the carotid endarterectomy (CEA) to best medical therapy, and CEA to carotid artery stenting (CAS) have only been based on the end points of stroke, myocardial infarction and death. Carotid revascularization procedures could result in a decline in cognitive function from microemboli causing ischemia from surgical dissection during CEA or from endovascular catheter and guide-wire manipulation during CAS. It could also occur from hypoperfusion during carotid clamping or balloon dilation and occlusion. Alternatively, cognitive dysfunction may be caused by a state of chronic hypoperfusion from the carotid stenosis that is corrected by revascularization, resulting in an improvement in cognition after CEA and CAS. It is still unclear whether these complex interactions ultimately result in a net improvement or a deterioration of cognitive function. Furthermore, it is not known whether the two methods of carotid revascularization have a differential effect on cognitive outcomes. It is becoming increasingly clear though, that there is a positive relationship between improvement in cognition and improvement in functional outcome of patients. This chapter reviews existing information on the affects of carotid stenosis, CEA and CAS on cognitive function.

INTRODUCTION

A decline in cognitive function from ischemic brain lesions has been termed vascular cognitive impairment.[1] Studies[2] have clearly shown that individuals with isolated cognitive deficits are at greater risk for employment problems, have difficulty with activities of daily living, may require personal assistance, and may be rendered unsafe drivers. Patients may experience problems in social situations, and the impact on family relationships is also significant. While the incidence of stroke after cardiac surgery has declined to almost 2%; nearly 30% of patients still experience some degree of cognitive impairment.[3] There has been extensive research to determine the best approaches to the prevention, management, testing and reporting of cognitive impairment after cardiac surgery.[4]

Fisher first proposed in 1951 that carotid artery disease could produce cognitive impairment.[5] He postulated that carotid occlusive disease could produce a dementia state, and proposed that restoration of blood supply could reverse the condition. This stimulated the first carotid artery reconstruction procedures on patients with stroke and internal carotid artery (ICA) stenosis. This established CEA as an important procedure in the management of stroke. Subsequently, stroke was recognized as a leading cause of death in the United States with about 20% attributable to atheroembolization from carotid artery stenosis. Therefore stroke prevention became the primary focus of carotid revascularization. The possibility that revascularization of carotid stenosis could alter cognitive function has only recently received attention again.

COGNITIVE VERSUS NEUROLOGIC FUNCTION

Cognitive function relates to how a person produces and controls behavioral processes such as thinking, learning, remembering, problem solving, and consciousness. Cognitive abilities are controlled by generally predictable areas of the brain although not quite as focal as motor and sensory abilities. For instance visual stimuli are initially received in the primary visual cortex while secondary processing for detection of direction, intensity, contrast, speed, and other combined attributes of the stimulus takes place in the surrounding higher-order visual cortex. Finally, the association cortex responds exclusively to a combination of two or more sensory inputs. Therefore cortical systems form a hierarchy based on the functions they participate in: primary, higher order, and association cortices. It is the interconnections and interactions within and between such systems that give rise to specific cognitive functions.

The major difference between the traditional neurologic deficit and a cognitive deficit is that the former is based on the loss of a localized sensory or motor function (such as movement of the left arm) whereas the latter is a loss of a system (such as ability to learn new facts). The two types of deficits may occur in isolation, or occur concurrently, depending on the nature and location of cerebral injury sustained. By-and-large, evidence for the coexistence of cognitive injury in patients with neurologic deficits from carotid stenosis is quite forthcoming. However, isolated cognitive deficits in patients without a stroke have not been looked for, and have therefore not been reported in any detail.

A subset analysis of the Cardiovascular Health Study (CHS) suggests that carotid stenosis may be a risk factor for cognitive impairment.[6] Of the 4006 patients followed in this study over 5 years, 32 patients were identified with an asymptomatic left carotid stenosis ≥75%. These patients, along with the rest of the cohort, were serially tested with a modified mini-mental state examination which measures cognitive function in the left brain hemisphere. There was a significant decline in 34% of the carotid stenosis patients (12/32) over 5 years. A decline was noted when patients with stenoses ≥50% were analyzed, but was not observed in the remaining cohort. However, this study was preliminary, sample size was small, and was limited to patients with left-sided stenosis due to the absence of an ideal cognitive battery that could test cognitive function in these patients.

While neurologic examinations aim at identifying specific sensory or motor deficits, a cognitive assessment consists of administering tests that examine a set of more-or-less independent functional domains that are controlled by brain systems. Most tests are designed to test individual domains, but some may examine combined categories. The major cognitive domains that are commonly tested include: attention and speed of information processing; working memory; learning; language; calculation; visuospatial perception and analysis; problem solving and judgment; abstract thinking; and executive functions. Most broadly accepted cognitive tests have standardized administration procedures with appropriate normative comparison groups. Guidelines for the assessment of cognition in clinical research have been published,[7] derived largely from cardiac surgery[8] and medical treatment outcomes studies.[9] However, a cognitive battery of tests specifically addressing the unique issues relating to carotid stenosis has not been devised.

The author's ongoing Asymptomatic Carotid Stenosis and Cognitive Function Study (ACCOF) is one of the first attempts to develop and validate a cognitive test battery that is comprehensive and responsive to the unique subset of carotid stenosis patients, and yet is clinically feasible (takes approximately 40 minutes). It will quantify the extent of cognitive impairment associated with carotid stenosis in a large sample of patients. It is also evaluating potential risk factors and etiologic mechanisms by which cognition may be affected by stenosis. Another study, CREST-2, is currently under review, and proposes to use this battery to compare cognitive outcomes between patients undergoing CEA versus CAS in a randomized setting.

POTENTIAL MECHANISMS FOR COGNITIVE CHANGES FROM CAROTID REVASCULARIZATION

Re-opening of a carotid stenosis by CEA or by carotid artery stenting (CAS) may have a salutary effect on cognition by enhancing cerebral perfusion.[5] Conversely, several mechanisms could lead to cognitive decline during the revascularization process. These mechanisms could be specific to the individual procedure used, or related to baseline characteristics of the patients. The net effect on cognitive function after revascularization may therefore relate to the type of procedure used or to intrinsic differences in the patients and their disease. Potential procedure-related factors include microembolization, new cerebral micro-infarctions, duration of carotid flow arrest, or incidence of systemic hypotension during revascularization. Potential patient-related factors include prior cerebral injury manifested as a stroke, prior cortical infarction that is silent, prior white matter injury, or carotid plaque morphology. The following sections outline the extent of our knowledge regarding how these multiple interactions may influence net cognitive outcome after carotid revascularization.

COGNITIVE OUTCOME AFTER CEA

The systematic reviews of Lunn et al[10] and Irvine et al[11] exemplify the current absence of consensus regarding cognitive outcome after CEA. They categorized 16 of 28 studies as demonstrating cognitive improvement after CEA. The remaining 12 studies showed no improvement or a decline. Sinforiani et al reported an *improvement* in 4 of 10 cognitive tests performed on 64 patients, before and 3 months after CEA.[12] However, this improvement may have been due to a practice effect since the same versions of cognitive tests were used during follow-up. Long-term outcomes and control groups were not included. In another study, Heyer et al, compared cognitive function in 80 patients undergoing CEA with controls undergoing lumbar spine surgery.[13] They found a *decline* in 1 of 4 cognitive tests, and when all tests were combined, there was a significant decline in the total cognitive score in the CEA group. This study was limited by a short and incomplete follow-up. Pearson studied 39 patients before and 3 months after CEA[14] and found that once age, education, and IQ were controlled for, there were *no changes* in cognitive function. Studies on cognitive performance after treatment of carotid stenosis have varied widely in the timing of assessment, specific tests performed, use of control populations, extent of follow-up, number of patients studied, and severity of stenosis. The inconsistent results prompted Irvine et al to conclude that while there were more reports of an improvement in cognition after CEA, reliable inferences could not be drawn due to the inadequacy of study designs.[11]

COGNITIVE OUTCOME AFTER CAS

There are even fewer studies addressing cognitive outcome after CAS. Crawley et al compared cognitive outcome in 20 patients undergoing carotid angioplasty without stenting, and 26 having CEA.[15] At 6 weeks, 5 patients in each group had an equivalent *decline* in cognitive performance. Another study based on the same cohort of patients also demonstrated no difference in cognitive performance between the two groups.[16] These early studies highlighted the likelihood of neurocognitive consequences from carotid angioplasty. CAS methodology has since evolved, and currently includes stenting with embolic protection devices (EPD). The most common form of protection used is a filter deployed in the distal ICA. The filter captures debris released during angioplasty and stenting, while still allowing blood flow to the brain through its micro-pores (approximately 120 μm in diameter). The filter is closed and withdrawn with the captured debris upon conclusion of the procedure. In a more recent study,[17] 40 patients underwent CAS with EPD protection. Based on a mini-mental state examination, the authors reported a trend towards *improvement* in cognitive outcome after CAS. However, as in studies related to CEA, limitations of study design and sample size preclude firm conclusions.

POTENTIAL MECHANISMS FOR CHANGES IN COGNITIVE FUNCTION

The clinical significance of silent cerebral microinfarction that does not manifest as a frank stroke has only recently been recognized. The Rotterdam scan study demonstrated that the presence of silent infarcts in healthy elderly people identified by MRI at base-line doubles the risk of developing dementia and decline in cognitive function on follow-up.[18] These findings were confirmed by the Atherosclerosis risk in communities study (ARIC)[19] and the Cardiovascular health study (CHS).[20] Baseline cerebral injury in the form of both, white matter lesions and cortical lesions have been correlated with poor cognition. Furthermore, people with silent infarcts are at a higher risk for additional silent or symptomatic infarcts during follow-up and cognitive decline is confined to such patients with additional infarcts during follow-up.[18] The cerebrovascular burden of new procedural microinfarction may worsen or accelerate Alzheimer's Disease progression.[21] These observations are mirrored in experimental studies where injection of 50μm microspheres into rat carotid arteries resulted in cerebral injury and reduced attentional performance.[22] Surgical[23] or catheter/guidewire[24] manipulation of the aorta during cardiac procedures also results in microembolic brain injury. While its etiology is likely multifactorial, postoperative cognitive decline in these patients has been correlated with silent microembolic cerebral injury.[25]

Manipulation of the carotid artery during surgical or endovascular revascularization causes atheroembolization with consequent silent cerebral microinfarction.[15] A combination of Diffusion Weighted Imaging (DWI) with ADC mapping and FLAIR sequences provides the optimal protocol to identify baseline cerebral injury and any new infarctions that may appear after carotid revascularization. Transcranial Doppler monitoring has identified approximately 1000 microemboli during CAS[26] while CEA is associated with 8 to 17 times fewer microemboli.[15] Consistent with the microembolization rates, CAS results in cerebral microinfarctions more frequently than CEA (54% vs. 17%).[27] This has prompted the routine use of embolic protection devices during CAS which have successfully captured atheroemboli[28] and reduced microinfarction rates (26% vs. 36% of unprotected CAS patients[29]). However, filters do not eliminate microembolic cerebral infarction completely, and protected CAS has continued to have over 1 log-fold higher microembolization than CEA.[30] This is not entirely unexpected, since filter pores are designed to allow continued cerebral perfusion when deployed. In the process, they also allow flow-through of particles<120 μm in size. Consequently, silent cerebral microinfarction still continues to be observed in more patients undergoing filter-protected CAS compared to CEA (43% vs. 9% in one representative study). Since these infarcts did not manifest as strokes in their study, Hauth et al[30] concluded that they were of no relevance. However, the potential neurocognitive consequences of the cerebral injury were not assessed. There are strong reasons to believe that despite the use of EPDs during CAS, silent microembolic cerebral injury may occur more frequently compared to CEA.

COMPARISON OF COGNITIVE FUNCTION AFTER CEA AND CAS

Only two studies have compared cognitive outcomes between surgical and endovascular carotid revascularization.[15,16] However, they used limited cognitive testing on a mixed cohort of symptomatic and asymptomatic patients, and a significant proportion of patients underwent angioplasty without stenting in the endovascular arm of the cohort. One other study compared stenting to CEA, but used a limited cognitive evaluation restricted to left-hemispheric functions alone (the Mini Mental State Examination) and did not find any differences.[31] The results of the above studies are difficult to interpret. Patients with prior stroke (vs. asymptomatic patients) or primary atherosclerosis (vs. smooth, post-CEA restenosis) have higher rates of atheroembolization; such patients were not equally distributed between treatment groups in the studies quoted above. Additionally, the prevalence of baseline cerebral injury (cortical or white matter) was not controlled for, and the reports varied widely in the timing of assessment, number of patients studied, imaging techniques, and methods used to identify and quantify microinfarction. Importantly, whether the reported differences in microinfarction between CEA and CAS translated into a differential cognitive outcome was not studied.

We have recently analyzed cognitive function in neurologically asymptomatic patients with primary atherosclerotic carotid stenosis undergoing CEA and CAS. Neurologic symptoms were evaluated by history, physical examination, and the NIH Stroke Scale. A 50-minute cognitive battery was performed 1–3 days before and 4–6 months after CEA or CAS. The tests (Trail Making Tests A/B, Processing Speed Index (PSI) of the Wechsler Adult Intelligence Scale - Third Edition (WAIS-III), Boston Naming Test, Working Memory Index (WMI) of the Wechsler Memory Scale - Third Edition (WMS-III), Controlled Oral Word Association & California Verbal Learning Test) for 6 cognitive domains (motor speed/coordination & executive function, psychomotor speed, language (naming), working memory/concentration, verbal fluency, and learning/memory) were conducted by a neuropsychologist.

Forty six patients underwent pre-post testing (CEA=25, CAS=21). Women comprised 36% of the cohort; mean pre-procedural stenosis was 84%; and 54% were right-sided lesions. All patients were successfully revascularized without peri-procedural complications. The scores for each test improved after CEA except WMI which decreased in 20/25 patients. Improvement occurred in all tests after CAS except PSI which decreased in 18/21 patients. In addition to comparing the changes in individual test scores, overall cognitive change was measured by calculating the change in composite cognitive score (CCS) post procedure vs. baseline. The composite score at baseline was then compared with that from the post-procedure testing. The CCS improved after both CEA and CAS, and the changes were not significantly different between the groups (0.51 vs 0.47, p=ns).

We therefore concluded that carotid revascularization results in an overall improvement in cognitive function. There are no differences in the composite scores of five major cognitive domains between CEA and CAS. When individual tests are compared, CEA results in a reduction in memory, while CAS patients show reduced psychomotor speed. Larger studies will help confirm these findings.

RISK FACTORS FOR CEREBRAL INJURY AND COGNITIVE IMPAIRMENT

Rapp et al[32] performed ex-vivo CAS on explanted human carotid plaques that were either fibrotic or calcific in composition. The microemboli released from the procedures were collected and separated by size. The particles were injected into the carotid arteries of rats and resulting cerebral infarctions were measured by histology. 100–200 μm particles caused infarctions in all animals, irrespective of their composition. However, 60–100 μm particles derived from calcified plaques caused infarctions in 58% of animals while only 9% of animals injected with fibrotic plaque fragments developed infarctions. They concluded that the composition of microembolic particles could influence the extent of ischemic cerebral injury. Furthermore, histological studies indicate that smooth homogeneous fibrous plaques are clinically stable and less prone to atheroembolization. Conversely, intraplaque hemorrhage, lipid core expansion, fibrous cap thinning and ulceration render a plaque heterogeneous, unstable, and prone to atheroembolization.[33] Endovascular or surgical manipulation of such unstable plaques could further increase atheroembolization and ischemic cerebral injury. Plaque composition can therefore be an important determinant of cerebral injury by influencing the quality and quantity of microemboli released, or the risk of plaque fragmentation during carotid instrumentation.

Our group[33,34] has demonstrated that the histological composition of carotid plaques can be inferred from non-invasive ultrasound imaging. Furthermore, non-invasive characterization of their composition can predict plaques that will generate more microemboli during ex-vivo CAS and patients that may develop peri-procedural stroke during CAS.[35] Plaques characterized as unstable correlate with the development of ipsilateral atheroembolic cerebral infarcts, stroke, or transient ischemic attacks (TIA). It is therefore likely that plaque heterogeneity may serve as an effect modifier and enhance the risk of atheroembolic cerebral injury and cognitive decline during carotid revascularization. We are currently testing this hypothesis in a longitudinal study evaluating plaque architecture versus cognitive function over time in patients with carotid stenosis.

OTHER RISK FACTORS FOR CEREBRAL INJURY AND COGNITIVE IMPAIRMENT

Carotid revascularization results in improved cerebral blood flow (CBF) which may translate into improved cognitive outcome.[36] This potential benefit would be derived by all patients irrespective of the method of revascularization used (CEA and CAS). However, each procedure also results in transiently reduced CBF. Patients undergoing carotid cross-clamping during CEA have EEG flattening when the CBF drops below 18 ml/100g/minute.[37] Progressive lowering of CBF is associated with initially transient, and then persistent attentional deficit.[36] CEA is generally associated with longer periods of ipsilateral carotid flow arrest from cross-clamping (mean 337 seconds) compared to the brief balloon inflations (mean 26 secs., p<0.001) associated with CAS.[38]

Cognitive dysfunction after cardiac surgery has been correlated with cerebral injury sustained from systemic hypotension during the bypass procedure. Systemic hypotension (reduction in systolic blood pressure by>30mmHg compared to baseline) occurs in up to 68% of patients undergoing CAS[39] and has been associated with elevated biochemical markers (S100B) of glial injury independent of embolization. Hemodynamic instability during CAS is associated with an increased likelihood of stroke (OR 3.05), MI (OR 3.34) and death (OR 3.6).[40] It has been surmised that the hypotension may cause watershed infarction or render an otherwise inconsequential peri-procedural embolic injury or other future insult to become relevant.[40]

While CAS involves shorter periods of carotid artery flow arrest it appears to have increased periods of systemic hemodynamic instability compared to CEA. The combined impact of these competing factors on cognitive outcome, if any, has not been evaluated.

RELEVANCE TO TRADITIONAL OUTCOMES OF CAROTID REVASCULARIZATION

In response to increasing enthusiasm for endovascular treatments of arterial occlusive disease, CAS has received increasing attention as an alternative to CEA in specific circumstances. Several randomized studies have recently compared CAS and CEA and arrived at different conclusions ranging from equivalence between, to superiority for CEA over CAS. No formal assessment of neurocognitive function has been made in prior or ongoing trials of revascularization for carotid stenosis. There is a strong need for such an evaluation because the largest clinical trial comparing CEA and CAS (Carotid Revascularization, Endarterectomy versus Stent Trial, CREST) failed to conclusively show a difference in stroke, MI and death rates between CAS and CEA. Therefore, the superiority of a procedure could be predicated on cognitive outcome. If stroke and cognitive outcomes are benefited by different procedures, then subgroups of patients at increased risk for cognitive dysfunction will have to be defined in order to prevent adverse outcomes. Either ways, it is to be anticipated that cognitive outcome will potentially guide future optimal treatment strategies in individual patients. This will stimulate the incorporation of cognitive testing in future clinical trials and in clinical practice.

REFERENCES

1. Roman GC. Vascular dementia: Distinguishing characteristics, treatment, and prevention. *J Am Geriatr Soc.* May 2003;51(5 Suppl Dementia):S296–304.
2. Chaytor N, Schmitter-Edgecombe M. The ecological validity of neuropsychological tests: A review of the literature on everyday cognitive skills. *Neuropsychol Rev.* Dec 2003;13(4):181–197.
3. Baker RA, Andrew MJ, Knight JL. Evaluation of neurologic assessment and outcomes in cardiac surgical patients. *Semin Thorac Cardiovasc Surg.* Apr 2001;13(2):149–157.
4. Murkin JM. Neurocognitive outcomes: The year in review. [Miscellaneous]. *Current Opinion in Anaesthesiology.* February 2005;18(1):57–62.
5. Fisher C. Senile dementia- A new explanation of its causation. *Arch of Neurol.* 1951;65(1):1–7.
6. Johnston SC, O'Meara ES, Manolio TA, et al. Cognitive impairment and decline are associated with carotid artery disease in patients without clinically evident cerebrovascular disease. *Ann Intern Med.* Feb 17 2004;140(4):237–247.
7. Lezak M. *Neuropsychological Assessment.* 3 ed. New York: Oxford University Press; 1995.
8. Murkin JM, Newman SP, Stump DA, et al. Statement of consensus on assessment of neurobehavioral outcomes after cardiac surgery. *Ann Thorac Surg.* May 1995;59(5):1289–1295.
9. Ryan CM, Hendrickson R. Evaluating the effects of treatment for medical disorders: Has the value of neuropsychological assessment been fully realized? *Appl Neuropsychol.* 1998;5(4):209–219.
10. Lunn S, Crawley F, Harrison MJ, et al. Impact of carotid endarterectomy upon cognitive functioning. A systematic review of the literature. *Cerebrovasc Dis. (Basel, Switzerland).* Mar-Apr 1999;9(2):74–81.
11. Irvine CD, Gardner FV, Davies AH, et al. Cognitive testing in patients undergoing carotid endarterectomy. *Eur J Vasc Endovasc Surg.* Mar 1998;15(3):195–204.
12. Sinforiani E, Curci R, Fancellu R, et al. Neuropsychological changes after carotid endarterectomy. *Funct Neurol.* Oct-Dec 2001;16(4):329–336.
13. Heyer EJ, Sharma R, Rampersad A, et al. A controlled prospective study of neuropsychological dysfunction following carotid endarterectomy. *Arch Neurol.* Feb 2002;59(2):217–222.
14. Pearson S, Maddern G, Fitridge R. Cognitive performance in patients after carotid endarterectomy. *J Vasc Surg.* Dec 2003;38(6):1248–1252; discussion 1252–1243.
15. Crawley F, Stygall J, Lunn S, et al. Comparison of microembolism detected by transcranial Doppler and neuropsychological sequelae of carotid surgery and percutaneous transluminal angioplasty. *Stroke.* Jun 2000;31(6):1329–1334.
16. Sivaguru A, Gains P, Beard J, et al. Neuropsychological outcome after carotid angioplasty: A randomized controlled trial. *J Neurol Neurosurg Psychiatry.* 1999;66 (suppl):262.

17. Grunwald I, Suppurian T, Politi M, et al. Cognitive Changes after Carotid Artery Stenting. *Neuroradiology*. 2006;48:319–323.
18. Vermeer SE, Prins ND, den Heijer T, Hofman A, Koudstaal PJ, Breteler MMB. Silent Brain Infarcts and the Risk of Dementia and Cognitive Decline. *New Engl J Med*. March 27, 2003;348(13):1215–1222.
19. Mosley TH, Jr, Knopman DS, Catellier DJ, et al. Cerebral MRI findings and cognitive functioning: The Atherosclerosis Risk in Communities Study. *Neurology*. June 28, 2005;64(12):2056–2062.
20. Longstreth WT, Jr., Bernick C, Manolio TA, et al. Lacunar infarcts defined by magnetic resonance imaging of 3660 elderly people: The cardiovascular health study. *Arch Neurol*. September 1, 1998;55(9):1217–1225.
21. Vinters HV. Cerebrovascular disease--practical issues in surgical and autopsy pathology. *Curr Top Pathol*. 2001;95:51–99.
22. Craft TKS, Mahoney JH, DeVries AC, et al. Microsphere embolism-induced cortical cholinergic deafferentation and impairments in attentional performance. *Eur J Neurosci*. 2005;21(11):3117–3132.
23. Braekken SK, Russell D, Brucher R, et al. Cerebral microembolic signals during cardiopulmonary bypass surgery. Frequency, time of occurrence, and association with patient and surgical characteristics. *Stroke*. Oct 1997;28(10):1988–1992.
24. Braekken SK, Endresen K, Russell D, et al. Influence of guidewire and catheter type on the frequency of cerebral microembolic signals during left heart catheterization. *AM J Cardiol*. Sep 1 1998;82(5):632–637.
25. Sylivris S, Levi C, Matalanis G, et al. Pattern and significance of cerebral microemboli during coronary artery bypass grafting. *Ann Thorac Surg*. Nov 1998;66(5):1674–1678.
26. Chen CI, Iguchi Y, Garami Z, et al. Analysis of Emboli during Carotid Stenting with Distal Protection Device. *Cerebrovasc Dis (Basel, Switzerland)*. Jan 27 2006;21(4):223–228.
27. Poppert H, Wolf O, Resch M, et al. Differences in number, size and location of intracranial microembolic lesions after surgical versus endovascular treatment without protection device of carotid artery stenosis. *J Neurol*. 2004;251(10):1198.
28. Ohki T, Roubin GS, Veith FJ, et al. Efficacy of a filter device in the prevention of embolic events during carotid angioplasty and stenting: An ex vivo analysis. *J Vasc Surg*. Dec 1999;30(6):1034–1044.
29. Cosottini M, Michelassi MC, Puglioli M, et al. Silent cerebral ischemia detected with diffusion-weighted imaging in patients treated with protected and unprotected carotid artery stenting. *Stroke*. November 1, 2005;36(11):2389–2393.
30. Hauth EAM, Jansen C, Drescher R, et al. MR and clinical follow-up of diffusion-weighted cerebral lesions after carotid artery stenting. *AJNR*. October 1, 2005;26(9):2336–2341.
31. ABCNews. Carotid artery stent procedure makes you smarter. http://abcnews.go.com/GMA/Health/story?id=1796304&page=1. 2006.
32. Rapp JH, Pan XM, Yu B, et al. Cerebral ischemia and infarction from atheroemboli<100 microm in size. *Stroke*. Aug 2003;34(8):1976–1980.
33. Lal BK, Hobson RW, 2nd, Hameed M, et al. Noninvasive identification of the unstable carotid plaque. *Ann Vasc Surg*. Mar 2006;20(2):167–174.
34. Lal BK, Hobson RW, 2nd, Pappas PJ, et al. Pixel distribution analysis of B-mode ultrasound scan images predicts histologic features of atherosclerotic carotid plaques. *J Vasc Surg*. Jun 2002;35(6):1210–1217.
35. Biasi GM, Froio A, Diethrich EB, et al. Carotid plaque echolucency increases the risk of stroke in carotid stenting: The Imaging in Carotid Angioplasty and Risk of Stroke (ICAROS) study. *Circulation*. Aug 10 2004;110(6):756–762.
36. Marshall RS, Lazar RM, Pile-Spellman J, et al. Recovery of brain function during induced cerebral hypoperfusion. *Brain*. Jun 2001;124(Pt 6):1208–1217.
37. Marshall RS. The functional relevance of cerebral hemodynamics: Why blood flow matters to the injured and recovering brain. *Curr Opin Neurol*. Dec 2004;17(6):705–709.

38. Crawley F, Clifton A, Buckenham T, et al. Comparison of hemodynamic cerebral ischemia and microembolic signals detected during carotid endarterectomy and carotid angioplasty. *Stroke.* Dec 1997;28(12):2460–2464.

39. Trocciola SM, Chaer RA, Lin SC, et al. Analysis of parameters associated with hypotension requiring vasopressor support after carotid angioplasty and stenting. *J Vasc Surg.* 2006;43(4):714.

40. Gupta R, Abou-Chebl A, Bajzer CT, et al. Rate, predictors, and consequences of hemodynamic depression after carotid artery stenting. *J Am Coll Cardiol.* Apr 18 2006;47(8):1538–1543.

Supra-aortic Trunk Disease

6

Current Management of Acute Spontaneous Carotid Dissections

Rudy J. Rahme, MD, Salah G. Aoun, MD, Tarek El Ahamdieh, MD, Yvonne Curran, MD, and Bernard R. Bendok, MD

INTRODUCTION

Extracranial internal carotid artery (ICA) and vertebral artery (VA) dissections are increasingly recognized as important causes of stroke. Although they account for only 2% of all ischemic strokes, they are responsible for approximately 20% of thromboembolic strokes in young patients under 45 years of age.[1] Their etiology can be categorized as either traumatic or spontaneous depending on the initiating event. In the absence of a preceding trauma, the dissection is deemed spontaneous. "Benign traumatic events" might sometimes be missed with the subsequent dissection therefore miscategorized as "spontaneous" (e.g. violent coughing or simple neck manipulations).

Carotid artery dissection can affect patients of all ages, with spontaneous dissections occurring primarily in middle-aged patients and traumatic dissections occurring in a slightly younger demographic. The yearly reported incidence of carotid dissection ranges between 2.5 and 3 per 100,000 although the real incidence might be higher due to the asymptomatic presentation of an unknown percentage of cases leading to under reporting of dissections. Spontaneous dissections, although mostly idiopathic, can be associated with connective tissue diseases such as fibromuscular dysplasia in up to 15% of cases, Marfan's syndrome, Ehler-Danlos syndrome type IV, and autosomal polycystic kidney disease.

PATHOPHYSIOLOGY

Carotid artery dissections are most likely due to a tear in the intima leading to a direct communication between the arterial lumen and the tunica media. It is also hypothesized that dissections could result from direct extravasation of blood from the vasa vasorum in to the media followed by extension of the hematoma within the arterial wall. In any case, the dissection is characterized by a longitudinal tear in the arterial wall within the tunica media. Potential narrowing of the arterial lumen can result from the formation intramural hematoma. Another potential complication is intraluminal thrombus formation with distal emboli due to the fact that the dissection exposes prothrombotic components of the subendothelial layer to the blood stream.

Whereas both the intracranial and the extracranial segments of the carotid artery are prone to dissection, the extracranial segments are more liable to injury then their intracranial counterparts. This is due to their greater mobility that puts them at an increased risk of injury through contact with surrounding bony structures such as the styloid process.[7]

NATURAL HISTORY

The true natural history of carotid artery dissection is not entirely clear. The reported mortality rate from carotid artery dissection is about 5%. Most dissections heal spontaneously with the objective of management being to decrease or prevent neurologic complications and sequelae. Stroke can be the presenting symptom in certain cases although it is often delayed in onset, sometimes as much as 31 days after the initial insult. Typically, the initial ischemic manifestation occurs within a few days following the dissection.

The majority of dissections heal spontaneously within 3 to 6 months with medical treatment, with the likelihood of spontaneous healing thereafter decreasing significantly.[1] The clinical implications of the arterial healing process is yet unclear though. In a prospective study, Kremer et al. revealed that the long-term rate of stroke in patients with carotid artery dissection is not related to the persistence of stenosis or occlusion. The risk of recurrence of spontaneous dissection is low. It is highest within the first month and reaches approximately 2%. It decreases thereafter to 1% a year. As for associated dissecting aneurysms, they tend to stabilize although they can in some cases either grow or decrease in size down to complete resolution.

CLINICAL PRESENTATION

Carotid artery dissections can in some cases be asymptomatic or can cause minor symptoms and therefore remain undiagnosed.[1] Typically though, the symptoms of a cervicocranial arterial dissection in general are thromboembolic or hemodynamic in nature. The intramural hematoma can cause a stenosis or occlusion of the intraluminal diameter and can therefore lead to a decrease in the distal blood flow. Also, the dissection can potentially leave the intraluminal blood exposed to the prothrombotic components of the subendothelial layer with subsequent platelet aggregation and potential release of distal emboli.[2] In addition, an intracranial extension of a dissection might also cause a subarachnoid hemorrhage although it is less common in carotid artery dissections than in vertebrobasilar dissections.

The typical clinical presentation of carotid artery dissection is present in less than a third of patients and is characterized by the triad of ipsilateral facial pain, partial Horner's syndrome, and ischemia. Patients presenting with 2 symptoms of the triad or with nonspecific neurologic symptoms, specifically in a post-traumatic setting, are highly suspect for an arterial dissection.

Headache, neck or facial pain is most frequently the initial symptom and can be the only symptom in less than 10% of cases.[1] Headaches are often gradual in onset, unilateral, constant, frontotemporal or frontoparietal, non-throbbing in nature. Occasionally, patients can also present with a severe "thunderclap" headache.[1,3] Orbital pain may also be present in half of the patients. Partial Horner's syndrome or oculosympathetic palsy is characterized with ptosis and miosis without anhidrosis. It is a typical symptom of internal carotid artery dissection and is found in 50% of cases. The sympathetic fibers innervating the facial sweat glands follow the external carotid artery and are therefore spared in cases of internal carotid artery dissection.[1] Patient presenting with a partial Horner's syndrome should be considered to have an internal carotid artery dissection until proven otherwise.[1,3]

In addition, due to its proximity to the carotid sheath, the hypoglossal nerve (XII) can also be injured in patients with carotid dissection.[4] Approximately 12% of patients with internal carotid artery dissection suffer cranial nerve palsies with the oculomotor (III), trigeminal (V) and the facial (VII) nerves mostly affected after the hypoglossal.[4] The clinical presentation of lower cranial nerve palsy associated with oculosympathetic impairment might therefore mimic a brain stem infarct.

Due to the potentially narrowed arterial lumen a pulsatile tinnitus can be heard in up to one fourth of the cases by the patients and can even sometimes be objectively present on auscultation.[3]

Ischemic manifestations are common with a reported frequency of 50% to 95%.[1,3] Although in 20% of cases it is the presenting symptom, stroke is often preceded by warning signs such as transient ischemic attacks and amaurosis fugax. The most common mechanism is thromboembolism. However, hemodynamic insufficiency can be the cause of ischemic complications when dissection results in acute severe stenosis or occlusion.[3] Due to increased early recognition of arterial dissections, added to the fact that ischemic symptoms often are a delayed manifestation of dissections the frequency of ischemic presentations has declined over the years.

DIAGNOSTIC IMAGING

The significant improvements in cerebral and vascular imaging over the last decade have changed the practice regarding the diagnostic approach to carotid dissection. The conventional gold standard is cerebral angiography.[1,3,5] However, the use of magnetic resonance imaging (MRI) technology and MR angiography (MRA) has increased significantly.[1,3,5] The major disadvantage of MR remains acquisition time limiting their use in emergency situations although this is rapidly evolving in positive ways. Computed tomography (CT) scans on the other hand can be obtained quickly, are widely available and can be used to assess for cerebral ischemia or bleeding.[1,3] Ultrasound is another non invasive imaging technique though it suffers from several limitations as it is highly operator dependent and has a low diagnostic performance with dissections at the level of the skull base. While the gray-scale ultrasound might reveal an intimal flap, an intramural hematoma, and in some cases a luminal narrowing,[6] the color Doppler on the other hand typically shows a high resistance flow.

Cerebral Angiography

A typical carotid artery dissection presents with a stenosis 2 to 3 cm above the carotid bulb extending distally without going past the petrous segment where the lumen reconstitutes precipitously. Aneurysmal dilation usually occurs in the cervical portion of the artery but can also occur intracranially.[7] They are fusiform in nature and occur in a third of the patients.

In broad terms, the most common finding of a dissection on conventional angiography is the segmental arterial stenosis also known as the "string sign".[3] It is not specific to dissection and is due to the narrowing of the vessel lumen. It can be seen in any other diseases that lead to narrowing of vessels such as atherosclerosis.[8] Other findings include: the "string and pearl sign" which is a fusiform dilation with proximal or distal narrowing, intimal flap, occlusion of the vessel usually tapered to a point, and double lumen with retention of the contrast in the false lumen well into the venous phase which is pathognomonic of arterial dissection.[1,3,5] The pathognomonic signs of dissection (e.g. double lumen and the intimal flap) are seen in less than 10% of patients.[6]

Based on presentation and imaging there is a risk of misdiagnosis with the differential diagnosis being either a saccular aneurysm when there is intracranial extension, atherosclerosis, or vasospasm following subarachnoid hemorrhage. Atherosclerotic patients are usually older, and have multiple diseased vessels, and the stenosis is usually irregular unlike the smooth stenosis in dissections. Regarding vasospasm, the history should clarify the diagnosis in most cases. In patients with dissection, unlike vasospasm, the stenotic appearance is present from the start. Patients presenting to the emergency room in delayed fashion might represent a diagnostic challenge.

Magnetic Resonance Imaging

The invasive nature of conventional angiography in addition to the significant advances in MR technology have led to the increasing use of MRI and MRA as a standard diagnostic tool for cervical and intracranial arterial dissection workups.[1,8] Different MR sequences allow for various visualizations of different aspects of the dissection. Whereas MRA is used to assess the luminal patency of the artery, T1-weighted, T2-weighted and proton density images allow direct evaluation of the vessel wall.[6,8,9] The most common finding on an MRI is the intramural hematoma.[9] The hematoma appearance follows a typical pattern of blood signal change on a MRI over time and can be viewed on different MR sequences. In the hyperacute phase, the hematoma appears hypointense on T1 and T2-weighted images. Due to hemoglobin breakdown overtime, the signal changes in the subacute phase to a characteristic hyperintense crescent shape around a flow void on T1-weighted images.[8,9] Fat saturation sequences might help differentiate small hematomas from surrounding soft tissue.[1] In addition, due to the stenosis and the intramural hematoma, the vessel might appear to have an increased external diameter with a decreased luminal diameter on the MR.

Computed Tomography

CT angiography (CTA) shows similar results to MR imaging with the added benefit of quick acquisition time making it the preferred modality in emergency situations and in cases of trauma.[1,3,5] CTA can typically show the stenosis and occlusion, a crescent-shaped mural thickening which is an image of the hematoma, the intimal flap, and potentially a dissecting aneurysm.[6]

TREATMENT

Most dissections heal spontaneously and therefore the treatment objective is to avoid or limit neurological complications.[1,3,5] Stroke is often delayed and preceded by warning signs such as transient ischemic attacks.[1,10] Therefore, the priority in managing these patients is determining whether medical management is sufficient or if there are any indications for microsurgical or endovascular interventions. In addition, it is important to detect the patients with acute arterial occlusion as these patients might need an aggressive therapeutic approach. Treatment options include thrombolysis, anticoagulation, endovascular interventions and surgical interventions. Unfortunately, there are no randomized trial comparing the various treatment options.

Medical Management

Thrombolysis

There is little evidence regarding the use of thrombolysis in patients with carotid artery dissections in the literature.[3] However, in cases of stroke due to acute blood flow blockage, intravenous or intra-arterial recombinant tissue plasminogen activator or urokinase could be warranted.[11] Thrombolysis could however potentially lead to certain complications including an increase in size of mural thrombus with worsening of the luminal stenosis, and mobilization of the mural thrombus with distal embolization. In case of intracranial dissection there is the theoretical risk of SAH due to leakage with potential subsequent development of a pseudoaneurysm. In a study by Georgiadis et al. 33 patients treated with IV thrombolysis for acute stroke post spontaneous cervical carotid artery dissection, none had new or worsening local signs, SAH or pseudoaneurysms. One meta-analysis of individual patient data of 180 patients from 14 retrospective series and 22 case reports revealed that the safety and outcome profile of thrombolysis for stroke in patients presenting with cervical dissections is similar to that of patients with all causes of stroke.[12] Therefore, although there a clear lack of data, we can conclude that thrombolysis appears to be a safe treatment modality but further studies are warranted to evaluate its efficacy.

Antithrombotic Therapy

In 2007, the Cervical Artery Dissection in Ischemic Stroke Patients (CADISP) study group published a summary of the pathophysiological hypothesis behind the ischemic manifestations of cervical artery dissections with an analysis of the clinical considerations regarding the use of antithrombotic agents.[2] The main questions that the CADISP group tried to answer were: what is the rationale behind antithrombotic therapy for cervical artery dissections? Which is better, anticoagulant or antiplatelet therapy?

The most commonly accepted hypothesis behind ischemia in arterial dissections is that of an embolic mechanism. Several observations support it and thus support the use of antithrombotic therapy: the infarct pattern on brain imaging,[13] the presence of distal branch occlusion and the observation of microemboli.[2] In addition, several reports using transcranial Doppler in both the posterior and anterior cerebral circulations have revealed findings suggestive of emboli in the intracranial circulation post vertebral and carotid dissections.[14] Finally, and at least theoretically, since most dissections heal and recanalize spontaneously, it could be construed that during the healing process the intramural thrombus might be mobilized into the blood stream therefore causing distal emboli and infarctions.[2]

The complication profile of antithrombotic therapy is similar to that of thrombolytics including increase in size of intramural thrombus with local compression symptoms (cranial nerve palsies, Horner's syndrome), and hemodynamic-induced infarcts.[2] Delayed occlusion of the internal carotid artery in the setting of carotid dissection have been reported with the use of heparin.[2] Finally, in cases where dissection caused a severe ischemic stroke, there is a potential risk of hemorrhagic transformation if anticoagulants are administered.

Unfortunately there are no randomized trials, and therefore no high level recommendations can be produced. Nonetheless, it is widely recommended that unless there are specific contraindications, antithrombotic therapy should be started in the acute phase of a carotid artery dissection (a large acute stroke could be an exception).[3,5,15,16]

Antithrombotic treatment consists of either anticoagulation with intravenous heparin followed by warfarin or antiplatelet therapy with aspirin.[3] Again, there is a lack of evidence as to the superiority of either one over the other although anticoagulation is typically preferred and more widely used.[3,15] A metaanalysis performed by the CADISP study group to compare the two treatment modalities,[2] included 26 studies and 327 patients and revealed no significant differences between both treatment modalities in terms of "death from all causes" and "death and disability".[2] Similarly, a Cochrane systematic meta-analysis of non-randomized studies found no difference between anticoagulants and antiplatelets in the treatment of arterial dissections.[17] However in both these metaanalyses, there was a distinct lack of data coming from randomized trials, therefore limiting the significance and the generalizability of their results. Typically, anticoagulation might be the preferred approach in patients with severe stenosis, occlusion or pseudoaneurysms, based on the fact that it is more effective in preventing thromboembolic complications.[3,15] Antiplatelets might be reserved for patients with poor prognosis or patients with large infarcts.[2,15,17]

Another topic of debate is duration of treatment. Dissections typically heal within 6 months of injury with a very low rate of recurrence.[1] Therefore treatment should be continued for 3 to 6 months.[15] Imaging findings could potentially be used as guidelines to continue or to stop anticoagulation but is not proven.

Endovascular Management

Indications

Endovascular interventions are not typically considered first line treatment for spontaneous carotid dissections. This is due to the high rate of spontaneous healing with low recurrence rates without the need for any invasive interventions.[3,16] However, in certain cases, a more invasive treatment option, endovascular or microsurgical, should at least be considered. Should a patient present with an intracranial extension of the dissection and subarachnoid hemorrhage, endovascular or microsurgical intervention may be warranted.[5,18] A diagnostic angiogram is first performed to look for a direct cause of the hemorrhage (e.g. pseudoaneurysm) and to better understand the vascular anatomy such as collateral circulation and length of the dissected segment.[5] Intracranial pseudoaneurysms and subarachnoid hemorrhages are more frequent in the posterior circulation and have a very high reported mortality rate that could reach 83% and a high rerupture rate.[5,19–21]

Usually the best treatment option with the lowest risk of rehemorrhage is to exclude the dissected segment from the circulation to avoid the risk of reruputure and further complications.[5,19] One option would be proximal occlusion although there is a risk of filling of the dissected segment through retrograde flow. The optimal approach would be to trap the dissected segment with or without a bypass depending on collateral circulation status. Both microsurgical and endovascular techniques may be needed.[5]

In addition, in patients presenting with acute occlusion of their carotid artery due to the dissection, hemodynamic insufficiency is the main mechanism behind the cerebral ischemia and not thromboembolism.[5] Therefore, in these patients, the primary treatment objective is to restore carotid patency. First, to preserve cerebral perfusion the patient should be kept normotensive or even slightly hypertensive and therefore started on a high-volume fluid resuscitation with strict monitoring of their volemic state through the placement of an arterial line and a Foley catheter, the objective again being a euvolemic or a slightly hypervolemic state.[5] Once the patient is stabilized, an endovascular intervention to restore normal carotid flow should be at least considered.[5] If the artery cannot be opened with a stent an extracranial to intracranial bypass can be considered.

Finally, endovascular therapy should be considered as a 2nd line treatment if medical management fails or if there is a contraindication of antithrombotic agents.[22] Although there is no agreed-upon definition for failure of medical therapy, progression of neurologic symptoms and new ischemic events despite adequate antithrombotic therapy generally warrant more invasive treatments.[22] Whether pseudoaneurysm enlargement can be considered as failure of medical therapy is debatable.[22]

Technical Nuances

In order to achieve optimal outcomes, thorough preoperative assessment of the radiological images is imperative. Various characteristics have to be carefully studied including length of the dissected segment, associated pseudoaneurysms, and location vis-à-vis perforators (relevant when the dissections extend intracranially). It is also important to analyze the images in the context of the clinical presentation, which might ultimately affect antithrombotic therapy strategy.

Once access has been achieved, typically through the femoral artery, the microcatheter should be advanced to the point of the dissection and then passed over the dissection as atraumatically as possible. Contrast material is then injected to confirm that the catheter is actually in the true lumen. Once the anatomy is confirmed, an exchange wire is left beyond the dissected segment. Ideally, wire access should not be lost until stenting is completed. Guidewires and catheters are foreign objects and as such are thrombogenic. Therefore, the procedure should be performed as fast and as efficiently as safely possible to avoid thromboembolic complications.

Different types of stents exist on the market and can be chosen depending on the location of the dissection and the needs of the patient. First, balloon-expandable stents have a high radial force in addition an increased metal-to-artery wall surface. Therefore, they may offer an advantage in patients with extracranial artery dissections,[23,24] where the high radial force would reappose the intimal flap as well as the thrombus on the vessel wall. Kinking of these stents has been an issue so the preference is usually for self-expanding stents. Self-expandable stents are also easier to deliver and intracranially.[22]

Finally, although there is a lack of evidence, distal embolic protection devices may not be needed in the endovascular treatment of dissections[22] Proximal protection devices might be a better option with less manipulation of the dissected segment but there is no evidence regarding their use in the current literature.[25]

Surgical Management

Surgical treatment of carotid arterial dissections has been largely replaced by endovascular management. It is mostly still used in dissection of the posterior circulation presenting with SAH where the microsurgical approach offers the benefit of visualizing the perforators and the PICA when trapping the dissected segment. In carotid dissections, microsurgery finds its use in thromboendarterectomy and in extracranial-intracranial bypass procedures for intracranial extensions of dissections with indications for trapping and flow replacement.

CONCLUSIONS

Carotid artery dissections are an important cause of stroke in the young population. Conservative medical management with antithrombotic therapy is the most widely accepted first line of treatment in most cases. Endovascular treatment still holds an important role in the management of these patients, either as a "back-up" option in case of failure of medical treatment or as a "first line" approach in patients with intracranial extension of the dissection and SAH presentation or severe flow limitation. Open surgical approach has largely been supplanted by the less invasive endovascular techniques. Even though there is a wide range of treatment options, management of this disease is mostly based on empirical evidence. Unfortunately, no level I evidence is available. Randomized trials are needed to validate the treatment modalities already in place and to innovate new management approaches in order to improve patient outcomes.

REFERENCES

1. Schievink WI. Spontaneous dissection of the carotid and vertebral arteries. *NEJM*. Mar 22 2001;344(12):898–906.
2. Engelter ST, Brandt T, Debette S, et al. Antiplatelets versus anticoagulation in cervical artery dissection. *Stroke*. Sep 2007;38(9):2605–2611.
3. Patel RR, Adam R, Maldjian C, et al. Cervical carotid artery dissection: current review of diagnosis and treatment. *Cardiol Rev*. May 2012;20(3):145–152.
4. Mokri B, Silbert PL, Schievink WI, et al. Cranial nerve palsy in spontaneous dissection of the extracranial internal carotid artery. *Neurology*. Feb 1996;46(2):356–359.
5. Amenta PS, Jabbour PM, Rosenwasser RH. Approaches to Extracranial and Intracranial Dissection. In: *Hemorrhagic and Ischemic Stroke: Medical, Imaging, Surgical, and Interventional Approaches*. Bendok BR, Naidech AM, Walker MT, Batjer HH, eds. NY: Thieme; 2011:461–472.
6. Flis CM, Jager HR, Sidhu PS. Carotid and vertebral artery dissections: clinical aspects, imaging features and endovascular treatment. *Eur Radiol*. Mar 2007;17(3):820–834.
7. Fisher CM, Ojemann RG, Roberson GH. Spontaneous dissection of cervico-cerebral arteries. *Can J Neurol Sci*. Feb 1978;5(1):9–19.

8. Rodallec MH, Marteau V, Gerber S, et al. Craniocervical arterial dissection: spectrum of imaging findings and differential diagnosis. *Radiographics*. Oct 2008;28(6):1711–1728.

9. Provenzale JM. MRI and MRA for evaluation of dissection of craniocerebral arteries: lessons from the medical literature. *Emer Radiol*. May 2009;16(3):185–193.

10. Biousse V, D'Anglejan-Chatillon J, Touboul PJ, et al. Time course of symptoms in extracranial carotid artery dissections. A series of 80 patients. *Stroke*. Feb 1995;26(2):235–239.

11. Kim YK, Schulman S. Cervical artery dissection: pathology, epidemiology and management. *Thromb Res*. Apr 2009;123(6):810–821.

12. Zinkstok SM, Vergouwen MD, Engelter ST, et al. Safety and functional outcome of thrombolysis in dissection-related ischemic stroke: a meta-analysis of individual patient data. *Stroke*. Sep 2011;42(9):2515–2520.

13. Benninger DH, Georgiadis D, Kremer C, et al. Mechanism of ischemic infarct in spontaneous carotid dissection. *Stroke*. Feb 2004;35(2):482–485.

14. Droste DW, Junker K, Stogbauer F, et al. Clinically silent circulating microemboli in 20 patients with carotid or vertebral artery dissection. *Cerebrovasc Dis*. 2001;12(3):181–185.

15. Debette S, Leys D. Cervical-artery dissections: predisposing factors, diagnosis, and outcome. *Lancet*. Jul 2009;8(7):668–678.

16. Shah Q, Messe SR. Cervicocranial arterial dissection. *Current treatment options in neurology*. Jan 2007;9(1):55–62.

17. Lyrer P, Engelter S. Antithrombotic drugs for carotid artery dissection. *Cochrane Database Syst Rev*. 2010(10):CD000255.

18. Uhl E, Schmid-Elsaesser R, Steiger HJ. Ruptured intracranial dissecting aneurysms: management considerations with a focus on surgical and endovascular techniques to preserve arterial continuity. *Acta neurochirurgica*. Dec 2003;145(12):1073–1083; discussion 1083–1074.

19. Boet R, Wong HT, Yu SC, et al. Vertebrobasilar artery dissections: current practice. *Hong Kong medical journal = Xianggang yi xue za zhi / Hong Kong Academy of Medicine*. Feb 2002;8(1):33–38.

20. Kitanaka C, Sasaki T, Eguchi T, et al. Intracranial vertebral artery dissections: clinical, radiological features, and surgical considerations. *Neurosurgery*. Apr 1994;34(4):620–626; discussion 626–627.

21. Mizutani T, Aruga T, Kirino T, et al. Recurrent subarachnoid hemorrhage from untreated ruptured vertebrobasilar dissecting aneurysms. *Neurosurgery*. May 1995;36(5):905–911; discussion 912–903.

22. Pham MH, Rahme RJ, Arnaout O, et al. Endovascular stenting of extracranial carotid and vertebral artery dissections: a systematic review of the literature. *Neurosurgery*. Apr 2011;68(4):856–866; discussion 866.

23. Ansari SA, Thompson BG, Gemmete JJ, et al. Endovascular treatment of distal cervical and intracranial dissections with the neuroform stent. *Neurosurgery*. Mar 2008;62(3):636–646; discussion 636–646.

24. Benndorf G, Herbon U, Sollmann WP, et al. Treatment of a ruptured dissecting vertebral artery aneurysm with double stent placement: case report. *AJNR. American Journal of Neuroradiology*. Nov-Dec 2001;22(10):1844–1848.

25. Fanelli F, Bezzi M, Boatta E, et al. Techniques in cerebral protection. *Eur J Radiol*. Oct 2006;60(1):26–36.

7

Effects of Renal Disease on Carotid Endarterectomy and Carotid Artery Stenting Outcomes

Ali F. AbuRahma, MD

INTRODUCTION

Stroke is the third leading cause of death in the United States after heart disease and cancer. The American Heart Association data showed that more than one-fourth of strokes were caused by recurrent events, advocating more improvement in secondary prevention, e.g. carotid endarterectomy (CEA) and carotid artery stenting (CAS).[1] Meanwhile, chronic renal insufficiency (CRI) is associated with advanced multiple vascular pathologies affecting various systems, e.g. cerebrovascular disease, coronary artery disease, and peripheral arterial disease, which may impact the operative outcome. The prevalence of chronic kidney disease in the general public (in the United States) has been estimated to be 9.6%.[2] Bax et al.[3] have shown that kidney failure is an important risk factor for adverse outcomes in patients with manifested arterial disease.

Patients with severe CRI have premature diffuse atherosclerosis in comparison to normal individuals.[4–6] The annual incidence of death in patients with chronic renal failure is approximately 10-30 times that of individuals without chronic renal failure and two-thirds of these deaths are due to cardiovascular disease.[4,7]

Patients with chronic kidney disease are at high risk for developing stroke, compared to the general population, even after adjusting for traditional risk factors like diabetes mellitus. Similarly, chronic kidney disease patients on renal replacement therapy also carry an elevated risk of stroke.[8,9] Stroke in dialysis patients has a 3–9% greater risk of hospitalization when compared with the general population.[10] Other associated co-morbidities in patients with chronic kidney disease, e.g. high blood pressure, advanced age, diabetes, malnutrition, and bleeding diathesis could increase the risk of stroke in these patients. Seliger et al. have shown that chronic kidney disease patients develop more severe atherosclerotic disease of the carotids than subjects with normal kidney function.[10] It has been speculated that this accelerated atherosclerosis could increase the risk of stroke in these patients.

Several studies have questioned the best treatment for patients with carotid stenosis concomitant with chronic renal failure, showing increased mortality and morbidity after CEA.[7,11–17] Some studies have only shown differences when patients are separated into mild (creatinine level of 1.6–2.9 mg/dL)[7,13,16,17] versus severe (creatinine level of ≥3 mg/dL) CRI, with increased stroke or death in patients with severe CRI after CEA. A few other studies have shown that CAS was associated with unacceptable risks in patients with CRI and questioned its effectiveness in these patients.[14,18]

The variations in the results of these publications can be explained, in part, by the definitions of CRI that were used. Most authorities use the plasma level of creatinine, while some believe creatinine clearance is better; meanwhile, others combine both functions. In addition, different levels of serum creatinine have been used to define the degree of CRI, and the methods used to calculate creatinine clearance may also differ. In most studies, either the Cockcroft-Gault or the Modification of Diet in Renal Disease (MDRD) methods was used.[13] This makes it difficult to compare the results of these studies and to determine the stage of CRI that may impact the results of carotid intervention. It is generally believed that creatinine is a late and insensitive marker, which can remain lower than 2.0 mg/dL, despite a significant reduction of the glomerular filtration rate (GFR) to as low as 15 ml/min/1.73 m². Because of these inaccuracies, the National Kidney Foundation Kidney Disease Outcomes Quality Initiative guidelines recommend the use of the GFR as a better indicator of chronic kidney disease.

OUTCOME OF CEA IN PATIENTS WITH CHRONIC KIDNEY DISEASE

Extracranial carotid artery disease accounts for about one-fourth of ischemic strokes. CEA has been considered the established gold standard for carotid revascularization in the general population,[19–23] meanwhile, CAS is continually developing into a safe and effective method of stroke prevention.

Severe CRI has been associated with an increased risk of death and shorter long-term survival, following abdominal aortic aneurysm repair and lower extremity vascular reconstruction procedures.[24,25] The influence of CRI on the short- and long-term outcome of CEA has mixed results, perhaps due to the associated low mortality and morbidity of this procedure.

Several retrospective and prospective studies have evaluated the perioperative outcome of patients with CRI after CEA. Some of these studies indicated a high perioperative morbidity and/or mortality in patients with chronic kidney disease undergoing CEA.[7,12–14,16,17,26–28] Although the perioperative outcomes, specifically stroke and myocardial infarction, are not consistent among these studies between normal patients and patients with severe renal insufficiency; most, if not all, of these studies, when they examined the outcome of patients with severe renal insufficiency as defined by a creatinine ≥3 mg/dL or a GFR of <30 ml/min/1.73 m², showed a significantly higher rate of 30-day mortality when compared to patients with normal renal function.[7,13,16,17]

Out of these previously reported studies, only three have examined the outcome of patients undergoing CEA using the Modification of Diet in Renal Disease (MDRD) formula to estimate renal function.[13,14,17] Sidawy et al.[17] reported the results of a multi-center Veterans Affairs study examining 20,899 patients utilizing the National Surgical Quality Improvement Program. Patients with moderate CRI, as defined by a GFR of 30-59 ml/min/1.73 m^2, were at increased risk for cardiac and pulmonary morbidity, but not mortality; in contrast to those with severe CRI, as defined by a GFR of <30 ml/min/1.73 m^2, who had a much higher operative mortality. There was no difference in the perioperative 30-day stroke or cardiac events. The incidence of neurological complications did not differ significantly (control 1.7%, moderate CRI 1.9%, severe CRI 2.7%). The moderate CRI group had significantly more cardiac events (1.7% versus 0.9% for the control, p<0.001) and higher rates of pulmonary complications (2.1% versus 1.3% control; p<0.001). Those with severe CRI had a much higher mortality (3.1% versus 1.0% control, p<0.001). Kretz et al.[13] found a similar outcome for CEA patients with normal and moderate CRI using the level of serum creatinine. In this analysis using the level of creatinine for renal function, there was no significant difference between the groups in the 30-day stroke and death rates (normal renal function 1.8%; moderate 2.7%; and severe 8.3%; p=0.21). However, when the analysis of renal function was calculated according to the creatinine clearance using the Cockcroft-Gault formula, it showed that in the severe CRI group, the stroke and death rates were higher than the other two groups (normal renal function 1.7%; moderate 1.4%, and severe 7.5%, p=0.004). Using the MDRD formula, similar differences occurred between the severe group and the other two groups, with a higher rate of 30-day stroke and death (normal renal function 1.4%, moderate 1.7%, and severe 12.5%; p<0.001).

Similarly, Protack et al. analyzed the influence of CRI on the outcome of 921 carotid interventions (750 CEAs and 171 CAS procedures)[14] The 30-day stroke rates were: 3% for patients with normal kidney functions, 2.7% for patients with moderate CRI, and 5.5% for patients with severe CRI (p=0.54). The 30-day mortality for these groups were: 0.66% (normal), 1.2% (moderate CRI), and 5.5% (severe CRI), p=0.005. There was no difference in freedom from stroke based on the level of renal function in patients who underwent CEA, however, CAS patients with severe CRI had significantly lower rates of freedom from stroke.

A recent study by van Lammeren et al.[15] concluded that patients with an estimated GFR of 30 to 59 have a 2.2-fold increased risk of cardiovascular death and a 1.9-fold increased risk for myocardial infarction during the three years after CEA, when compared to patients with an estimated GFR of 60 or more, independent of other cardiovascular risk factors.

Other studies have reported similar findings, i.e. a negative impact on the clinical outcome of CEA in patients with CRI using serum creatinine levels. Rigdon et al.[7] reported an incidence of 30-day postoperative stroke and death of 43% (3/7 CEAs) in six patients with severe CRI (>2.9 mg/dL) versus 6% stroke and 1% mortality in 264 CEAs in patients with normal renal function (p<0.001 and <0.001, respectively). The authors concluded that CEA can be justified only for carefully selected symptomatic carotid artery disease patients with severe CRI. They also felt that CEA in patients with mild CRI (1.5-2.9 mg/dL) is associated with low-risk. Plecha et al.[11] evaluated the medical and operative risk factors and surgical outcome of CEA patients at the Cleveland Clinic and found that patients requiring chronic hemodialysis had a significant increase in stroke and death after CEA. Similarly, Tarakji,[12] who analyzed 143 patients with CRI, found that the 30-day combined stroke/death rate was 9%, whereas the stroke/death rate for 150 control patients without CRI was 2.6% (p=0.032). The stroke/death rate for patients with severe CRI (serum creatinine ≥3) was 19%. The authors also felt that CRI was associated with an increased incidence of stroke, myocardial infarction, and death after CEA.

Ascher et al.[16] also reported their results in analyzing 675 consecutive CEAs where 166 patients had a serum creatinine level of ≥1.5 mg/dL and 443 patients had normal creatinine levels. There was no significant difference in the stroke rate between the CRI group and the control group (1.2% versus 0.5%). However, the mortality rate for the CRI group was 3% versus 0% for the control group (p<0.002). Patients with creatinine levels between 1.5 to 2.9 mg/dL had a 0.7% mortality rate versus 17% for patients with serum creatinine levels of ≥3 mg/dL (p<0.01). The stroke rate for the former group was 0.7% and 4.3% for the latter group (nonsignificant). The authors concluded that a high mortality rate was observed in patients with serum creatinine levels of ≥3 mg/dL after CEA, and they recommended nonoperative treatment in asymptomatic carotid artery stenosis in patients with CRI (serum creatinine ≥3 mg/dL).[16]

Similar outcomes were noted by Debing et al[27] where the perioperative mortality rate was specifically higher in patients with CRI (3.9% versus 1%, p=0.013). A multivariate logistic regression analysis showed a significant association between CRI and 30-day death rates (an odds ratio of 3.76, p=0.032). The authors felt that the mortality risk in this group may be related to the increased rate of perioperative coronary artery disease and/or perioperative hypertension and myocardial infarction.

Other studies have shown that patients with preoperative renal dysfunction can safely undergo CEA. Reil et al.[28] analyzed 398 CEAs done on 370 patients. Patients were categorized by preoperative creatinine levels as normal (creatinine ≤1.5) or abnormal (creatinine >1.5). They concluded that CEA can be safely performed in patients with renal dysfunction with no increase in perioperative stroke or death rates. However, they noted an increased rate of myocardial infarction in their series, and they recommended preoperative cardiac evaluations in patients with renal insufficiency. Similarly, Amin et al.[29] analyzed 28 patients requiring dialysis who underwent CEA and reported no perioperative complications. They concluded that patients undergoing dialysis were not at any greater risk for complications when undergoing CEA than the general population. Sternbergh et al.[30] analyzed 1,081 patients who had CEA; 51 of these were performed in 44 patients with CRI (32 in 27 patients) and end-stage renal disease (19 in 17 patients). There were no perioperative strokes in the patients in the CRI and end-stage renal group, but one patient died 29 days postoperatively because of myocardial infarction; for a combined stroke and death rate of 2%. This was in contrast to the control group, who had a 2.6% stroke/death rate. Long-term survival analysis showed a four year survival rate of 12% for patients with end-stage renal disease and 54% for patients with CRI, compared to 72% for the control (p<0.05). They concluded that CEA can be performed safely in patients with CRI or end-stage renal disease with perioperative stroke and death rates equivalent to that of patients with normal renal function. However, they felt that the benefit of long-term stroke prevention in asymptomatic patients with end-stage renal disease is in question because of the high four-year death rate in these patients.

OUTCOME OF CAROTID ARTERY STENTING (CAS) IN PATIENTS WITH CHRONIC KIDNEY DISEASE

Several multicenter prospective randomized studies have been conducted to evaluate the efficacy of CAS for both low-risk and high-risk patients, with mixed results. These included the Carotid Revascularization with Endarterectomy or Stent Trial (CREST) that compared CEA and CAS in patients with symptomatic and asymptomatic significant carotid stenosis;[31] the International Carotid Stenting Study (ICSS),[32] which is a multi-national prospective randomized trial comparing CAS or CEA for symptomatic patients; the Endarterectomy Versus Angioplasty in Patients with Symptomatic Severe Carotid Stenosis (EVA-3S) trial;[33] the Stent-Protected Angioplasty versus Carotid Endarterectomy trial (SPACE);[34] and the Stenting and Angioplasty with Protection in Patients at High-Risk for Endarterectomy trial (SAPPHIRE).[35] There were also numerous carotid registries that analyzed the outcome of CAS in both symptomatic and asymptomatic patients, which include: the Carotid Artery Revascularization using the Boston Scientific FilterWire EX/EZ and the EndoTex NexStent trial (CABERNET),[36] ACCULINK for Revascularization of Carotids in High-Risk patients trial (ARCHeR),[37] Carotid Revasularization with ev3 Arterial Technology Evolution trial (CREATE),[38] Carotid Acculink/Accunet Post Approval Trial to Uncover Unanticipated or Rare Events trial (CAPTURE),[39] and Boston Scientific EPI: A Carotid Stenting Trial for High-Risk Surgical Patients trial (BEACH).[40]

Unfortunately, most, if not all, of the clinical trials that analyzed the outcome of CAS excluded patients with chronic kidney disease from their study population. In addition, dialysis patients are prone to bleeding, and, hence, require close observation if dual antiplatelets or anticoagulation is initiated during or after CAS. The use of contrast during CAS, may also potentially induce contrast-induced nephropathy and exaggerate the chronic kidney disease.

A few studies have shown that CAS was associated with unacceptable risks in patients with CRI and question its effectiveness.[14,18]

Saw et al.[18] conducted a retrospective analysis of patients who underwent CAS at the Cleveland Clinic between 1998 and 2003, who had their baseline creatinine and weight recorded. Creatinine clearance was calculated using the Cockcroft-Gault equation, which inputs the patient's weight, age, gender, and serum creatinine level to estimate the GFR.[41] Patients were grouped according to the presence or absence of chronic kidney disease (GFR <60 ml/min/1.73 m²). These patients were divided into four groups, according to their creatinine clearance quartiles. Of 641 patients who underwent CAS, 581 patients had information available for creatinine clearance. The presence of chronic kidney disease was associated with a higher combined event rate (stroke, death, and myocardial infarction) at seven days (6.8% versus 2.7%, p=0.023) and at six months (14.7% versus 5.6%, p<0.001), compared with the absence of chronic kidney disease. The presence of chronic kidney disease was also associated with a higher patient endpoint of death rate (8.4% versus 3.4%, p=0.015) and stroke (4.2% versus 0.8%, p=0.009) at six months compared without chronic kidney disease. The six-month Kaplan-Maier event free (death, stroke, or myocardial infarction) survival was significantly higher among those without chronic kidney disease versus those with chronic kidney disease (p<0.001). When the results were analyzed according to the creatinine clearance quartiles, the highest creatinine clearance quartile (4th quartile) was associated with a significantly lower combined event rate at both seven days (1.4% versus 6.2%, p=0.049) and at six months (4.1% versus 14.5%, p=0.004), compared with the lowest creatinine clearance quartile. A Cox regression analysis showed chronic kidney disease, prior myocardial infarction, diabetes, age, and baseline hemoglobin as univariate predictors of six-month combined death, stroke, or myocardial infarction event rates; however a multivariate analysis identified only chronic kidney disease and diabetes as independent predictors of six-month combined event rates.

Similar findings were noted by Protack et al.[14] They found that patients with severe CRI undergoing CAS exhibited higher 30-day stroke, death, and combined stroke, death, and myocardial infarction rates when compared to those with normal renal function. A long-term analysis revealed no difference in five-year rates for freedom from stroke, myocardial infarction, death, or major adverse events between patients with normal and moderate CRI, however patients with severe CRI had significantly lower rates at five years for freedom from stroke, death, and major adverse events, compared to those with normal renal function.

OUR CLINICAL EXPERIENCE

Impact of Chronic Renal Insufficiency on Clinical Outcome of CEA

Nine hundred and fifty-three CEAs (881 patients, who had both serum creatinine levels and GFR using the MDRD equation) during a recent two-year period were analyzed. Patients were classified according to serum creatinine levels and MDRD into three groups: normal (serum creatinine <1.5 mg/dL or GFR ≥60 ml); moderate CRI (serum creatinine ≥1.5–2.9

TABLE 7-1. A AND B PERIOPERATIVE MAJOR COMPLICATIONS/RENAL FUNCTIONS
(ALL CEA PATIENTS)

Complication	Serum Creatinine <1.5 mg/dL No.=818	Serum Creatinine 1.5–2.9 mg/dL No.=113	Serum Creatinine >3 mg/dL No.=9	P value
Stroke	16 (2%)	4 (3.5%)	1 (11.1%)	0.0914
Death	4 (0.5%)	1 (0.9%)	0	0.5018
Myocardial infarction	12 (1.5%)	4 (3.5%)	0	0.245
Major adverse events	27 (3.3%)	6 (5.3%)	1 (11.1%)	0.146

Complication	GFR (MDRD) ≥60 No.=614	GFR (MDRD) 30–59 No.=274	GFR (MDRD) <30 No.=37	P value
Stroke	7 (1.1%)	10 (3.7%)	2 (5.4%)	0.0176
Death	1 (0.2%)	4 (1.5%)	0	0.0572
Myocardial infarction	7 (1.1%)	7 (2.6%)	2 (5.4%)	0.0519
Major adverse events	14 (2.3%)	15 (5.5%)	3 (8.1%)	0.0159

or GFR ≥30–59), and severe CRI (serum creatinine ≥3 or GFR < 30). Major adverse events ([MAE] stroke/death/MI) were compared for all groups. Univariate and multivariate regression analyses were used to compare clinical outcomes.

Results

Patients with moderate and severe CRI were older (p<0.001) and had significantly more comorbidities: hypertension (p=0.006), diabetes mellitus (p=0.0005), and coronary artery disease (p=0.01). Using serum creatinine levels, the perioperative stroke and MAE rates for normal, moderate, and severe CRI were: 2%, 3.5%, and 11.1% (p=0.091) and 3.3%, 5.3%, and 11.1% (p=0.146), respectively. This was in contrast to perioperative stroke rates of 1%, 3.7%, and 5.4% (p=0.018) and perioperative MAE rates of 2.3%, 5.5%, and 8.1% (p=0.016) using MDRD. A subgroup analysis using serum creatinine showed perioperative stroke rates for symptomatic patients were 2.8% and 2.6% (p=1) for normal and moderate CRI; and 1.6%, 4.1% and 11.1% (p=0.045) for asymptomatic patients with normal, moderate, and severe CRI, respectively. This was in contrast to 1.6%, 4.7%, and 9.1% for symptomatic patients (p=0.09) and 1%, 3.2%, and 3.9% for asymptomatic patients (p=0.07) using MDRD. The perioperative MAE rates for symptomatic patients using serum creatinine levels were 3.6% (normal patients) and 2.6% (moderate CRI) (p=1); and for asymptomatic patients 3.2%, 6.8%, and 11.1% (p=0.09); in contrast to 2.1%, 5.9%, and 9.1% (p=0.112) for symptomatic patients and 2.4%, 5.3%, and 7.7% (p=0.09) for asymptomatic patients using MDRD

TABLE 7-2. A AND B PERIOPERATIVE MAJOR COMPLICATIONS/RENAL FUNCTIONS (FOR SYMPTOMATIC AND ASYMPTOMATIC CEA PATIENTS)

Complication	Serum Creatinine <1.5 mg/dL	Serum Creatinine ≥1.5–2.9 mg/dL	Serum Creatinine >3	P value
Symptomatic Patients (292)	No.=253	No.=39	No.=0	----
Stroke	7 (2.8%)	1 (2.6%)	----	1
Major adverse events	9 (3.6%)	1 (2.6%)	----	1
Asymptomatic Patients (648)	No.=565	No.=74	No.=9	
Stroke	9 (1.6%)	3 (4.1%)	1 (11.1%)	0.0453
Major adverse events	18 (3.2%)	5 (6.8%)	1 (11.1%)	0.093

Complication	GFR (MDRD) ≥60	GFR (MDRD) 30–59	GFR (MDRD) <30	P value
Symptomatic Patients (288)	No.= 192	No.=85	No.=11	
Stroke	3 (1.6%)	4 (4.7%)	1 (9.1%)	0.090
Major adverse events	4 (2.1%)	5 (5.9%)	1 (9.1%)	0.112
Asymptomatic Patients (637)	No.=422	No.=189	No.=26	
Stroke	4 (1%)	6 (3.2%)	1 (3.9%)	0.0737
Major adverse events	10 (2.4%)	10 (5.3%)	2 (7.7%)	0.0906

(Tables 7-1 and 7-2). Moderate CRI had more cardiac complications, 5.5% versus 1.9% (p=0.004) and respiratory complications, 2.5% versus 0.2% (p=0.018).

Impact of Chronic Renal Insufficiency on Clinical Outcome of CAS

We analyzed the impact of CRI on clinical outcomes of 313 CAS patients who had both serum creatinine levels and GFR (MDRD). Again, patients were classified according to serum creatinine levels and MDRD into three groups, as previously described.

Patients with moderate and severe CRI had significantly more comorbidities: hyperlipidemia (p=0.026), congestive heart failure (p=0.039), and smoking (p=0.025). Using serum creatinine levels, the perioperative stroke and MAE rates for normal, moderate, and severe CRI were 4.9%, 0%, and 25% (p=0.05) and 4.9%, 2.1%, and 25% (p=0.179), respectively. This was in contrast to a perioperative stroke rate of 4.6%, 3.7%, and 11.1% (p=0.44) and a perioperative MAE rate of 4.6%, 4.6%, and 11.1% (p=0.666) using MDRD. A subgroup analysis using serum creatinine showed the perioperative MAE rates for symptomatic patients using serum creatinine levels were 9.3% and 0% (p=0.355) and 2% and 5.9% for asymptomatic patients (p=0.223 in patients with normal versus moderate/severe CRI, respectively). In contrast to 8.1% and 7.8% for symptomatic patients and 2.5% and 3% (p=1) for asymptomatic patients using MDRD (Tables 7-3 and 7-4).

At a mean follow-up of 21 months (range: 1-78 months), the late MAE rates in normal patients versus moderate/severe CRI patients were 8% and 14% (p=0.247) using the serum creatinine level versus 6.6% and 13.3% (p=0.05) using MDRD. The late MAE rates for symptomatic patients in normal versus moderate/severe CRI were 8.7% versus 27% (p=0.06) using creatinine levels and 5.7% versus 19% (p=0.026) using MDRD

TABLE 7-3. A AND B PERIOPERATIVE MAJOR COMPLICATIONS/RENAL FUNCTIONS (ALL CAS PATIENTS)

Complication	Serum Creatinine <1.5 mg/dL No.=262	Serum Creatinine 1.5–2.9 mg/dL No.=47	Serum Creatinine >3 mg/dL No.=4	P value
Stroke	13 (5%)	0	1 (25%)	0.0555
Death	1 (0.4%)	0	0	1
Myocardial infarction	0	1 (2.1%)	0	0.1629
Major adverse events	13 (5%)	1 (2.1%)	1 (25%)	0.1789

Complication	GFR (MDRD) ≥60 No.=196	GFR (MDRD) 30–59 No.=108	GFR (MDRD) <30 No.=9	P value
Stroke	9 (4.6%)	4 (3.7%)	1 (11.1%)	0.44
Death	0	1 (0.9%)	0	0.3738
Myocardial infarction	0	1 (0.9%)	0	0.3738
Major adverse events	9 (4.6%)	5 (4.6%)	1 (11.1%)	0.6666

TABLE 7-4. A AND B MAJOR ADVERSE EVENTS/RENAL FUNCTIONS (FOR SYMPTOMATIC AND ASYMPTOMATIC CAS PATIENTS)

Complication	Serum Creatinine <1.5 mg/dL	Serum Creatinine ≥1.50 mg/dL	P value
Symptomatic Patients (125)	No.=108	No.=17	
Major adverse events	10 (9.3%)	0	0.355
Asymptomatic Patients (188)	No.=154	No.=34	
Major adverse events	3 (2%)	2 (5.9%)	0.226

Complication	GFR (MDRD) ≥60	GFR (MDRD) <60	P value
Symptomatic Patients (125)	No.=74	No.=51	
Major adverse events	6 (8.1%)	4 (7.8%)	1
Asymptomatic Patients (188)	No.=122	No.=66	
Major adverse events	3 (2.5%)	2 (3%)	1

and for asymptomatic patients 7.8% versus 7.1% (p=1) using creatinine and 7.1% versus 8.8% (p=0.76) using MDRD. Late death rate was 0.55% in normal patients versus 7.6% (p=0.0017) in moderate/severe CRI.

CONCLUSIONS

In conclusion, and based on studies that have been published to date, it could be argued that the risk of carotid intervention (CEA or CAS) can be justified only for carefully selected symptomatic carotid disease patients with severe CRI who have an acceptable operative risk and a good long-term life expectancy. CEA in patients with mild CRI is generally associated with lower risk and may be treated with the same consideration as patients with normal kidney function. Patients with severe CRI and asymptomatic carotid stenosis should be offered optimal medical therapy. Dialysis patients with asymptomatic carotid stenosis should probably not undergo intervention since they are nearing the end of their life span. However, others may argue that the quality of their remaining life is a concern, and the addition of a neurological deficit in these patients can be more devastating. This should be carefully weighed after discussing all options with these patients before offering carotid intervention.

REFERENCES

1. Thom T, Haase N, Rosamond W, et al. Heart Disease and Stroke Statistics – 2006 Update: A report from the American Heart Association Statistics Committee and Stroke Statistics Subcommittee. *Circulation.* 2006; 113:e85–e151.
2. Coresh J, Byrd-Holt D, Astor BC, et al. Chronic kidney disease awareness, prevalence, and trends among U.S. adults, 1999 to 2000. *J Am Soc Nephrol.* 2005; 16:180–188.

3. Bax L, Algra A, Mali WP, et al. Renal function as a risk indicator for cardiovascular events in 3216 patients with manifest arterial disease. *Atherosclerosis*. 2008; 200:184–190.

4. Porter GA. Cardiovascular complications in end-stage renal disease patients. In: Cummings NB, Klahr S, eds. *Chronic Renal Disease: Causes, Complications and Treatment*. New York: Plenum Medical Book Co., 1985; pp 219–223.

5. Hellerstedt WL, Johnson WJ, Ascher N, et al. Survival rates of 2,728 patients with end-stage renal disease. *Mayo Clin Proc*. 1984; 59:776–783.

6. Ritz E, Wiecek A, Gnasso A, et al. Is atherogenesis accelerated in uremia? *Contrib Nephrol*. 1986; 52:1–9.

7. Rigdon EE, Monajjem N, Rhodes RS. Is carotid endarterectomy justified in patients with severe chronic renal insufficiency? *Ann Vasc Surg*. 1997; 11:115–119.

8. McCullough PA, Li S, Jurkovitz CT, et al. CKD and cardiovascular disease in screened high-risk volunteer and general populations: The Kidney Early Evaluation Program (KEEP) and National Health and Nutrition Examination Survey (NHANES) 1999–2004. *Am J Kidney Dis*. 2008; 51:S38–S45.

9. Seliger SL, Gillen DL, Tirschwell D, et al. Risk factors for incident stroke among patients with end-stage renal disease. *J Am Soc Nephrol*. 2003; 14:2623–2631.

10. Seliger SL, Gillen DL, Longstreth WT Jr, et al. Elevated risk of stroke among patients with en-stage renal disease. *Kidney Int*. 2003; 64:603–609.

11. Plecha EJ, King TA, Pitluk HC, et al. Risk assessment in patients undergoing carotid endarterectomy. *Cardiovasc Surg*. 1993; 1:30–32.

12. Tarakji A, McConaughy A, Nicholas GG. The risk of carotid endarterectomy in patients with chronic renal insufficiency. *Current Surgery*. 2006; 63:326–329.

13. Kretz B, Abello N, Brenot R, et al. The impact of renal insufficiency on the outcome of carotid surgery is influenced by the definition used. *J Vasc Surg*. 2010; 51:43–50.

14. Protack CD, Bakken AM, Saad WE, et al. Influence of chronic renal insufficiency on outcomes following carotid revascularization. *Arch Surg*. 2011; 146:1135–41.

15. van Lammeren GW, Moll FL, Blankestijn PJ, et al. Decreased kidney function: An unrecognized and often untreated risk factor for secondary cardiovascular events after carotid surgery. *Stroke*. 2011; 42:307–312.

16. Ascher E, Marks NA, Schutzer RW, et al. Carotid endarterectomy in patients with chronic renal insufficiency: A recent series of 184 cases. *J Vasc Surg*. 2005; 41:24–9.

17. Sidawy AN, Aidinian G, Johnson ON, et al. Effect of chronic renal insufficiency on outcomes of carotid endarterectomy. *J Vasc Surg*. 2008; 48:1423–30.

18. Saw J, Gurm HS, Fathi RB, et al. Effect of chronic kidney disease on outcomes after carotid artery stenting. *Am J Cardiol*. 2004; 94:1093–1096.

19. Barnett HJM, Taylor DW, Eliasziw M, et al. Benefit of carotid endarterectomy in patients with symptomatic moderate or severe stenosis. *N Engl J Med*. 1998; 339:1415–1425.

20. North American Symptomatic Carotid Endarterectomy Trial Collaborators. Beneficial effect of carotid endarterectomy in symptomatic patients with high-grade carotid stenosis. *N Engl J Med*. 1991; 325:445–453.

21. European Carotid Surgery Trialists' Collaborate Group. MRC European Carotid Surgery Trial: Interim results for symptomatic patients with severe (70–99%) or with mild (0–29%) carotid stenosis. *Lancet*. 1991; 337:1235–1243.

22. Mayberg MR, Wilson SE, Yatsu F, et al. Carotid endarterectomy and prevention of cerebral ischemia in symptomatic carotid stenosis. Veterans Affairs Cooperative Studies Program 309 Trialist Group. *JAMA*. 1991; 266:3289–3294.

23. Executive Committee for the Asymptomatic Carotid Atherosclerosis Study. Endarterectomy for asymptomatic carotid artery stenosis. *JAMA*. 1995; 273:1421–1428.

24. Chang BB, Paty PSK, Shah DM, et al. Results of infrainguinal bypass for limb salvage in patients with end-stage renal disease. *Surgery*. 1990; 108:742–746.

25. Cohen JR, Mannick JA, Couch NP, et al. Abdominal aortic aneurysm repair in patients with preoperative renal failure. *J Vasc Surg*. 1986; 3:867–870.

26. Hamdan AD, Pomposelli FB. Renal insufficiency and altered postoperative risk in carotid endarterectomy. *J Vasc Surg*. 1999; 29:1006–11.
27. Debing E, van den Brande P. Chronic renal insufficiency and risk of early mortality in patients undergoing carotid endarterectomy. *Ann Vasc Surg*. 2006; 20:609–13.
28. Reil T, Shekherdimian S, Golschet P, et al. The safety of carotid endarterectomy in patients with preoperative renal dysfunction. *Ann Vasc Surg*. 2002; 16:176–80.
29. Amin A, Golarz S, Scanlan B, et al. Patients requiring dialysis are not at risk of greater complication after carotid endarterectomy. *Vascular*. 2008; 16:167–70.
30. Sternbergh WC III, Garrard L, Gonze MD, et al. Carotid endarterectomy in patients with significant renal dysfunction. *J Vasc Surg*. 1999; 29:672–7.
31. Mantese VA, Timaran CH, Chiu D, et al. The Carotid Revascularization Endarterectomy versus Stenting Trial (CREST): stenting versus carotid endarterectomy for carotid disease. *Stroke*. 2010; 41:S31–4.
32. International Carotid Stenting Study Investigators. Carotid artery stenting compared with endarterectomy in patients with symptomatic carotid stenosis (International Carotid Stenting Study): an interim analysis of a randomised controlled trial. *Lancet*. 2010; 375:985–997.
33. EVA-3S Investigators. Endarterectomy vs. Angioplasty in Patients with Symptomatic Severe Carotid Stenosis (EVA-3S) Trial. *Cerebrovasc Dis*. 2004; 18:62–65.
34. SPACE Collaborative Group; Ringleb PA, Allenberg J, Bruckmann H, et al. 30-day results from the SPACE trial of stent-protected angioplasty versus carotid endarterectomy in symptomatic patients: a randomized non-inferiority trial. *Lancet*. 2006; 368:1239–1247.
35. Yadav JS, Wholey MH, Kuntz RE, et al. Protected carotid-artery stenting versus endarterectomy in high-risk patients. *J Engl J Med*. 2004; 351:1493–1501.
36. Hopkins LN, Myla S, Grube E, et al. Carotid artery revascularization in high surgical risk patients with the NexStent and the Filterwire EX/EZ: 1-year results in the CABERNET trial. *Catheter Cardiovasc Interv*. 2008; 71:950–60.
37. Gray WA, Hopkins LN, Yadav S, et al. Protected carotid stenting in high-surgical-risk patients: The ARCHeR results. *J Vasc Surg*. 2006; 44:258–68.
38. Safian RD, Bacharach JM, Ansel GM, et al. Carotid stenting with a new system for distal embolic protection and stenting in high-risk patients: the carotid revascularization with ev3 arterial technology evolution (CREATE) feasibility trial. Catheter Cardiovasc Interv. 2004; 63(1):1–6.
39. Gray WA, Yadav JS, Verta P, et al. The CAPTURE registry: Predictors of outcomes in carotid artery stenting with embolic protection for high surgical risk patients in the early post-approval setting. *Catheter Cardiovasc Interv*. 2007; 70:1025–33.
40. White CJ, Iyer SS, Hopkins LN, et al. **Carotid** stenting with distal protection in high surgical risk patients: the **BEACH trial** 30 day results. Catheter Cardiovasc Interv. 2006; 67:503–12.
41. Eknoyan G, Levin N, K/DOQI clinical practice guidelines for chronic kidney disease: evaluation, classification, and stratification. *Am J Kidney Dis*. 2002; 39:S1–246.

8

Vertebral Artery Stenting

Biraj M. Patel, MD and Sameer A. Ansari, MD, PhD

INTRODUCTION

The vertebrobasilar system supplies the posterior intracranial circulation including the cerebellar hemispheres, medulla, pons, midbrain, thalami, and occipital lobes. Various major branches of the vertebrobasilar system include the posterior inferior cerebellar artery (PICA), anterior inferior cerebellar artery (AICA), superior cerebellar artery (SCA), and posterior cerebral artery (PCA). Thromboembolic occlusions of these vessels result in posterior circulation ischemia which, unlike anterior circulation ischemia, commonly present with nonspecific symptoms such as nausea, vomiting, vertigo, dizziness, nystagmus, dysarthria, dysphagia, dysmetria, ataxia, Horner's syndrome (with brainstem involvement), or visual disturbances (with occipital lobe involvement). Therefore, prompt diagnosis of vertebrobasilar insufficiency is important to prevent further progression of devastating neurological deficits.

Ischemia involving the posterior circulation is less common compared to the anterior circulation, accounting for approximately 25–30% of all cerebrovascular ischemic events.[1] However, when posterior circulation ischemia is symptomatic, it is accompanied by higher morbidity and mortality with reported mortality rates approaching 80–100% associated with vertebrobasilar occlusions and a 5–11% risk of stroke or death at 1 year associated with medically refractory vertebral artery stenosis.[2] Furthermore, patients that present with vertebrobasilar TIA symptoms and atherosclerotic disease within the vertebral arteries carry a 30–35% risk of stroke over a 5-year period.[3]

ATHEROSCLEROTIC DISEASE

Approximately 20–30% of all the cerebrovascular ischemic disease involves the posterior circulation. The most common cause of posterior circulation ischemia is thromboembolism secondary to atherosclerotic disease.

In a reported series of 260 patients, the most common site of stenosis or occlusion in the posterior circulation due to atherosclerotic disease involves the extracranial vertebral artery (43.5%), most frequently at its origin, followed by the basilar artery

(41.8%), and the intracranial vertebral artery (41.5%). Other less common sites include the PCA (15%), subclavian artery (1.9%) and innominate artery (0.7%).

ARTERIAL DISSECTION/TRAUMATIC PSEUDOANEURYSM

Vertebral artery dissections are spontaneous or traumatic events related to blunt/penetrating forces to the cervical region such as MVAs or sports injuries. However, iatrogenic etiologies are also well documented due to chiropractic manipulation, catheter angiography, or endovascular/surgical intervention. Non-traumatic, spontaneous vertebral artery dissections have been associated with underlying arteriopathy leading to poor vascular integrity from etiologies such as hypertension, migraine, fibromuscular dysplasia, arteritides (i.e. Takayasu's arteritis, polyarteritis nodosa) or connective tissue disorders such as Ehler-Danlos syndrome type IV and Marfan syndrome. Cases of vertebral artery dissections have also been reported in patients with neurofibromatosis type 1 and osteogenesis imperfecta type 1.

The intradural vertebral artery is more susceptible to rupture than the extradural segments because histologically the intradural segment has a thicker internal elastic lamina, absence of the external elastic lamina, a thinner adventitia, and fewer elastic fibers in the media.[4]

The extracranial cervical arteries may be more susceptible to traumatic injury due to their mobility within the neck soft tissues along the cervical spine and tethering at the skull base; hence, the potential for direct injury from the adjacent bony structures.[4] The most common location of vertebral artery dissections is at the C1-C2 level or V3 segment where there is redundancy of the vertebral arteries, with cervical mobility may predispose to rotational injuries. Intracranial complications include intradural propagation of a dissection beginning at this level, formation of an intracranial dissecting aneurysm at risk for rupture and subarachnoid hemorrhage, or distal thromboemboli arising from the dissection flap or a pseudoaneurysm. Very rarely, extracranial pseudoaneurysms may rupture in the neck resulting in a hematoma leading to significant mass effect, arteriovenous fistulas, and hemodynamic compromise.

DIAGNOSIS

Digital Subtraction Angiography

The gold standard modality for evaluating vertebrobasilar disease is digital subtraction angiography (DSA) performed via transfemoral approach, and occasionally transradial or brachial approaches. Typically a 4-Fr or 5-Fr catheter is used to perform the diagnostic angiogram. For adults, injection rates for diagnostic angiography are 12–30 mL/s for total volume of 30–40 mL for aortogram, 5–8 mL/s for total volume of 10–16mL in the subclavian artery, and 4–5 mL/s for total volume of 8–10 mL with a 0.5–1 second rate rise in the vertebral artery. It may be wise to perform a hand injection in the setting of a hypoplastic vessel, suspected arterial dissection, or recently ruptured aneurysm.

First and foremost, an aortic arch or subclavian artery angiography is performed to evaluate the origins of the vessels for patency and anatomic variance. Next, a complete cervical and cerebral angiogram is performed to evaluate the bilateral internal carotid/external arteries, vertebral arteries and thyrocervical/costocervical trunks to identify circle of Willis (posterior communicating artery), external carotid (occipital C1/C2 or ascending pharyngeal odontoid arcade), and superficial and deep cervical artery collaterals to the vertebral-basilar circulation in the setting of proximal compromise. Meticulous technique and caution is required during catheterization, particularly of the vertebral arteries to minimize risk of disturbing atherosclerotic plaque and causing distal emboli as well as minimizing the risk of iatrogenic arterial dissection. Heparin anticoagulation is recommended in the setting of both atherosclerotic disease and cervical arterial dissections unless there are intracranial complications or associated traumatic injuries. Depending on the tortuosity of the vessel, a 20–30 degree contralateral anterior oblique projection is often required to visualize the origin of the vertebral artery. Additional cranial obliquity may also be helpful in certain cases. The cervical segment of the vertebral artery can be best imaged with direct AP or ipsilateral 20-degree obliquity. The intracranial segment is best seen on AP projection with cranial angulation of 20–40 degrees, also known as the Townes view, and a concurrent lateral projection.

While DSA remains the gold standard modality for evaluation of the extracranial and intracranial vasculature, it if often preceded by computed tomographic angiography (CTA) or magnetic resonance imaging/angiography (MRI/MRA) studies due to their noninvasive nature and additional cross-sectional evaluation of the vessel wall. At our institution the typical quoted risk of complications for conventional angiography including stroke is approximately <1%.

The V1 and V3 segment at the points of entry (C6–C7) and exit (C1–C2 loops) from the foramen transversarium appear to be common locations for cervical dissections. Location of the pathology and involvement of long segments in cervical dissections helps in differentiation from atherosclerotic disease.[4] Other angiographic findings may include distal thromboembolic branch occlusions of the intracranial arteries that may be difficult to appreciate on cross-sectional imaging. In addition, DSA accurately depicts flow directionality and intracranial transit time, and remains the best modality to assess the collateral intracranial circulation despite evolving time resolved MRA techniques. DSA is superior to cross-sectional imaging studies in evaluating flow-limiting dissections, dissections complicated by arteriovenous fistulas, and flow remodeling after stent placement.

Although DSA is the optimal technique to assess the arterial lumen, its major limitation is its inability to directly image the vessel wall. Therefore, it may be inferior to cross-sectional techniques in the evaluation of nonstenotic dissections with benign intramural hematomas or thrombosed pseudoaneurysms. Another disadvantage of DSA is its invasiveness, radiation and potential for ischemic complications. However, the incidence of major neurologic complications from DSA is low when performed by an experienced physician. Since multiple vessel dissections occur in up to 25% of patients, careful diagnostic analysis should include bilateral carotid and vertebral artery injections with proximal catheter positioning (proximal common carotid or subclavian arteries) to prevent further injury of a dissected vessel segment and to visualize the entire cervical course and intracranial vasculature.

Computed Tomography Angiography (CTA)

CTA is a commonly used non-invasive modality to evaluate the vasculature of the head and neck, particularly in an emergent setting such as ischemia or trauma. Multidetector scanners allow for improved contrast resolution and faster scanning times, compared to MRA. Furthermore, sensitivity for significant (>50%) stenosis is excellent, upwards of 100%. Specificity for atherosclerotic disease or arterial dissection is also very high for CTA.

Multi-detector CT scanners have the ability to image at the peak contrast enhancement yielding excellent detail to evaluate the vessel lumen in addition to the vessel wall. Furthermore, axial thin-section imaging with advanced post-processing capabilities allow for acquisition of multiplanar reformatted images, 3D reconstructions, and curved maximum intensity projections in virtually any orientation of the vessel. In a study comparing CTA and MRA, Virtinsky et al showed CTA to be the preferred cross-sectional modality to delineate the imaging features of cervical dissections, especially for vertebral artery dissections.[5] CTA provides accurate measurements of the vessel lumen diameter and dissection length, which are important adjuncts for endovascular treatment planning and stent reconstruction.

In the carotid or vertebral arteries, CTA findings of an irregular, narrowed contrast enhancing lumen are indicative of dissection. Vessel wall thickening is often identified on CTA from a subintimal or intramural hematoma and it frequently corresponds with a methemoglobin crescent sign on MRA.[5] A discrete intimal flap or patent double lumens are rarely seen findings. Dissecting aneurysms may be readily identified as focal outpouchings of the enhancing arterial lumen, with or without associated thrombus, and often in an orientation parallel to the vessel.[5]

A relative limitation of CTA imaging is difficulty in its interpretation when extensive atherosclerotic calcifications are present along the arterial wall, obscuring stenotic segments. Furthermore, streak and beam hardening artifact from a patient's dental hardware may limit evaluation of the mid-cervical segments. Despite recent advances in dynamic CTA with 256 and 320 multiline CT scanners, which are able to capture both arterial and venous phases, flow directionality and transit times are best analyzed on DSA. Other limitations of CTA is the exposure of the patient to ionizing radiation and limited contrast resolution of intramural blood products in comparison to MRI.

Magnetic Resonance Angiography (MRA)

MRA is another non-invasive modality to evaluate extracranial and intracranial vasculature. Unlike CTA, there is no patient exposure to ionizing radiation and it is relatively insensitive to arterial calcification. Sensitivity of MRA for significant stenosis is in the range of 90–95%. With addition of axial fat saturated T1 imaging through the neck, the specificity for arterial dissection is excellent.

MRI/MRA is typically an initial screening modality of choice to evaluate patients with suspected cervical dissections. MR imaging with fat-saturated axial T1- and T-2 weighted or proton density sequences provide a sensitive technique to identify subtle dissections where no significant luminal narrowing or mural thickening may be appreciated on DSA or CTA. In fact, subintimal or intramural hematoma can be readily identified on MRI in the subacute stage (3–14 days).

While MR imaging exhibits excellent contrast resolution, spatial and temporal resolution is relatively lower compared to CTA and DSA studies. Increased scanning times are also required in TOF MRA, perhaps explaining a decreased sensitivity for vertebral artery dissections with this technique.[5] Phase-contrast MRA and newer dynamic time-resolved MRA techniques allow assessment of flow directionality, velocity, and even transit times to detect flow limiting dissections. Nevertheless, flow patterns remain better appreciated qualitatively with DSA.

Ultrasound/Duplex

Ultrasound has traditionally been the initial modality of choice for evaluation of extracranial carotid and vertebral artery disease because it is noninvasive, fast, inexpensive, and does not utilize ionizing radiation. However, unlike CTA and MRA, direct evaluation of the vascular lumen is limited and severity of stenosis is based on elevated velocities rather than direct measure of lumen diameter. It has been shown to have good sensitivity for of mid-cervical dissections, but its ability to assess the proximal carotid and vertebral arteries and distal cervical/intracranial vasculature is limited due to interference from the thoracic inlet, mandible, and skull base. Additionally, evaluation of the vertebral arteries is challenging as they course through the foramen tranversarium.

Although flow pattern abnormalities may be identified because of dissection-related stenosis in more than 90% of patients, these are nonspecific findings demonstrating either decreased velocity with high resistance (stenosis), a biphasic pattern (occlusion), or compensatory elevated velocities. More specific findings include segmental dilatation, double lumen with echogenic flap, eccentric echogenic hematoma surrounding a narrowed arterial lumen, and low or absent flow velocity in the dissected false lumen. However, these findings are observed in less than one third of cases and most, if not all, patients will require further noninvasive cross-sectional imaging or conventional angiography for definitive diagnosis.[4]

ANATOMY

Prior to any endovascular intervention, it is imperative to obtain a full diagnostic evaluation for treatment planning and to identify variant anatomy in advance. The vertebral artery most commonly arises from the superoposterior aspect of the proximal subclavian artery. In approximately 2–6% of patients, the left vertebral artery arises directly off the aortic arch between the left common carotid artery and left subclavian artery. Rare right vertebral artery variations include anomalous origin directly from the aorta, carotid arteries, or brachiocephalic artery.

The vertebral artery is divided into 4 segments (3 extracranial and 1 intracranial). From proximal to distal: The V1 segment extends from the origin to the entrance of the C5 or C6 foramen transversarium. The V2 segment extends within the intervertebral foramina to the C2 atlas. The V3 segment extends out of the C2 foramen transversarium, courses posteriorly and horizontally along the superior surface of the posterior arch of C2 and skull base to the level of the foramen magnum. The V4 (intracranial) segment pierces the dura at the foramen magnum and extends to the vertebrobasilar junction.

A single vertebral artery is dominant (larger caliber than the contralateral side). The left vertebral artery is more commonly the dominant artery, in approximately 60% of the patients. Conversely, a vertebral artery may be hypoplastic and may terminate in the PICA (<5%). This variant is important to recognize on the distal runoff from the vertebral artery because direct full volume injection into a hypoplastic artery can result in vessel injury or even infarction in the respective territory.

TREATMENT

Medical Management

Current guidelines for medical management of extracranial carotid and vertebral artery atherosclerotic disease recommend antihypertensive control (goal: <140/90 mmHg), and statin anticholesterolemic therapy with (goal LDL: </=100 mg/dL; or </=70 mg/dL in diabetic patients). Thus far, no proven benefit has been shown in primary prevention of

stroke with aspirin therapy. However, after stroke or TIA, there has been proven benefit of antiplatelet therapy with aspirin, clopidogrel, or combination of aspirin and extended-release dipyrimadole.[6]

Approximately 85% of extracranial arterial dissections and at least 36% of dissecting aneurysms heal spontaneously. It is estimated that greater than 90% of dissection-related infarcts are caused by thromboembolic rather than hemodynamic causes with transcranial Doppler studies confirming passage of microemboli.[7]

Despite a lack of randomized prospective studies, interval treatment with anticoagulation therapy is advocated to prevent thromboembolic complications.[8,9] Anticoagulation therapy with intravenous heparin followed by oral warfarin therapy with a target international normalized ratio of 2.0 to 3.0 is the standard treatment for 3 to 6 months. Follow-up MRI/MRA or CTA imaging is performed at 3 months and 6 months with an expected high rate of dissection healing and recanalization at 3 months (Figure 8-1). If a dissection-related abnormality persists at 6 months, warfarin treatment is usually discontinued in preference for antiplatelet therapy. The majority of dissecting aneurysms that persist either remain stable or decrease in size with a relatively benign course, hence treatment of dissecting aneurysms is not indicated unless they are symptomatic (pain, cranial neuropathies, arteriovenous fistula) enlarging, or ruptured.[8,9] Antiplatelet therapy may be substituted for anticoagulation to avoid iatrogenic hemorrhagic complications in patients with asymptomatic cervical dissections, bleeding diathesis intracranial extension, or recent large infarcts at risk for hemorrhagic transformation.

Endovascular Management

Early surgical or endovascular treatment is recommended in symptomatic patients refractory to medical treatment to prevent further thromboembolic complications. Endovascular treatment may also be considered in patients with contraindications to anticoagulation in favor of antiplatelets, severe flow limiting dissections with impending infarct, symptomatic or enlarging/ruptured dissecting aneurysms, and intracranial dissection/pseudoaneurysm presenting with severe intracranial or subarachnoid hemorrhage. In some cases, asymptomatic dissections with persisting stenosis, hemodynamic flow limiting stenosis, or unstable intimal flaps at risk for complete occlusion may also be aggressively treated.[8,9,10] Since the incidence of thromboembolic complications from persistent stenosis or nonhealing dissections is approximately doubled (0.7% versus 0.3%), an argument can be made to treat these lesions,[8] though there are no established criteria to intervene prior to the failure of medical management.

Cervical dissections may be treated with surgical ligation to deconstruct the vertebral arteries with or without extracranial to intracranial bypass techniques. However, high complication rates of ischemic injury or cranial nerve deficits have been reported due to technically demanding skull base exposure in high cervical. Furthermore, most dissecting aneurysms are fusiform and rarely amenable to surgical clipping with vessel reconstruction and salvage.[11]

Vessel deconstruction or parent vessel occlusion may also be performed with endovascular coils or the Amplatzer plug (AGA Medical, Plymouth, MN), with the risk of delayed ischemia caused by thrombus propagation, emboli, or hemodynamic insufficiency similar to surgical ligation. An endovascular balloon test occlusion study is recommended to assess the patient's collateral circulation and cerebrovascular reserve (or requirement for bypass) to prevent a hemodynamic infarct after vessel sacrifice, especially if the contralateral vertebral artery is hypoplastic. Despite a successful

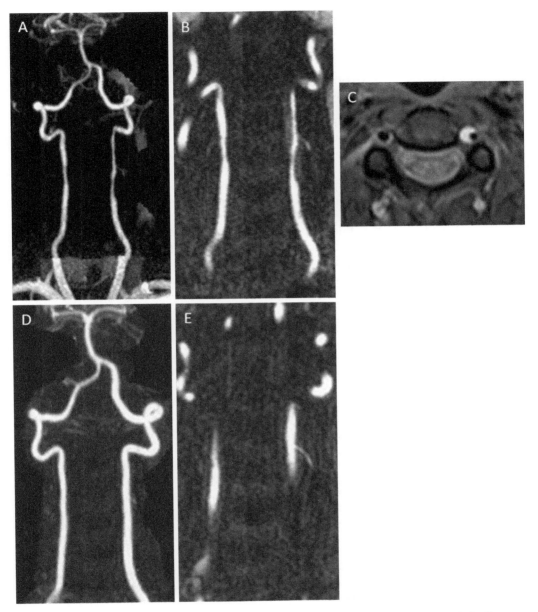

Figure 8-1. Medical management of vertebral artery dissection. 31-year-old female presented with severe left head and neck pain. A and B) CE-MRA axial and MIP coronal images through the neck demonstrate long segment arterial dissections involving the V2 segment of the left vertebral artery, with associated moderate stenosis. Subacute intramural methemoglobin is subtly noted within the wall of the vessel (arrows). Short segment arterial dissection involving the V2 segment of the right vertebral artery, with associated mild stenosis is also present. The lack of T1 hyperintense signal in the wall suggests either hyperacute or chronic dissection of this segment. C) Axial T1 fat-saturated image demonstrates cresentic hyperintense T1 signal involving the V2 segment of the left vertebral artery, corresponding to methemoglobin present within the subacute intramural hematoma. The patient was acutely treated with heparin anticoagulation and bridges to warfarin for 3 months, and subsequently antiplatelet therapy with aspirin 325 mg daily. D and E) Follow up CE-MRA coronal MIP images demonstrates complete resolution of the bilateral vertebral artery dissections at 7 weeks, with resorption of the subintimal/intramural hematomas and normalization of the vessel caliber.

balloon test occlusion study, a small risk of infarction remains, and therefore, preservation of intracranial blood flow is the preferable alternative.[12] Endovascular stent reconstruction is the primary interventional option over endovascular/surgical vessel deconstruction or surgical bypass. It is an effective and relatively safe technique, but studies have been limited to multiple case reports and retrospective small case series involving both the carotid and vertebral arteries.

The procedure is typically performed under conscious sedation after acquiring an arterial line for constant neurological and hemodynamic monitoring. Hemodynamic paramenters must be strictly controlled and altered as needed, balancing adequate cerebral perfusion pre-stenting versus the risk of hyperperfusion post-stent reconstruction. The technique involves placement of a 6 French guide sheath or 8 French guide catheter proximal to the level of dissection in the subclavian-vertebral arteries. Cervical and intracranial angiograms are performed as part of treatment planning to confirm the degree of stenosis, arterial diameter measurements and length of dissection, though exact measurements are deferred to cross-sectional CT/MR studies if available. Additionally, the presence of flow-limitation, mural thrombus, dissecting aneurysm, and the baseline intracranial vasculature can be evaluated. Through the guide sheath or catheter, a microwire-microcatheter complex is carefully advanced across the narrowed arterial segment utilizing fluoroscopic roadmap guidance. It is imperative to advance across the dissection cautiously, remaining within the true vessel lumen. Intermittent proximal check angiograms or microcatheter angiograms with gentle contrast hand injections are used to confirm access through the true lumen, opacifying the normal distal vessel and intracranial vasculature. As currently utilized in peripheral interventions, intravascular ultrasound may have a future role in directing intraluminal wire placement.

Distal filter protection devices or proximal flow arrest/reversal techniques are not typically warranted in the treatment of cervical dissections, unlike atherosclerotic lesions which have a greater propensity for thromboemboli during carotid pre- and post-stent angioplasty. If used in the treatment of dissections, there is a risk of further intimal injury or dissection propagation during advancement and deployment of a rigid filter protection device. New flow reversal strategies may be theoretically intuitive alternatives. Similarly, the indications for angioplasty in the treatment of dissections are very limited, usually to obtain access across the stenosis or salvage an incompletely expanded stent. In previously reported rare cases, angioplasty alone has been shown to achieve sufficient luminal expansion in symptomatic, cervical and intracranial vertebral dissections.

Stent selection is based on size criteria, vessel tortuosity, and specific stent characteristics (flexibility, radial force, metal-mesh ratio, deployment mechanism). The stent is advanced across the dissection flap or dissecting aneurysm and deployed using rapid exchange or over-the wire techniques. As important as they are for pretreatment planning, post-treatment cervical and intracranial angiograms assess the vessel wall post-stent reconstruction: adequacy of luminal expansion, uniform stent apposition to the vessel wall, improvement in flow dynamics, and complications of in-stent thrombus formation, dissection progression, or distal intracranial thromboemboli. Stent placement expands the true lumen of a dissected vessel to reestablish blood flow, realigning the intimal flap, and trapping the subintimal hematoma. Over the next several weeks to months, hematoma resorption, intimal healing, and stent endothelialization reconstructs the parent artery. Furthermore, flow remodeling through the stent may promote pseudoaneurysm thrombosis secondary to intimal apposition, reduced porosity through the stent mesh (decreased intra-aneurysmal inflow velocity and vorticity), and eventual stent endothelialization based on aneurysm flow models and animal experiments.[13] Alternatively, the stent provides scaffolding for pseudoaneurysm treatment with coil embolization if needed, to protect the parent artery.

In the vertebral arteries, lower profile self- or balloon-expanding (coronary stents) may be required. Balloon-expanding stents possess advantageous properties in the treatment of cervical dissections generally exerting greater radial force and a higher metal-mesh ratio than self-expanding stents. Adequate radial force is necessary to maintain patency of the dissected artery, expanding the true lumen and tacking up the intimal flap. The higher metal-mesh ratio allows for decreased porosity across the inflow zone to allow intimal healing and help secure preexisting thrombus along the dissected vessel wall, preventing intracranial emboli. Several case reports have shown the spontaneous thrombosis of dissecting vertebral artery aneurysms after placement of overlapping balloon-expanding stents using the double stent or stent-within-a stent technique,[14] presumably due to the combined radial force against the intimal flap and decreased porosity through the interstices of two stents. In fact, spontaneous healing of a few dissecting fusiform and even true saccular/fusiform intracranial aneurysms have been reported using a single balloon-expanding stent.[15,16]

Conversely, balloon-expanding stents are relatively inflexible and difficult to advance across tortuous or redundant vessel segments. Although somewhat improved with newer delivery systems, balloon-expanding stents are inherently noncompliant and can exert excessive radial force during deployment in dissected or fragile distal cervical/intracranial vasculature leading to vessel dissection or rupture. Using these rigid closed cell stents at the craniocervical junction and skull base may lead to crimping of the stent or kinking of the parent vessel during neck flexion or extension with grave consequences. Furthermore, the greater metal matrix of balloon expanding stents may predispose to increased foreign body reaction and platelet aggregation resulting in thromboembolic complications or myointimal proliferation, especially in the setting of preexisting endothelial injury. A new generation of self-expanding stents are 4–5F sheath compatible, range from 3–8 mm in diameter, and are deployed over an .018 in wire (eg Xpert, Abbott Vascular, Abbott Park, IL). Improved vessel sizing, low profile and stable delivery are ideal for vertebral artery stenting, providing alternatives to the rigid balloon-expanding coronary stents or higher profile carotid stents.

In tortuous anatomy, redundant vessels, or high cervical/skull base segments, self-expanding nitinol intracranial stents may be a safer option due to their inherent low profile and flexible thin-strut properties for optimum trackability. Intracranial stents have been shown to provide adequate radial force and atraumatic expansion in successfully treating distal cervical/intracranial dissections, but their open cell design and low metal-mesh ratio may require overlapping multiple stents for optimum stent reconstruction and flow remodeling.[17] More importantly, this is an off-label application for intracranial stents, strictly approved for intracranial aneurysm treatment and monitored through the Humanitarian Device Exemption (HDE) program, and would require either emergent notification or pre-approval by an Institutional Review Board (IRB) prior to their use.

Covered stent grafts are considered salvage devices in the simultaneous treatment of dissections and dissecting aneurysms, in excluding giant pseudoaneurysms or AVFs, or for emergent hemostasis in frank arterial rupture [18,19] The utilization of covered stent grafts in the vertebral arteries could be challenging due to their rigid and high profile delivery platforms (6–8F compatibility) as well as the risk of excluding a radiculomedullary, artery of cervical enlargement with supply to the anterior spinal artery. Although lower profile self-expanding covered stent grafts for the coronary vasculature are available, literature favors uncovered balloon or self-expanding stents for the treatment of arterial dissections with subsequent coil embolization through the stent interstices to manage dissecting aneurysms.[10] Covered stent grafts may be a rare option in the traumatic setting of a symptomatic vertebral artery dissection/pseudoaneurysm; either when traditional stent reconstruction and coil embolization would be inadequate, or there is hesitation for parent vessel occlusion of a dominant vertebral artery and a balloon test occlusion study cannot be performed.

Thromboembolic complications and intimal hyperplasia causing hemodynamically significant in-stent stenosis are well-documented following metallic stent placement in the cervical and intracranial vasculature. The common practice of systemic heparinization (activated clotting time 2.0–2.5 times baseline) is crucial for prevention of acute thromboemboli during endovascular procedures. The platelet aggregation properties of metallic stents mandates antiplatelet therapy as a pre- and post-procedure supplement to procedural heparinization. In addition, we recommend patient specific assessment of both aspirin and P2Y12 resistance assays prior to stent placement. Common protocols include an antiplatelet regimen (75 mg clopidogrel and 81 mg ASA daily) for 5 days or a loading bolus (300 mg clopidogrel and 325–650 mg ASA) 1 day before stent placement and dual antiplatelet therapy (75 mg clopidogrel and 81 mg ASA daily) after stent placement for at least 12 weeks. In emergent situations, a loading bolus of 400–600 mg clopidogrel approximately 2 to 5 hours before an endovascular procedure has also be shown to achieve maximum platelet inhibition. Routine Doppler ultrasound and clinical follow-up is recommended at 3-month intervals for 1–2 years to detect complications of intimal hyperplasia, in-stent stenosis, or thrombosis.

Three major trials evaluating the efficacy of cervical vertebral artery stenting for atherosclerotic disease have been performed or are ongoing. The Carotid And Vertebral Artery Transluminal Angioplasty Study (CAVATAS) is the only completed randomized controlled trial to compare the efficacy of percutaneous transluminal angioplasty and stenting (PTAS) versus medical management for extracranial vertebral atherosclerotic disease. Out of a cohort of 520 patients, only 16 were identified with vertebral artery disease for randomization. While this small sample size (n=8) failed to prove any benefit of endovascular treatment with a 25% periprocedural risk, it suggested the importance of addressing concomitant carotid and coronary artery disease to reduce the risk of death from stroke and myocardial infarction respectively in this population.[20]

The Stenting of SYmptomatic atherosclerotic Lesions in the Vertebral or Intracranial Arteries (SSYLVIA) trial was prospective, multicenter, non-randomized trial that reported 6-month restenosis (>50%) rates of 32% (12/37) in the intracranial arteries and 43% (6/14) in the extracranial vertebral arteries, including 67% (4/6) restenosis of vertebral ostial lesions.[21] Recurrent stenoses were symptomatic in 39% of cumulative intracranial and vertebral artery cases.[21] Since in-stent restenosis is often attributed to neointimal hyperplasia, several investigators subsequently attempted PTAS of vertebral ostial lesions with drug-eluting stents (DES) as opposed to bare metallic stents, analogous to the coronary literature (Figure 8-2).[22,23] A study by

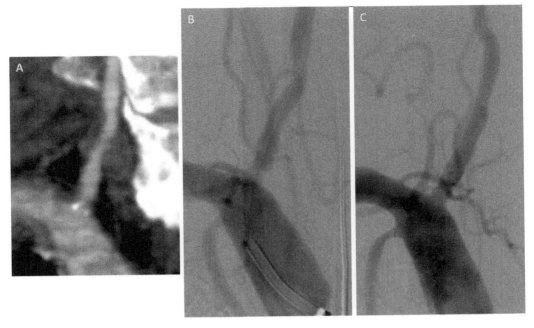

Figure 8-2. Extracranial vertebral artery stenting. 67-year-old male presented with left-sided hemiparesis and transient episodes of vision loss. MRI/MRA head identified a severe stenosis of the the right vertebral artery (RVA) origin as well as the right V4 intracranial segment. MR brain perfusion study demonstrated elevated transit times in the right posterior circulation territory. A) Pre-stenting coronal CTA reconstruction and B) DSA images show a severe 60–70% ostial stenosis of the RVA with atherosclerotic irregularity extending 1–2 cm distally in the V1 segment. C) Post-stenting DSA image demonstrates successful deployment of a balloon-mounted coronary DES (Taxus, Boston Scientific, Natick, MA) with significant interval improvement at the ostium.

Vajda et al studied 48 patients with 52 vertebral ostial stenoses reporting no periprocedural complications or post-procedure TIAs/strokes (midterm follow-up 7.7 months), and a remarkably low restenosis (>50% diameter) rate of 12%, of which all were asymptomatic.[22] Another similar study by Ogilvy et al reported a decreased incidence of in-stent restenosis (>50% diameter) (36 patients with mean follow-up 21 months), from 38% in 9/24 patients who received non-drug eluting stents (bare metal and heparin-coated stents) to 17% in 2/12 patients receiving DES. In addition, 7/9 patients with bare metal stents versus 0/2 patients in the DES group with restenosis required re-angioplasty.[23]

The Vertebral Artery Stenting Trial (VAST) is a randomized clinical trial designed to assess feasibility and safety (primary aim) of PTAS in patients with a symptomatic atherosclerotic stenosis (≥50% diameter) of the cervical vertebral artery and the rate of new vascular events in the territory of the vertebrobasilar arteries (secondary aim) on best medical management with and without PTAS. VAST is an on-going trial in which medical treatment is left to the discretion of the neurologist, although a statin and at least one antiplatelet drug is recommended. Likewise, the type of stent and use of distal protective devices is left to the discretion of the interventionalist.[24]

Furthermore, there has been no convincing data obtained from the intracranial stenting trials. The latest Stenting and Aggressive Medical Management for

Preventing Recurrent stroke in Intracranial Stenosis (SAMMPRIS) trial attempted to assess the role endovascular management (angioplasty/stenting) in the setting of a symptomatic (>70%) intracranial stenoses, including the vertebral-basilar arteries. In the SAMMPRIS trial there was randomization to optimum medical management with dual antiplatelets (ASA and clopidogrel) and statin therapy versus endovascular treatment with Gateway balloon angioplasty/Wingspan stenting (Boston Scientific, Maple Grove, MN) (Figure 8-3). This trial stopped enrollment after randomization of 451 patients demonstrating a 30-day rate of stroke or death of 14.7% in the angioplasty/stenting group versus 5.8% in the medical management group and 1 year rate primary endpoint of (20.0%) versus 12.2% respectively.[25]

The pending VAST trial will need to be studied in the context of the failed, but limited CAVATAS and SSYLVIA trials and the promising application of DES in symptomatic vertebral ostial stenoses. Despite the small sample sizes of vertebral artery atherosclerotic lesions in each of these trials, one cannot advocate for endovascular management with PTAS for *all* symptomatic vertebral artery stenoses at this time. A prudent interpretation of the current data suggests maximum medical therapy with either single or dual antiplatelet agents and a statin should be the primary treatment paradigm, with endovascular PTAS therapy reserved for specific patients exhibiting refractory symptoms and failing aggressive medical management. Identification of susceptible high risk populations that will fail medical management and may benefit from earlier intervention is a field of ongoing research encompassing flow velocity analysis across the stenosis, distal intracranial CT/MR brain perfusion imaging, and high resolution atherosclerotic plaque imaging.

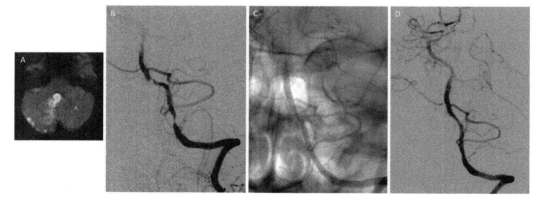

Figure 8-3. Intracranial vertebral artery stenting. 57-year-old male with hypertension, diabetes, and hyperlipidemia presents with acute right posterior inferior cerebellar artery (PICA) territory infarct as well as smaller infarcts in the left PICA territory on MR-DWI (A). MRA head examination demonstrated occlusion of the right vertebral artery (RVA) and two tandem segments of severe stenoses involving the intracranial V4 segment left vertebral artery (LVA), confirming intracranial atherosclerotic disease on DSA(B). Due to the global hypoperfusion of the posterior fossa on MR brain perfusion study and risk for brainstem infarction despite maximum medical management, the patient underwent intracranial angioplasty/stenting. C and D) Post-angioplasty and stenting DSA images demonstrate deployment of 2 tandem intracranial stents (Gateway-Wingspan, Boston Scientific, Natick, MA) obtaining vessel reconstruction and significant improvement in the dissection related stenoses (arrows).

REFERENCES

1. Stayman AN, Nogueira RG, Gupta R. A Systematic Review of Stenting and Angioplasty of Symptomatic Extracranial Vertebral Artery Stenosis. *Stroke.* 2011;42:2212–6.
2. Jenkins JS, Patel SN, White CJ et al. Endovascular stenting for vertebral artery stenosis. *J Am Coll Cardiol.* 2010;55:538–42.
3. Lee CJ and Morasch MD. Endovascular management of vertebral artery disease. *Expert Review of Cardiovasc Ther.* 2011;9(5):575
4. Schievink WI. Spontaneous dissection of the carotid and vertebral arteries. *N Engl J Med.* 2001;344(12):898–906.
5. Vertinsky AT, Schwartz NE, Fischbein NJ, et al. Comparison of multidetector CT angiography and MR imaging of cervical artery dissection. *AJNR Am J Neuroradiol.* 2008;29(9):1753–60.
6. Brott TJ, Halperin JL, Abbara S et al. 2011 ASA/ACCF/AHA/AANN/AANS/ACR/ASNR/CNS/SAIP/SCAI/SIR/SNIS/SVM/SVS Guideline on the Management of Patients with Extracranial Carotid and Vertebral Artery Disease. *J Am Coll Cardiol.* 2011;57:e16–94.
7. Srinivasan J, Newell DW, Sturzenegger M et al. Transcranial Doppler in the evaluation of internal carotid artery dissection. *Stroke.* 1996;27(7):1226–30.
8. Kremer C, Mosso M, Georgiadis D et al. Carotid dissection with permanent and transient occlusion or severe stenosis: long-term outcome. *Neurology.* 2003;60(2):271–5.
9. Touze E, Randoux B, Meary E et al. Aneurysmal forms of cervical artery dissection: associated factors and outcome. *Stroke.* 2001;32(2):418–23.
10. Kadkhodayan Y, Jeck DT, Moran CJ et al. Angioplasty and stenting in carotid dissection with or without associated pseudoaneurysm. *AJNR Am J Neuroradiol.* 2005;26(9):2328–35.
11. Muller BT, Luther B, Hort W et al. Surgical treatment of 50 carotid dissections: indications and results. *J Vasc Surg.* 2000;31(5):980–8.
12. van Rooij WJ, Sluzewski M, Slob MJ et al. Predictive value of angiographic testing for tolerance to therapeutic occlusion of the carotid artery. *AJNR Am J Neuroradiol.* 2005;26(1):175–8.
13. Lieber BB, Stancampiano AP, Wakhloo AK. Alteration of hemodynamics in aneurysm models by stenting: influence of stent porosity. *Ann Biomed Eng.* 1997;25(3):460–9.
14. Benndorf G, Herbon U, Sollmann WP et al. Treatment of a ruptured dissecting vertebral artery aneurysm with double stent placement: case report. *AJNR Am J Neuroradiol.* 2001;22(10):1844–8.
15. Lylyk P, Cohen JE, Ceratto R et al. Endovascular reconstruction of intracranial arteries by stent placement and combined techniques. *J Neurosurg.* 2002; 97(6):1306–13.
16. Vanninen R, Manninen H, Ronkainen A. Broadbased intracranial aneurysms: thrombosis induced by stent placement. *AJNR Am J Neuroradiol.* 2003; 24(2):263–6.
17. Ansari SA, Thompson BG, Gemmete JJ et al. Endovascular treatment of distal cervical and intracranial dissections with the neuroform stent. *Neurosurgery.* 2008;62(3):636–46.
18. Saket RR, Razavi MK, Sze DY et al. Stent-graft treatment of extracranial carotid and vertebral arterial lesions. *J Vasc Interv Radiol.* 2004;15(10): 1151–6.
19. Felber S, Henkes H, Weber W et al. Treatment of extracranial and intracranial aneurysms and arteriovenous fistulae using stent grafts. *Neurosurgery.* 2004;55(3):631–8.
20. Coward LJ, McCabe DJ, Ederle J et al. Long-Term Outcome After Angioplasty and Stenting for Symptomatic Vertebral Artery Stenosis Compared With Medical Treatment in the Carotid And Vertebral Artery Transluminal Angioplasty Study (CAVATAS): A Randomized Trial. *Stroke.* 2007;38:1526–30.
21. SSYLVIA study investigators. Stenting of symptomatic Atherosclerotic Lesions in the vertebral or intracranial Arteries (SSYLVIA): study results. *Stroke.* 2004;35:1388–92.
22. Vajda Z, Miloslavski E, Güthe T et al. Treatment of stenoses of vertebral artery origin using short drug-eluting coronary stents: improved follow-up results. *AJNR Am J Neuroradiol.* 2009;30:1653–6.

23. Ogilvy CS, Yang X, Natarajan SK et al. Restenosis rates following vertebral artery origin stenting: does stent type make a difference? *J Invasive Cardiol.* 2010;22:119–24.
24. Compter A, van der Worp HB, Schonewille WJ et al. VAST: vertebral Artery stenting Trial. Protocol for a randomized safety and feasibility trial. *Trials.* 2009;9:65.
25. Chimowitz MI, Lynn MJ, Derdeyn CP et al. Stenting versus Aggressive Medical Therapy for Intracranial Arterial Stenosis. *N Engl J Med.* 2011;365:993–1003.

9

Aortic Arch Debranching for TEVAR: Open Surgical Options

Christopher J. Kwolek, MD and Virendra I. Patel, MD

Thoracic aortic endovascular stent graft repair (TEVAR) has been shown to decrease both the short and long term morbidity and mortality associated with the management of descending thoracic aortic pathology.[1,2] Thus it is not surprising that skilled interventionalists have sought to apply this technology to treat more proximal pathology involving the aortic arch.[3,4,5] While isolated aneurysms of the aortic arch are uncommon, many patients will have involvement of the aortic arch and branch vessels in conjunction with either ascending or descending thoracic aortic disease.

While these patients are often asymptomatic when discovered by incidental CT scan or chest x-ray, they can present with symptoms of local compression or expansion in the chest leading to back or retrosternal pain, on the trachea leading to stridor or shortness of breath, on the recurrent laryngeal nerve leading to hoarseness, on the esophagus leading to dysphagia or reflux, on the veins leading to SVC syndrome, and on the sympathetic chain leading to Horner's syndrome. There can also be complications directly related to pathology of the vessel wall leading to rupture, with hypotension, back pain and bleeding into the chest and mediastinum. These patients can also present with dissection into the arterial wall leading to branch vessel occlusion or atheroembolization leading to stroke, upper or lower extremity ischemia, and visceral and renal malperfusion.

Treatment has traditionally been performed using open surgical repair with hypothermic circulatory arrest. However this is usually reserved for good surgical risk patients and carries with it a 10–20% risk of Mortality, 10% stroke risk and 5% risk of dialysis dependent renal failure in some series.[5,6]

Total endovascular repair has also been reported using combinations of snorkel or chimney grafts placed in retrograde fashion via the arch vessels, or more recently by burning holes directly through the main body of a stent graft placed in the aortic arch and placing a PTFE covered stent graft directly through the graft to create a fenestration.[7–10] However the number of patients treated by these methods are small and while initial results seem promising, there is no data about long–term durability.

The use of branched endografts has also been reported for the treatment of complex arch and thoracoabdominal aortic aneurysms by selected centers both in and outside the United States. However despite recent advances in design, these are currently limited in availability to selected centers and are currently custom designed for each patient.[11–12] The availability of "off the shelf" designs which can be customized In-Situ will greatly increase the utility of these systems. However currently these grafts require 8 weeks to make, involve multiple complex catheter and wire manipulations and may have an increased risk of embolization with stroke.

Currently the most common method for the endovascular treatment of complex aortic arch pathology is through the use of hybrid arch debranching procedures. This technique can be used to treat isolated arch aneurysms, thoracoabdominal aortic aneurysms involving the arch vessels, and ascending aortic pathology which extends into the aortic arch. By directly bypassing the arch vessels, thoracic stent grafts can then be placed in zone 0 and zone 1 (Figure 9-1).[13] Three types of hybrid options exist depending on the underlying patient anatomy. Type I involves starting a graft directly from the ascending aorta with direct bypass to the arch vessels. This is performed through a median sternotomy but does not require cardiopulmonary bypass since a sidebiting clamp can be placed directly on the native aorta. Typically an 8 or 10 mm Dacron graft is taken directly from the native aorta and anastomosed in end-to end fashion to the innominate artery. An additional 6 or 8mm limb can then be anastomosed directly to the left common carotid artery or a carotid to carotid bypass can be performed directly in the neck. Since the left subclavian artery is difficult to reach from the anterior approach, we usually choose to revascularize this via a left carotid to subclavian bypass to preserve antegrade left vertebral flow and minimize the chance of spinal chord ischemia.

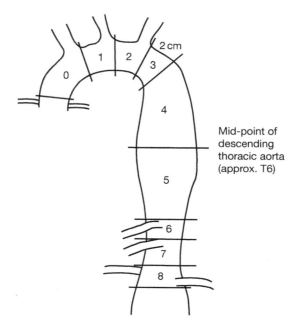

Figure 9-1. Landings zones in Arch and descending thoracic aorta.

The thoracic aortic stent graft is then deployed in antegrade fashion into the aortic arch via a 10mm Dacron conduit. The conduit is sewn onto the hood of the previously placed bypass graft to the arch vessels at the time of initial placement (Figures 9-2–9-4). After graft deployment in the arch, retrograde injection is then performed via a left brachial approach to evaluate for blood flow from the left subclavian artery into the aneurysm sac. Coil or amplatzer plug embolization can then be

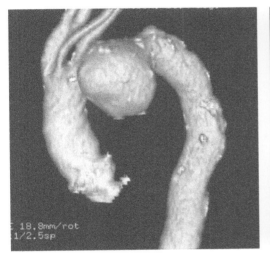

Figure 9-2. CT angiogram of arch aneurysm.

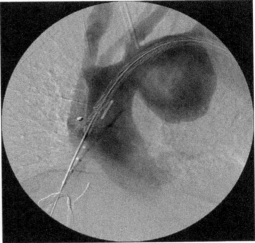

Figure 9-3. Intraop angiogram showing ascending aorta to innominate, left common carotid bypass graft with stent graft ready to deploy with coverage of left subclavian.

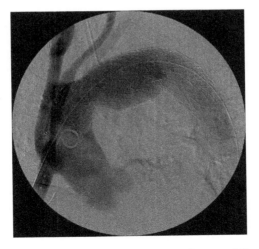

Figure 9-4. Deployment of stent graft across left subclavian with patent innominate, left CCA bypass.

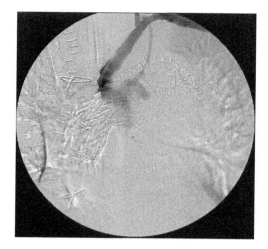

Figure 9-5. Retrograde angiogram from left arm demonstrating endoleak from subclavian into aneurysm sac.

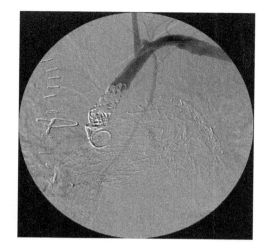

Figure 9-6. Retrograde angiogram showing successful coil embolization of left subclavian artery with resolution of endoleak.

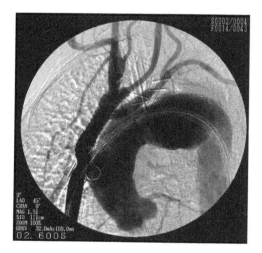

Figure 9-7. Arch aortogram showing Ascending aorta to innominate, left common carotid and left subclavian bypass graft with stent graft ready to deploy via antegrade 10 mm Dacron conduit in ascending aorta.

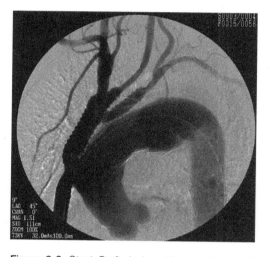

Figure 9-8. Stent Graft deployed just past origin of ascending aorta to innominate artery, left common carotid and left subclavian bypass graft.

performed in the proximal left subclavian artery, taking care to preserve flow to the left vertebral, the left internal mammary and the thyrocervical trunk (Figures 9-5–9-6). Occasionally a direct bypass can be performed to the left subclavian artery as seen in (Figures 9-7–9-8). Postoperative CT angiograms are performed at 1 and 6 months and then annually to assess for any endoleaks and for suitable exclusion of the aneurysm sac (Figures 9-9–9-10).

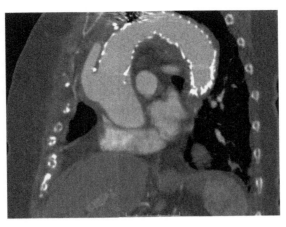

Figure 9-9. Completion CT Angiogram with multiplanar reconstruction demonstrating stent graft positioned just distal to origin of debranching bypass graft.

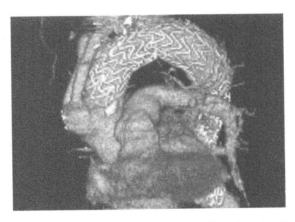

Figure 9-10. Spiral CT 3d reconstruction demonstrating relative position of stent graft and debranching bypass graft.

Type II pathology involves replacing the ascending aorta with a Dacron graft and then bringing the arch vessel bypass off the new graft. The stent graft is then landed directly into the ascending aortic graft proximally while distally the graft lands in the proximal descending thoracic aorta. Type III anatomy involves a mega aorta within the arch and descending thoracic aortic. After replacing the aorta and bypassing the great vessels directly, the stent graft is landed in the normal aorta just above the celiac axis.[5,14] Both Type II and III pathology require circulatory arrest in addition to the stent graft procedure.

The results of a recent multicenter study evaluated the results of TEVAR with total arch debranching with stent graft landing in zone 0. Sixty six patients were treated across 5 sites between 2003–2011.[15] Forty eight patients were treated for aneurysm, 6 for Type B dissection, 6 for Type B dissection after a previous Type A dissection, and 1 for an anastomotic pseudoaneurysm. Only 12 percent of patients were considered suitable for standard open repair due to their complex anatomy and multiple medical co-morbidities. 79% of patients had type I anatomy with bypass from the native aorta and 21% had Type II anatomy with the ascending aorta being replaced.

Overall mortality was 9% with a 5% incidence of stroke and 3% incidence of paralysis. There were no Type I or Type II endoleaks. Mean follow-up was 25 months with a 5 year survival of 72% and 5 year freedom from aneurysm related mortality of 96%.

The University of Pennsylvania group recently reported their single institutions experience with arch reconstruction as well. Between 2000 and 2009, 1196 open arch procedures were performed. During that time 45 Total arch replacements were performed and 27 hybrid arch procedures were performed for comparison. The hybrid patients were significantly older 71 vs 63 years old, and had more severe COPD (44% vs 11%). However despite these risk factors, the perioperative mortality between open and hybrid endovascular repair was no different (Open –16% vs Endo –11% p=.739), the stroke rate was no different (Open – 9% vs Endo 4% p=.644) and the incidence of renal failure requiring dialysis was no different (Open – 7% vs Endo –11% p=.665).

Multiple small series have also been published evaluating the outcomes of hybrid versus standard open repair for treatment of aortic arch disease. A recent publication summarized the recent series in the literature. TEVAR had a mortality range of 9–14% while total open repair was 10–22%. Periprocedural stroke rate was 0–9% in the TEVAR group and 7–10% in the Open repair group.[16]

Thus in summary, TEVAR in association with hybrid arch debranching provides a useful alternative to open surgical repair for aneurymal disease of the aortic arch. The perioperative morbidity and mortality are equal to or better than open repair in most series. This has occurred despite the fact that most of the TEVAR patients are significantly older and less healthy than their Open surgical candidates. While total branched endovascular solutions are on the horizon, they still remain limited in their availability at this time.

REFERENCES

1. Stone DH, Brewster DC, Kwolek CJ, et al. Stent-graft versus open surgical repair of the thoracic aorta: mid-term results. *J Vasc Surg*. 2006;44:1188–1197.
2. Conrad MF, Ergul EA, Patel VI, et al. Management of disease of the descending thoracic aorta in the endovascular era: a Medicare population study. *Ann Surg*. 2010;252:603–610.
3. Murphy EH, Stanley GA, Ilves M, et al. Thoracic Endovascular Repair (TEVAR) in the management of Aortic Arch Pathology. *Ann Vasc Surg*. 2012;26:55–66.
4. Bergeron P, Mangialardi N, Costa P, et al. Great vessel management for endovascular exclusion of aortic arch aneurysms and dissections. *Eur J Vasc Endovasc Surg*. 2006;32:38–45.
5. Milewski RK, Szeto WY, Pochettino A, et al. Have hybrid procedures replaced open aortic arch reconstruction in high-risk patients? comparative study of elective open arch debranching with endovascular stent graft placement and conventional elective open total and distal aortic arch reconstruction. *J Thorac Cardiovasc Surg*. 2010;140:590–597.
6. Sundt TM, Orszulak TA, Cook DJ, et al. Improving results of open arch replacement. *Ann Thorac Surg*. 2008;86:787–796.
7. Criado FJ. A percutaneous technique for preservation of arch branch patency during thoracic endovascular aortic repair (TEVAR): retrograde catheterization and stenting. *J Endovasc Ther*. 2007;14:54–58.

8. Larzon T, Gruber G, Friberg O, et al. Experiences of intentional carotid stenting in endovascular repair of aortic arch aneurysmse two case reports. *Eur J Vasc Endovasc Surg.* 2005;30:147–151.
9. Hiramoto JS, Schneider DB, Reilly LM, et al. A double-barrel stent-graft for endovascular repair of the aortic arch. *J Endovasc Ther.* 2006;13:72–76.
10. Ohrlander T, Sonesson B, Ivancev K, et al. The chimney graft: a technique for preserving or rescuing aortic branch vessels in stent-graft sealing zones. *J Endovasc Ther.* 2008;15:427–432.
11. Chuter TA, Schneider DB, Reilly LM, et al. Modular branched stent graft for endovascular repair of aortic arch aneurysm and dissection. *J Vasc. Surg.* 2003; 38: 859–63.
12. Stanley BM, Mylankal KJ, Tibbalis J, et al. Branch thoracic stent graft repair for arch aneurysm. *ANZ J Surg.* 2012;82:348–351.
13. Fillinger MF, Greenberg RK, McKinsey JF, et al. Reporting Standards for Thoracic Aortic Endovaascular repair (EVAR) *J Vasc Surg.* 2010;52:4:1022–1033.
14. Brinkman WT Szeto WY, Bavaria JE. Stent graft treatment for transverse arch and descending thoracic aorta aneurysms. *Curr Opin Cardiol.* 2007;22:510–516.
15. Czerny M, Weigang E, Sodeck G, et al. Targeting Landing Zone 0 by Total Arch Rerouting and TEVAR: Midterm Results of a Transcontinental Registry. *Ann Thoracic Surg.* 2012, e-publish ahead of print.
16. Ferrano E, Ferri M, Viazzo, et al. Is total debranching a safe procedure for extensive aortic arch disease? A single center experience. *Eur J CardioThoracic Surg.* 2012;41(1):177–182.

10

Aortic Arch Debranching for TEVAR: Endovascular Options

Shonak B. Patel, MD and William D. Jordan, Jr., MD

INTRODUCTION

Conventional open surgery for TAAA is known to be associated with a high morbidity and mortality, mainly attributed to its major surgical exposure and aortic cross-clamping. Consequently, post-operative complications are frequently severe and include myocardial infarction, acute renal failure, and respiratory insufficiency. The role of debranching in thoracic endovascular aortic aneurysm repair (TEVAR) has emerged over the last ten years as an alternative in patients who are poor candidates for open surgery and their anatomy is not suitable for currently available endografts.[1] As increasing data demonstrates that TEVAR has several short-term advantages over open repair, including lower peri-operative morbidity and mortality,[2] TEVAR is emerging as the preferred treatment strategy in majority of patients. Though TEVAR offers a potentially less invasive means of thoracic aortic aneurysm (TAA) repair, several factors continue to limit the application of endovascular approaches. Complex aortic arch anatomy such as, a short neck, involvement of supra-aortic or visceral vessels, and steep angulation of the aortic arch represent a unique challenges for endovascular therapy. In addition, the thoracic aorta has unique physiologic properties including rotational pulsation and high shear stress that must be considered when placing endovascular grafts and when evaluating the long term durability this repair. Traditionally, open repair has been suited to address the complexity of these aneurysms; however, the open method is associated with prolonged operative time, increased blood loss, increased visceral ischemia due to aortic cross clamping, and greater physiologic stress. As new devices are continued to being introduced, hybrid and total endovascular techniques offer treatment for these complex aneurysms with logical apparent advantages open repair.

PRE-OPERATIVE PLANNING

Detailed preoperative knowledge of the radiological anatomy is essential for endoluminal stent grafting. Prerequisites for endovascular repair include ideal proximal and distal

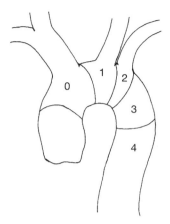

Figure 10-1. Proximal endovascular landing zones of the thoracic aorta. Zone 0 is defined as the ascending aorta, which covers all the arch vessels. Zone 1 includes coverage of the left carotid and subclavian arteries. Zone 2 covers the left subclavian artery. Zone 3 encroaches upon, but does not cover the left subclavian artery. Zone 4 is limited to the descending thoracic aorta beyond any of the origins of the arch vessels.

landing zones and its relation to critical branch vessels, length of the aorta that needs coverage, as well as, the suitability of femoral and iliac access vessels for endograft introduction. Preprocedural CTA or MRI to assess the aortic landing zone is essential to identify secure landing zones for the endograft. Conventional TEVAR seals zones (as described by Ishimaru's group)[3] (Figure 10-1) generally extend from zone 2 just distal to the left common carotid artery (CCA), and zone 4 to the level of the celiac axis. Celiac axis coverage has shown to be safe provided demonstration of good flow from mesenteric collaterals.[4] Considering some of these lessons learned from endovascular repair including these visceral vessels, these principles can be applied to endovascular aortic arch reconstruction. Proximal landing zones are usually near the left subclavian artery (SCA) and can even cover the subclavian origin when the anatomy permits. However, as more data emerges regarding neurologic complications, there has been increased interest in preserving antegrade flow into the SCA. Additionally, the proximal landing zone has continued to "creep" into the more proximal aortic arch (Zone 0 and 1). Careful consideration of aortic diameter, angulation, and calcification will ultimately guide the optimal proximal seal zone. When TAAs involve more proximal sealing zones or complex anatomy would not safely allow ≥2 cm seal, debranching should be considered. These options include: open debranching, snorkel/chimney techniques, and branched/fenestrated endografts. The endovascular options will then comprise the focus of this review.

THE SNORKEL/CHIMNEY TECHNIQUE

The "snorkel" or "chimney" technique is an advanced endovascular technique to maintain branch vessel perfusion when intentional endograft coverage is employed to gain additional neck length. The concept of chimney graft was first introduced by Greenberg et al[5] in relation to renal artery stenting to depress the proximal edge of endograft material that was protruding a few millimeters over the renal ostia. Ohrlander et al further described the use of a chimney graft for treatment of juxtarenal aneurysms with chimney grafts placed in the SMA and renal arteries. Their technique included cannulating the renal arteries and the SMA in an antegrade fashion with an Amplatz Super Stiff (Boston Scientific, Natick, MA, USA) wire, followed by placing a long sheath containing the covered stent into the side branch. The aortic endograft is then deployed and the covered stent is subsequently deployed into the visceral branch as a chimney graft.[6] These same principals can then be used in the supra-aortic branches of the arch. Indication for chimney grafts include preservation of flow in aortic branches accidently or intentionally covered during aneurysmal repair, in cases unsuitable for branched/fenestrated EVAR due to anatomical tortuosity or graft availability, and as a "bail-out" procedure after inadvertent coverage of a branch vessel.[7,8]

The technique involves placing peripheral stents into a branch-artery before or after fully deploying the aortic endograft. The approach may involve either an antegrade or retrograde cannulation of the branch vessels via a brachial, carotid, or femoral approach[9] (Figure 10-2). After deploying the aortic endograft, the branch vessel stent is then deployed in a parallel orientation to the endograft. Ultimately, the stent maintains patency of the partially or totally covered branch vessel in conjunction to extending the proximal landing zone of the endograft. Baldwin et al[8] described a double-barrel technique to maintain patency of aortic arch branches that were either inadvertently covered or as a planned procedure intended to maintain patency of an aortic arch branch during TEVAR. Demonstrating that endograft coverage of all the aortic branches (zone 0) with double-barrel stent is feasible without median sternotomy for arch debranching.

There are many unknowns regarding chimney/snorkel grafts. These include, mechanism of sealing, optimal stent type (ie self-expanding vs balloon-expandable and covered vs uncovered stents), and maximal number of chimney stents that can be used. Bruen et al[10] describe a funnel-shape neck as suitable anatomy to allow

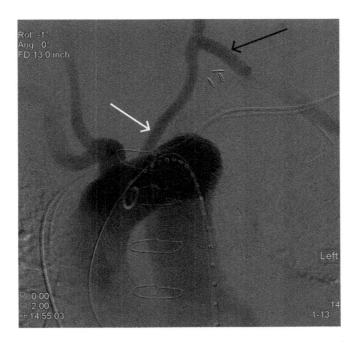

Figure 10-2. Preservation of antegrade flow in the left subclavian artery using a snorkel graft (black arrow). White arrow represents carotid-subclavian bypass.

a "sealing ring" for optimal seal. The mechanism of sealing chimney stents is still unclear; however, early rate of type IA endoleaks are low in most series, but may well be expected due to chimney stent deforming the main aortic graft. The competition for the seal zone can then form "gutters" (Figure 10-3) between the chimney stent and the endograft creating an endoleak. Therefore, a balance reduces the chance of a type IA endoleak. There are no studies indicating the optimal length of the gutter or the best choice for graft interaction and size. Furthermore, there is no data to suggest the maximum number of chimney grafts that can be used though some operators have successfully used 3 or more stents.[11] Overall, the use of chimney/snorkel grafts is shown to be feasible and safe, though long-term outcomes still need evaluation.[12]

Regardless, we have faced certain clinical circumstances that require utilization of these endovascular techniques to treat complex arch anatomy:

Case 1: A 9 year old boy presented with signs of tamponade after suppurative pericarditis from methicillin-sensitive *Staphylococcus aureus*. Mediastinal washout was performed but required re-exploration 1 day later due to a ruptured mycotic aneurysm of the distal ascending aorta repaired with a homograft patch. A third operation was required for final washout of his chest and subsequent closure. Approximately two months later, he presented with an infection of that site in addition to further expansion of the aneurysm (Figure 10-4). He was referred for endovascular management of the mycotic aneurysm after two cardiac surgeons deemed open surgical reconstruction too risky with the understanding for delayed removal of the stent graft due to the high risk of continued infection. A two-staged procedure was performed. He first underwent a left carotid-subclavian transposition and returned one week later for endovascular repair of the mycotic aortic aneurysm. Right brachial, right common femoral, and left iliac artery access sites were obtained. Next, intravascular ultrasound was used to determine the

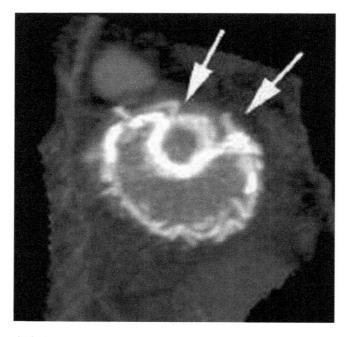

Figure 10-3. Arrows depict "gutters" which can be a source for potential endoleak..

diameters of the innominate artery as well as the proximal and distal landing zones. Two 11 × 5 Viabahn (W.L. Gore & Associates, Flagstaff, Arizona) stents in the innominate artery via the brachial site as a snorkel graft and a 26 × 10 Gore TAG (W.L. Gore and & Associates) device across the aortic arch were placed simultaneously. A 10 × 37 ICAST (Atrium Medical Corporation, Hudson, New Hampshire) stent was then placed to assist with proximal expansion of the Viabahn stent graft near the aortic root. (Figure 10-5). Follow-up carotid duplex and CT angiogram done 2 years later show adequate

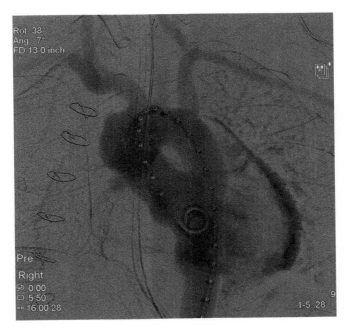

Figure 10-4. Arch angiogram demonstrating irregular aneurysm of the cranial ascending aorta.

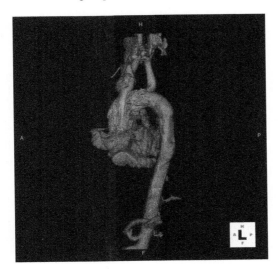

Figure 10-5. 3D reconstruction demonstrates chimney graft within the innominate artery with Zone 0 TEVAR. The left common carotid has been transposed to the subclavian artery.

positioning of the stent grafts with no abnormalities on duplex ultrasonography. Furthermore, duplex ultrasound following total arch replacement can be technically challenging. The snorkel technique provided adequate sealing and coverage of this aneurysm and he cleared his infection. The challenges for this case included using a 10cm endograft and the need to shift the left common carotid to a more distal site on the subclavian. An additional periscope graft was planned but the endograft landed just proximal to the subclavian and a periscope stent was not needed.

Case 2: A 78 year old male was referred for a large saccular thoracic aortic aneurysm. (Figure 10-6). The aneurysm originated on the inner curve of the arch opposite the left subclavian artery. He underwent a two-staged procedure. The first stage involved creation of a left common carotid to subclavian artery bypass with an 8mm PTFE graft (history of LIMA-LAD bypass). In addition to this, we placed an 8 × 38 left common

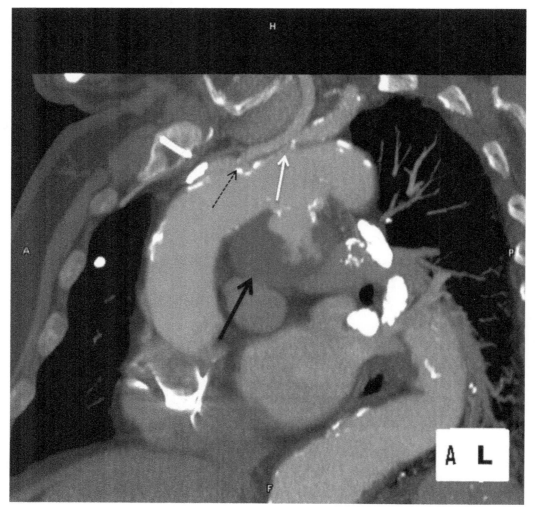

Figure 10-6. CTA demonstrating large saccular aortic arch aneurysm (black arrow). Note the origins of the LCCA (dashed arrow) and LSCA (white arrow)

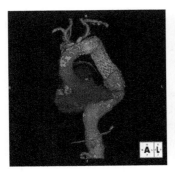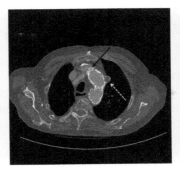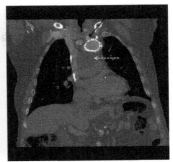

Figure 10-7. Zone 1 endograft with snorkel graft in LCCA. Follow-up CTA demonstrates intact LCCA stent graft (black arrow) and endograft with no endoleak (dashed arrow).

carotid ICAST (Atrium Medical Corporation, Hudson, New Hampshire) stent in antici-pation for stent graft placement close to the origin of the carotid ostium. The second stage of the procedure involved placement of a thoracic aortic endograft. Right femoral artery exposure was performed for our access. Intravenous ultrasound was used to measure the diameters of the proximal and distal seal zones. A 37 × 10 Gore TAG (W.L. Gore and & Associates) device was placed up to the level of the common carotid stent that was protruding slightly into the aorta, which functioned as a chimney graft. He recovered well with aneurysm shrinkage until three years later when he was found to have an enlarging aneurysm and endoleak. Left femoral and left brachial exposure was used for the secondary procedure access sites. Angiography demonstrated both a type 2 endoleak from the subclavian artery and possible type IA endoleak. A 10 mm Amplatzer plug (St. Jude Medical, Inc. St. Paul, MN) was deployed at the origin of the left subclavian artery. We then dilated a 9 × 40 balloon in the left common carotid stent while we deployed an additional 37 × 20 Gore TAG (W.L. Gore and & Associates) endograft at the level of the common carotid stent graft. (Figure 10-7). Completion angiogram showed no endoleak. For patients such as this who require deployment across the left subclavian artery and the origin of the left CCA (Zone 1), it is helpful to use the LCCA chimney graft as a marker for endograft deployment along with pro-tection for potential ostial coverage. This "marker" for endograft deployment aids in accurate visualization of the arch when landing the leading edge of the endograft over the CCA origin (Zone 1) or immediately adjacent to the CCA origin (Zone2).

BRANCHED AND FENESTRATED GRAFTS

The advent of branched and fenestrated endografts has now allowed complex aortic arch repair to be addressed via endovascular techniques. Branched devices incorporate side arm branches originating from the main device. Branch characteristics include internal/external or both, caudally or cranially directed, and axial/helical positioning. These characteristics allow the possibility of "off-the-shelf" use in many patients. In the largest series compar-ing endovascular and open TAAA repair, Greenberg et al[13] demonstrated that endovascu-lar repair was feasible though mortality and spinal cord ischemia were not insignificant. However, most of these reports are related to branched technology around the paravisceral aorta. There are limited case reports using these same concepts for the aortic arch. Chuter et al[14] placed of the first branched arch device via the right common carotid artery in 2003.

It consisted of using a proximal bifurcated component, with a wide proximal trunk and two distal limbs, one large diameter and one small diameter. The small diameter limb lands in the innominate artery and the larger diameter extends distally into the arch. After delivery, a distal component is deployed via femoral access. In addition, an extra-anatomic bypass was necessary for cerebral perfusion.

Fenestrated branch devices are combined with balloon expandable stent grafts, which are positioned via fenestrations directed at the location of the branch vessel(s). This customization of endografts with fenestrations for the visceral vessels allows the use of more proximal portion of the aorta as a sealing zone for the graft. These fenestrations come in three basic types: small (6mm in diameter), large (8mm in diameter), and scallop fenestrations located at the proximal portion of the device.[15] After the graft orientation and partial deployment of the proximal tubular graft, the target vessels are cannulated through the fenestrations. Construction of these devices requires customizing them to fit individual patient anatomy. This current manufacturing process for the paravisceral branches usually takes 6 to 12 weeks. An example of this is the Zenith fenestrated graft by Cook Medical (Bloomington, IN) which is only commercially available fenestrated graft outside the United States.[16] This delay limits their use in a small group of patients with stable aneurysms. To counteract this, many operators have also employed a "back-table" modification of standard commercially available endografts to construct their own version of a fenestrated graft.[17]

Notable limitations for branched and fenestrated grafts include visceral vessel stenosis and access vessel or aortic calcification and tortuosity.

FUTURE

Many of these same branch and fenestrated principles can be applied to the aortic arch repair. This advancement will encompass a multimodal process of not only the manufacturing of the device, but the advancement of techniques, preoperative imaging, and off the shelf availability of the devices.

Current experimental models for the aortic arch include: Zenith internal branches, and side branches by Gore and Medtronic (Minneapolis, MN). Next generation thoracic stent grafts are involving branch technology with the potential to treat aortic arch disease without compromising branch vessel flow. Zenith aortic arch branch device (Figure 10-8): provides branches for two great vessels, the innominate and left carotid arteries that includes cannulation via the brachial approach. The graft is mounted on a pre-curved nitinol cannula that helps align it along the outer curvature of the aortic arch. The ascending aorta should not be larger than 40 mm and the proximal diameter of the stent graft can be up to 46mm in diameter to obtain good seal. The branch diameters for the innominate and left carotid arteries are 12 mm and 8 mm in diameter respectively. Carotid subclavian bypass is utilized for branch delivery and the proximal vessel can then be embolized after aneurysm exclusion if the artery is not ligated at the time of the bypass. The Gore branched aortic stent graft (Figure 10-9) is an off-the-shelf device adaptable to a variety of aortic anatomy. This device has two configurations: Left subclavian artery and Brachiocephalic artery configuration. These configuration help eliminate the need for surgical bypass or transposition. The steps for implantation include femoral artery access with guidewire insertion into the aorta and its branch vessels. After introduction of the aortic component over both

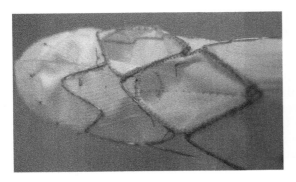
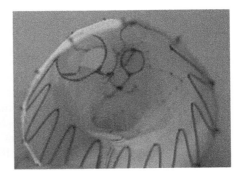

Figure 10-8. Zenith Aortic Arch Branch Device. Permission pending.
TEVAR: State of the Art an Unmet Need; Michael D. Dake, M.D.; Professor, Department of Cardiothoracic Surgery; Stanford University School of Medicine.

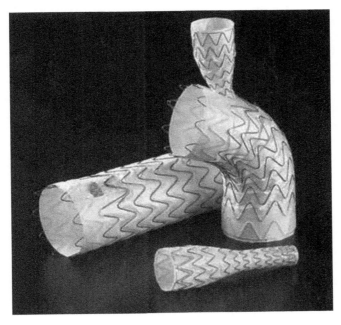

Figure 10-9. Gore Branch Device. The device has a single arch branch and additional cervical bypasses are necessary for complete arch exclusion. Permission pending.

the guidewires into position within the aortic arch, it is deployed. Finally, the custom sheath and dilator are advanced within the branch vessel and then the branch component is advanced and deployed.

In-situ fenestration was first applied by McWilliams et al[18] for reperfusion of the left subclavian artery after it had been intentionally over-stented during a TEVAR. Their technique involved modifying a 36-mm Zenith TX1 thoracic stent-graft (William Cook Europe, Bjaeverskov, Denmark), which is delivered via the femoral artery. The left subclavian artery is also exposed into which a 6-Fr sheath was introduced into the arch. After deploying the main thoracic endograft, a 7-mm balloon is inflated and the fabric is punctured with the reversed end of a SV-5, 0.018-inch guidewire

(Cordis Endovascular, Miami, FL, USA) introduced through the guidewire lumen of the balloon. After withdrawing the balloon, a cutting component of a 21.5-cm 2-part needle from a multipurpose drainage set is used, which was passed over the wire and rotated as it reached the fabric of the stent-graft. Once an opening is created, a 3.5 mm cutting balloon (Interventional Technologies Europe Ltd, Letterkenny, Ireland) is inflated at the fabric level creating an in-situ fenestration. The wire was then passed into the arch and snared via the femoral artery access. After placement of an 11-Fr sheath, a larger cutting balloon is used to widen the fenestration and the fenestration is then stented with a covered stent as a chimney graft. The short-term follow-up indicates that the technique is successful, but long-term stability still remains uncertain.

This technique has been applied successfully to perfuse the proximal supra-aortic branches in high-risk patients. In situ laser fenestration has been described by Panneton and Arko et al.[19,20] Panneton et al[19] describe the use of in-situ laser fenestration for revascularization of the left subclavian artery, which is intentionally covered during emergent TEVAR. This technique involves retrograde brachial access with a 0.018-inch wire placed at the ostium of the LSA followed by laser catheter fenestration of the graft. After creating the fenestration, a covered stent is then deployed to traverse the endograft and LSA. Midterm outcomes in their series show laser fenestration to be feasible and an effective option for LSA revascularization during emergent TEVAR. Ohki et al have also shown the feasibility of in-situ fenestration techniques with the use of a spinal needle to create a fenestration which can subsequently be stented. Other experimental studies involve total endovascular aortic arch reconstruction via in-situ fenestration. Numan el al[21] have shown successful arch reconstruction in animals using novel fenestration devices and simultaneous cerebral circulation. They create fenestrations in a Valiant stent graft (Medtronic CardioVascular, Santa Rosa, CA) using prototype balloon centered and anchored needle puncture catheter, in addition to radiofrequency (RF) plasma puncture catheter (Figure 10-10).

Overall, without long-term data to support the use of in-situ fenestration this approach is largely used in emergency situations and in high risk patients. Factors such as the durability of seal between the margins of the fenestration and the branch stent, risk of cerebral ischemia associated with supra-aortic vessel occlusion or embolization secondary to catheter manipulation, and durability of the chimney/snorkel graft in a state of constant strain from the arch physiology in conjunction with the main endograft body itself need to be addressed.

CONCLUSION

Endovascular options for TAAA though technically demanding have been shown to be feasible with acceptable morbidity and mortality. However, most of these reports are related to the paravisceral aorta. Endovascular options for aortic arch reconstruction are limited and present a new challenge for treating this tortuous anatomy along with major aortic branches. While a variety of techniques have been described, none have shown long term, large series durability. Further engineering modifications likely will be required before the arch can be consistently and successfully treated with these devices. Meanwhile, off-label techniques can be used for unusual circumstances when endovascular options have a better risk-benefit profile than open surgery or natural history. With

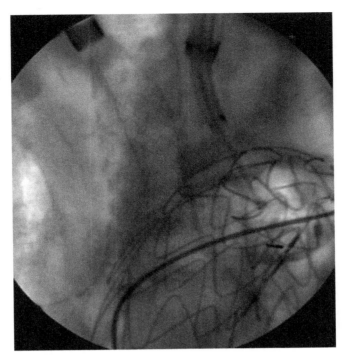

Figure 10-10. Fenestration through the left carotid artery using the RF plasma catheter. Permission pending.
Furuzan Numana, Harun Arbatlib,*, Walter Bruszewskic, Mustafa Cikirikcioglud Total endovascular aortic arch reconstruction via fenestration in situ with cerebral circulatory support: an acute experimental study. Interactive CardioVascular and Thoracic, Surgery 7 (2008) 535–538.

careful patient selection and ongoing graft designs, fenestrated and branch grafts will have an important role in endovascular treatment for high-risk patients and those with complex aortic anatomy.

REFERENCES

1. Criado FJ, Barnatan MF, Rizk Y, et al. Technical strategies to expand stent-graft applicability in the aortic arch and proximal descending thoracic aorta. *J Endovasc Ther.* 2002;9(suppl II):II32–II38

2. Dake MD, Miller DC, Semba CP, et al. Transluminal placement of endovascular stent-grafts for the treatment of descending thoracic aortic aneurysms. *N Engl J Med.* 1994;331:1729–1734.

3. Mitchell RS, Ishimaru S, Ehrlich MP, et al. First International Summit on Thoracic Aortic Endografting: roundtable on thoracic aortic dissection as an indication for endografting. *J Endovasc Ther.* 2002;9/suppl II:98–II105.

4. Vaddineni SK, Taylor SM, Patterson MA, Jordan WD. Outcome after celiac artery coverage during endovascular thoracic aortic aneurysm repair. *J Vasc Surg.* 2007;45(3):467.

5. Greenberg RK, Clair D, Srivastava S, et al. Should patients with challenging anatomy be offered endovascular aneurysm repair? *J Vasc Surg.* 2003;38:990–996.

6. Ohrlander T, Sonesson B, Ivancev K, et al. The chimney graft: a technique for preserving or rescuing aortic branch vessels in stent-graft sealing zones. *J Endovasc Ther.* 2008;15:427–432.

7. Criado FJ. A percutaneous technique for preservation of arch branch patency during thoracic endovascular aortic repair (TEVAR): retrograde catheterization and stenting. *J Endovasc Ther.* 2007 Feb;14(1):54–58

8. Baldwin ZK, Chuter TAM, Hiramoto JS, et al. Double-Barrel technique for preservation of aortic arch branches during thoracic endovascular aortic repair. *Ann Vasc Surg.* 2008; 22:703–709

9. Larzon T, Gruber G, Friberg O, et al. Experiences of intentional carotid stenting in endovascular repair of aortic arch aneurysms—two case reports. Eur J Vasc Endovasc Surg. 2005 Aug;30(2):147–151.

10. Bruen KJ, Feezor RJ, Daniels MJ, et al. Endovascular chimney technique versus open repair of juxtarenal and suprarenal aneurysms. *J Vasc Surg.* 2011 Apr;53(4):895–904; discussion -5.

11. Brechtel K, Ketelsen D, Endisch A, et al. Endovascular Repair of Acute Symptomatic Pararenal Aortic Aneurysm With Three Chimney and One Periscope Graft for Complete Visceral Artery Revascularization. *Cardiovasc Intervent Radiol.* 2011 Jun 18.

12. Donas KP, Torsello G, Austermann M, et al. Use of abdominal chimney grafts is feasible and safe: short-term results. *J Endovasc Ther.* 2010 Oct;17(5):589–593.

13. Greenberg et al. Branched endografts for thoracoabdominal aneurysms. *J Thorac Cardiovasc Surg.* 2010; 140(6 Suppl):S171–178.

14. Chuter TA, Schneider DB, Reilly LM, Lobo EP, Messina LM. Modular branched stent graft for endovascular repair of aortic arch aneurysm and dissection. *J Vasc Surg.* 2003;38(4):859–63. Epub 2003/10/16.

15. Faruqi RM, Chuter TA, Reilly LM, et al. Endovascular repair of abdominal aortic aneurysm using a pararenal fenestrated stent-graft. *J Endovasc Surg.* 1999;6(4):354e8.

16. Amiot S, Haulon S, Becquemin JP, et al. Fenestrated endovascular grafting: the French multicentre experience. *Eur J Vasc Endovasc Surg.* 2010;39:537–544.

17. Oderich GS, Ricotta JJ 2nd. Modified fenestrated stent grafts: device design, modifications,implantation, and current applications. *Perspect Vasc Surg Endovasc Ther.* 2009;21:157–167.

18. McWilliams RG, Murphy M, Hartley D, et al. In situ stent-graft fenestration to preserve the left subclavian artery. *J Endovasc Ther.* 2004;11:170–174.

19. Ahanchi SS, Almaroof B, Stout CL, et al. In situ laser fenestration for revascularization of the left subclavian artery during emergent thoracic endovascular aortic repair. *J Endovasc Ther.* 2012 April; 19(2):226–230.

20. Murphy EH, Dimaio MJ, Arko FR, et al. Endovascular Repair of Acute Traumatic Thoracic Aortic Transection With Laser-Assisted In-Situ Fenestration of a Stent-Graft Covering the Left Subclavian Artery. *J Endovasc Ther.* 2009 August; 16(4):457–463.

21. Numan F, Arbatlib H, Bruszewski W, et al. Total endovascular aortic arch reconstruction via fenestration in situ with cerebral circulatory support: an acute experimental study. Interactive *CardioVasc Thorac Surg.* 2008;7:535–538.

SECTION **III**

Lower Extremity
Arterial Disease

11

Technical Tips to Improve Outcomes of Distal Lower Extremity Bypass Surgery

Michael S. Conte, MD

INTRODUCTION

Since first reported by Kunlin in 1951,[1] the use of autogenous vein as a bypass conduit to treat peripheral artery occlusive disease has become an established method of lower extremity revascularization. Despite advances in catheter-based therapies, an autogenous vein graft remains the gold standard for distal arterial reconstruction, superior in durability and versatility to alternative conduits or endovascular interventions for advanced ischemia. Yet there remains great heterogeneity in the utilization, techniques, and outcomes associated with lower extremity vein bypass (LEVB) in current practice. Despite improvements in surgical technique and postoperative surveillance, vein graft failure remains a significant clinical problem affecting 30–50% of patients within 5 years. Experience, clinical judgment, creativity and technical precision are required to optimize long-term results. Many factors, including comorbidities and biologic responses in the venous conduit, influence the ultimate outcome of the bypass graft. Technical factors, however, play a dominant role in determining clinical success in LEVB surgery.

Long term (5–10 year) data have demonstrated functional patency of vein grafts to tibial and pedal targets in significant percentages (up to 50%) of patients, validating the biologic capacity of vein as a small caliber artery substitute. The factors responsible for the variability in outcomes of LEVB are only partially understood. Traditionally surgeons have divided the causes of vein graft failure along temporal lines, based on clinical and pathologic observations. Early failure (30 days) is generally ascribed to technical factors, mid-term failure (up to 24 months) to the biologic response in the graft (neointimal hyperplasia), and late failure to atherosclerosis within the conduit or native arteries. However this delineation is somewhat artificial as technical factors such as conduit injury may manifest later as accelerated neointimal formation, and neointimal disease may be a critical substrate for subsequent atherosclerosis.

A focus on technical considerations is useful for the surgeon because it stresses the importance of anatomic and procedural variables that may potentially be modified by the operative strategy and its execution. Technical elements and postoperative care offer the best current opportunity to broadly improve the outcomes for patients undergoing LEVB. The availability of contemporary multi-center trial data (PREVENT-III[2]) allows for the assessment of variables affecting bypass surgery outcomes that transcends individual surgeon and institutional biases. Each surgeon should seek to incorporate key lessons from the available evidence to optimize their own approach to LEVB.

CONDUIT ASSESSMENT AND QUALITY

The quality of the conduit used is the single greatest factor in determining the outcome of lower extremity bypass grafts. Optimal planning therefore requires preoperative knowledge of the location and quality of available vein. The availability of good quality ipsilateral saphenous vein is recognized as a limitation of LEVB surgery, and may be lacking in as many of 40% of patients needing revascularization.[3] Quality of the venous conduit encompasses a range of attributes including lumen diameter, wall compliance, and absence of pathologic changes such as sclerosis, calcification, and varicosities.[4,5] Ultrasound vein mapping allows for accurate, objective evaluation prior to surgery and should be standard. Vein diameter, patency, and wall thickness may be estimated noninvasively. Mapping facilitates placement of harvest incisions to avoid wound complications, allows for planning of alternative vein options, and reduces operating time. Intraoperative assessment of the vein is crucial to technical success in LEVB. The same features are evaluated by direct inspection, and gentle distension with vein harvesting solution allows the surgeon to determine venous distensibility. If sclerotic or non-distensible segments are encountered, it is far better to excise the segment and splice together two healthy ends of vein rather than retain a marginal segment that may increase the likelihood of graft failure.

The great saphenous vein (GSV) is the optimal conduit for distal bypass, with alternative veins (lesser saphenous, arm) or spliced veins being a secondary option. A number of studies have demonstrated the strong influence of vein diameter on graft patency.[6,7] Data from the PREVENT-III trial (N = 1,404 vein bypass grafts for critical limb ischemia [CLI] performed at 83 North American institutions), which included ultrasound surveillance and clinical follow-up to one year, has confirmed the strength of this relationship.[8] Vein diameter was a strong predictor of early (30-day) graft failure; loss of primary patency within 30 days was observed in 14%, 10% and 7% of grafts <3 mm, 3–3.5 mm, and >3.5 mm respectively. More impressively, profound differences in primary and secondary patency across these diameter groupings were observed within the first year after surgery (Figure 11-1). On multivariable analysis, the strongest predictor for loss of primary, primary assisted, or secondary vein graft patency at one year was a vein diameter <3 mm. Of note, in the PREVENT III trial of exclusively CLI patients, 43% of the LEVB were completed using a single segment GSV (SSGSV) graft with diameter >3.5 mm, and these grafts demonstrated 72% primary and 87% secondary patency at one year. Tibial/pedal grafts using such good quality vein (SSGSV, > 3.5 mm) performed equally as well as popliteal outflow grafts in PREVENT III (Figure 11-2). Thus, two key principles of LEVB surgery: first, don't compromise on the conduit quality—and second, select a suitable distal target that is as disease-free as possible, rather than choosing a more proximal diseased artery for outflow.

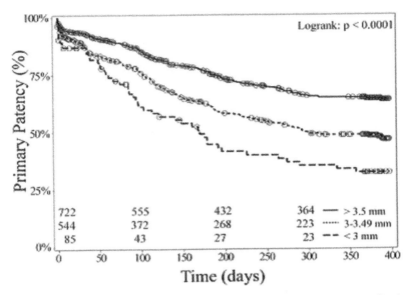

Figure 11-1. Influence of vein diameter on primary patency of vein bypass grafts at one year in the PREVENT III trial of 1,404 operations for critical limb ischemia. (from Schanzer, et al.[8] by permission of Elsevier).

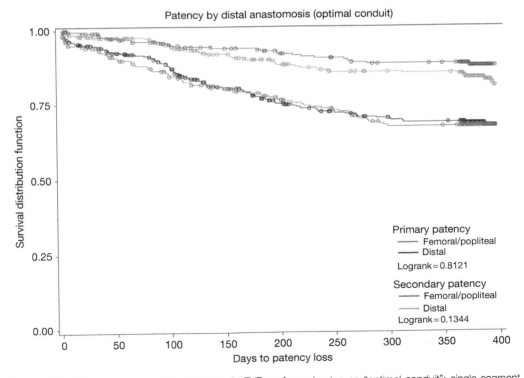

Figure 11-2. Primary and secondary patency of LEVB performed using an "optimal conduit": single-segment great saphenous vein (SSGSV) conduit with diameter >3.5 mm, in the PREVENT III trial. No difference was seen in graft performance by level of the distal anastomosis.

SURGICAL HARVESTING AND PREPARATION

As the quality of the conduit is the most important, and yet the most variable, determinant of a successful operation, our preference in LEVB surgery is to expose the vein first. Ultrasound mapping, repeated by the surgeon in the operating room just prior to draping, facilitates planning of incisions. The skin is opened directly over the course of the saphenous vein with a scalpel, taking care not to create long subcutaneous flaps. Flaps may undermine skin perfusion and subcutaneous ischemia may lead to wound necrosis. Large flaps, and therefore larger potential spaces, are also more likely to develop hematomas or seromas. We often leave one or more bridges of intact skin (2–3 cm) along the course of the exposure to facilitate closure. A minimal touch technique of handling saphenous vein is used, as even minor manipulation of the vein has been shown to traumatize the underlying endothelium. Electrocautery is avoided in direct proximity to the vein, as uncontrolled discharge of current can result in injury to the vein.

Surgical harvesting of the vein results in mechanical injury, endothelial disruption, and vasospasm. Excised veins undergo a period of warm ischemia followed by reperfusion upon implantation. Compounded by the acute hemodynamic stresses of arterialization, these insults lead directly to inflammation, platelet adhesion, and the initiation of a vascular injury response. It has long been known that careful handling of the vein, avoiding overdistension, and minimizing ischemic time results in less endothelial loss and a reduced early inflammatory response.[9] Maintenance of the vasa vasorum and avoidance of harvest ischemia were originally postulated as benefits of the in-situ approach, however this has not translated into a definable clinical advantage versus excised vein grafts. Recently there has been interest in endoscopic techniques for vein harvesting to minimize harvest wound complications,[10] however recent data suggests the performance of such grafts may be less than optimal.[11,12] Further studies are needed before making conclusions on the utility of this technique.

The optimal solution for vein harvesting and storage has been a subject of investigation albeit with limited clinical translation.[13] Most of this work derives from cardiac surgery where the conduct of coronary bypass surgery often requires a longer period of ischemia for the harvested veins. Some vascular surgeons prefer heparinized blood but most employ a crystalloid based solution. A buffered, balanced salt solution such as Plasmalyte is recommended here as it has a neutral pH in comparison to saline solutions which are quite acidic. The use of a vasodilator such as papaverine (60 mg/500 ml) reduces reactive spasm during harvesting, and heparin (1000 units/500 ml) is added for its anticoagulant properties. The Plasmalyte is kept refrigerated and the additives applied to the chilled solution on the table at the start of the case. Importantly, while the vein is fully mobilized and exposed early in the case we leave it in-situ to minimize ischemia time as much as possible. The distal end of the vein is never divided until the inflow and outflow sites have been confirmed and the length determined, always harvesting an additional 2–3 cm. Once divided distally, the vein is cannulated and then gently flushed and distended with the Plasmalyte solution as it is harvested in distal to proximal fashion.

GRAFT CONFIGURATION, LENGTH, AND LOCATION

Lower extremity vein grafts may be implanted in reversed, non-reversed (excised), or in-situ bypass configurations. Large single center series demonstrate comparable results for mid and long-term patency.[14–16] A single, small randomized trial showed no difference in outcomes between reversed and in-situ grafts.[17] In PREVENT III, all grafts were excised in accordance with the study protocol, and no difference in patency was observed between reversed and non-reversed conduits.[8] In specific circumstances there may be technical advantages to select one configuration over the other, such as optimizing the artery-vein size match at anastomoses and minimizing graft length. For these reasons I most commonly employ a non-reversed, translocated GSV configuration for crural bypass.

Valve lysis is a critical technique for non-reversed bypass, and can be a major source of technical errors and inadvertent vein injury. A retrograde valvulotome (Mills) is preferred by the author, with direct visualization of the entire length of the conduit. Lysis can be done either while flushing vein solution by hand or after creating the proximal anastomosis—regardless the vein must be kept distended whenever the valvulotome is employed (Figure 11-3A). Careful positioning of the valvulotome is essential, as branch points can be inadvertently torn. The valvulotome may be inserted via serial side branches and finally from the distal end of the vein to achieve lysis of the full length. Successful lysis is demonstrated by vigorous pulsatile flow through the end of the graft—if this is not the case, then a retained valve is likely and the entire graft should be re-interrogated.

Several studies have suggested that graft length is a factor that influences patency.[18,19] It is difficult to separate the influence of graft length from that of choice of arterial inflow/outflow sites, since these variables are intrinsically related. In PREVENT III, multivariable analysis demonstrated that graft length had a significant influence on primary patency, even when controlling for the location of the proximal and distal anastomosis in addition to graft diameter and vein type.[8] Compared to grafts less than 40 cm in length, grafts that were 50–60 cm and >60 cm long had an increased risk for loss of primary patency at one year. If the surgeon has choices of appropriate inflow and outflow vessels that meet the hemodynamic and anatomic criteria described below, the shorter length graft appears to offer better primary patency.

Lower extremity bypass grafts using excised vein may be placed in either a deep, anatomic position or more superficially. There is no data to suggest that graft location influences patency. In-situ GSV grafts have demonstrated excellent long-term durability in the subcutaneous location. In addition, superficial location facilitates Duplex surveillance and greatly simplifies surgical revisions (e.g. patch or interposition grafts) when needed. The primary advantage of placing the graft in a deeper position is improved soft tissue coverage and a reduced chance of having a wound complication that threatens the bypass. When there are concerns about acute or chronic skin conditions, soft tissue quality, or increased likelihood of wound breakdown or infection, deeper tunneling of the graft is preferred.

ALTERNATIVE AND SPLICED VEINS

In the absence of an adequate ipsilateral GSV, the best available substitute for infrainguinal bypass is contralateral GSV if it is of good quality and the source limb is not at near-term vascular risk.[20] I tend to avoid contralateral vein harvest in the presence of symptomatic disease or an ABI <0.5 in the donor limb. Lesser saphenous vein is difficult to harvest, and therefore I generally prefer good caliber arm vein as the next choice in a patient lacking GSV. The performance of alternative (arm, lesser saphenous vein) and spliced vein grafts is known to be inferior to that of SSGSV, but is still significantly better than prosthetic grafts for patients with CLI, or those requiring bypass to distal targets.[21-23] Venovenostomy is performed in end to end fashion, beveling the ends at 45 degrees and using continuous 6–0 or 7–0 polypropylene sutures (Figure 11-3B). Gentle distension as the suture line is completed and tied reduces purse-stringing. These grafts require intensive surveillance and have a higher reintervention rate, yet long term patency may be gratifyingly achieved in a large percentage of cases.[24]

INFLOW

A fundamental principle of bypass surgery is the requirement for unimpeded arterial inflow at the proximal end. In the ideal circumstance, the proximal anastomosis is performed to a disease-free vessel with a widely patent native system upstream. However, treatment of inflow disease by either endovascular or surgical means has been a successful strategy in infrainguinal bypass surgery. The durability of these interventions for aortoiliac disease is generally as good if not superior to that of isolated distal bypass, although more liberal use of endovascular treatment for diffuse iliac disease must be considered carefully. Distal origin grafts, defined as bypasses originating at the superficial femoral, popliteal, or distal vessels, have performed well in selected patients particularly in diabetics.[25] The

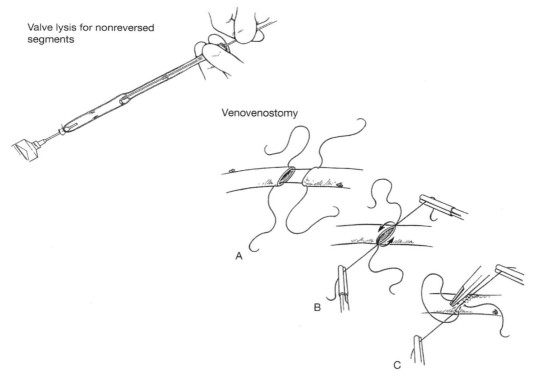

Figure 11-3. Conduit handling in LEVB surgery.
A. Valve lysis of an excised vein segment for use in a nonreversed orientation requires gentle distension using vein preparation solution and serial engagement of the valve cusps with a Mills valvulotome.
B. Technique of venovenostomy.

use of angioplasty of focal superficial femoral artery (SFA) disease to support inflow of a distally placed vein graft has also shown success, albeit in small numbers of carefully selected cases.[26] It is not recommended for more extensive (TASC C/D) SFA disease. In these cases postoperative surveillance should always include the upstream area of arterial intervention as well.

There is little objective evidence that the selection of arterial inflow site influences vein graft patency. One randomized trial demonstrated no difference between common femoral and distal origin grafts.[19] One can conclude that shorter grafts based on hemodynamically normal inflow are an excellent strategy to both preserve conduit and optimize performance. The greater versatility of excised (as opposed to in-situ) vein grafts allows this strategy to be more completely explored.

OUTFLOW

Selection of the outflow artery requires considerable surgical judgment, correlating several anatomic and hemodynamic factors. In general, the most proximal vessel that provides continuous runoff to the foot is the primary target. Extensively calcified tibial and pedal arteries should be avoided if possible, but can be used with success. For patients with extensive tissue loss, there is controversy regarding the choice between peroneal, pedal, and plantar targets.[27-29] The relationship between runoff and graft performance is somewhat unclear. Although some studies have suggested that poor runoff is an important factor,[30] many others have not found strong correlations and measurement of graft runoff per se is not straightforward. The implication from the available data is that conduit quality, graft length, and adequate inflow appear as stronger predictors of vein graft patency than level of the distal anastomosis per se. However it is understood that this mostly retrospective data is intrinsically flawed by careful selection, and the technical challenges associated with anastomosis to small, diseased vessels with poor runoff can be a significant cause of early and late graft failure.

GENERAL POINTS AND ADDITIONAL TIPS

The anesthetic technique is largely dependent upon the patients underlying comorbid conditions and operator preference. In patients with significant pulmonary disease, epidural anesthesia can help attenuate postoperative pulmonary complications. Regional anesthesia has the additional benefit of facilitating post-operative pain control, and a continuous epidural is preferred by the author. For patients in whom there are questions regarding the quality of lower extremity veins, general anesthesia is preferred should there be need for harvesting arm vein. The addition of an epidural to a general anesthetic provides excellent perioperative analgesia for lower extremity surgery.

There are few "short-cuts" of value in the performance of lower extremity vein bypass surgery, however errors in planning, judgment, and technique can greatly lengthen the operation, increase the risk of complications, and reduce the long-term benefit for the patient. Few operations in vascular surgery are as technically demanding, or require as much creativity. As in all surgical procedures, minimizing intraoperative surprises and having well thought out primary and secondary strategies correlate directly with success. The major unknown, and the most critical element, is the conduit. If there is concern about the GSV from either clinical evaluation or preoperative vein mapping, the next best available vein should be identified prior to starting the operation, and that extremity prepped. When an issue of vein quality is unexpectedly encountered, the surgeon must weigh the options carefully based on knowledge of alternative veins available and other factors. In general, a spliced vein graft made of good quality segments is preferred over retaining a segment of poor/marginal quality within the bypass. Small diameter, sclerotic, or non-distensible vein segments are the source of both early failure and subsequent reinterventions, and are better excised.

Completion imaging is an essential component in distal bypass surgery. Duplex ultrasound is a highly sensitive tool for conduit assessment at the completion of the bypass, and provides the baseline for postoperative surveillance. A normal intraoperative scan is highly predictive of early technical success while abnormalities associated with increased velocity (ratio >2) or low flow (velocity <45 cm/s) should be addressed pre-emptively.[31,32] Contrast arteriography is complementary in that it demonstrates the runoff bed; however duplex is likely more sensitive for abnormalities within the conduit itself. The use of completion imaging, incorporating one or both of these modalities, is highly recommended.

Techniques of anastomosis vary widely among surgeons, and cannot be directly correlated with outcome. My strong preference is to perform the proximal anastomosis first in all cases. This allows the graft to be tunneled while under arterial pressure, minimizing the chance of kinks or twists. Furthermore, it allows for greater flexibility in case of unsuspected issues arising at the distal target artery, leaving excess distal vein length in place until after the artery is opened and prepared for anastomosis. Calcified arteries pose a technical challenge particularly for the distal anastomosis. Tourniquet control in the thigh or calf is an excellent approach in general, minimizing manipulation of the target artery, and greatly facilitating re-do bypass surgery. In cases of extensive arterial calcification it may or may not be adequate. In such cases, intraluminal balloon control or microvascular clamps are the remaining options. Sometimes circumferential ("egg-shell") calcification can be gently cracked with forceps without producing extensive intimal disruption, but this must be done with great care and any loose debris removed from the lumen. Limited endarterectomy is sometimes needed and if a longer arteriotomy is required, then a primary vein patch angioplasty is recommended. In all cases, direct visualization of an unobstructed downstream lumen is required to execute the distal anastomosis with precision. "Parachuting" at the distal anastomosis is an excellent technique for tibial/pedal bypass, allowing for full visualization of all of the sutures at the critical heel and toe of the suture line.

CONCLUSIONS

Technical factors are strong determinants of the short and long-term success of infrainguinal bypass using autogenous vein. Knowledge of the impact of key factors such as vein diameter, quality and handling informs preoperative planning and the conduct of the operation. Furthermore, knowledge that certain factors have limited impact on outcomes—such as level of inflow and graft orientation—allows surgeons to be more flexible and creative in their approach. LEVB grafts, when executed properly, continue to provide the most versatile, effective and durable solution for patients with advanced peripheral artery occlusive disease.

REFERENCES

1. Kunlin J. [long vein transplantation in treatment of ischemia caused by arteritis.]. *Rev Chir.* 1951;70:206–235.
2. Conte MS, Bandyk DF, Clowes AW, et al. Results of PREVENT III: A multicenter, randomized trial of edifoligide for the prevention of vein graft failure in lower extremity bypass surgery. *J Vasc Surg.* 2006;43:742–751; discussion 751.
3. Taylor LM, Jr., Edwards JM, Brant B, et al. Autogenous reversed vein bypass for lower extremity ischemia in patients with absent or inadequate greater saphenous vein. *Am J Surg.* 1987;153:505–510.
4. Panetta TF, Marin ML, Veith FJ, et al. Unsuspected preexisting saphenous vein disease: An unrecognized cause of vein bypass failure. *J Vasc Surg.* 1992;15:102–110; discussion 110–102.
5. Marin ML, Veith FJ, Panetta TF, et al. Saphenous vein biopsy: A predictor of vein graft failure. *J Vasc Surg.* 1993;18:407–414; discussion 414–405.
6. Towne JB, Schmitt DD, Seabrook GR, et al. The effect of vein diameter on patency of in situ grafts. *J Cardiovasc Surg (Torino).* 1991;32:192–196.
7. Wengerter KR, Veith FJ, Gupta SK, et al. Influence of vein size (diameter) on infrapopliteal reversed vein graft patency. *J Vasc Surg.* 1990;11:525–531.
8. Schanzer A, Hevelone N, Owens CD, et al. Technical factors affecting autogenous vein graft failure: Observations from a large multicenter trial. *J Vasc Surg.* 2007;46:1180–1190; discussion 1190.
9. LoGerfo FW, Quist WC, Cantelmo NL, et al. Integrity of vein grafts as a function of initial intimal and medial preservation. *Circulation.* 1983;68:II117–124.
10. Jordan WD, Jr., Voellinger DC, Schroeder PT, et al. Video-assisted saphenous vein harvest: The evolution of a new technique. *J Vasc Surg.* 1997;26:405–412; discussion 413–404.
11. Pullatt R, Brothers TE, Robison JG, Elliott BM. Compromised bypass graft outcomes after minimal-incision vein harvest. *J Vasc Surg.* 2006;44:289–294; discussion 294–285.
12. Lopes RD, Hafley GE, Allen KB, et al. Endoscopic versus open vein-graft harvesting in coronary-artery bypass surgery. *N Engl J Med.* 2009;361:235–244.
13. Adcock OT, Jr., Adcock GL, Wheeler JR, et al. Optimal techniques for harvesting and preparation of reversed autogenous vein grafts for use as arterial substitutes: A review. *Surgery.* 1984;96:886–894.
14. Shah DM, Darling RC,III, Chang BB, et al. Long-term results of in situ saphenous vein bypass. Analysis of 2058 cases. *Ann Surg.* 1995;222:438–446; discussion 446–438.
15. Taylor LM, Jr., Edwards JM, Porter JM. Present status of reversed vein bypass grafting: Five-year results of a modern series. *J Vasc Surg.* 1990;11:193–205; discussion 205–196.
16. Belkin M, Knox J, Donaldson MC, et al. Infrainguinal arterial reconstruction with nonreversed greater saphenous vein. *J Vasc Surg.* 1996;24:957–962.
17. Wengerter KR, Veith FJ, Gupta SK, et al. Prospective randomized multicenter comparison of in situ and reversed vein infrapopliteal bypasses. *J Vasc Surg.* 1991;13:189–197; discussion 197–189.
18. Ascer E, Veith FJ, Gupta SK, et al. Short vein grafts: A superior option for arterial reconstructions to poor or compromised outflow tracts? *J Vasc Surg.* 1988;7:370–378.
19. Ballotta E, Renon L, De Rossi A, et al. Prospective randomized study on reversed saphenous vein infrapopliteal bypass to treat limb-threatening ischemia: Common femoral artery versus superficial femoral or popliteal and tibial arteries as inflow. *J Vasc Surg.* 2004;40:732–740.
20. Chew DK, Owens CD, Belkin M, et al. Bypass in the absence of ipsilateral greater saphenous vein: Safety and superiority of the contralateral greater saphenous vein. *J Vasc Surg.* 2002;35:1085–1092.
21. Londrey GL, Bosher LP, Brown PW, et al. Infrainguinal reconstruction with arm vein, lesser saphenous vein, and remnants of greater saphenous vein: A report of 257 cases. *J Vasc Surg.* 1994;20:451–456; discussion 456–457.

22. Faries PL, Arora S, Pomposelli FB, Jr., et al. The use of arm vein in lower-extremity revascularization: Results of 520 procedures performed in eight years. *J Vasc Surg*. 2000;31:50–59.

23. Chew DK, Conte MS, Donaldson MC, et al. Autogenous composite vein bypass graft for infrainguinal arterial reconstruction. *J Vasc Surg*. 2001;33:259–264; discussion 264–255.

24. Armstrong PA, Bandyk DF, Wilson JS, et al. Optimizing infrainguinal arm vein bypass patency with duplex ultrasound surveillance and endovascular therapy. *J Vasc Surg*. 2004;40:724–730; discussion 730–721.

25. Reed AB, Conte MS, Belkin M, et al. Usefulness of autogenous bypass grafts originating distal to the groin. *J Vasc Surg*. 2002;35:48–54; discussion, 54–45.

26. Schanzer A, Owens CD, Conte MS, et al. Superficial femoral artery percutaneous intervention is an effective strategy to optimize inflow for distal origin bypass grafts. *J Vasc Surg*. 2007;45:740–743.

27. Pomposelli FB, Jr., Jepsen SJ, Gibbons GW, et al. Efficacy of the dorsal pedal bypass for limb salvage in diabetic patients: Short-term observations. *J Vasc Surg*. 1990;11:745–751; discussion 751–742.

28. Raftery KB, Belkin M, Mackey WC, et al. Are peroneal artery bypass grafts hemodynamically inferior to other tibial artery bypass grafts? *J Vasc Surg*. 1994;19:964–968; discussion 968–969.

29. Bergamini TM, George SM, Jr., Massey HT, et al. Pedal or peroneal bypass: Which is better when both are patent? *J Vasc Surg*. 1994;20:347–355; discussion 355–346.

30. Seeger JM, Pretus HA, Carlton LC, et al. Potential predictors of outcome in patients with tissue loss who undergo infrainguinal vein bypass grafting. *J Vasc Surg*. 1999;30:427–435.

31. Bandyk DF, Mills JL, Gahtan V, et al. Intraoperative duplex scanning of arterial reconstructions: Fate of repaired and unrepaired defects. *J Vasc Surg*. 1994;20:426–432; discussion 432–423.

32. Johnson BL, Bandyk DF, Back MR, et al. Intraoperative duplex monitoring of infrainguinal vein bypass procedures. *J Vasc Surg*. 2000;31:678–690.

12

Hybrid Approaches for Ilio-femoral Arterial Occlusive Disease

Michele Piazza, MD and Joseph J. Ricotta II, MD, MS

INTRODUCTION

Ilio-femoral occlusive disease (IFOD) can often manifest in a debilitating condition for patients, and be challenging to manage because multiple levels of the arterial tree are involved. The gold standard for treatment of extensive occlusive disease of the ilio-femoral segment is open surgical reconstruction with either aorto-bifemoral (ABF) or iliofemoral (IF) bypass depending on the extent and laterality of the lesions. Excellent durability has been demonstrated for these open surgical reconstructions, however, they require a laparotomy or flank incision and often aortic cross-clamping, which are associated with increased morbidity, and can be challenging particularly in patients at high operative risk.[1] In the last decade, less invasive endovascular procedures such as iliac balloon angioplasty (PTA) and stenting, have gained popularity as an alternative to open surgery for the treatment of focal iliac occlusive disease. Rapid evolution of techniques and materials has also allowed operators to treat more extensive and severe iliac lesions in an endovascular fashion.

In hybrid reconstructions, patients are treated using both endovascular and open revascularization techniques simultaneously, most often at different levels of the arterial tree. These multilevel hybrid reconstructions have been used increasingly more often, and have become a popular technique for vascular surgeons who have mastered both open and endovascular revascularization techniques.

According to the recently modified guidelines from the Trans-Atlantic Society Consensus (TASCII) document, endovascular management is preferred to open surgery in the presence of TASC A and B iliac lesions, and surgical reconstruction is the recommended treatment for TASC D lesions and TASC C lesions in good-risk patients.[2] Femoral endarterectomy for occlusive disease of the common femoral artery (CFA) has been standard practice for more than 50 years.[3,4] Patch arterioplasty with either autogenous vein, or more recently prosthetic or bovine pericardial patch material is generally used, providing satisfactory results with low surgical risk. In the presence of severe IFOD, hybrid repair (HR) combining endovascular iliac stenting and common femoral endarterectomy (CFE), may represent an alternative to open ilio-femoral surgical reconstruction (OR), with shorter length of hospitalization and less resource utilization.[5]

In this chapter, we describe the techniques used for ilio-femoral hybrid revascularization with particular attention to technical aspects and required materials depending on the type and extension of obstructive lesions. Furthermore, we report the results from our published experience comparing open surgical reconstruction and the hybrid approach for treatment of IFOD as well as provide a current review of the literature.

TECHNIQUE

It is our preference to perform hybrid procedures in a dedicated endovascular suite. However, they can also be routinely performed in a standard operating room with a mobile C-arm for intraoperative fluoroscopy. We routinely perform endovascular iliac PTA and stenting following the completion of the femoral endarterectomy and patch angioplasty. Once the CFE is performed, its proximal and distal endpoints are secured with tacking sutures and the femoral artery is closed with patch angioplasty using a standard elliptical bovine pericardial, Dacron, or rarely venous patch. Upon completion of patch closure, blood flow is restored to the leg. Access to the iliac arteries is performed through a center patch puncture with a 18 gauge needle and subsequent placement of a 7Fr sheath over the wire and through the center of the patch (Figure 12-1).

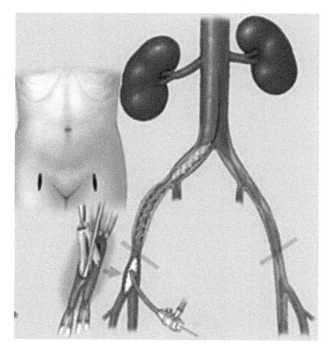

Figure 12-1. Example of our preferred technique during hybrid approach to iliac-femoral occlusive disease. The first step is common femoral endarterectomy followed by patch angioplasty. Subsequently, through a center puncture in the patch, endovascular access is performed to reach the iliac segment.

Our preference is to perform the endarterectomy and patch prior to iliac stenting because it can be difficult to access the true lumen in a severely stenotic or occluded common femoral artery. Once the endarterectomy is performed, it is important to tack down the proximal endpoint so as not to raise a dissection flap with needle entry through the patch.

In addition, placing stents into the distal iliac arteries prior to CFE and patch often precludes the ability to use a clamp for proximal control of inflow into the CFA because of concern over crushing the stent and necessitates placement of a balloon for inflow control which can make the CFE and patch closure more cumbersome. The authors prefer to avoid this by performing the CFE and patch first followed by stenting of the iliac arteries.

In general, primary stenting of severe iliac stenosis is predominantly performed with self-expanding nitinol stents except in cases of common iliac artery orificial lesions, where balloon expandable stents are used. In some cases, long occlusive segments can be treated with stent-graft placement following recanalization (Figure 12-2). For lesions involving the external iliac artery, it is our practice to extend our treatment zone down (PTA or stenting) to the superior border of the inguinal ligament if necessary, with great care not to cross the inguinal ligament to avoid kinking of the stent with hip and waist flexion. In cases with extensive bilateral iliac disease involving the origin of both arteries, the aortic bifurcation can be reconstructed using two covered stent ballooned in a kissing fashion through a bilateral groin access (Figure 12-3).

In cases were the plaque in the CFA is extended to the EIA, it is possible to perform remote endarterectomy of the external iliac artery. In this case, the proximal end of the blinded endarterectomy could result in a short dissection. Therefore, in this situation, we extend our treatment zone down (PTA or stenting) to the superior border of the inguinal ligament in order to cover the limit of remote endarterectomy, again with great care not to cross the inguinal ligament to avoid kinking of the stent with hip and waist flexion (Figure 12-4).

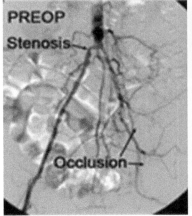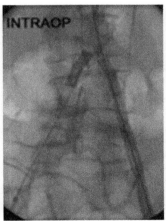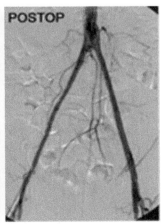

Figure 12-2. Case of a 74 yo M, with severe short stenosis of the right common iliac artery and long segment occlusion of the left common femoral and external iliac arteries. The patient underwent first to left common femoral endarterectomy followed by subintimal iliac recanalization; percutaneous access at the level of the right common femoral artery. PTA and stenting of both side iliac lesions (From Mayo Vascular and Endovascular Clinic, Rochester MN Archives).

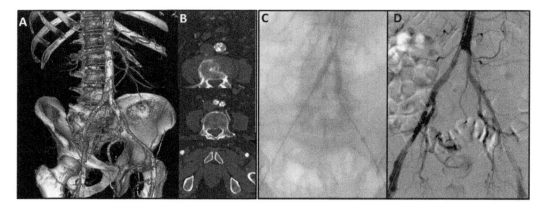

Figure 12-3. Case of a 81 yo M, with aorto-iliac and femoral obstructive disease (**A** and **B**). To guarantee safety and efficacy of aortic bifurcation reconstruction, a double barrel technique with two covered Viabahn stent was performed; subsequently the aortic bifurcation and both iliac branches were ballooned simultaneously in "kissing" fashion(**C**). (**D**) Final angiography showing reconstitution of the aortoiliac and femoral arteries (From the Clinic of Vascular and Endovascular Surgery, Padova University, Archives).

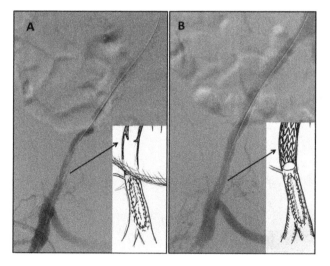

Figure 12-4. Case of a 73 yo M, with bilateral iliac and femoral obstructive disease (TASC D on the left side). Bilateral common femoral endarterectomy+ GSV patch angioplasty; subsequently a fem-fem (right to left) bypass was performed. Through a center puncture at the origin of the right superficial femoral artery, access to the right iliac axis was obtained with a 0.035 hydrophilic J wire; particular attention was applied in crossing the proximal flap of the remote femoral endarterectomy (**A**). Finally right iliac stenting was performed from the common iliac artery till the distal portion of the external iliac artery just before the inguinal ligament. (From the Clinic of Vascular and Endovascular Surgery, Padova University, Archives).

OUR EXPERIENCE

A retrospective review was performed of all consecutive patients admitted at Mayo Clinic who underwent HR or OR for severe chronic IFOD between January 1, 1998 and December 31, 2008. Forty-eight patients were classified as TASC A–B (59 limbs treated) and

114 patients as TASC C–D (189 limbs treated). During this time, 92 patients underwent OR with aorto-bifemoral ($n = 72$) or iliofemoral bypass ($n = 20$, all unilateral) supplying blood flow to 164 limbs, and 70 patients underwent HR supplying blood flow to 84 limbs (14 bilateral and 56 unilateral). Stenting in the HR group was selectively performed in the common iliac artery in 20 limbs (23.8%), external iliac artery in 41 limbs (48.8%) and combined common and external iliac artery in 23 limbs (27.4%). In the OR group, patients requiring ABF or IF bypass were included in this study only if simultaneous CFE was performed on at least one limb side. In the HR group, all patients with both focal and extensive iliac obstructive disease that underwent endovascular iliac revascularization were included only if concomitant CFE was performed.

In recent years, HR has surpassed OR as the preferred treatment for severe chronic IFOD. In the first three years of this experience, more than 90% of the revascularizations were performed with OR. With improvement in techniques and materials for endovascular procedures, HR has become more popular. Most of the HR have been performed in the last five years, especially those with bilateral or extensive iliac disease, precluding a meaningful contemporary comparison. (Figure 12-5)

Operative comorbidity risk was evaluated using the Society for Vascular Surgery (SVS) comorbidity grading system,[6] the America Society of Anesthesiology score (ASA) and the Eagle criteria.[7] Chronic limb ischemia was classified by symptoms at presentation using SVS/AAVS reporting standards.[8] TransAtlantic Inter-Society Consensus (TASC) classification[2] was used to evaluate iliac and femoro-popliteal occlusive disease extent in both groups of patients. The severity of stenosis and therefore the decision to perform CFE was based on CT imaging. CFE was performed when the femoral artery stenosis was ≥50%. Common femoral artery runoff was evaluated according to SVS/AAVS reporting standards in a decimal scoring system that ranges from 1–2 (patent) to >9 (minimal/absent)[8]. Early outcomes (≤30 days from surgery) were evaluated comparing peri-procedural data, associated morbidity, and mortality between the two groups. Criteria for evaluating improvement after surgery were: absolute difference between pre and post operative ankle brachial index (ABI), and SVS/AVSS post operative clinical improvement score.[8] Average length of follow-up was 3.54 years (range 30 days to 11.5 years) (OR = 4.41 ± 3.26 yrs; HR = 1.54 ± 1.56 yrs). Primary, primary assisted, and secondary patency were determined in concordance with the SVS/AAVS guidelines[8] after meticulous stratification by TASC A–B and C–D.

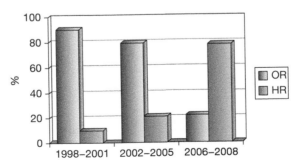

Figure 12-5. Evolution in the treatment of iliac and femoral obstructive disease at Mayo Clinic, from 1998 to 2008 between hybrid repair (HR) and open repair (OR).

The overall cohort of patients undergoing OR were younger (61 ± 14 vs 68 ± 12 years; p = .003), and this was maintained even after stratifications by TASC category (A–B, p = .02; C–D, p = .01); age less than 60 at the time of surgery was significantly higher in the OR group than HR group for TASC A–B lesions (p = .004). Patients in TASC C–D undergoing HR had significantly higher cardiac comorbidities at presentation including NYHA class III and IV (p = .047), Eagle criteria (p = .004), SVS cardiac score (<.001) and often presented with a previous history of CABG (p < .001), current home oxygen therapy (p = .015); moreover perioperative risk score assessment was greater for patients who underwent HR, with significantly higher Eagle criteria score, mean ASA score and SVS sum comorbidity score compared to OR. Patients in TASC A–B undergoing HR had only significant higher rate of smoking history and higher SVS cardiac score. All others risk factors and perioperative risk assessment are shown in Table 12-1 stratified by TASC category.

59% of HR patients were categorized as TASC A, B (limbs = 50), while 94.5% of OR patients presented in TASC C and D (limb = 155). The majority of patients in both groups presented with disabling claudication (74.4% OR and 60% HR) and this was maintained after TASC subdivision, but tissue loss at presentation was higher in the HR group than in the OR group for TASC C–D (26% HR and 10% OR, p = 0.04) (Figure 12-6).

The overall rate of severe occlusive disease of the common femoral artery was significantly higher in HR group (98% vs 64%, p < .001) than in OR group and this was maintained even after TASC subdivision (p = < .001 for A–B and p = < .002 for C–D). No significant difference in CFA runoff or femoro-popliteal TASC classification between the two groups and after stratification by TASC category were identified.

Patients undergoing HR had significantly shorter intensive care unit (0.14 vs 2 days, p = .04) and hospital stay (3.9 vs 8.3 days, p = .005) compared to the OR group for TASC C–D, but interestingly no difference were noted for TASC A–B.

HR was more often associated with deep femoral artery revascularization even for TASC A–B than for TASC C–D (p < .001 for both), and greater than 80% of iliac

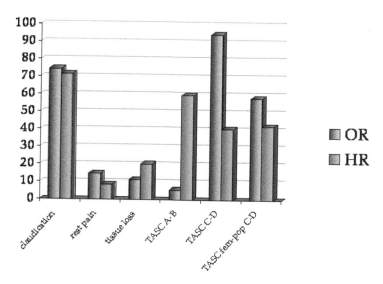

Figure 12-6 Distribution of clinical presentation.

endovascular procedures were performed using PTA + stenting (mean number of stents per patient 1.12 for TASC A–B and 1.42 for TASC C–D). No significant difference in overall long-term patency was identified after stratification for site of stent placement (EIA 88.1%, CIA 94.4% and both CIA-EIA 95.7%, $p = 0.97$) and type of stent used (uncovered stent 88.3% and stent-graft 100% $p = 0.47$). The incidence of associated outflow revascularization procedures in the femoral-popliteal segment was not significantly different between OR and HR group (3% and 5% respectively $p = 0.42$).

Overall technical success was 100% for OR group and 99% for HR group. Postoperatively, the mean ABI increased significantly from 0.48 to 0.77 in the OR patients and from 0.52 to 0.77 in the HR patients ($p = .001$ for both group). After stratification by TASC only patients underwent open repair with A and B lesions had a significant increase in ABI compared to HR ($p = .031$). Evaluation of lower limb clinical status at 30 days from surgery described similar improvement between HR and OR for TASC A–B (99% vs 100%), but higher improvement for OR (96% vs 91%) in TASC C–D even if this was not significant ($p = .06$). Major medical postoperative complications occurred with similar incidence in both groups, with an overall rate of 5% in the OR group and 3% in the HR group ($p = 0.55$). Surgical-related complications were not statistically different between either group, and mortality at 30 days was 1% for both groups. Limb salvage related to the ilio-femoral revascularization was 100% for both groups.

There were no statistically significant differences in overall primary (91% vs 98%, $p = 0.3$), assisted primary (93% vs 98%, $p = 0.5$), or secondary patency (97% vs 100%, $p = 0.11$) at 3 years between hybrid or open repair. This held true even after stratifying for aorto-iliac TASC A–B primary patency, (HR 89% vs 100% OR, $p = 0.38$), secondary patency (HR 95% vs OR 100%, $p = 0.54$) and TASC C–D primary patency (95% v 97%, $p = 0.54$), secondary patency (100% vs. 100%, $p = 0.79$). We carefully explored multivariate modeling for patency, which demonstrated that the only negative predictor for patency was major tissue loss (Rutherford Class 6) at presentation in patients undergoing HR. Moreover the presence of an high grade of CFA stenosis or occlusion did not represent a significant factor for long term patency as well. Interestingly, even though associated profundoplasty was significantly more often performed during HR, this was not a positive predictor of patency in the multivariate analysis. Overall survival was significantly higher for patients undergoing OR than for patients undergoing HR (88% vs 73%, $p = .007$).

Multivariate analysis for survival was performed to evaluate the association with patient demographics, risk factors, risk score, and operative characteristics. Despite the fact that the HR group had a higher mortality rate (hazard ratio = 1.965), multivariate analysis did not demonstrate HR to be an independent risk factor for mortality ($p = 0.18$). Rutherford class 5 (minor tissue loss) and 6 (major tissue loss) at presentation, ASA score 3–4, and an SVS score >15 were negative predictors of survival ($p = 0.02$, p = 0.02, $p = 0.01$) with hazard ratios of 2.3, 4.5 and 3.0 respectively. Interestingly, age less than 60 at the time of intervention did not have an effect on mortality ($p = 0.79$).

In recent years, we have adopted a preferred strategy of hybrid repair with combined common femoral endarterectomy and iliac artery stenting rather than traditional open repair with aorto-femoral or ilio-femoral bypass for the treatment of severe ilio-femoral occlusive disease. The treatment of IFOD with HR has obvious appeal. Decreased hospital and ICU length of stay, less surgical morbidity, and more recently, patient preference dictating a "minimally invasive" approach are all factors that have helped popularize HR.

Despite the non-randomized nature of this study, the two groups undergoing OR or HR were well matched for risk factors, and other salient clinical variables.

Thirty-day mortality and morbidity were similar between the two groups, however, overall survival at 3 years was significantly higher for patients who underwent OR rather than HR. Using the multivariate model, we investigated whether the reduced long-term survival with HR was related to the procedure itself. This analysis demonstrated that hybrid repair was not an independent predictor of mortality, but that high SVS comorbidity and ASA scores were predictive of reduced long-term survival as was Rutherford classes 5 and 6. The decreased survival seen in patients undergoing HR is likely related to the fact that those patients have greater comorbidities and overall worsened medical condition than those who underwent open surgery, but not related to the hybrid procedure itself. Consequently, HR could be a valid alternative to OR for high-risk patients, eliminating the invasiveness and physiologic stress that result from aortic cross-clamping, as well as shortening ICU and hospital stays and potentially reducing perioperative morbidity.

The TASC consensus statement provides a framework to assess the treatment of aortoiliac lesions by stratifying lesion length and morphology[2]. In this series, aortoiliac TASC classification as well as severity of CFA disease was different between the two groups, with HR having the majority of patients in TASC A or B lesions and OR with TASC C and D lesions. In addition, HR had a greater preponderance of severe stenosis or occlusion of the CFA compared to OR. Although this may bias the results in this study, multivariate analysis for patency did not show any statistically significant difference for CFA grade of stenosis or iliac TASC classification between the two groups. The only negative predictor of patency was Rutherford class 6 ischemia, suggesting that clinical presentation may be a more accurate predictor of patency rather than the specific location or severity of stenosis in the presence of ilio-femoral occlusive disease. In our study, patients with bilateral iliac TASC C and D lesions were preferentially treated with OR and patients with focal and unilateral iliac disease with associated severe common femoral occlusive disease were treated with HR. During the last three years of this study, the number of patients with bilateral TASC C and D lesions treated with HR increased significantly, particularly for high-risk patients. This is a reflection of advancement in techniques and materials, as well as increased skill and comfort level of the operators. It is important to note, however, that even in the presence of concomitant CFA disease, the recommendations put forth from the TASC document can be applied.

Another important determinant of long-term patency after iliac endovascular treatment and CFE is the adequacy of distal runoff of the CFA and femoral-popliteal segment. Even though in the multivariate model, associated profundoplasty and associate distal revascularization were not predictive of increased patency, approximately 60% of HR procedures were associated with profundoplasty even for TASC A−B than C−D. Differently associated profundoplasty in OR had much lower rate varying from 14% for TASC A−B to 34% in TASC C−D. Additional profundoplasty to CFE in a patient with femoral-popliteal disease could allow sufficient clinical improvement and critical outflow to the lower extremity. Previously, it has been demonstrated that treating deep femoral artery orificial lesions leads to improvement in ABF bypass patency.[9] Similarly, we can suppose that CFE and associated profundoplasty during HR, when indicated, may contribute to improved patency of the revascularized ilio-femoral segment.

LITERATURE REVIEW

Recently the European Society of Vascular Surgery,[10] published guidelines for the treatment of critical limb ischemia. With regard to the hybrid approach for aorto-ilio-femoral occlusive disease, the guidelines state that the hybrid technique is an acceptable alternative treatment in patients requiring open surgical repair (Recommendation of Level 3b; Grade C). Furthermore, they also report that the use of stent-grafts compared to bare-metal stents in the iliac segment is likely associated with better outcomes, but this requires confirmation by future prospective studies (Recommendation Level 4 G; Grade C).

The first reports of combined endovascular and open surgical procedures are from the 1970s.[11] Since then, most reports have dealt with femoral endarterectomy or femoro-femoral bypass combined with iliac PTA and stenting. Primary success rates have been high: 93%–100%.[12,5,13] The long-term results in such inflow endovascular procedures have been shown to be comparable to those of open surgical procedures, with lower or equal morbidity and mortality rates and with primary patency rates of 60%–91%.[5,14,12,15,16] In some reports, morbidity has been higher in hybrid procedures as compared to only endovascular procedures, possibly due to the patient having a more generalized atherosclerosis,[12] the more common use of general anesthesia, and frequent need for a groin incision. Yet there are no randomized studies involving comparisons between hybrid and open procedures. Such studies may be very difficult to conduct due to the complexity of and variations in the outflow and inflow anatomy of these patients with multilevel disease and various clinical presentations.

The proportion of hybrid procedures among all revascularizations has increased steadily during the last decade and is estimated to constitute between 5%–20% of all vascular reconstructions.[12,17] Technical aspects regarding target vessel recanalization, wire and catheter placement, stent placement and the timing or order of an endovascular and open procedure usually involve femoral endarterectomy and patching with iliac stenting. The stent materials and brands used vary in all of the reports and reflect the complex and versatile nature of vascular disease.

Chang et al.[4] in their experience with hybrid procedures reported a technical success higher than 98% with more than 90% of patients reporting clinical improvement; similar results have been reported by Piazza et al.[15] after stratification for iliac lesion TASC classification, and by Nelson et al.[16] who reported their experience with selective external iliac artery stenting plus common femoral endarterectomy. These results of these studies are summarized in Table 12-1. This tabular review includes all reports, published between 2000 and 2012, of patients treated with hybrid repair for extensive aortoiliac and femoral occlusive disease. The main concern in reviewing all previous clinical experiences is the problem of mixed series. Reports on Hybrid repair tend to blend together TASC a–b with TASC c–d lesions. Furthermore, results are biased by the use of different techniques and materials to perform this procedure. In our analysis of the literature, weighted ranges have been calculated when possible, and when data could be considered of iliac stenting plus common femoral endarterectomy only. The clinical data extracted from the selected reports are allocated as they appear in crude percentages with ranges of presentation. The tabular data include clinical presentation, post operative technical and clinical success as ABI increase. Thirty-day mortality and survival as patency are reported when available.

TABLE 12-1. TABULAR REVIEW OF EARLY AND LONG TERM OUTCOMES FOR HYBRID PROCEDURES IN THE TREATMENT OF ILIO-FEMORAL ARTERIAL OBSTRUCTIVE DISEASE

Variable	(%)	Range	References
Clinical presentation			
Claudication	43	41–70	5,14,15
Rest pain	33	8–59	5,14,15
Tissue loss	21	20–22	5,14,15
Anatomical location			
CIA + CFE	42	24–61	5,14,15
EIA + CFE	62	48–100	5,14,15
CIA-EIA + CFE	44	28–61	5,14,15
Type of stent for iliac			
Stent graft	30	20–41	5,14
Stent	75	65–88	5,14,15
Operative outcomes			
Technical success	98.5	98–100	5,14,15,18
Clinical improvement	94	92–97	5,14,15
ABI increase (mean)	0.35	0.34–0.38	5,14,15
Lenght of stay (mean)	3	2–4	5,14,15
30 day mortality	1.8	1–2.3	5,14
Survival			
3 year	60	-	14
5 year	60	-	5
Patency			
Primary (1y)	84*	-	15
Primary assisted (1y)	97*	-	15
Primary (3 y)	91	-	14
Primary assisted (3 y)	95	-	14
Secondary (3y)	98	-	14
Primary (5y)	60	-	5
Primary assisted (5 y)	97	-	5
Secondary (5 y)	98	-	5

CONCLUSION

In recent years, the frequency of hybrid repair for the treatment of iliac and common femoral artery obstructive disease has progressively increased and has been demonstrated to be a valid and safe technique with acceptable early and long-term results. The results of our experience clearly demonstrates that IFOD can be treated using HR with shorter hospitalization and similar early and long term efficacy when compared to OR. Hybrid repair should be considered for all patients with IFOD and particularly for those at high surgical risk. Long-term patency is similar in both groups regardless of severity of TASC classification. However, when deciding between HR or OR, one must consider that major tissue loss at presentation is a negative predictor of long-term patency in patients undergoing hybrid repair. New advances in materials used and technical approaches will probably allow this technique in the future to be the first line approach for these patients.

REFERENCES

1. de Vries SO, Hunink MG. Results of aortic bifurcation grafts for aortoiliac occlusive disease: a meta-analysis. *J Vasc Surg*. 1997;26(4):558–69.
2. Norgren L, Hiatt WR, Dormandy JA, et al. Inter-society consensus for the management of peripheral arterial disease. *Int Angiol*. 2007;26(2):81–157.
3. Cardon A, Aillet S, Jarno P, et al. [Endarteriectomy of the femoral tripod: long-term results and analysis of failure factors]. *Ann Chir*. 2001;126(8):777–82.
4. Kang JL, Patel VI, Conrad MF, et al. Common femoral artery occlusive disease: contemporary results following surgical endarterectomy. *J Vasc Surg*. 2008;48(4):872–7.
5. Chang RW, Goodney PP, Baek JH, et al. Long-term results of combined common femoral endarterectomy and iliac stenting/stent grafting for occlusive disease. *J Vasc Surg*. 2008;48(2):362–7.
6. Chaikof EL, Fillinger MF, Matsumura JS, et al. Identifying and grading factors that modify the outcome of endovascular aortic aneurysm repair. *J Vasc Surg*. 2002;35(5):1061–6.
7. Eagle KA, Coley CM, Newell JB, et al. Combining clinical and thallium data optimizes preoperative assessment of cardiac risk before major vascular surgery. *Ann Intern Med*. 1989;110(11):859–66.
8. Rutherford RB, Baker JD, Ernst C, et al. Recommended standards for reports dealing with lower extremity ischemia: revised version. *J Vasc Surg*. 1997;26(3):517–38.
9. Brewster DC, Darling RC. Optimal methods of aortoiliac reconstruction. *Surgery*. 1978;84(6):739–48.
10. Setacci C, de Donato G, Teraa M, et al. Chapter IV: Treatment of critical limb ischaemia. *Eur J Vasc Endovasc Surg*. 2011 Dec;42 Suppl 2:S43–59.
11. Porter JM, Eidemiller LR, Hood RW, et al. Transluminal angioplasty and distal arterial bypass. *Am Surg*. 1977 Nov;43(11):695–702.
12. Dosluoglu HH, Lall P, Cherr GS, Harris LM, Dryjski ML. Role of simple and complex hybrid revascularization procedures for symptomatic lower extremity occlusive disease. *J Vasc Surg*. 2010 Jun;51(6):1425–1435.e1.
13. Simó G, Banga P, Darabos G, Mogán I. Stent-assisted remote iliac artery endarterectomy: an alternative approach to treating combined external iliac and common femoral artery disease. *Eur J Vasc Endovasc Surg*. 2011 Nov;42(5):648–55. Epub 2011 Jun 24.
14. Kashyap VS, Pavkov ML, Bena JF, et al. The management of severe aortoiliac occlusive disease: endovascular therapy rivals open reconstruction. *J Vasc Surg*. 2008;48(6):1451–7, 7 e1-3.
15. Piazza M, Ricotta JJ 2nd, Bower TC, et al. Iliac artery stenting combined with open femoral endarterectomy is as effective as open surgical reconstruction for severe iliac and common femoral occlusive disease. *J Vasc Surg*. 2011 Aug;54(2):402–11. Epub 2011 Apr 30.
16. Nelson PR, Powell RJ, Schermerhorn ML, et al. Early results of external iliac artery stenting combined with common femoral artery endarterectomy. *J Vasc Surg*. 2002 Jun;35(6):1107–13.
17. Ebaugh JL, Gagnon D, Owens CD, et al. Comparison of costs of staged versus simultaneous lower extremity arterial hybrid procedures. *Am J Surg*. 2008 Nov;196(5):634–40.
18. Sharafuddin MJ, Kresowik TF, Hoballah JJ, et al. Combined direct repair and inline inflow stenting in the management of aortoiliac disease extending into the common femoral artery. *Vasc Endovascular Surg*. 2011 Apr;45(3):274–82.

13

Sutureless Anastomosis in Femoral-Popliteal Bypass for Lower Extremity Revascularization

Syed M. Hussain, MD and Nabeel R. Rana, MD

Peripheral arterial disease (PAD) affects approximately eight to ten million Americans, of which 30% are over the age of 65 years.[1-3] Approximately 30% of patients have classic PAD symptoms such as claudication, rest pain, or pedal ulcers. The remainder (70% of patients) are asymptomatic or demonstrate atypical exertional symptoms. The U.S. Census bureau predicts the population to be 350 million persons by 2030. Of this number, over 50% of people will be over the age of 55 years. The continued rise of cardiovascular disease along with an aging population will only increase the incidence of PAD.

Atherosclerosis is the cornerstone of PAD. Multiple revascularization modalities exist for the treatment of PAD such as angioplasty and stent placement, atherectomy, surgical endarterectomy, and bypass procedures. It has been predicted that approximately 1.7 million vascular interventions will occur in the next 15 years of which 1.2 million will be operative.[3]

For lower extremity PAD, options for bypass conduit include prosthetic grafts or autologous vein. Although vein conduit is considered to be superior in patency rates to prosthetic material, it is limited by its availability. With the rise of cardiac disease, end stage renal disease and dialysis, vein conduit has often already been harvested or is of poor quality. It is well documented in the literature that a vein diameter less than 3.5 mm when used as a bypass conduit results in a 2.1 fold increase in graft failure at 30 days.[4] Thus, the use of prosthetic grafts has risen, specifically in the femoral-popliteal artery location. The purpose of this chapter is to briefly discuss the role of a specific prosthetic graft, expanded polytetraflourethylene (ePTFE - W.L. GORE), in femoral-above knee popliteal artery bypass procedures, limitations of currently available PTFE grafts, techniques and outcomes of the new HYBRID PTFE graft in femoral popliteal artery bypass, and finally, future directions of lower extremity bypass involving prosthetic conduits.

CHANGING FACES OF ePTFE

The use of ePTFE for above knee femoral-popliteal bypass has been well documented in the literature. Initially receiving a reputation for poor outcomes when compared to vein conduit in the 1980's, ePTFE has regained significant ground in patency rates and limb salvage since its origin in 1976. In 1986, Veith et al reported 4-year primary patency results for ePTFE and vein conduits to infrapopliteal arteries at 12% and 49%.[5] Since this large study, few studies were published comparing PTFE grafts to vein conduit grafts. However, due to lack of any or quality vein conduits, a renewed interest has been sparked in ePTFE.

Dairaku et al reviewed 145 patients who had undergone either an above knee or below knee popliteal artery bypass with vein, ePTFE, or ePTFE combined with the Linton patch. The one and three year results for the three groups were not statistically significant for above knee popliteal artery bypass. However, for below knee popliteal work, primary patency rates at 5 years were 75%, 42%, and 93% respectively.[6]

Sala and co-workers conducted a nonrandomized prospective trial comparing vein to ePTFE for above knee popliteal artery bypass procedures. Forty-eight cases used vein conduit and 27 cases were performed with ePTFE. Four year primary patency rates were 82% and 81% respectively, with a 96% limb salvage rate.[7] This study suggested no difference between the two conduits for above knee popliteal bypass grafting.

Although standard ePTFE demonstrates comparable results to vein conduits in above knee popliteal arteries, it has repeatedly demonstrated suboptimal results in below knee blood vessels. This led to the advent of the heparin bonded ePTFE graft (GORTEX PROPATEN, W.L.GORE). A heparin-bonded graft was hypothesized to demonstrate decreased thrombogenicity when compared to standard ePTFE, thereby increasing the patency in below knee bypass procedures. The PROPATEN graft uses a CARMEDA Bioactive Surface (CBAS). CBAS technology involves the covalent bonding of heparin to a polymer on the inner surface of the Gortex graft.

Bosiers et al performed a clinical study evaluating the use of Propaten in the above knee popliteal artery, below knee popliteal artery, and crural vessels. The trial demonstrated a 1-year patency of 84% for above knee popliteal artery, 81% for below knee popliteal artery, and 74% for crural vessel bypass.[8] This study showed very promising results when compared to a pooled meta-analysis of 40 trials utilizing standard ePTFE reported an abysmal 59% patency at 1 year.[9] The Scandinavian Propaten Trial reported a 37% decrease in bypass graft failure when Propaten was utilized compared to standard ePTFE in above knee popliteal bypass procedures.[10] This again confirmed that heparin bonded ePTFE grafts increase the patency and longevity of the bypass graft in the lower extremity.

Our own experience with the use of Propaten for above knee and below knee popliteal artery bypass has been quite encouraging. We have performed 72 bypass grafts to the above knee popliteal artery and 74 grafts to the below knee popliteal artery in our practice. The four-year patency for above knee popliteal artery bypass grafts is 92% and the four-year patency for below knee popliteal artery grafts is 86%. In our opinion, in light of these results, Propaten is well on its way to becoming our standard graft for above knee and below knee popliteal artery bypass work.

HYBRID BYPASS GRAFT

The HYBRID bypass graft (W.L. GORE) was initially developed on the platform of the Propaten graft and the heparin coated VIABAHN stent graft (W.L. GORE). The graft combines the strengths of both technologies. The proximal 45 cm is a non-ringed ePTFE heparin coated graft and the last 5 cm is a heparin coated nitinol-reinforced stent graft (Figure 13-1). The graft was initially developed for use in arterio-venous (AV) grafts for dialysis access. It is thought that AV grafts fail because of intimal hyperplasia at the venous anastamosis. If a sutureless anastomosis could be performed at the graft-venous attachment, a more hemodynamically favorable flow dynamic (provided by the nitinol reinforced segment) should potentially decrease the chance for AV graft thrombosis, resulting in a longer lifespan for the dialysis graft. The technique involves suturing the hood of the HYBRID graft to the brachial artery; the nitinol-reinforced segment of the HYBRID graft is placed into the vein either directly through a small venotomy or by utilizing an over the wire technique. No anastomotic sutures are required to create the venous anastomosis; the hemodynamics become more fluid, and the chance of developing intimal hyperplasia and graft failure is decreased.

Based on this concept, the HYBRID graft can also be utilized in other applications beyond dialysis access. For example, the Achilles heel of the femoral popliteal artery bypass graft is the distal anastomosis. The distal anastomosis is typically constructed in an end to side beveled fashion resulting in an "acute angle" between the graft and

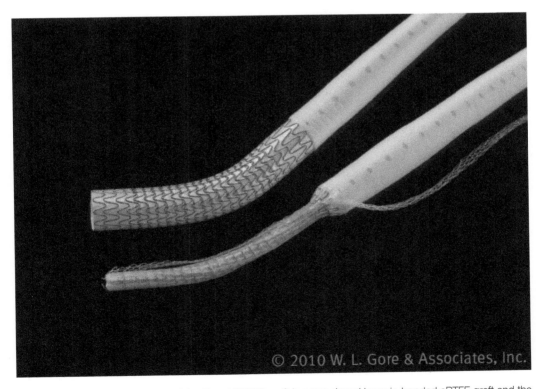

Figure 13-1. The proximal 45 cm of the Gore HYBRID graft is a non-ringed heparin-bonded ePTFE graft and the distal 5 cm is a heparin-bonded nitinol-reinforced stent graft.

the artery (Figure 13-2). Hemodynamic studies have shown that there are irregular oscillating flow patterns rather than laminar blood flow at the distal anastomosis due to this anastamotic geometry.[11,12] These flow dynamics create low wall shear stress at the arterial wall, which ultimately stimulates intimal hyperplasia (Figure 13-3). This, in turn, causes narrowing at the distal anastomosis resulting in eventual thrombosis and failure of the bypass graft if left unchecked.

Our practice decided to use the HYBRID graft specifically in the femoral to above knee popliteal artery bypass application. Since the graft is a standard nonringed 6 mm ePTFE graft with nitinol-reinforced segment sizes ranging from 6–9 mm, all popliteal arteries were not considered candidates for the use of this graft. Careful assessment of the popliteal artery diameter is crucial when embarking on the use of this graft in

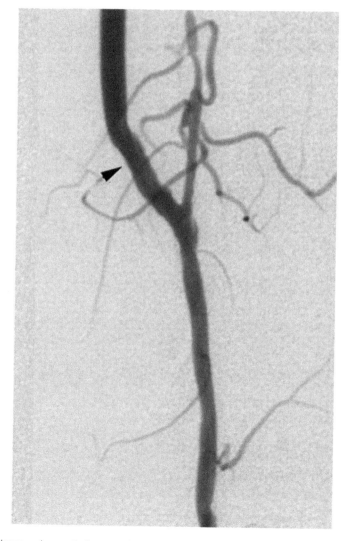

Figure 13-2. Arteriogram demonstrating angulation at the interface between a bypass graft and native vessel using a standard end-to-side distal anastomosis.

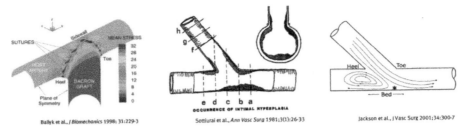

Figure 13-3. End-to-side anastomoses result in turbulent non-laminar flow dynamics and variations in wall shear stress resulting in intimal hyperplasia.

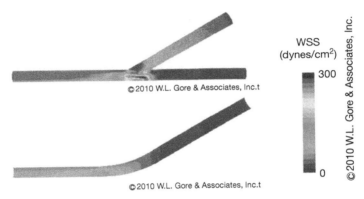

Figure 13-4. Sutureless distal anastomosis with a nitinol-reinforced stent graft allows for more laminar flow dynamics when compared to tradition end-to-side sutured anastomosis.

this application. It is clear from previously published Viabahn data that oversizing can result in stent-graft failure. This concept must be considered when using this graft in the lower extremity bypass application as well.

There are many advantages in utilizing the HYBRID graft in femoral-popliteal bypass procedures. Smaller incisions are needed to do the bypass since only a small portion of the popliteal artery needs to be exposed. It allows for a sutureless distal anastomosis, decreasing the anastomotic suture burden, which itself can stimulate scarring and intimal hyperplasia. In addition, the nitinol-reinforced segment allows a more laminar flow pattern and eliminates the acute angle at the distal anastomosis (Figure 13-4). Furthermore, the graft technology gives patients the option to undergo an above knee popliteal bypass even though the above knee popliteal artery may not be ideal for accommodating a distal anastomosis. The nitinol-reinforced segment of the HYBRID graft can be used to cover or reline the suboptimal portion of the above knee popliteal artery, thus creating a laminar flow pattern at the distal landing zone, which may be within the below knee popliteal artery and adjacent to the crural vessel(s).

There are a few disadvantages in considering the HYBRID graft, as well. The most pronounced is the lack of adequate sizing and the lack of rings in the current configuration of this graft. The graft is a standard 6 mm ePTFE Propaten with no rings. In our practice, we routinely implant either a 7 mm or 8 mm Propaten graft to accommodate the proximal femoral anastomoses. Furthermore, the sizes for the nitinol-reinforced segment of the HYBRID graft begin range from 6 mm to 9 mm. The length of the nitinol-reinforced segment is 5 cm. In our opinion, a 5 mm diameter nitinol-reinforced segment is a much needed addition to the graft's current design; we also would be interested in having more choices in terms of the length of the nitinol-reinforced segment (perhaps a 7 cm length and a 10 cm length). The distal end of the nitinol-reinforced segment does risk covering collateral flow into the popliteal artery at the level of the knee provided by the profunda femoral artery. These collaterals are often considered the most important source of "back-up" flow if the traditional end-side anastomosis of the graft were to fail. It is imperative that the anatomy be studied carefully on digital subtraction angiography to ensure that the distal nitinol-reinforced segment of the HYBRID bypass does not inadvertently cover the geniculate artery collateral flow.

IMPLANTATION TECHNIQUE

The procedure is ideally performed in a HYBRID endovascular suite with modern imaging capabilities. The utilization of a C-arm is an option if the imaging is of acceptable quality. The patient is placed under general anesthesia and the procedure is begun in the standard fashion one would perform a femoral-popliteal artery bypass. Our practice is to make a small vertical groin incision to expose the common femoral artery; we make a small incision above the knee on the medial thigh to expose the popliteal artery. Only a small portion of the popliteal artery needs to be exposed to function as an access site; we use vessel loops to encircle the artery (Figure 13-5). This allows for smaller skin incisions to be performed resulting in a lower incidence of wound breakdown and infection.

Once the arteries are adequately exposed, a subsartorial tunnel is made and a large umbilical tape is passed through the tunnel. Heparin is administered systemically.

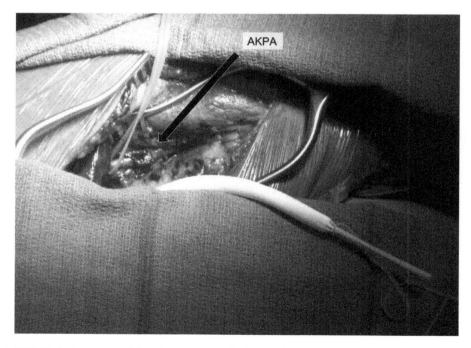

Figure 13-5. Limited exposure of the above knee popliteal artery (controlled here with a vessel loop) is required for sutureless anastomosis of the distal nitinol-reinforced segment of the hybrid graft.

The popliteal artery is punctured with a 21-gauge needle and under fluoroscopy; a .018 wire is advanced into the distal arterial vasculature. A 5 French (F) micro-sheath (Cordis Company) is advanced over the wire and into the artery. On table angiography of the popliteal artery is performed to ensure the wire is not in a dissection plane and that the artery is suitable for the HYBRID graft. The .018 wire is removed and a .035 stiff angled Glidewire (Terumo Inc.) is advanced into the below knee popliteal artery. The 5F micro-sheath is then removed and an 11 French × 11 cm peel away sheath is inserted into the popliteal artery for a short distance (Figure 13-6a). The HYBRID graft is loaded onto the wire, leading with the nitinol-reinforced segment (NRS) (Figure 13-6b). As the surgeon advances the NRS, the assistant peels away the sheath until the sheath is removed and approximately 1 cm of the stent is outside the artery (Figure 13-6c). The deployment string for the NRS is pulled and

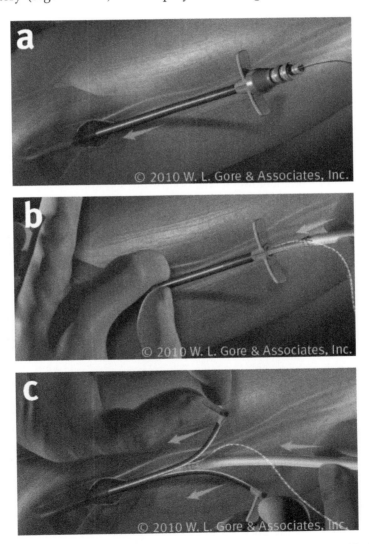

Figure 13-6. (a) 11-french peel-away sheath in inserted into popliteal artery over a wire **(b)** NRS of HYBRID graft is inserted into the peel-away sheath over the wire **(c)** sheath is peeled away as the NRS is advanced into the popliteal artery, leaving about a 1 cm segment of the stent outside the artery.

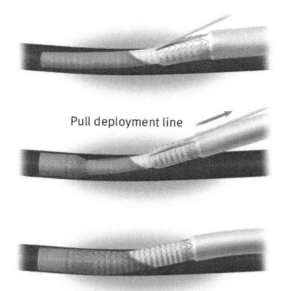

Pull deployment line

Figure 13-7. Pulling the deployment string opens the stent graft segment completely in a radial fashion.

the graft is deployed completely (Figure 13-7). An appropriate sized balloon catheter is then loaded onto the wire and used to angioplasty the distal NRS anastomosis. There is minimal or no bleeding at this point from the entry site at the popliteal artery (Figure 13-8). Three 6-0 prolene stay sutures (ETHICON Inc) at the nine-, twelve-, and three-o'clock positions. The wire is removed.

The umbilical tape is tied around the proximal HYBRID graft, and the graft is pulled through the tunnel into the groin. A simple end-side beveled anastomosis is created, and the graft is flushed in the standard fashion. An on table angiogram is then

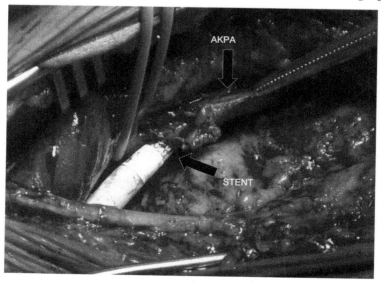

Figure 13-8. Following balloon dilation of the NRS, there is no residual narrowing and no bleeding around the stent segment at the above knee popliteal artery (AKPA) entry site.

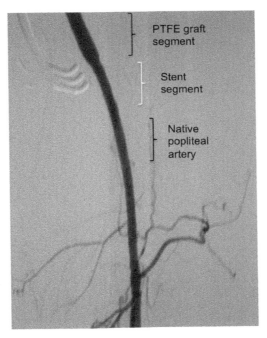

PTFE graft
segment

Stent
segment

Native
popliteal
artery

Figure 13-9. Completion on-table arteriogram shows smooth transition at the distal anastomosis allowing laminar flow dynamics.

performed with a 20 gauge butterfly needle inserted into the common femoral artery above the proximal anastomosis or into the hood ePTFE graft itself to assess the final result of the distal sutureless anastomosis (Figure 13-9). Incisions are closed per the surgeons' discretion.

RESULTS

Modifications of the HYBRID graft have been performed around the world. Ferreto et al have performed the VIPS (Viabahn Padova Sutureless) technique in Europe. This involves the transection of the popliteal artery above the knee, an end to end anastomosis of a Propaten graft to a partially deployed VIABAHN stent graft, placement of the non-deployed stent graft into the popliteal artery and subsequent deployment of the stent graft within the artery and adjunctive balloon catheter angioplasty of the stent. A total of five patients have undergone this procedure for Rutherford class 5 diseases. Operative time was under 60 minutes and blood loss was minimal for the case. At three-week follow-up, all 5 grafts were patent and all of the pedal ulcers had healed completely.[13]

The HYBRID bypass graft was initially approved for dialysis access in the United States in late August 2010. The graft was released on a limited-access basis to 16 centers in the country. Our center was the first to utilize this device for the indication of lower extremity arterial occlusive disease in September 2010. Our goal was to prospectively analyze the patency rates for femoral-above knee popliteal artery bypass using this HYBRID graft technology. A total of 9 patients received the graft for this procedure from September 2010 to May 2011. Follow-up occurred at 1-month post implantation with an arterial duplex and every 6 months thereafter. At present, 7 of 9 patients have patent grafts. The longest patency is 21 months and the shortest patency is 13 months. One graft occluded after 3 months of implantation due to new onset atrial fibrillation and clot embolization to the external iliac artery. As a result, graft thrombosis occurred in the patient. The second failure occurred 2 weeks after implantation due to graft infection. The graft was explanted and patient has had stable claudication since that time. In addition, he was diagnosed with a hypercoagulable disorder after the bypass graft was removed.

From this early experience, it is encouraging to note that this graft can perform well in the short term. Of course, we will continue to follow these patients to observe long-term outcomes.

FUTURE DIRECTIONS

The HYBRID graft is a promising new technology for femoral popliteal artery bypass procedures. It has also been applied in other areas such as de-branching procedures for thoracoabdominal aneurysms and renal artery bypass procedures in hybrid cases involving aortic endograft placement. Since the graft was not developed for these applications, anatomy and size of the blood vessels as well as limited sizes of the graft currently limit its use. Our hope is that the manufacturer will implement new modifications to the graft (wider range of diameters and lengths) to accommodate its multifaceted use in vascular hybrid procedures.

Acknowledgements

I would like to thank my colleagues and friends, Dr. Nabeel Rana MD, Dr. Jennifer Ash MD, Sherri Morrison PAC, Katherine Tetrault PAC, and my colleagues at OSF/HeartCare Midwest. With their support and dedication, we will continue to advance vascular care not only in our community but globally.

REFERENCES

1. Roger VL, Go AS, Lloyd-Jones DM, et al. Heart disease and stroke statistics—2011 updated: a report from the American Heart Association. *Circulation*. 2011 Feb 1;23(4):e18–e209.
2. Thom T, Haase N, Rosamond W, et al. Heart disease and stroke statistics—2006 updated: a report from the American Heart Association Statistics Committee and StrokeStatistics Subcommittee. *Circulation*. 2006 Feb 14;113(6):e85–151.
3. McDermott MM, Mehta S, Greenland P. Exertional leg symptoms other than intermittent claudication are common in peripheral arterial Disease. *Arch Intern Med*. 1999 Feb 22;159(4):387–92.
4. Schanzer A, Hevelone N, Owens CD, et al. Technical factors affecting autogenous vein graft failure: observations from a large multicenter trial. *J Vasc Surg*. 2007 Dec;46(6):1180–90.
5. Veith FJ, Gupta SK, Ascer E, et al. Six-year prospective multicenter randomized comparison of autologous saphenous vein and expanded polytetrafluoroethylene grafts in infrainguinal arterial reconstructions. *J Vasc Surg*. 1986 Jan;3(1):104–14.

6. Dairaku K, Fujioka K, Yamashita A, et al. Experimental and clinical studies investigating the efficacy of distal anastomosis with patch plasty in bypass operations with expanded polytetrafluoroethylene grafts. *Surg Today*. 2003;33(5):349–53.

7. Sala F, Hassen-Khodja R, Lecis A, et al. Long-term outcome of femoral above-knee popliteal artery bypass using autologous saphenous vein versus expanded polytetrafluoroethylene grafts. *Ann Vasc Surg*. 2003 Jul;17(4):401–7.

8. Bosiers M, Deloose K, Verbist J, et al. Heparin-bonded expanded polytetrafluorothylene vascular graft for femoropopliteal and femorocrural bypass grafting: 1-year results. *J Vasc Surg*. 2006 Feb;43(2):313-8; discussion 318–9.

9. Albers M, Battistella VM, Romiti M et al. Meta-analysis of polytetrafluoroethylene bypass grafts to infrapopliteal arteries. *J Vasc Surg*. 2003 Jun;37(6):1263–9.

10. Lindholt JS, Gottschalksen B, Johannesen N, et al. The Scandinavian Propaten® trial — 1-year patency of PTFE vascular prostheses with heparin-bonded luminal surfaces compared to ordinary pure PTFE vascular prostheses- a randomised clinical controlled multi-centre trial. *Eur J Vasc Endovasc Surg*. 2011 May;41(5):668–73.

11. Jackson ZS, Ishibashi H, Gotlieb AI, et al. Effects of anastomotic angle on vascular tissue responses at end-to-side arterial grafts. *J Vasc Surg*. 2001 Aug;34(2):300–7.

12. Ojha M, Cobbold RS, Johnston KW. Influence of angle on wall shear stress distribution for an end-to-side anastomosis. *J Vasc Surg*. 1994 Jun;19(6):1067–73.

13. Ferretto L, Piazza M, Bonvini S, et al. ViPS (Viabahn Padova Sutureless) technique: preliminary results in the treatment of peripheral arterial disease. *Ann Vasc Surg*. 2012 Jan;26(1):34–9.

14

Update on Clinical Trials Evaluating the Effect of Biologic Therapy in Patients with Critical Limb Ischemia

Richard J. Powell, MD

ABSTRACT

Critical limb ischemia (CLI) represents the most severe degree of peripheral arterial disease and is associated with significant morbidity and mortality. In patients with CLI who do not have revascularization options major amputation or death occurs within one year in as many as 40% of patients. Biological therapies which include gene therapy and cellular therapy offers the potential to promote wound healing and prevent amputation in patients who otherwise have poor options for revascularization. Several recent phase 2 trials have shown acceptable safety and suggest that these biologic therapies have the potential to improve outcomes in patients with "no-option" CLI. Phase 3 trials are now in progress. This report summarizes the recent results of gene and cellular therapy clinical trials in patients with CLI.

INTRODUCTION

Critical limb ischemia (CLI) represents the most severe degree of peripheral arterial disease manifesting as either ischemic rest pain or tissue loss. In patients with CLI who do not have revascularization options major amputation is required within one year in as many as 40% of patients and mortality is as high as 20%. The one year amputation rate varies depending on whether a patient presents with rest pain which carries a 10–15 % incidence of amputation at one year or with tissue loss which is associated a 35% incidence of major amputation. Biological therapies which include gene therapy and cellular therapy offers the potential to promote wound healing and prevent amputation in patients who otherwise have no options for revascularization. This report summarizes the results of recent gene and cellular therapy clinical trials in patients with CLI.

GENE THERAPY CLI TRIALS

Therapeutic angiogenesis which is the growth of blood vessels from pre-existing blood vessels in response to growth factor stimulation has been shown to occur in animal models of hind limb ischemia. This concept was introduced into the clinical realm by Dr Jeffery Isner in the early 1990's. Various growth factors such as vascular endothelial growth factor (VEGF), hepatocyte growth factor (HGF) and fibroblast growth factor (FGF) have been shown to promote angiogenesis in animal models. Because of the short half-life of these proteins gene therapy has been used to maintain sustained expression in the ischemic limb. Most trials have utilized intramuscular injection of either the plasmid or adenoviral mediated transfection. Expression of the protein is maintained from 2–6 weeks. General concerns regarding gene therapy safety have been related to the potential for "off-target " angiogenesis that could result in promotion of occult tumor growth or accelerated progression of diabetic proliferative retinopathy. To date these concerns have not occurred in gene therapy trials that have been completed.

Fibroblast Growth Factor (FGF) has been extensively studied in the context of CLI. The TALISMAN Phase 2 trial (Clinicaltrials.gov NCT00798005) enrolled 125 patients and reported a significant improvement in amputation free survival of 52% in placebo treated patients with no options for revascularization compared to 73% in patients treated with FGF plasmid ($p = .009$).[1] In this trial which was conducted entirely in Europe there was a decrease in major amputation at one year from 34% in placebo treated patients to 16% in NV1FGF treated patients ($p = 0.015$). In addition mortality was 12% in the treated patients compared to 23% in placebo treated patients. The 34% major amputation rate in placebo treated patients was unusually high compared to previous no-option CLI trials. It is also unclear why a limb sparing therapy would have such a dramatic effect on mortality. In a separate study these investigators proved proof of concept of gene therapy when they identified the FGF plasmid, mRNA and protein in the amputation specimens in patients with CLI who received FGF plasmid injections prior to amputation.[2] These findings led Sanofi-Aventis to complete a Phase 3 pivotal trial; The TAMARIS trial (NCT 00566657). Unlike the earlier phase 2 trial the TAMARIS trial failed to show a difference in AFS (amputation free survival) when compared to placebo in patients with CLI.[3] (see Table 14-1). This trial enrolled 525 patients at 170 sites in over 30 countries with either hemodynamically confirmed ischemic ulcer or minor gangrene. Major amputation or death at one year occurred in 33% of placebo treated patients and 36% of treated patients. The amputation free survival for both groups was similar to the FGF treated patients in the phase 2 TALISMAN trial. The likely explanation for the different results observed in the phase 2 TALISMAN and Phase 3 TAMARIS trials is a type II error.

The only remaining gene therapy under late phase clinical evaluation is hepatocyte growth factor (HGF) plasmid. Early phase 2 trials (NCT00189540, NCT00060892) have shown that HGF plasmid gene therapy can improve TcPO2 and pain scores in

TABLE 14-1. TAMARIS TRIAL NV1FGF PLASMID vs PLACEBO IN CLI PIVOTAL TRIAL

12 month Endpoint	AFS	Amputation	Death
NV1FGF	63%	26%	18%
Placebo	67%	21%	15%
p	.48	.31	.53

• n = 525

patients with CLI compared to placebo.[4,5] A simultaneous trial in Japan was stopped early by the data safety monitoring board due to an improvement in ulcer size in 100% of the HGF plasmid-treated patients compared to an improvement in 40% of the pacebo-treated patients ($p = 0.014$).[6] Based on these data the sponsoring company, AnGes, plans to begin a pivotal phase III trial . This trial plans to enroll 560 poor option patients with critical limb ischemia manifested as either tissue loss or rest pain. Poor option is defined as patients who are not endovascular candidates and are suboptimal candidates for surgical bypass. This would include patients who have significant co morbid risk, the need for synthetic below the knee bypass, or vein bypass with either non great saphenous vein or a great saphenous vein <3 mm in diameter. Patients will undergo multiple intramuscular injections of HGF plasmid over a 6 month period. The primary end point is amputation free survival at 18 months. This trial though currently not registered with clinicaltrials.gov will be registered prior to an expected start date in 2012.

Additionally an HGF plasmid phase 2 trial in no option CLI patients using a plasmid that codes for two separate HGF isoforms sponsored by ViroMed is currently enrolling and is expected to be completed by March 2013 (Viromed, NCT01064440).

STEM THERAPY CLI TRIALS

Preclinical studies using animal hind limb ischemia models have shown that stem cells injected intramuscularly into the hind limb can promote improved blood flow via an angiogenic mechanism. Early studies in humans have similarly shown improved vascularity in the treated extremity as measured by ankle brachial index though the mechanism by which this occurs in humans is unknown. Cellular therapies can be divided into autologous and allogeneic. Several phase 1/2 trials have been recently completed including Harvest Technologies (NCT00498069) and Biomet both of whom have reported promising early results of phase 2 trials using autologous bone marrow mononuclear cells (BMNC) in the treatment of CLI.[7–8] Both companies have developed point of care cell preparation systems that following bone marrow harvest of 240–300 ml allows separation of the cells and extraction of the BMNC component for direct intramuscular injection into the ischemic limb. Based on promising early results both companies have begun phase III trials and are performing these trials through Investigator Device Exemptions (IDE) from the Center for Device and Radiologic Health (CDRH) of the Food and Drug Administration. Based on their phase 2 trial in which major amputations occurred in 18% of treated patients compared to 29% in placebo treated (see Table 14-2) patients Harvest Technologies has initiated a phase 3 trial (NCT01245335) that plans to

TABLE 14-2. HARVEST TECHNOLOGIES PHASE 2 TRIAL BONE MARROW ASPIRATE CONCENTRATE IN CLI

End Point at 3 Months	Bone Marrow Concentrate (34)	Control (14)
Major Amputation	17.6%	28.6% ($p = .45$)
Improved Pain	44%	25% ($p = .54$)
Improved ABI	32%	7% ($p = .08$)
Improved Rutherford Classification	35%	14% ($p = .18$)

• 48 patients

enroll 210 no-option CLI patients with only tissue loss and is expected to be completed by June 2014. Murphy and coworkers have shown amputation free survival of 86% in an open label trial using autologous bone marrow cells in patients with rest pain or ischemic ulcers.[8] Biomet plans to enroll 152 no-option CLI patients with either minor tissue loss or rest pain and is expecting completion of the study by May 2014(NCT01049919).

Aastrom recently published the analysis of their phase 2 trial utilizing expanded autologous stem cells, ixmyelocel-T, in the treatment of no-option CLI patients.[9] In the RESTORE-CLI trial 50 ml of bone marrow aspirate from the patient was sent to the sponsor and the cells cultured in a bioreactor and expanded over a two week period. The cell population which when expanded is enriched with mesenchymal precursors and alternatively activated macrophages is then returned to the trial site for intra muscular injection into the ischemic limb of the patient. This trial enrolled 72 patients with either ischemic rest pain or tissue loss. Those treated with cellular therapy, ixmyelocel-T, experienced overall treatment failure defined as death, major amputation, doubling of wound size from baseline or new onset gangrene in 40% of patients compared to 67% of placebo treated patients at 12 months (log rank $p = 0.003$)[10] (see Figure). These differences were especially pronounced in patients who presented with tissue loss at baseline. In the subgroup of patients presenting with wounds 45% ixmyelocel-T-treated patients compared to 88%% of control patients experienced a treatment failure event ($p = 0.01$). For AFS 21% ixmyelocel-T-treated patients with baseline wounds and 44% of control patients with baseline wounds experienced a major amputation of the injected leg or death ($p = 0.169$). Currently Aastrom has begun a phase III trial, REVIVE, (NCT01483898) through the Center of Biologic Evaluation and

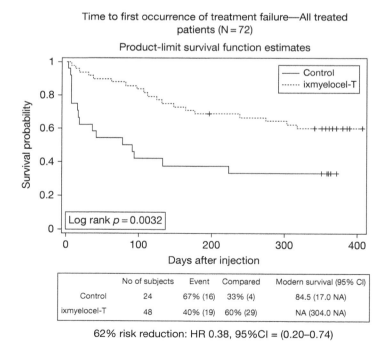

Time to first occurrence of treatment failure—All treated patients (N = 72)

	No of subjects	Event	Compared	Modern survival (95% CI)
Control	24	67% (16)	33% (4)	84.5 (17.0 NA)
ixmyelocel-T	48	40% (19)	60% (29)	NA (304.0 NA)

62% risk reduction: HR 0.38, 95%CI = (0.20–0.74)

Research (CBER) of the FDA to assess the efficacy of this therapy on amputation free survival in no-option CLI patients with tissue loss. Completion of this trial is expected in mid-2015.

When comparing the two different stem cell techniques currently in phase 3 trials the advantage of the Harvest Technologies system includes point of care therapy where by patients can be treated at one setting; a disadvantage is that the amount of bone marrow removed from the patient is not trivial. Potential advantages of the Aastrom technique include a significantly smaller bone marrow aspirate and the potential to expand cell lines important in the anti-inflammatory/angiogenic/healing process prior to injection. The main disadvantage is the 2 week delay between bone marrow harvest and cell therapy injection.

The recently completed phase I allogeneic cell therapy trial sponsored by Pluristem(NCT00951210) has shown promising safety and potential efficacy. This open label trial of allogeneic placental stem cells (PLX-PAD cells) will be entering phase II placebo controlled trials. PLX-PAD cells are mesenchymal-like stromal cells derived from the full-term placenta and are expanded in the Sponsor's proprietary bioreactor. The cells are reportedly immune privileged and would offer a potentially "off the shelf" treatment option.

CLI trials face multiple hurdles that have resulted in delays in completion. Early concerns over off-target angiogenesis and the potential for progression of diabetic proliferative retinopathy or occult tumor growth had resulted in significant restrictions in the inclusion and exclusion criteria for entry into the study. As early studies demonstrated an acceptable safety record for this therapy and potential concerns over off-target angiogenic complications have lessened these restrictions have decreased. An additional complicating factor is the overall comorbid burden of the CLI patient population results in a high incidence of adverse events throughout the conduct of the study. The heterogenous nature of CLI results in highly variable natural history. Patients with ischemic tissue loss have a major amputation rate at one year of up to 35% compared to less than 10% in patients with rest pain. In addition the FDA suggests that amputation free survival (AFS) should be the primary efficacy end-point in a phase 3 CLI trial. This has resulted in studies with an expectant enrollment of at least 500 patients. The reason for the large number of patients in a phase 3 trial is that because biologic treatment of CLI is a limb sparing procedure it is not expected to significantly influence mortality even though mortality is a component of the primary end-point. Because of the nonspecific nature of the AFS endpoint, the selective inclusion/exclusion criteria, and the heterogenous and frail nature of the CLI patient population large numbers of patients are needed to complete a clinical trial to detect any potential efficacy on amputation at one year. This requires a dedicated group of site investigators willing to deal with these issues to complete such trials within a reasonable time frame.

In summary there have been promising early safety and efficacy trial data for both gene and cellular therapies in patients with CLI. Despite these early promising results there have been no phase III trials that have shown this therapy to be effective. Current trial design has improved and there are currently many phase III clinical trials that are either actively enrolling or are in early stages of development. These are potentially disruptive technologies that if proven effective could dramatically alter how we care for patients with CLI in the future.

REFERENCES

1. Nikol S, Baumgartner I, Van Belle E, et al. Therapeutic angiogenesis with intramuscular NV1FGF improved amputation-free survival in patients with critical limb ischemia. *Molecular Therapy*. 2008;16:972–978.
2. Baumgartner I, Chronos N, Camerota A, et al. Local gene transfer and expression following intramuscular administration of FGF-1 plasmid DNA in patients with critical limb ischemia. *Molecular Therapy*. 2009;17:914–921.
3. Belch J, Hiatt WR, Baumgartner I, et al. Effect of fibroblast growth factor NV1FGF on amputation and death: a randomized placebo-controlled trial of gene therapy in critical limb ischaemia. *Lancet*. 2011;377:1929–37.
4. Powell RJ, Goodney P, Mendelsohn FO, et al. Safety and efficacy of patient specific intramuscular injection of HGF plasmid gene therapy on limb perfusion and wound healing in patients with ischemic lower extremity ulceration: Results of the HGF-0205 Trial. *J Vasc Surg*. 2010;52:1525–1530.
5. Powell RJ, Simons M, Mendelsohn FO, et al. Results of a double-blind, placebo-controlled study to assess the safety of intramuscular injection of hepatocyte growth factor plasmid to improve limb perfusion in patients with critical limb ischemia. *Circulation*. 2008;118:58–65.
6. Shigematsu H, Yasuda K, Iwai T, et al. Randomized, double-blind, placebo-controlled clinical trial of hepatocyte growth factor plasmid for critical limb ischemia. *Gene Ther*. 2010;17(9):1152–61.
7. Iafrati MD, Hallet JW, Geil G, et al. Early results and lesions learned from a multicenter randomized, double-blind trial of bone marrow aspirate concentrate in crtical limb ischemia. *J Vasc Surg*. 2011;54:1650–8.
8. Murphy MP, Lawson JH, Rapp BM, et al. Autologous bone marrow mononuclear cell therapy is safe and promotes amputation-free survival in patients with critical limb ischemia. *J Vasc Surg*. 2011 Jun;53(6):1565–74.e1. Epub 2011 Apr 22.
9. Powell RJ, Comerota AJ, Berceli SA, et al. Interim analysis results from the RESTORE-CLI, a randomized, double-blind multicenter phase II trial comparing expanded autologous bone marrow-derived tissue repair cells and placebo in patients with critical limb ischemia. *J Vasc Surg*. 2011;54(4):1032–41.
10. Powell RJ, Marston WA, Berceli SA, et al. Cellular Therapy with Ixmyelocel-T to Treat Critical Limb Ischemia: The Randomized, Double-Blind, Placebo-Controlled RESTORE-CLI Trial. *Molecular Therapy*, Accepted 2012.

15

Liquid Cast Arterial Stents: Stents of the Future

Melina R. Kibbe, MD and Guillermo A. Ameer, ScD

INTRODUCTION

Despite being a highly efficacious treatment for coronary and peripheral artery disease, the use of arterial stents has clinically significant limitations. The restenosis of stents secondary to neointimal hyperplasia and stent thrombosis because of delayed artery healing remain the leading limitations. Drug-eluting stents (DES) have dramatically reduced the neointimal response. However, DES elute antiproliferative agents that slow down re-endothelialization and worsen endothelial function. To overcome these challenges, pre-formed biodegradable stents are being developed and evaluated. However, these stents pose their own set of challenges mostly related to preservation of stent integrity and mechanical properties after deployment from a small caliber delivery catheter. Thus, we proposed a radically different way to stent an artery using a methodology that will overcome the above mentioned challenges. Specifically, we have developed a novel liquid cast nitric oxide (NO)-eluting biodegradabe stent. This chapter serves to describe the challenges faced by conventional bare metal stents, DES, and pre-formed biodegradable stents, as well as describe our novel technology, the barriers faced in developing this technology, and potential use thereof.

RESTENOSIS

Atherosclerosis is the leading cause of death and disability in the United States. An estimated $475 billion per year is spent in the United States on cardiovascular disease, with a significant portion being attributed to the cost of repeat interventions.[1] One of the current therapeutic modalities for severe arterial atherosclerosis, whether it is from coronary or peripheral arterial disease, consists of balloon angioplasty and stenting. In fact, in 2006 more than 1.3 million Americans underwent coronary angioplasty and more than 90% of these patients received an arterial stent.[1] While stent technology has improved over the years, including the development of DES, failure rates remain high. The long-term durability of this procedure is limited due to the development of neointimal hyperplasia, which results from an aggressive growth of the cells that form the arterial wall, and results in restenosis at the site of intervention. For example, approximately 31–46% of balloon angioplasty sites develop angiographic restenosis at 6 months.[2] By two years, 20% of patients require repeat balloon angioplasty.[3] DES have slightly reduced the need for re-intervention.[4] However, long-term data now suggest equal or higher mortality rates with DES compared to bare-metal stents.[4] Moreover, the recent COURAGE trial reported that 21% of patients who underwent balloon angioplasty and stenting still required subsequent revascularization within a median time of 10 months.[5] Thus, neointimal hyperplasia is an alarming problem that causes significant morbidity and mortality. Currently, no effective therapeutic modality exists to prevent neointimal hyperplasia.

NEOINTIMAL HYPERPLASIA

The classic description by Clowes and Ross of the arterial injury response that leads to the development of neointimal hyperplasia involves injury to the arterial wall leading to endothelial denudation.[6–10] The underlying internal elastic lamina and vascular smooth muscle cells (VSMC) are exposed to circulating blood elements. Platelets immediately aggregate and adhere to the site of injury.[11] An inflammatory response follows, with the infiltration of neutrophils, macrophages, and leukocytes.[12,13] Twenty-four hours following injury, under the influence of growth factors and cytokines, medial VSMC convert from a contractile to a synthetic phenotype and begin to proliferate.[14] VSMC migration to the neointima where they continue to proliferate for weeks.[6,15,16] Concurrently, endothelial cell regeneration occurs through the stimulation of basic fibroblast growth factor (bFGF) within 24 hours after injury, and can continue for 6–10 weeks.[17] Lastly, transforming growth factor beta (TGFβ) stimulates extracellular matrix deposition.[18,19]

However, the classic arterial injury response described above includes no mention of the adventitia. The adventitia is now thought to be more of a driving force in the development of neointimal hyperplasia than the media. Couffinhal et al and Wilcox et al have both characterized the proliferative response following arterial injury in rat and pig arteries.[20,21] Common to both is that the proliferative response in the adventitia is much greater at almost all time points compared to the intima and media. While Couffinhal et al reported 1.5-2-fold more proliferation in the adventitia compared to the media in rat carotid arteries, Wilcox reported nearly 7-fold more proliferation in the adventitia than the media in pig coronary arteries. Furthermore, upon examining early time points, Couffinhal et al found that proliferation in the adventitia actually occurred before proliferation in the media, at time points as early as 4 hours. It has also been recognized that the adventitia is host to many cell types, resident and circulating, that regulate or participate in the development of the neointima. Thus, any current description of the formation of neointimal hyperplasia following arterial injury should include a description of the cells that populate the adventitia.

ARTERIAL STENTS

While the percutaneous treatment of severe atherosclerosis has evolved over the years, it is still fraught with difficulty and challenges. In 1977, the concept of percutaneous transluminal coronary angioplasty was introduced.[22] Yet, concerns over elastic recoil or dissections secondary to balloon angioplasty led to the development of the bare metal stent in 1986. Originally, placement of the bare metal stent was seen as a bailout procedure when recoil or dissection was present and/or severe. However, over the years, stenting became more commonplace even though implantation of a permanent metal stent led to in-stent restenosis. In fact, in-stent restenosis due to the development of neointimal hyperplasia was worse than that induced from the barotrauma of angioplasty alone.[23,24] To combat in-stent restenosis, DES were introduced in 1999 using cytostatic or cytotoxic drugs (i.e., sirulimus, paclitaxel, etc) in combination with polymers. However, it was later found that these drugs not only inhibit proliferation of VSMC and fibroblasts, effectively limiting neointimal hyperplasia, but also indiscriminately inhibit endothelial cell proliferation. This creates a significant problem with arterial healing, leaving a collagen-exposed surface in contact with circulating blood elements, leading to late in-stent thrombosis. To combat this problem, patients are now maintained on aspirin and Plavix for extended durations of time following placement of DES. This practice has led to a variety of bleeding complications and difficult situations for patients requiring other operations for which antiplatelet agents are contraindicated. Thus, there is a great need to develop new technology for the treatment of severe atherosclerosis that will promote vascular healing and not prevent it.

PRE-FORMED BIODEGRADABLE STENTS

Pre-formed drug-eluting biodegradable polymer stents attempt to address late in-stent thrombosis and other shortcomings associated with bare metal and DES, such as the persistent proinflammatory environment created by the permanent placement of metal into the vasculature. The ideal biodegradable stent should include: 1) sufficient physical support, 2) acceptable hemodynamic and biocompatibility profiles, 3) safe degradation characteristics, 4) ease of use, 5) simplicity with the manufacture and sterility process, and 6) cost-efficiency with production. With respect to physical characteristics, the stent must have sufficient external radial strength to resist elastic recoil and other compressive forces, maintain self-expandability, and anchor itself to the surrounding tissue. In addition, the pre-formed stent must be designed so that it can be collapsed into a delivery device with a small profile (2–3 millimeters), be flexible in order to negotiate curves during the delivery process, and be structurally sound enough to withstand balloon expansion during deployment and not undergo strut fracture. Lastly, the stent should inhibit thrombosis and neointimal hyperplasia and stimulate endothelialization. To date, no pre-formed biodegradable stent has met all these challenges.

Thus, biodegradable stents are a novel approach to arterial revascularization that provide transient vessel support with drug delivery capability without the long-term limitations of current bare metal or drug eluting stents (DES) such as persistence of inflammatory substrates (e.g., metallic scaffold and/or durable polymer) that may lead to restenosis and delayed re-endothelialization.[24–26] A few biodegradable stents with some of the above described qualities have been fabricated and even placed in humans.[25,26] This includes the first biodegradable stent fabricated from poly-L-lactic acid (PLLA). Since these initial zigzag designs, many more biodegradable stents have been developed and are in various phases of evolution. This includes the poly(ethylene amide) stent designed by MediVas, the BVS stent fabricated from PLLA by Abbott (formerly Guidant), the REVA slide and lock stent made of a tyrosine-derived polycarbonate material by REVA Medical, and the absorbable magnesium alloy stent by Biotronik. In clinical trials, pre-formed biodegradable stents performed favorably to current DES, and may even reduce stent thrombosis.[27,28] However, current biodegradable stents demonstrate a similar neointimal response as 2nd generation DES.[29] Failure to outperform DES may be related to utilization of anti-proliferative agents in the biodegradable polymer, and persistence of intraluminal polymeric masses that may induce persistent inflammatory responses.[30] To date, no pre-formed biodegradable stent has overcome the mechanical and biologic limitations of current bare metal and DES.

LIQUID CAST BIODEGRADABLE STENT

We plan to solve the problems related to bare metal and DES by developing a stent unlike any other stent that has been used in the healthcare arena: we developed a solid stent that forms *in the body* from a liquid phase. This technology represents the first dramatic change in stent design since the first stent was placed in the coronary artery in 1986. Our stent technology will provide sufficient and tailorable external radial force to resist recoil, inhibit thrombosis, inhibit neointimal hyperplasia, stimulate re-endothelialization, and biode-grade over time, thereby allowing for complete healing of the arterial site. Furthermore, our polymer will release NO, a potent vasodilator, thereby combating elastic recoil. Below follows a description of the approach our research team has taken to develop this novel stent technology as well as the specialty catheter required to cast this stent *in vivo*.

OUR APPROACH

In order to develop a liquid cast biodegradable DES, we followed a series of step-wise approaches over the past several years to demonstrate feasibility of our concept. First, we identified the appropriate drug (i.e., NO), and appropriate polymer (i.e., PDC). Second, we demonstrated the biocompatibility of our PDC polymer *in vitro* and *in vivo*. Third, we formulated an acrylated version of our polymer that could undergo photo-polymerization. Fourth, we demonstrated extended release of NO from our polymer. Fifth, we confirmed feasibility of our concept by casting solid cylindrical stents from our liquid prepolymer. Sixth, we developed, fabricated, assembled, and tested our specialty catheter with industry engineers and demonstrated success at photo-polymerization using both an LED and laser blue light source. Seventh, we measured the mechanical properties of our stent and dem-onstrated that the mechanical properties are tunable, and in alignment with commercially available bare metal stents.

Nitric Oxide

A promising therapeutic strategy to prevent neointimal hyperplasia has centered on the use of NO, a molecule normally produced in endothelial cells that serves to protect the vessel wall. NO has been shown to possess many different vasoprotective properties, including vasodilation, inhibition of platelet aggregation, leukocyte adherence, VSMC pro-liferation, VSMC migration, stimulation of VSMC apoptosis, and endothelial cell growth.[27] All of these properties of NO serve to maintain vascular homeostasis by affecting all the key components in the injury response. Since the normal source of NO is lost following vascular injury due to denudation of the endothelial cells, if NO were restored at the site of injury, the development of neointimal hyperplasia should be prevented. Furthermore, NO is a far more attractive candidate for drug delivery compared to the drugs used in the FDA-approved DES given all the beneficial properties of NO toward the vasculature.

Indeed, many investigators have shown that supplementation of NO at the site of injury prevents the development of neointimal hyperplasia. These forms of NO-based approaches have included systemic delivery of L-arginine or NO donors, inhalational NO, local application of NO donors, gene therapy of one of the nitric oxide synthase (NOS) enzymes, NO-releasing prosthetic materials, and NO-eluting metallic stents. Using the standard rat carotid artery injury model, we evaluated the efficacy of several different NO-based approaches at inhibiting neointimal hyperplasia.[28,29] We found that all of the NO donors evaluated inhibited neointimal hyperplasia, but the NO donor PROLI/NO was most effective at inhibiting the neointimal (91.2% inhibition of intimal area versus injury alone $p < 0.05$). The NO donors were also effective at inhibiting neointimal hyperplasia following balloon arterial injury in different animal models of diabetes, as well as in both sexes, regardless of hormone status.[30-32] Thus, these studies support the highly effective nature of NO at inhibiting neointimal hyperplasia as well as the feasibility of an intralumenal stent-based delivery approach.

Poly(diol citrate) Elastomers

With an effective drug identified, next we focused our attention on an appropriate polymer for the vasculature. Realizing that we needed to develop a polymer that will release NO and be mechanically compatible with blood vessels, Dr. Ameer developed a family of biodegradable and biocompatible elastomers referred to as poly(diol citrates) (PDC). The properties of PDC (i.e. mechanical properties, biodegradation rate, hemocompatibility) can be tailored in several ways by simply changing the diol used for the polycondensation reaction or the feed monomer ratio. The hemocompatible and elastic properties make it an ideal candidate for use in the vasculature. In particular, two polyesters have been investigated, poly(1,8 octanediol citrate) (POC) and poly(1,12 dodecanediol citrate) (PDDC). PDDC is a more hydrophobic version of POC due to the longer, less water-soluble aliphateic diol, 1,12 dodecandiol. In addition, we have shown that PDC can be used as a drug delivery vehicle for a NO donor. Thus, we followed a methodical approach to first evaluate the biocompatibility of PDC in the vasculature *in vitro* and *in vivo* before developing the NO-releasing PDC pre-polymer.

Biocompatibility of PDC Elastomers

To assess the biocompatibility of PDC *in vitro*, primary human aortic endothelial cells (HAEC) were seeded onto POC coated surfaces and processed for SEM. HAEC attached in significant numbers to the POC-coated ePTFE samples and not the uncoated ePTFE samples.[33] To assess the phenotype, endothelial cells were cultured on POC and stained for VE-cadherin and von Willibrand factor. Cells stained positive for both.[33] Endothelial cells grown on POC also released NO and prostacyclin.[34] The degree of platelet adhesion on POC, ePTFE, and POC-coated ePTFE was assessed using a modified lactate dehydrogenase assay. There were significantly fewer platelets attached to POC-ePTFE compared to ePTFE, suggesting reduced thrombogenicity. On SEM, platelets that attached to ePTFE formed aggregates and flattened out on the node surface, suggesting platelet activation. In contrast, the platelets that attached to the POC-coated ePTFE surface tended to be isolated, had fewer pseudopodia-like extensions, and were rounded in morphology. We also evaluated platelet activation via detection of soluble P-selectin using an enzyme-linked immunosorbent assay (ELISA) kit. Exposure of platelets to glass and poly(lactic-co-glycolic acid) resulted in significantly more soluble P-selectin release relative to POC and ePTFE. These data demonstrate the biocompatible and favorable nature of PDC *in vitro*.[33,35]

Using our established pig ePTFE bypass model,[36] we implanted control and POC-coated ePTFE grafts into 4 male pigs and assessed thrombogenicity and inflammation at 7 days.[35] Prior to euthanasia, grafts were imaged for blood flow using time-of-flight and contrast-enhanced magnetic resonance angiograms (MRA). All grafts were patent. POC-ePTFE grafts were found to have more than 10-fold less fibrocoagulum adherent to the luminal surface of the graft compared to the ePTFE grafts, as measured by SEM. Upon immunohistochemical analysis, POC-coated grafts were found to have less macrophage infiltration compared to control ePTFE grafts. Furthermore, and surprisingly, POC supported endothelialization of the graft. This is an added benefit for this technology given that creation of an intact endothelial cell monolayer on foreign material placed in the vasculature should in theory behave similar to native tissue.

Next, we evaluated the POC-coated ePTFE grafts at 28 days in 5 conventional pigs using the same model to further assess the biocompatibility of PDC in the vasculature.[36,37] At 4 weeks, all grafts were found to be patent with no hemodynamically significant stenoses detected by ultrasonography, angiography, and MRA. Upon morphometric analysis, POC-ePTFE grafts resulted in a similar extent of neointimal hyperplasia compared to control ePTFE grafts. These data reveal that POC, without any additional drug release, did not result in worse neointimal hyperplasia, and that POC is biocompatible, supporting the notion that POC may be a good vehicle for drug delivery. Assessment of von Willibrand staining revealed that, similar to the data obtained at 7 days, POC supported endothelial cell growth. These data were confirmed with SEM, demonstrating coverage of the lumen of the POC-coated grafts with an endothelial cell monolayer. Lastly, since POC is known to be biodegradable over time, SEM was performed on segments of graft removed at 28 days and confirmed the presence of POC on the ePTFE grafts. Thus, these data reveal that surface modification of blood-contacting surfaces with POC results in a biocompatible surface that does not induce any untoward effects in the vasculature. These findings are important as they serve as the foundation for the development of a biocompatible and biodegradable drug-eluting arterial stent.

Synthesis of the NO-Releasing PDC Liquid Prepolymers

After demonstrating the biocompatibility of our polymer with the vasculature *in vitro* and *in vivo*, we then synthesized a NO-releasing PDC liquid prepolymer that is capable of polymerization using light. To demonstrate the feasibility of our approach to form a solid cylindrical stent from the liquid PDC prepolymers, we demonstrated that PDC and PDDC can polymerize into cylindrical structures *ex vivo* using photo-polymerization (470 nM wavelength). Furthermore, we demonstrated that we can uniformly coat the inner surface of a harvested porcine artery with the PDC prepolymer and form a solid stent from our liquid material *ex vivo*. The PDC polymer adhered to the inner wall of the artery, thereby increasing its resistance to deformation.

Next, we measured the NO release profile from PDDC and POC cast stents using the Griess reaction. Upon incorporation of the NO donor DEDETA/NO into the polymeric matrix, NO release under physiological conditions was significantly delayed. This delayed release process is attributed by degradation of the polymer, diffusion of water into the polymer matrix, and the subsequent diffusion of NO from the polymer matrix. The more hydrophilic the polymer matrix is, the quicker the polymer degrades, the easier the water diffusion proceeds, and the quicker the NO releases due to hydrolysis of the NO donor. Thus, we compared NO release from both PDDC and POC, and found, as expected, that the more hydrophobic material, PDDC, exhibited the more extended NO release profile. The NO release rate can also be altered by varying the quantity of the NO donor. Increasing the content of NO donor in the polymer matrix increased the release rate. Photo-polymerizing PDDC/NO on the lumen of fresh porcine aorta resulted in a similar prolonged NO release profile from the coating on the lumen surface.

Specialty Catheter Development

In order to deliver the liquid PDC prepolymer to the intravascular space and polymerize it into a solid stent, a specialty catheter is required that can do the following: 1) occlude flow at the desired target site, 2) deliver the liquid prepolymer, 3) allow for polymerization, 4) cast the polymer into a cylindrical stent shape with desired thickness and no edge effect, 5) aspirate nonreacted prepolymers, and 6) prevent distal embolization. Thus, the delivery catheter we envisioned would need to consist of a typical over-the-wire double-balloon occlusion catheter that has a third balloon in the middle that will both deliver the NO-releasing PDC liquid prepolymer to the enclosed space created from the occlusion balloons while simultaneously forming the cylindrical cast. The distal end of the catheter would need to be translucent, allowing a fiberoptic light cable to be passed down a central lumen to initiate photo-polymerization. Lastly, the catheter should be able to aspirate and irrigate the space of interest. With these requirements in mind, we hired the services of Synectic, Inc to collaborate with us to develop a prototype catheter. Synectic is a company that specializes in design, development, and fabrication of specialty catheters. They employ a variety of engineers, including design engineers, mechanical engineers, and electrical engineers.

Our specialty catheter was designed for effective use in the clinical arena. Thus, while 6 lumens were required, our goal was to maintain the outer diameter of the catheter at 6F, as this is the common size used for most cardiac and peripheral interventions. We were successful with this goal. The catheter is fabricated from flexible polyether block amide (PEBAX). The zone of catheter between the occlusion balloons is transparent, allowing light to pass through the catheter to polymerize the polymer. The wire lumen is 0.7 mm in diameter, allowing the use of a 0.018 guidewire. The light lumen is 0.64 mm in diameter. The inflation balloon lumens are 0.3 mm in diameter. The polymer aspiration/irrigation lumens are 0.5 mm in diameter. The current inter-balloon distance is 7 cm, and the middle inflation balloon is 4 cm in length. The occlusion balloons are made from Yule, a very compliant material. The casting balloon is made from Nylon, a non-compliant material. To initiate polymerization, we will use a fiberoptic cable of 0.64 mm diameter from Schott with fused ends and a 120 degree output. We have successfully used one of two different power sources: 1) a blue light emitting LED power source from Schott with a 445 center wavelength, and 2) a blue light emitting laser power source from Nescel with a 463–469 nm wavelength. With this specialty catheter, light fiber, and power source, we have successfully cast and polymerized a solid cylindrical stent from our liquid NO-releasing PDC polymer.

Mechanical Properties of the Liquid Cast Stent

Lastly, we have measured the mechanical properties of our liquid cast NO-releasing stents and compared them to a commercially available self-expanding bare metal stent from Cordis (Precise, 5 mm diameter by 30 mm length [N530SB]). We measured the radial compression of our stents by exerting a fixed load and measuring the degree of compression. We found that the radial compression of the PDC stents vary according to diameter of the cast stent (thickness kept constant), with the small diameter stents being less compressible, and the large diameter stents being more compressible. Of note, the radial resistance of our PDC stents was in the range of that exhibited by the commercially available stent from Cordis. We then measured the radial compression of stents cast with different wall thickness. Similarly, the radial compression varied by wall thickness, with the thick walled stents (5.88 mm) exhibiting the least compression by a fixed load, and the thin walled stent (2.54 mm) exhibiting the greatest compression by a fixed load. We measured flexibility (i.e., ability to tolerate bending) of the stents and found that flexibility varied by stent wall thickness and stent diameter, and that the flexibility measurements were consistent with the Cordis bare metal stent. We measured axial compression, as there are places in the body where an axial load is projected onto stents (i.e., the superficial femoral artery). Axial compression varied by stent wall thickness as well as stent diameter, and was consistent with the Cordis bare metal stent. Lastly, we measured radial compression of a porcine artery coated with a PDC stent and compared this to an uncoated porcine artery and porcine artery with the Cordis bare metal stent. The PDC-stented artery displayed similar mechanical characteristics as the porcine artery with the metal stent.

CONCLUSION

This chapter serves to summarize the process of developing a novel stent technology. To date, our research has lead to the development of a drug-eluting biodegradable stent that forms from liquid, demonstration of its biocompatibility *in vitro* and *in vivo*, development of a specialty catheter, and demonstration of adequate stent mechanical properties. However, much remains to be done. Our multidisciplinary team of investigators is now well positioned to evaluate the stent technology in a preclinical animal model. After successful stent implantation and demonstration of the safety and efficacy of our technology, first-in-man studies will be in the near future.

Acknowledgements

The research described in this chapter was supported by an award #5 RC1 HL100491-02 from the National Institutes of Health Recovery act limited competition: NIH Challenge Grants in health and Science Research and funded in part by the Northwestern Memorial Foundation Dixon Translational Research Grant Initiative and the Northwestern Memorial Foundation Priority Program Collaborative Development Initiative: Center for Limb Preservation.

REFERENCES

1. Lloyd-Jones D, Adams R, Carnethon M, et al. Heart disease and stroke statistics—2009 update. A report from the American Heart Association Statistics Committee and Stroke Statistics Subcommittee. *Circulation.* 2009 Jan 27;119(3):480–486.
2. Smith SC, Jr., Dove JT, Jacobs AK, et al. ACC/AHA guidelines of percutaneous coronary interventions—executive summary. A report of the American College of Cardiology/American Heart Association Task Force on Practice Guidelines. *J Am Coll Cardiol.* 2001;37(8):2215–2239.
3. Unger F, Serruys PW, Yacoub MH, et al. Revascularization in multivessel disease: Comparison between two-year outcomes of coronary bypass surgery and stenting. *J Thorac Cardiovasc Surg.* 2003;125(4):809–820.
4. Lagerqvist B, James SK, Stenestrand U, et al. Long-term outcomes with drug-eluting stents versus bare-metal stents in Sweden. *N Engl J Med.* 2007;356(10):1009–1019.
5. Boden WE, O'Rourke RA, Teo KK, et al. Optimal medical therapy with or without PCI for stable coronary disease. *N Engl J Med.* 2007;356(15):1503–1516.
6. Clowes AW, Reidy MA, Clowes MM. Kinetics of cellular proliferation after arterial injury. I. Smooth muscle growth in the absence of endothelium. *Lab Invest.* 1983;49(3):327–333.
7. Clowes AW, Reidy MA, Clowes MM. Mechanisms of stenosis after arterial injury. *Lab Invest.* 1983;49(2):208–215.
8. Clowes AW, Clowes MM, Reidy MA. Kinetics of cellular proliferation after arterial injury. III. Endothelial and smooth muscle growth in chronically denuded vessels. *Lab Invest.* 1986;54(3):295–303.
9. Ross R, Glomset J, Kariya B, et al. Platelet-dependent serum factor that stimulates proliferation of arterial smooth-muscle cells in vitro. *P Natl Acad Sci. USA* 1974;71(4):1207–1210.
10. Ross R, Bowenpope DF, Raines EW. Platelets, macrophages, endothelium, and growth-factors—their effects upon cells and their possible roles in atherogenesis. *Ann N Y Acad Sci.* 1985;454:254–260.
11. Fingerle J, Johnson R, Clowes AW, et al. Role of platelets in smooth muscle cell proliferation and migration after vascular injury in rat carotid artery. *Proc Natl Acad Sci USA.* 1989;86(21):8412–8416.
12. Davies MG, Hagen PO. Pathobiology of intimal hyperplasia. *Br J Surg.* 1994;81(9):1254–1269.
13. Libby P, Schwartz D, Brogi E, et al. A cascade model for restenosis. A special case of atherosclerosis progression. *Circulation.* 1992;86(6 Suppl):III47–III52.
14. Lindner V, Lappi DA, Baird A, et al. Role of basic fibroblast growth factor in vascular lesion formation. *Circ Res.* 1991;68(1):106–113.
15. Bendeck MP, Zempo N, Clowes AW, et al. Smooth muscle cell migration and matrix metalloproteinase expression after arterial injury in the rat. *Circ Res.* 1994;75(3):539–545.
16. Hasenstab D, Forough R, Clowes AW. Plasminogen activator inhibitor type 1 and tissue inhibitor of metalloproteinases-2 increase after arterial injury in rats. *Circ Res.* 1997;80(4):490–496.
17. Lindner V, Majack RA, Reidy MA. Basic fibroblast growth factor stimulates endothelial regrowth and proliferation in denuded arteries. *J Clin Invest.* 1990;85(6):2004–2008.
18. Nabel EG, Shum L, Pompili VJ, et al. Direct transfer of transforming growth factor beta 1 gene into arteries stimulates fibrocellular hyperplasia. *Proc Natl Acad Sci U S A.* 1993;90(22):10759–10763.
19. Majesky MW, Lindner V, Twardzik DR, et al. Production of transforming growth factor beta 1 during repair of arterial injury. *J Clin Invest.* 1991;88(3):904–910.
20. Couffinhal T, Dufourcq P, Jaspard B, et al. Kinetics of adventitial repair in the rat carotid model. *Coron Artery Dis.* 2001;12(8):635–648.

21. Wilcox JN, Okamoto EI, Nakahara KI, et al. Perivascular responses after angioplasty which may contribute to postangioplasty restenosis: a role for circulating myofibroblast precursors? *Ann N Y Acad Sci.* 2001;947:68–90.

22. Serruys PW, Garcia-Garcia HM, Onuma Y. From metallic cages to transient bioresorbable scaffolds: change in paradigm of coronary revascularization in the upcoming decade? *Eur Heart J.* 2012 Jan;33(1):16–25b.

23. Serruys PW, de Jaegere P, Kiemeneij F, et al. A comparison of balloon-expandable-stent implantation with balloon angioplasty in patients with coronary artery disease. Benestent Study Group. *N Engl J Med.* 1994;331(8):489–495.

24. Fischman DL, Leon MB, Baim DS, et al. A randomized comparison of coronary-stent placement and balloon angioplasty in the treatment of coronary artery disease. Stent Restenosis Study Investigators. *N Engl J Med.* 1994;331(8):496–501.

25. Stack RS, Califf RM, Phillips HR, et al. Interventional cardiac catheterization at Duke Medical Center. *Am J Cardiol.* 1988;62(10 Pt 2):3F–24F.

26. Tamai H, Igaki K, Kyo E, et al. Initial and 6-month results of biodegradable poly-l-lactic acid coronary stents in humans. *Circulation.* 2000;102(4):399–404.

27. Ahanchi SS, Tsihlis ND, Kibbe MR. The role of nitric oxide in the pathophysiology of intimal hyperplasia. *J Vasc Surg.* 2007;45 Suppl A:A64–A73.

28. Pearce CG, Najjar SF, Kapadia MR, et al. Beneficial effect of a short-acting NO donor for the prevention of neointimal hyperplasia. *Free Radic Biol Med.* 2008;44(1):73–81.

29. Kapadia MR, Chow LW, Tsihlis ND, et al. Nitric oxide and nanotechnology: a novel approach to inhibit neointimal hyperplasia. *J Vasc Surg.* 2008;47(1):173–182.

30. Ahanchi SS, Varu VN, Tsihlis ND, et al. Heightened efficacy of nitric oxide-based therapies in type II diabetes mellitus and metabolic syndrome. *Am J Physiol Heart Circ Physiol.* 2008;295(6):H2388–H2398.

31. Varu VN, Ahanchi SS, Hogg ME, et al. Insulin enhances the effect of nitric oxide at inhibiting neointimal hyperplasia in a rat model of type 1 diabetes. *Am J Physiol Heart Circ Physiol.* 2010;299(3):H772–H779.

32. Hogg ME, Varu VN, Vavra AK, et al. Effect of nitric oxide on neointimal hyperplasia based on sex and hormone status. *Free Radic Biol Med.* 2011;50(9):1065–1074.

33. Motlagh D, Allen J, Hoshi R, et al. Hemocompatibility evaluation of poly(diol citrate) in vitro for vascular tissue engineering. *J Biomed Mater Res A.* 2007;82(4):907–916.

34. Allen J, Khan S, Serrano MC, et al. Characterization of porcine circulating progenitor cells: Toward a functional endothelium. *Tissue Eng Part A.* 2008;14(1):189–194.

35. Yang J, Motlagh D, Allen JB, et al. Modulating expanded polytetrafluoroethylene vascular graft host response via citric acid-based biodegradable elastomers. *Adv Mater Adv Mater.* 2006;18(12):1493.

36. Kapadia MR, Aalami OO, Najjar SF, et al. A reproducible porcine ePTFE arterial bypass model for neointimal hyperplasia. *J Surg Res.* 2008;148(2):230–237.

37. Kibbe MR, Martinez J, Popowich DA, et al. Citric Acid-Base elastomers provide a biocompatible interface for vascular grafts. *J Biomed Mater Res A* 2010 Apr;93(1):314–24.

Lower Extremity Venous Disease

Management of Venous Trauma: Civilian and Military Injuries

Xzabia A. Caliste, MD and Colonel (ret) David L. Gillespie, MD

INTRODUCTION/BACKGROUND HISTORY

Treatment of venous injury dates back to the 19th Century. In 1879, the Russian surgeon Eck was the first to successfully accomplish the permanent union of two blood vessels. He created a lateral anastamosis between the portal vein and the vena cava.[1] The first successful reported repair of a major vein was by Schede in 1882.[2] He successfully repaired a femoral vein via lateral suture venorrhaphy. In 1899, Kummel reported a successful end to end anastamosis of a vein.[2] Despite these early advances during the 19th Century, in World War I and II, the mainstay of treatment of major venous injury was ligation of the vessel. Advances in modern surgical technology and medical care have ensued, nonetheless, ligation continues to be a predominant method of treating venous injury in both civilian and military centers even today. Thus, the management of venous injury remains a topic of controversy.

Most techniques currently in practice have evolved from experiences during military conflict and most agree that there has been a gross underestimation of the rate of venous injury in early and current wartime. The discovery of venous injury, in many instances, occurs at the time of arterial repair. Ligation was the mainstay of therapy and advocates for ligation of major veins believed that the consequences of ligation were few. Concern for Deep Vein Thrombosis (DVT) and subsequent Pulmonary Embolism (PE) as a potential consequence of repair was purported, despite a lack of robust documentation supporting this.[3] There have been several reports in both animal and human studies indicating increased morbidity associated with ligation of major veins. Most concerns are related to the sequelae of venous insufficiency: venous hypertension, phlegmasia of the extremities, compromise of arterial flow, stasis ulceration, and potential contribution to early amputation rates.[2,4,5] It was not until the Korean and Vietnam Wars that repair of venous injury began to be reported. During the Korean War upwards of 90% of venous injuries continued to be treated with ligation and the remainder underwent repair. Rich and colleagues evaluated the Vietnam Registry and determined that of the 4,500 patients registered, over 1,000 had venous injuries. Approximately one third of these patients underwent repair of venous injuries and the remaining patients underwent ligation. Rich reported a low incidence of complications associated with repair of injured veins, and therefore advocated repair.[5] Advocates of venous repair cite the advantage of this method in avoiding the possibility of early limb loss from venous hypertension or the long term disability associated with chronic edema. Others believe that the durability of complex venous repair is poor and often leads to occlusion. Some theorize that a period of patency allows for collateral flow to develop which in turn decreases the complications of venous insufficiency. In our recent wartime experience in Iraq and Afghanistan, management of venous trauma parallels management during the Vietnam War.[2] Only about one third of injuries to major venous vessels are treated by lateral venorrhaphy or interposition grafts. In the civilian world, there have been sporadic reports by surgeons using prosthetic interposition grafts and temporary intravascular shunts.[4] Currently ligation of major veins in patients in extremis remains the most common modality of treatment. Under compromising circumstances, it is quick and efficient, thereby allowing management of concomitant issues in a patient that may quickly become acidotic, coagulopathic and hypothermic.[4]

ANATOMIC PATTERN OF INJURY

The anatomic patterns of venous injury sustained by patients in the military and the civilian world differ. Injury to the extremities delineates the most common anatomic pattern of injury for both. The rate of extremity injury, however, was higher in the U.S. Armed forces compared to the civilian population. The civilian population accounts for a higher incidence of truncal injury. The rate of military truncal injury is significantly less than that of the civilian population due in large part to modern body armor.[6–7] In both the military and civilian worlds, the rate of lower extremity vascular injury is higher compared to upper extremity venous trauma.[8]

MECHANISM OF INJURY

Venous trauma during military conflicts is most commonly due to blast injury or high velocity weapons. As a result, concomitant injuries generally occur in the form of arterial, orthopedic, soft tissue injury, head or torso injury, or associated full or partial thickness burns.[9,10]

Penetrating trauma also accounts for the majority of venous injuries in the civilian realm. Gunshot wounds (GSW) are the most common, followed by stab wounds (SW), lacerations, rifles and blunt traumatic injury. These mechanisms of injury are less often accompanied by other injuries. The exception is close range shotgun injuries which often have associated arterial injury, soft tissue damage, nerve damage, and bony fractures.[9,10]

DIAGNOSIS

Venous injuries can be difficult to detect. In fact, a majority of venous injuries are discovered incidentally while exploring an arterial injury. A majority of venous injuries in previous wars and currently in the Global War on Terrorism, do occur in conjunction with arterial injury. Isolated venous injuries are less common and generally are elucidated due to hemodynamic instability of the patient. Injuries to the Inferior Vena Cava (IVC), iliac veins, jugular veins in the neck or lower extremity veins may be associated with uncontrolled hemorrhage. The true difficulty in diagnosis lies in a patient with venous injury in whom extrinsic signs of injury are subtle, but in whom a venous injury may be suspected. Clinical signs of extremity venous injury may include swelling or pain. In these circumstances a duplex ultrasound, arteriogram or contrast venogram may play a role in delineating injury.[2,10,11]

MANAGEMENT OPTIONS

In the management of venous trauma, several factors must quickly be assessed. First, the hemodynamic stability of the patient must be addressed and patients in extremis must be managed according to standard Advanced Trauma Life Support (ATLS) guidelines. Patients exhibiting critical hypothermia, acidosis or coagulopathy are managed with Damage Control Surgery which includes minimization of operating room time and allowance of correction of the aforementioned triad of death. Once hemodynamic stability is obtained, the surgeon is faced with further management decisions. The decision to ligate, temporarily shunt or repair a venous injury must be determined.

Venous Ligation

In some circumstances, the option of venous ligation is appropriate. Most would agree that ligation is a valuable tool that should be employed in the hemodynamically unstable patient. In their retrospective review of 184 civilian patients sustaining major venous injury, Timberlake and colleagues did not determine any permanent sequelae of venous ligation. In this study, 30 of the 43 patients (70%), sustaining isolated venous injury, underwent management via ligation. The remaining 141 patient sustained both arterial and venous injury and 117 patients (83%) underwent venous ligation. Of the isolated venous injury, the mechanism of injury was predominantly penetrating trauma, and the location of injury was femoral (23), popliteal (9), iliac (8) and inferior vena cava (3). In patients sustaining both arterial and venous injury, the majority experienced predominantly upper extremity injury followed by popliteal injury. There were nine isolated popliteal vein injuries, five of which were primarily repaired and three of five underwent lower extremity fasciotomies. None of the 5 patients had venous sequelae, however, in surveillance studies, the venous repair was noted to be occluded. The remaining 4 popliteal vein injuries were ligated and three of four also had fasciotomies. Two of the four ligations experienced post operative occlusion of the veins and 2 had edema which resolved within 6 weeks. One third of patients, all of which sustained lower extremity venous trauma, developed a transient edema which resolved completely within 12 weeks post injury. In this study in which the majority of venous injury was managed with ligation, according to the authors no patient experienced persistent edema and no extremity was lost after ligation or repair. Although no detailed assessment of edema or lower extremity swelling is expressed by the authors. Aggressive management after vein ligation can minimize complications by implementation of limb elevation, compression and early fasciotomy when indicated. This study supports the conclusion that repair of venous injury is not mandatory for limb salvage or prevention of long term morbidity. However, despite the findings in their own cohort, Timberlake and colleagues do recommend an aggressive approach to venous repair specifically with injury to the popliteal vein.[12]

Venous Repair

The underlying condition of the patient, the severity of other injuries and the complexity of repair versus ligation must be considered. Information gathered from our military experience, advances in surgical technique and judicious use of antibiotics have significantly impacted the argument advocating surgical repair of traumatic venous injury. Most agree that if a venous repair can be performed quickly and safely in an otherwise stable patient, then it should be accomplished. There are a variety of different modalities of venous repair: primary repair, lateral repair, end to end anastamosis, autogenous vein patching, interposition autogenous vein graft, or paneled autogenous vein graft. In a study evaluating the patency and management of lower extremity venous injury with various types of repair, Parry and colleagues evaluated the results of 86 major lower extremity venous injuries, 27 of which underwent primary repair, 37 complex repair with autogenous vein and PTFE, 18 patients had temporary intraluminal shunts, and 20 patients undergoing ligation. They found an overall patency rate of 73.8%. Of this overall patency rate, patients undergoing primary repair had a patency rate of 76.5%, autogenous vein graft was 66.7% and PTFE 73.7%. They concluded that irrespective of the type of venous repair, the short term patency rates were similar.[13] Although Timberlake and colleagues advocate venous ligation, they do support an aggressive approach to management of popliteal vein injuries via repair as the one venous bed they believe this is beneficial in.

Meyer et al. performed a study of 36 patients to determine the patency of venous repair and to assess the accuracy of various methods used to evaluate patency. 34/36 patients had concomitant arterial injuries requiring repair, 22% had repair of upper extremity venous injuries and 78% lower extremity using a variety of repair methods. Using clinical exam, impedence plethysmograpohy, doppler US, and contrast venography, they determined that 39% of the venous repairs had thrombosed, and 61% remained patent. Local venous repair had a lower thrombosis rate than interposition vein grafting. Compared to venography, the clinical accuracy rate was 67% and the noninvasive exam had an accuracy rate of 53%. They concluded that a substantial number of venous repairs thrombosed although the limb salvage rate was not adversely affected. They recommend that contrast venography be the gold standard for evaluation of the integrity of the venous system to assess for patency after venous repair. Their data also supports the idea that maintenance of outflow from the extremity via the main venous conduit is not essential for limb salvage.[14]

There are several methods used to assess the patency and durability of a venous repair. These include duplex ultrasound, contrast computed tomography (CT), impedance plethysmography, and contrast venography. Meyer and colleagues recommend use of routine post op venography as they found that the clinical and non-invasive evaluation of venous repair patency to be inaccurate.[14] Most other authors however use standard color flow duplex to assess the long term patency of venous repairs with great accuracy.

Temporary Intra-Vascular Shunts

Vascular shunts are an adjunct to damage control surgery and are used as a method of stabilizing and moving patients in extremis. The goal is to re-establish perfusion prior to definitive repair. In patients with both an arterial and venous injury, a shunt placed in a vein allows for drainage and thereby decreases venous hypertension which can exacerbate tissue ischemia and bleeding. There have been a few small series published from civilian centers reporting the use of temporary intravascular shunts. Despite these reports, the use of shunts in civilian centers remains sporadic and somewhat controversial. In one civilian series, Parry and colleagues reported the use of intra-luminal venous shunts in 18 extremities, 16 of which went on to definitive repair. Half of the shunts were placed to allow for management of complex orthopedic injuries and the remaining were placed during damage control surgery. All of the venous injuries were accompanied by arterial injuries and 15 injuries underwent fasciotomies. Venous flow was confirmed with Doppler transducer and on average, shunts were in place for approximately 22 hours. In this study they recommend the use of temporary intraluminal shunts over venous ligation in proximal lower extremity veins for unstable extremities and for damage control surgery.[13]

The present day military vascular experience using shunts was evaluated by Rasmussen and colleagues. Data collected during Operation Iraqi Freedom (OIF) at a Level III echelon facility was recorded in the Balad Vascular Registry. The anatomic location of the shunt, shunt related complications, type of shunt, and the patency of the shunt at the time of exploration of injury was reported. The primary endpoint was shunt patency, and shunt related complications were defined as dislodgement and hemorrhage. During the 12 consecutive month period of this study in 2004–2005, there were 30 temporary shunts placed, four of which were venous. Three shunts were placed in the femoral vein and one in the popliteal vein. On average, shunts remained in place for less than 2 hours and all were patent at the time of exploration. No shunt related complications were noted and there was no decrease in early limb viability. The temporary use of intra-vascular shunts as an adjunct measure to damage control surgery is a safe and effective technique.[10,15] Woodward and colleagues agree that femoropopliteal shunts do well in patients in war that are being evacuated to higher levels of care.[7]

SELECT VENOUS BEDS

Renovascular Injuries

A firm understanding of anatomy is critical in the management of venous renovascular injury. The renal veins lie anterior to the renal arteries. The left renal vein is longer than the right and its course is anterior to the aorta. The left renal vein has collateral branches from the left adrenal vein superiorly, the left gonadal vein inferiorly and the lumbar vein posteriorly.

If feasible, lateral venorrhaphy can be used to manage renovascular injury. Patients with extensive injury or who are hemodynamically unstable, should undergo ligation. Ligation of the left renal vein near the IVC is well tolerated secondary to the remaining venous drainage via the left gonadal vein, the left adrenal vein, and via lumbar veins. If ligation of the right renal vein is required however, nephrectomy is recommended. This is due to the lack of collateral drainage for the right kidney as the right gonadal and right adrenal vein drain directly into the inferior vena cava.[16]

Iliac Venous Injury

Management of iliac vein injuries can be extremely challenging and life threatening. The common iliac veins converge at the level of L5, below the aortic bifurcation and underneath the right common iliac artery. Midline laparotomy provides rapid exposure to this area. Hemorrhage control is usually obtained with abdominal packing. Once the patient has stabilized with resuscitation from anesthesia a rapid exploration of the iliocaval confluence can be undertaken. In instances of injury to the common iliac veins, either direct exposure or transection of the overlying right common iliac artery can be performed. Once exposure of the injured iliac vein is obtained, the decision must be made to ligate or to repair. Repair of the iliac vein is advocated only if severe stenosis of the vessel can be avoided. The most often used method of repair is lateral venorrhaphy. The consequences of stenosis include thrombosis and PE. Ligation is preferred to a repair that produces major stenosis. Complex reconstruction in a hemodynamically unstable patient is not recommended. The consequences of ligation can include transient leg edema, and some may experience massive LE edema and compartment syndrome requiring fasciotomy. In patients sustaining both iliac artery and vein injury, complex venous reconstruction is not advocated because patients with combined injury are likely in critical condition and procedures which prolong the operation should be avoided. The mortality associated with isolated iliac venous injury is about 10% and ranges from 25–40% in those with concomitant injury.[16]

Inferior Vena Cava (IVC)

The IVC lies to the right of the aorta and ascends to course behind the liver, across the diaphragm into the thoracic cavity where after 2–3 cm it drains into the right atrium of the heart. As the IVC ascends towards the heart, it receives 4–5 pairs of lumbar veins, the right and left renal veins, the right gonadal vein, the right adrenal vein, the hepatic veins, and the phrenic veins. The IVC is the most commonly injured abdominal vessel and represents approximately 25% of abdominal vascular injuries. The most common mechanism of injury is penetrating trauma and blunt injury accounts for about 10%. Although blunt injury is rare, it has the potential to be very lethal. Mortality rates upwards of 50% have been reported.[17]

Acceleration and rapid deceleration injuries coupled with the mobility of the heart can lead to lacerations of the IVC. Injuries secondary to blunt trauma generally occur at regions where the vasculature is fixed and therefore vulnerable to sheer forces, like at the diaphragm. This can result in retrohepatic IVC and hepatic vein injuries. Also, downward deceleration of the liver may produce a laceration of the IVC. In patients sustaining extensive injuries to the retro-hepatic vena cava aggressive resuscitation without exploration is attempted first. In the rare case where the patient with a retrohepatic venous cava injury does not stabilize with nonoperative management operative exploration may be attempted. The techniques of atrial-caval shunt or cardiopulmonary bypass may be needed in these cases.[16,17]

Penetrating injury to the inferior vena cava is certainly more common and the location of injury, more unpredictable. In those with penetrating injury, approximately 18% have an associated arterial injury. Upon presentation, over 50% of patients with IVC injury are hypotensive. Hemorrhage control is most often obtained by spongestick control. Repair of the injured IVC can usually be accomplished using lateral venorrhaphy with 3-0 or 4-0 suture. Posterior vena cava injuries can be technically challenging. In this case the injury can be exposed by rotating the IVC. A posterior injury may also be accessed when repairing an anterior injury by extending the anterior wound, thereby exposing the posterior wound from inside the vein. Ligation of the IVC is a feasible option in patients in extremis with severe infra-renal injuries or when repair is likely to result in major stenosis. It is not advised to perform ligation of the supra-renal

IVC as that would lead to renal failure. In those instances, repair may be attempted with a patch or ringed prosthetic graft. Postoperative management of patients subject to ligation of the IVC should include aggressive management with bilateral lower extremity elevation and compression therapy. A majority of patients will likely experience at least temporary edema. Some patients may progress to more significant complications of venous outflow obstruction such as phlegmasia.[16,17]

Sullivan and colleagues conducted a small retrospective review of the outcomes of ligation of the IVC. They reviewed 100 patients sustaining injury to the inferior vena cava, of which 25 underwent ligation. In this series they did not directly compare ligation to repair, they simply reported the outcomes of the patients who underwent ligation. Of the 100 IVC injuries 22 of 54 infra-renal injuries were ligated, 3/21 supra-renal injuries were ligated, 15 sustained retro-hepatic injury and 10 supra-hepatic. 10/13 patients with infrarenal IVC injuries had fasciotomies, and one out of three with suprarenal injury survived and had normal renal function post operatively. Overall, 10/25 ligations survived to discharge. Not surprisingly, patients undergoing ligation of the inferior vena cava are more hemodynamically unstable than the majority of their counterparts undergoing repair. The ISS score, transfusion requirements and length of stay, as well as mortality were higher. Ligation of the infra-renal IVC is an acceptable method of gaining hemostasis during damage control surgery of the critically ill patient. Supra-renal ligation is generally utilized as a last ditch effort to aid in survival of an exsanguinating patient. It generally results in near 100% mortality and significant renal dysfunction in the few that do survive. Only seven patients had follow up information and none of them had significant long term edema or extremity dysfunction at the average follow up time of 42 months.[18]

Extremity Venous Injury

In both the military and civilian realms, lower extremity venous injury occurs at a significantly more frequent rate than upper extremity venous trauma. The most common lower extremity veins injured are the superficial femoral vein (42%), popliteal vein (23%) and the common femoral vein (14%). When the patient is hemodynamically stable and the injury is localized, repair of major venous injury via end to end or lateral venorrhaphy is advocated. In instances of extensive venous injury, placement of an interposition, panel or spiral graft may be considered for repair. If the patient is hemodynamically unstable or the repair is complex, simple ligation of the vessel may also be considered. With ligation, postoperative edema may be minimized with elevation of the extremity and elastic wrapping. Patency is monitored via hand held Doppler or duplex scan.[9]

Quan & Gillespie evaluated the experiences in the Global War on Terrorism and evaluated 82 patients sustaining 103 venous injuries. The majority of which were blast injuries, followed by GSWs and motor vehicle accidents (MVA). Patients were evaluated for limb edema and phlegmasia. Patency of venous repairs was evaluated by CT, ultrasound, contrast venography or a combination of these. Management of venous injury was via ligation only, venous repair only or both ligation and venous repair. Clinical outcomes were DVT, PE, thrombosis of injured vein after surgical repair and phlegmasia. Of note, DVT in this study was defined by thrombosis of a vein not involved in ligation or repair. Thrombosis at the site of vein repair was categorized as a thrombosis complication after surgical repair. The most common MOI was blast injuries, accounting for 65.9%, followed by high velocity GSWs, 30.5%, and rollovers while in combat, 3.5%. The majority of patients sustained both venous and arterial injuries (65.9%), 34.1% had isolated venous injury, 19.5% sustained multiple venous injuries. The majority of venous injuries were in the extremities (67%), 57.3% of which were of the lower extremities. Ligation occurred in 63.1% and open surgical repair in 36.9%. Of those undergoing repair, two thirds had primary repair which consisted of lateral venorrhaphy, vein patch and vein graft. There was some use of temporary arterial shunts in 8 of the 54 patients sustaining combined arterial and venous injury. One patient received a venous shunt. In regards to the outcomes: the incidence of DVT unrelated to the site of venous repair, DVT occurred in 6.9% of patients in the repair only group, 14.6% of patients undergoing ligation only and 20% of those in the ligation + repair group. The differences amongst the groups were not noted to be statistically significant. The presence of DVT was confirmed by duplex ultrasound or contrast CT. All patients with venous injury were noted to have edema of the affected extremity. The presence of phlegmasia occurred in 2.4% of patients ligated and in no patient in the venous repair group. Despite this, no group had a statistically higher risk of phlegmasia. Thrombosis after injury did occur in 15.8% of those sustaining venous repair only. In this series, three patients developed PE: one patient after surgical repair only and two patients after ligation only, no patient in the ligation + surgical repair group developed PE. No statistically significant difference was found in these numbers. The patency of LE vein repair was 84.6%. In this study, 39% of venous injuries were repaired, a figure that runs in close parallel to that seen in the management of venous injury in the Vietnam war. In this study, the authors concluded that ligation is advocated for patients in extremis, and prophylactic fasciotomy is also recommended to prevent phlegmasia. There is not a higher incidence of PE associated with venous repair, it is equivalent to ligation. Ideally, if the patient can tolerate it, repair of traumatic venous injury is advocated. This is particularly important in watershed regions that are responsible for significant venous outflow like the ileofemoral, popliteal, and internal jugular systems.[4]

Woodward and colleagues evaluated their experiences in management of femoro-popliteal injury during OIF. They were aggressive in repair of venous injuries unless the physiologic state of the patient precluded that attempt. Repair techniques included lateral suture repair, saphenous vein interposition grafting or panel grafting for size mismatch. In this registry there were 86 femoropopliteal venous injuries, 10 of which were isolated to the femoral vein only, 47 cases were a combination of femoral vein and artery injury. 12 of these injuries were subject to ligation. 28 patients had combination popliteal arterial and venous injuries, and 1 patient had an isolated popliteal vein injury. 12 injuries were treated with ligation. Overall 62/86 (72%) of femoropopliteal injuries underwent venous repair. In patients that did lose limbs, all had combined venous and arterial injury. They believe that repair of injury is improved from the Vietnam war, because rapid evacuation, use of shunts and early fasciotomy are effective methods assisting in definitive repair.[7]

An evaluation of in-theater management of vascular injury from the Balad registry supports the idea that most venous trauma occurs in the LE and incidences in the upper body tend to occur in the neck, particularly the internal jugular vein. The subclavian-axillary veins account for the second most common location. There were 107 venous injuries noted over a 24 month period. The internal jugular vein is often managed by ligation. In fact, of the 24 IJ injuries documented in this study, 20 were managed by ligation. In the LEs the most common venous injuries occurred in the femoropopliteal region. Management of the LE injuries was predominantly managed by repair, either primary or autogenous vein graft or patch angioplasty. The authors of this article support the management of venous repair when feasible and cite the fact that all limbs lost in the series occurred in patients with arterial and venous injury.[8]

CONCLUSION

Venous trauma is common. The management of injured veins depends on the location of injury, associated injuries and the stability of the patient. The use of ligation, repair and temporary intravascular shunts, all have their place. Minor associated injured veins can be ligated with impunity. In the hemodynamically unstable patient even major venous ligation in an effort to save life is prudent. At other times, control of hemorrhage may be gained and placement of a temporary shunt is the appropriate temporizing management option. Whether using a shunt or not, most would agree that definitive repair of a major venous injury of the vena cava, iliac, femoral or popliteal vein, if feasible, is recommended.

REFERENCES

1. Guthrie CC. History of Blood Vessel Surgery. In: Hill L, Bulloch W, eds. *Blood-Vessel Surgery and Its Applications*. New York: Longmans, Green & Co.;1912 p.2
2. Quan RW, Adams ED, Cox MW, et al. The management of trauma venous Injury: civilian and wartime experiences. *Perspect Vasc Surg Endovasc Ther*. 2006:18(2):149–158.
3. Bermudez KM, Knudson MM, Nelken NA, et al. Long-term results of lower-extremity venous injuries. *Arch Surg*. 1997;132:963–968.
4. Quan RW, Gillespie DL, Stuart RP, et al. The effect of vein repair on the risk of venous thromboembolic events: A review of more than 100 traumatic military venous injuries. *J Vasc Surg*. 2008:47(3):571–577.
5. Rich NM, Hughes CW, Baugh JH. Management of venous injuries. *Ann Surg*. 1970:171(5):724–730.
6. Rasmussen TE and Fox CJ. Vascular Trauma: Military*. In: Cronenwett JL and Johnston KW, eds. *Rutherford's Vascular Surgery 7th edition, Volume 2*. Philadelphia: Saunders Elsevier;2010:2374–2388.
7. Woodward EB, Clouse WD, Eliason JL, et al. Penetrating femoropopliteal injury during modern warfare: Experience of the Balad Vascular Registry. *J Vasc Surg*. 2008:47(6):1259–1265.
8. Clouse WD, Rasmussen TE, Peck MA, et al. In-theater management of vascular injury: 2 years of the Balad Vascular Registry. *J Amer Coll Surg*. 2007:204(4):625–632.
9. Patel KR and Rowe VL. Vascular Trauma: Extremity. In: Cronenwett JL and Johnston KW, eds. *Rutherford's Vascular Surgery 7th edition, Volume 2*. Philadelphia: Saunders Elsevier;2010:2361–2373.
10. Qi Y and Gillespie DL. Venous trauma: new lessons and old debates. *Perspect Vasc Surg Endovasc Ther*. 2011:23(2):74–79.
11. Levy RM, Alarcon LH, Frykberg ER. Peripheral Vascular Injuries. In: Peitzman AB, Rhodes M, Schwab CW, Yealy DM and Fabian TC, eds. *The Trauma Manual: Trauma and Acute Care Surgery*. Third edition. Philadelphia: Lippincott Williams & Wilkins; 2008:35:355–369.
12. Timberlake GA, O'Connell RC, Kerstein MD. Venous injury: To repair or ligate, the dilemma. *J Vasc Surg*. 1986:4(6):553–558.
13. Parry NG, Feliciano DV, Borke RM, et al. Management and short-term patency of lower extremity venous injuries with various repairs. *Am J Surg*. 2003;186:631–635.

14. Meyer J, Walsh J, Schuler J, etal. The early fate of venous repair after civilian vascular trauma: A clinical, hemodynamic, and venographic assessment. *Ann Surg.* 1987;206(4):458–462.

15. Rasmussen TE, Clouse WD, Jenkins DH, et al. The use of temporary vascular shunts as a damage control adjunct in the management if wartime vascular injury. *J Trauma.* 2006;61(1):8–12.

16. Demetriades D and Inaba K. Vascular Trauma: Abdominal. In: Cronenwett JL and Johnston KW, eds. *Rutherford's Vascular Surgery 7th edition, Volume 2.* Philadelphia: Saunders Elsevier;2010:2343–2360.

17. Brinkman WT and Bavaria JE. Vascular Trauma: Thoracic. In: Cronenwett JL and Johnston KW, eds. *Rutherford's Vascular Surgery 7th edition, Volume 2.* Philadelphia: Saunders Elsevier;2010:2330–2342.

18. Sullivan PA, Dente CJ, Patel S, etal. Outcome of ligation of the inferior vena cava in the modern era. *Am J Surg.* 2010:199:500–506.

17

Iatrogenic Venous Injuries

Charles L. Mesh, MD and Creighton B. Wright, MD

"I am sure that the mistake of that time will not be repeated; we shall probably make another set of mistakes."

- Sir Winston Churchill

Iatrogenic venous trauma has been altered with the movement from open surgery to endovascular therapy. As modes of therapy have changed, so too have modes of injury. Iatrogenic venous injury causes partial or complete disruption in venous mural integrity. The clinical end-result of partial injury is frequently thrombosis while that of complete injury may be either rupture or thrombosis. Thrombosis develops according to Virchow's triad with even relatively mild venous injury being the constant, and varying degrees of hyper-coagulability and stasis completing the equation. Thrombosis may cause clinical symptoms that are not immediately life- or limb- threatening. Subsequent venous scarring can cause late symptoms due to chronic venous hypertension. Rupture invariably occurs due to application of undue force to the thin venous wall (usually endovascular) or direct penetrating injury (generally open surgical misadventure). In contrast to thrombosis, rupture, particularly within a body cavity, is an emergent problem which requires immediate intervention.

This review will initially discuss venous mural structure in order to provide a context in which to understand the mechanisms of venous injury and healing. We will then examine upper extremity (including intra-thoracic), intra-abdominal and lower extremity iatrogenic venous injuries. Focus will be on venous injuries in the adult population (open surgical or endovascular) that fully disrupt venous integrity and those in which partial disruption is thought to be the primary cause for thrombosis and/or chronic stenosis. The most frequent injury scenarios that usually require vascular surgical expertise will be presented. Finally the principles of therapy for thrombosis and rupture for each anatomic region will be considered.

VENOUS STRUCTURE AND RESPONSE TO OCCLUSION

Venous histologic structure, like that of the artery, has intimal, medial and adventitial layers. The main difference between arteries and veins is that venous media is less developed in terms of elastin-smooth muscle cell lamellar units and thus is much thinner. The fact that the main strength-providing layer of the venous wall is thin explains why the normal veins are more prone to balloon rupture or catheter/guidewire perforations than arteries. Venous compliance and capacitance is large until the vein is fully distended. The vein then becomes more rigid, and like the artery, must rely on collagen for strength.

The cellular and molecular biology of the vein wall is beyond the scope of this chapter but has been discussed in a number of excellent reviews.[1] The venous response to thrombosis reflects this extensive biology and involves coagulation, thrombolysis, inflammation and scarring. The latter results in chronic venous hypertension. The physiologic effects of acute venous occlusion have been studied in animal models by Wright et al.[2] Sudden increases in venous outflow resistance cause significant reductions in arterial inflow. The inflow recovers over a period of days as venous pressure falls with the recruitment of venous collaterals. Experimental studies have documented that after DVT the vein wall cellular milieu is shifted to a profibrotic state with increases in MMP 2 and 9 and increased expression of Type I and III collagen. This change appears to be mitigated, at least in part, by thrombus. In an experimental model of stasis and thrombosis the levels of vein wall protein gene expression, proteinases and their mediators all increased over time. In contrast, models of limited stasis, non-stasis, and non-thrombotic injury showed markedly reduced inflammatory response suggesting the importance of both stasis and thrombus in directing venous wall response to injury.

The clinical importance of the aforementioned findings has been supported both in observational and interventional investigations.[1] In patients with deep venous thrombosis (DVT) studied with serial ultrasound observations over a mean time of 55 months, the severity of chronic venous disease independently correlated with the rate of thrombus resolution. This finding indirectly implied the potentiating effect of thrombus contact on venous mural scarring after DVT. Recognition of the role of thrombus in venous scarring and the ultimate effect of venous fibrosis itself are reflected in contemporary therapy of acute and chronic DVT. The former has resulted in early, aggressive thrombolysis as a first line therapy of proximal DVT. The latter may allow for aggressive application of endovascular recanalization techniques without rupture.[3]

VENOUS TRAUMA: INCIDENCE AND RISK FACTORS

Iatrogenic venous injury occurs in particular settings. Catheter-related venous thrombosis is a common problem seen in both the adult and pediatric populations because of the extensive utilization of indwelling central venous catheters. In contrast, catheter-associated venous rupture and perforation are less common. Direct venous injury at the time of surgery occurs in the context of open, laparoscopic, and robotic surgery. Although often accompanied by arterial injury, venous problems are potentially more life-threatening due to the difficulty encountered in their control and repair.

UPPER EXTREMITY

Acute Thrombosis

Acute DVT of the upper extremity is commonly associated with central venous catheterization as a risk factor. It carries the risk of pulmonary embolization[1,4] and thus may become a life-threatening problem. These catheters, inserted either centrally or peripherally, even when done correctly, represent a venous injury and have been described as "a stress test for the coagulation system".[4] Studies have demonstrated development of a fibrin sleeve around catheters as early as 24 hours after placement. Factors that are associated with development of catheter-related mural thrombus and/or clinical DVT include malignancy, thrombophilia, composition of infusion, catheter composition, catheter size, and catheter location within the central veins.

Reports of catheter-associated upper extremity deep vein thrombosis are plentiful, but determination of accurate incidence and prevalence is limited by lack of reporting standards.[4] Retrospective studies have confirmed DVT with clinical exam, venography, or autopsy. Clinical incidence ranging from 0.3 to 46% and symptomatic DVT rates of 0 to 35% have been reported. In general, higher rates reflect either populations with increased risk factors for DVT or studies in which diagnostic investigations were liberally performed. On average upper extremity DVT may be seen in approximately 24% of all patients with central lines while only 4% of these patients will present with symptoms. A contemporary review in which all patients underwent venographic studies after central line placement noted that 41% developed DVT(range 12% to 74%) with a 12% rate of symptoms(range 5% to 54%).[4] Frizzelli et al.[5] performed prospective duplex examination in 810 cardiac surgery patients with internal jugular triple lumen catheters 5 to 7 days after open heart surgery. They found evidence of DVT (thrombus adhering closely to vessel wall on one side) in 48%. Five developed pulmonary emboli, and all had central line-associated DVT. Of the patients with proven DVT, 33% had thrombus described at high risk for pulmonary embolus (clot occupying at least half of the lumen or echogenic strip > 2 cm in length, attached to the wall at one end and free-floating at the other). Admittedly, in a high risk group, this study emphasizes the very real incidence of catheter-induced upper extremity DVT and its potential for pulmonary embolization.

The hazards of pneumothorax, major arterial injury, and infection associated with central line insertion prompted the appearance of peripherally-inserted central catheters (PICC) as a safer, simpler alternative. Most studies of PICC-associated DVT are retrospective and utilize duplex surveillance for diagnosis.[6] Many are limited by non-uniform definition of DVT—some without any specification and some including only DVT of the brachiocephalic and subclavian veins. Because PICCs are placed via superficial veins, the development of superficial phlebitis (SVT) further confounds upper extremity DVT reports in that many authors group SVT and DVT together as one. Risk factors associated with PICC-associated upper extremity DVT include catheter size, number of puncture attempts, specific vein used for entry, number of previous PICCs, catheter tip location, catheter material, malignancy, anticoagulation, and female sex. Liem et al.[7] reviewed 831 upper extremity duplex scans performed over a 12 month period. During the same time frame 2056 PICCs were placed in their institution. While the incidence of PICC-associated upper extremity DVT was calculated at 2.6%, 35% of all upper extremity DVTs were associated with PICCs. Although retrospective design underestimates incidence, this study demonstrated the important role of PICCs in upper extremity DVT. In smaller prospective studies, the incidence of PICC-associated upper extremity DVT is higher and ranges from 9.3 to 19.4%.

The symptoms of upper extremity DVT almost always include extremity pain and/or swelling. While there are myriad causes for these symptoms, the diagnosis of DVT must always be taken seriously because of the risk of pulmonary embolization. In general, central venous thrombosis causes more significant edema than peripheral thrombosis simply due to more extensive outflow obliteration. Pain is variable in that it may range from aching and a feeling of fullness to localized tender cords from associated superficial phlebitis. Prominent superficial veins may be seen in the shoulder and pectoral regions and reflect collateral development. With profound outflow obstruction, edema, bullae, and even venous gangrene may be observed.

CHRONIC OBSTRUCTION

The omnipresence of non-occlusive thrombus associated with central venous catheters over long periods may cause central venous stenosis (CVS). This clinical combination may be reflected in the 50% rate of CVS seen in patients with pacemaker and defibrillator leads.[8] Another example of chronic, perhaps milder, venous injury that can result in CVS is the PICC. Although of smaller caliber and generally in place for shorter periods than pacemaker leads, prospective venography before and after PICC placement has shown a 7% incidence of CVS.[8]

CVS is clinically recognized with the onset of characteristic arm edema. These symptoms represent an imbalance between upper extremity blood flow volume and upper extremity outflow resistance. At resting blood flow levels symptoms are unusual in the absence of severe central venous narrowing. However, more moderate lesions can cause significant symptoms in the context of increased upper extremity blood flow. Since arteriovenous fistulae and arteriovenous grafts for hemodialysis are the most common reason for persistently increased upper extremity blood flow, central venous stenosis is frequently unmasked in renal failure patients. In this population the incidence of CVS ranges from 25 to 40%.[8] Significantly, 27% of hemodialysis patients with central venous stenosis have a history of a previous central venous catheter.[8] Further studies have demonstrated central venous stenosis rates of 42% and 10% for the subclavian and internal jugular positions respectively.[8] This data has prompted preferential use of the internal jugular as the initial site for temporary hemodialysis access. Interestingly, the internal jugular location is now being recognized as a cause of CVS in a much higher proportion of hemodialysis patients.[8]

Symptoms of chronic central venous obstruction, like those of acute DVT, include pain and/or swelling. While these symptoms may develop in a more insidious manner than with DVT, they are frequently seen shortly after either creation of upper extremity AV access or placement of a relatively large central venous catheter. The former increases extremity blood flow while the latter obscures an underlying silent stenosis. Depending on the site of obstruction, swelling may be limited to the extremity (axillo-subclavian), include a side of the face and neck (brachiocephalic), or involve both upper extremities and the entire head and neck (superior vena cava). These findings are variable in that brachiocephalic vein and SVC stenosis may show themselves only as arm swelling. The presence of edematous conjunctiva, upper airway edema, and headaches indicate a more severe form of central venous stenosis described as superior vena cava syndrome. In the absence of swelling, high venous pressures or inefficient dialysis due to recirculation may signify an occult central venous stenosis.

RUPTURE

Peripheral Venous Rupture

Intimal hyperplasia in the venous outflow tract is the most common cause of access failure. Traditional surgical therapy of these lesions consists of open patch angioplasty or segmental bypass of the obstructing lesion. Contemporary first-line therapy is now catheter-based and takes the form of angioplasty, stents and stent grafts.[9] Due to the fibrous, resistant nature of the inciting lesions, ultrahigh pressure (20 atmospheres) noncompliant balloons are utilized. Not uncommonly venous rupture is the end result with an incidence that ranges from 0.9 to 4.5%.[10,11] The use of cutting balloons, oversized balloons (> 2mm), fistulae as compared to grafts, transposed as compared to non-transposed fistulae, and female sex have all been associated with higher risk of rupture.[10]

Recognition of transmural injury is based on radiographic signs, clinical signs or both. Pain is common during angioplasty, but is usually limited to the period of balloon inflation. Pain that persists or worsens after balloon deflation should alert the operator to the possibility of rupture. While the physical finding of a mass in the area of angioplasty is diagnostic, this sign may not appear immediately. Therefore, the presence of persistent or worsening extremity pain should prompt immediate completion angiography to confirm venous integrity. Angiographic classification is based on the appearance of contrast extravasation: grade I is a non-flow-limiting hematoma, grade II is flow-limiting (Figure 17-1), and grade III shows pulsatile extravasation.[10]

The peripheral location of this form of venous rupture allows for rapid recognition and control of hemorrhage. The latter usually takes the form of simple angioplasty

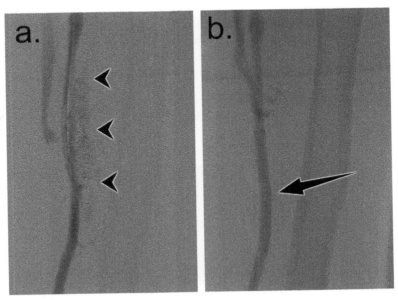

Figure 17-1. Angioplasty-induced rupture of hemodialysis access stenosis. **a.** Grade II contrast extravasation (arrowheads) in to hematoma causing flow limitation in fistula. **b.** Placement of stent (arrow), alleviating stenosis and allowing sealing of venous injury.

balloon inflation within the fistula at the site of rupture. If this technique is unsuccessful or cannot be achieved due to loss of wire access, direct manual pressure on the fistula or graft will control bleeding until emergent, definitive repair can be safely accomplished. Provided that access is adequate, prolonged balloon inflation and stent placement can manage low grade injury. Larger defects require stent grafts. This technique, while elegant and efficient, has 2 drawbacks: it is not ideal for injuries that cross the elbow joint due to the extreme flexion forces and it may not control all bleeding. In either case standard open surgical repair with interposition grafting can stem hemorrhage and salvage the access. Mortality is limited due to simple hemorrhage-control maneuvers. Morbidity takes the form of hemodialysis access failure which can be seen in 12 to 80 % of cases at one month. Primary patency with endovascular repair runs from 26 to 67% at 180 days and from 17 to 48% at one year. Secondary patency is much better with rates of 65 to 89% at 6 months and 69 to 87% at one year.[10,11]

Central Venous Rupture

Prior to the endovascular era, central venous rupture was encountered only in the context of central line placement. Although the incidence of this problem is low (0.25 to 0.4%), it remains important because over 6 million central venous catheters are placed annually (Figure 17-2). Angioplasty is a cause of iatrogenic central venous rupture that has appeared with the emergence of endovascular therapy. While only 13 superior vena cava (SVC) perforations have been described,[12] since first line therapy of central venous stenosis is now catheter-based, for both malignant and benign lesions,[13,14] it is likely that this complication is under-reported.

Virtually all central venous perforations are associated with pain. In the case of balloon angioplasty, pain that persists after balloon deflation is highly suspicious. Further manifestations reflect the anatomic location of the injury. Hemorrhage into the open space of the thoracic cavity or the trachea-bronchial tree or into the closed space of the mediastinum or pericardium can cause cardiovascular collapse. Open space hemorrhage produces profound hypotension that may respond temporarily to volume administration. Closed space hemorrhage into the mediastinum is limited by the mediastinal boundaries, and cardiovascular collapse is less common unless there has been rupture into the thoracic cavity. Bleeding into the pericardium

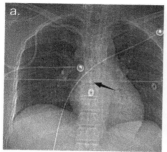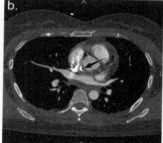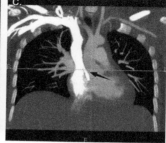

Figure 17-2. Plasmapharesis catheter injury of the superior vena cava causing cardiac tamponade. **a.** Plain chest x ray demonstrates globular cardiac shadow and catheter (arrow) in apparently good position. **b.** Axial CT image delineates extra-caval and intra-pericardial location of catheter (arrow). **c.** Coronal CT image showing intrapericardial position of catheter between the superior vena cava and ascending aorta (arrow).

causes cardiac tamponade if the right side of the heart is compressed. The classic findings of hypotension, jugular venous distension and muffled heart sounds, known as Beck's triad, will be present. This form of hypotension is unresponsive to fluid administration. Subclavian and brachiocephalic perforations are mediastinal as are those of the distal, medial SVC. Lateral rupture of the distal SVC in proximity to the right atrium uniformly bleeds into the right thoracic cavity. In patients with bronchogenic carcinoma, brachiocephalic and superior vena cava injuries can involve the trachea and right main stem bronchus and present as massive hemoptysis. Intrapericardial SVC injuries hemorrhage into the pericardium. A high index of suspicion can be life-saving when unexpected hypotension develops during central line placement or central venous intervention. Prompt chest x-ray can demonstrate new pleural effusions consistent with hemothorax, widened mediastinum associated with mediastinal hemorrhage, and the enlarged, globular cardiac silouette of tamponade. If echocardiography is available, this can rapidly and reliably diagnose pericardial effusion and tamponade. Subxyphoid aspiration of non-clotting blood from the pericardium can also swiftly diagnose cardiac tamponade, and provide temporary improvement.

DIRECT INJURY

Thoracic Outlet Syndrome

Direct injury to the subclavian vein can be encountered during trans-axillary first rib resection. This injury is infrequently reported, but all descriptions of operative technique emphasize its potential for uncontrollable hemorrhage. Distal injuries, when promptly recognized, can be easily managed with judicious placement of vascular clamps for venorrhaphy. More proximal injuries are problematic because mechanical control may be difficult or impossible due to overlying osseous structures, and are most likely to occur when the vein is decompressed by division of the subclavius muscle. Immediate proximal control may be achieved by increasing PEEP (positive end-expiratory pressure) in the ventilator circuit, thus increasing intrathoracic pressure to levels greater than central venous pressure. This effect may however be limited by impaired ventricular filling. As an initial maneuver, PEEP may staunch hemorrhage enough to allow proximal intravascular balloon placement. Ultimately, more proximal injuries may require clavicle resection or thoracotomy for definitive repair.

Hemodialysis Access Venous Pseudoaneurysm

Hemodialysis access pseudoaneurysms develop as a result of repeated single-site cannulation. They are reported to occur in 2 to 30% of hemodialysis accesses, and are more common in AV grafts (2–10%) than in autogenous fistulae.[15] These lesions present as painful or non-painful masses over the fistula that may be pulsatile or non-pulsatile. Larger pseudoaneurysms can cause skin erosion and hemorrhage. Intervention is reserved for expanding or painful lesions and for those associated with infection, skin erosion, or hemorrhage. Prevention takes the form of cannulation techniques that involve either sequential "rope-ladder" or localized "button-hole" needle placement in the fistula. Repair is straightforward and can be accomplished with stent grafts, localized open surgical interposition grafting, or more proximal transposition of the fistula anastomosis.

ABDOMINAL CAVITY

Vena Cava Filter Thrombosis

Vena cava interruption is a common method for prevention of pulmonary embolism when anticoagulation is either inadequate or unsafe. Expanded relative indications and the development of percutaneous delivery systems have been paralleled by a 25 fold increase in vena cava filter placement between 1979 and 1999.[1] While filters clearly prevent PE, they are also associated with increased rates of recurrent DVT as compared to standard anticoagulation. Since filters trap thrombus before it reaches the pulmonary circulation, it is not surprising that vena cava thrombosis develops following 2 to 30% of filter placements. This condition may manifest itself with symptoms of massive bilateral lower extremity edema and pain. Lack of lower extremity venous outflow and subsequent congestion may result in blue skin discoloration or phlegmasia cerulea dolens. This is a sign of threat to limb viability and can lead to irreversible venous gangrene. Diagnosis can be confirmed with abdominal duplex scan, computed tomographic venography, or magnetic resonance imaging. Conservative measures of lower extremity elevation, compression and full anticoagulation can provide significant symptomatic relief. Prior to the advent of thrombolysis these measures were the extent of therapy. Significant numbers of surviving patients were left with chronic lower extremity edema and many developed post-phlebitic skin changes. Contemporary therapy includes aggressive pharmacologic or mechanical thrombolysis in order to avoid both the acute limb loss associated with phlegmasia cerulea dolens as well as the late sequelae of post-phlebitic syndrome.

DIRECT INJURY

Iatrogenic venous injury is a rare component within a busy trauma practice. In a 30-year experience from a large metropolitan city reported by Mattox et al., it accounted for only 0.06% vascular injuries.[16] Timberlake et al. reported the largest series of isolated major venous injuries with 85 patients.[17] In their experience, 23% of damaged veins were intra-abdominal (17 iliac and 3 vena cava), and there was no limb-loss regardless of chosen therapy (repair versus ligation). The Walter Reed Army Medical Center reviewed 212 patients with iatrogenic vascular trauma during the period from 1966 to 1982.[18] In this experience 17 isolated venous injuries were identified. Eleven were intra-abdominal, of which 7 involved the iliac veins. Venous injuries are more likely to be encountered in oncologic resections, difficult anatomic exposures, and repeat surgeries and are associated with a mortality rate of up to 18%.[19] In contrast to young, relatively healthy trauma patients, the population suffering iatrogenic vascular injury is generally older and undergoing procedures for accompanying morbidities. Interestingly, a Swedish population-based study has documented higher mortalities associated with iatrogenic vascular injury as compared to those from non-iatrogenic causes.[20]

Spine Surgery

The anterior approach to the spine is used to manage degenerative disc disease, scoliosis spondylolisthesis, and spinal instability from a number of etiologies. The risk of vascular injury exists because of the coverage of the spine by the great vessels. This confluence of major arteries and veins stretches across the L4 and L5 vertebral bodies and becomes more complex in the presence of venous anomalies such as duplicated or left sided vena cava. A review of 88 articles regarding anterior lumbosacral surgery noted that venous injuries ranged from 0 to 18.1% and were much more common than arterial injuries.[21] Recognition is straightforward as a sudden rush of blood into the operative field. This generally occurs during vascular exposure or vessel retraction for hardware placement. The left common iliac vein, the inferior vena cava, and the iliolumbar vein are damaged most frequently. Risk factors are L4-L5 approach, revision surgery, use of threaded interbody devices, trans-peritoneal exposure, and laparoscopic technique. Repair, although generally accomplished with simple suture placement, can be treacherous. Mortality can reach 4% and is uniformly associated with massive blood loss. Endovascular hemorrhage control with balloons can be life-saving,[22] and treatment with endografts has been described.[23]

The posterior approach to the spine is a minimally invasive method for decompression of disc herniation. Vascular injury occurs in less than 1% of cases. For the same anatomic reasons as the anterior approach, 75% of injuries occur to the aortoiliac or iliocaval vessels. Disc debridement with either a curette or pituitary rongeur can penetrate the anterior spinal ligament and blindly tear the posterior surface of overlying veins, arteries, or both. These injuries may not be immediately recognized in the operating room as hemorrhage may occur either directly posteriorly into the operative field or anteriorly into the relatively large retroperitoneal space. In combined arterial and venous injuries, a similar pattern of initial bleeding may be seen followed by sudden cessation as "decompression" results in a traumatic arteriovenous fistula.

Hypotension and tachycardia are the most frequent manifestations of unrecognized, isolated arterial or venous damage. The presence of abdominal distension or a new palpable abdominal mass immediately after posterior spine surgery is highly suggestive of vascular injury. Once the patient is awake, non-specific signs of possible retroperitoneal hematoma include undue flank or abdominal pain, nausea, or vomiting. The signs and symptoms of traumatic arteriovenous fistula are the same whether the injury is recognized early or late. Dyspnea, orthopnea, tachycardia, and leg edema indicate high output congestive heart failure and elevated regional venous pressures. A continuous bruit may be auscultated over the abdomen or flank. In the patient with stable hemodynamics, the diagnosis can be easily confirmed with contrast-enhanced CT scan. In the presence of hemodynamic instability, the possibility of vascular injury mandates intervention, either open[24] or endovascular.[24,25]

Laparoscopic Surgery

Laparoscopy is an extremely safe procedure with an estimated death rate of 0.007%. Vascular trauma during standard laparoscopy occurs in less than 0.04% of cases but accounts for the majority of deaths. The aorta, inferior vena cava, and iliac vessels are the most commonly injured vessels.[26] Seventy-five percent of injuries occur during trocar or Veress needle placement. Higher vascular injury rates, up to 3.5%, are noted with more complex procedures such as laparoscopic nephrectomy, ureteral diversion, ureterolysis and retroperitoneal lymph node dissection.[27] Iatrogenic trauma associated with complex procedures is predominantly venous and occurs during dissection as opposed to needle entry. While most injuries result in hemorrhage, inadvertent division or narrowing of major venous structures can also occur due to disorientation of landmarks.[28]

Laparoscopic procedures begin with either Veress needle entry or open access (Hassan Technique) to the abdominal cavity for pneumoperitoneum. When the abdominal wall is relaxed, the entry point is just below the umbilicus and only a few centimeters from the great vessels. As such, any factor that produces uncontrolled passage may result in vascular injury. Early indicators are blood return from the needle or the presence of a retroperitoneal hematoma with minimal intraperitoneal blood after laparoscope insertion. Either finding should prompt immediate preparation for laparotomy. During the course of a complex laparoscopic procedure, as with open surgery, most vascular misadventures occur during dissection. The disturbing finding of the vascular injury is the rapid filling of the operative field with blood. This may be due to direct vascular damage, clip slippage from a ligated vessel, or misplacement or malfunction of a vascular stapling device. Maintenance of pneumoperitoneum is important during injury assessment as it may decrease venous bleeding. Advanced laparoscopic surgeons may add additional trocars for retraction and exposure. Aspiration of blood with one hand and the use of an angled or curved grasper with the other, for occlusion or compression, may allow visualization for clip placement. If the surgeon has the least bit of discomfort with laparoscopic management or rapid control, conversion to open management should not be delayed.

Oncologic Surgery

Surgery for tumor resection carries its own risk factors that may predispose to iatrogenic injury. These patients are likely to have distorted anatomy due to malignancy, prior surgery, previous radiation, or a combination of these factors.[19,29] Published reports do not include minor injuries as these are likely repaired without incident. In a large series from the Mayo Clinic[19] Whipple procedure, colon resection, and tumor debulking were the most common operations with injury. Six of 7 portal vein injuries occurred during Whipple operation, 7 of 8 partial internal iliac vein lacerations arose in pelvic oncologic surgery patients, and 3 of 6 inferior vena cava injuries were in patients undergoing surgery for retroperitoneal masses. Mortalities of 28%, 25%, and 17% respectively were noted. While accompanying arterial injury was not unusual, all deaths occurred in the context of venous injury with massive blood loss. These mortality rates are significantly better than the mortality rates of 48% with IVC injury and 41% with portal vein injury in trauma reports.

Vascular Surgery

Direct venous injury to the left renal vein and iliac veins can be encountered in open aortic aneurysm surgery due to proximal aortic and distal iliac clamp placement respectively. In both elective and emergent situations unanticipated venous anomalies may increase the chance of such injuries. Circumaortic left renal vein, retroaortic left renal vein, and abnormalities of the IVC are noted in 6%, 3.3% and 2.4% of patients respectively and often may not be appreciated until after they are damaged.[30] Currently, since almost all aortic aneurysms are investigated with CT scan to assess suitability for endovascular repair, these variations should be identified prior to most open aneurysm operations. In the context of aneurysm rupture, clamp placement is treacherous, even with foreknowledge of anomalous anatomy, due to obscured anatomy from hematoma. In ruptured aortic aneurysm repair venous injury is the most important technical misstep that can lead to massive uncontrollable hemorrhage and subsequent mortality. Careful dissection and clamp application at the proximal infrarenal aorta, utilization of intraluminal occluding balloons and application of the principles of endoaneurysmorraphy can minimize inadvertent venous injury.

RUPTURE

Vena Cava Filter Penetration

Instrumentation of the inferior vena cava has increased geometrically during the last 4 decades simply from the increased availability and placement of vena cava filters. With the advent of catheter-based interventions for acute and chronic iliocaval thromboses, these numbers continue to grow. Fortunately the incidence of cava or iliac vein disruption is rare and consequences are self-limited in many cases. Vena cava filters rarely rupture the vena cava, but frequently penetrate this vessel. The Greenfield stainless steel filter has the highest rate of 40% due to the wire leg hook tips. Newer filters with different wire structure have rates of less than 10%. Most patients are asymptomatic from penetration, but transgression of the abdominal aorta, iliac artery and duodenum have been reported. It is disruption of adjacent structures that necessitates vascular surgical intervention for removal (Figure 17-3). Standard proximal and distal control of the vena cava allows for vena cavotomy. The filter legs are then divided with wire cutters and removed from inside the vessel. Simple venorrhaphy is used for repair.

Angioplasty-induced Iliac Vein Rupture

Iliac and vena cava angioplasty and stenting is now first line treatment for lower extremity iliofemoral chronic venous occlusive disease and May-Thurner syndrome. Reports of large and small series note no perforations or retroperitoneal hemorrhage.[3,31] There is, however, a case report of 2 instances of iliac venous rupture that occurred during angioplasty.[32] Both patients were female. The etiology of occlusion was a surgical staple from prior gynecologic surgery in one and venous stricture from a prior lower limb hemodialysis catheter in the other. Both patients required covered stents for successful treatment. Since large iliac

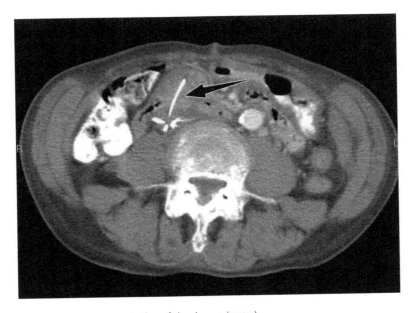

Figure 17-3. Vena cava filter limb penetration of duodenum (arrow).

venoplasty/stent series include only chronic DVT and no surgical stricture or hemodialysis catheter as etiology, one can speculate that the lack of rupture may be due to chronic peri-venous scarring associated with DVT.

LOWER EXTREMITY

Thrombosis

Lower extremity deep venous thrombosis is a potential complication that exists with any catheter-based or open lower extremity intervention. The incidence of this problem after vascular access for coronary or peripheral intervention is low. However, because of the prevalence of groin access and the increasing utilization of the femoral vessels for cardio-pulmonary bypass in robotic heart surgery, it will continue to be encountered with relative frequency. Similarly, the femoral vein can be injured during conventional open hernia surgery. DVT identification in either situation is predicated on a high index of suspicion, and duplex imaging provides confirmation. Conventional anticoagulation is indicated when DVT is present. Because these DVTs are "provoked by surgery," anticoagulation duration of 3 months is recommended.[33]

Radiofrequency or laser-assisted ablation of the greater saphenous vein for venous insufficiency creates a thrombotic process within the greater saphenous vein(GSV). The risk of proximal thrombus propagation into the deep venous system after GSV ablation is well-recognized and surveillance duplex scanning is recommended at 72 hours post-procedure. Selective, full-dose anticoagulation for GSV thrombus is commonly utilized. Singh et al. recently described ligation and division of the saphe-nofemoral junction concomitant with GSV ablation as a safe alternative that eliminates the need for post-operative duplex surveillance.[34]

DIRECT INJURY

Direct iatrogenic trauma to lower extremity veins occurs from the same sources that result in thrombosis—percutaneous catheter-based interventions and open surgery. Direct venous injuries caused by catheters that do not result in thrombosis may be associated with concomitant arterial injury and form arteriovenous fistulae (AVF). These lesions develop in 0.2% to 2% of groin arterial access cases, and are associated with female gender, hypertension and ongoing anticoagulation[35] Diagnosis in the post-procedure period is made either by duplex investigation of a bruit, thrill, or groin mass suspicious for pseudoaneurysm or, less commonly, when secondary venous hypertension causes leg swelling or pulmonary edema. Catheter-induced, iatrogenic AVF will resolve spontaneously in up to 67% of cases.[35] Indications for intervention include leg edema, painful mass, pulmonary edema, and leg ischemia. Traditional therapy is surgical closure of arterial and venous defects and reconstruction as necessary. While reliable, this approach is associated with relatively significant morbidity and even mortality, particularly in the infirm patient population likely to suffer such injury. Less invasive methods such as ultrasound-guided compression, plug embolization and covered stenting have had success in selected cases. Stent graft repair is ideal for discrete catheter lesions and can be applied to the superficial femoral and iliac vessels. Coverage of profunda femoris vasculature, although feasible and indicated in dire circumstances, is to be generally avoided in order to preserve this important lower extremity collateral. Similarly, stent graft placement in the distal external iliac and common femoral vessels is unfavorable due to risk of stent compression from extreme joint flexion as well as the potential for interference with subsequent catheter-based procedures that may require groin access.

Venous laceration during open surgery is usually recognized due to sudden bleeding and corrected with simple suture techniques. When unrecognized or when repair compromises venous outflow these injuries can result in DVT. Anatomic abnormalities, due either to prior surgery or developmental variance, provide the setting for most of these injuries. Direct venous injury occurs with open hernia surgery—most commonly as the transition suture is placed in the femoral sheath. If bleeding is encountered with this maneuver suture removal, as opposed to tying, will minimize the risk of venous narrowing and subsequent DVT. Gentle application of pressure will usually arrest any subsequent low pressure venous bleeding. Venous injury can also be encountered in urologic surgery with blind tunneling for penile prosthesis placement. Anatomic variants are seen frequently during ligation and division of the saphenofemoral junction. Inconsistent junctioning branches can occur in up to 63% of patients and can lead to inadvertent division of the common femoral or femoral vein. In either situation, primary repair is the rule. As noted above, any suspicion of venous luminal compromise should prompt duplex scan. DVT, if identified, requires anticoagulation.

SURGICAL AND CATHETER-BASED THERAPIES

Acute Venous Thrombosis

Vascular surgical consultation is frequently called for upper extremity deep venous thrombosis in the presence of either a central line or vena cava thrombosis associated with a vena cava filter. The approach to these situations should be systematic. Upper or lower extremity central venous thrombosis in the active, otherwise healthy individual, should be mechanically and/or chemically lysed to avoid the sequelae of untreated venous hypertension and post-thrombotic syndrome. Offending catheters should be removed, if possible, with subsequent anticoagulation for 3 months.[33] Prolonged anticoagulation is indicated if the offending catheter must remain in place and in the case of vena cava filters.[33] In debilitated patients, those at risk for hemorrhage, and those who are relatively symptom-free, anticoagulation alone with extremity compression is appropriate.[33] There is no compelling evidence for prophylactic anticoagulation in patients with either centrally or peripherally inserted central lines.[36]

VENOUS INJURIES: OPEN SURGERY

The principles for management of venous trauma are hemorrhage control, repair of the vascular defect, and preservation of critical venous outflow. In open surgery, hemorrhage control is achieved with direct access to the injured vessel. Standard median sternotomy, right lateral thoracotomy and midline laparotomy incisions provide wide access to the mediastinal and intrapericardial great veins, the extra-pericardial superior vena cava, and all major abdominal veins respectively. After evacuation of clotted blood, initial venous control can be achieved with digital and sponge stick pressure, followed by precise application of vascular clamps. If simple maneuvers do not allow adequate visualization to perform safe repair, arterial inflow control can be useful. For inferior vena cava injuries, aortic cross clamping at the infrarenal position can allow for resuscitation and reduce lower extremity venous return enough to allow identification of the injury. For portal venous trauma a similar effect can be provided by application of a supraceliac aortic or superior mesenteric artery clamp. Retrohepatic vena cava injury can be controlled with a combination of portal triad clamping (Pringle maneuver), and suprarenal and suprahepatic inferior vena cava clamping. The latter may be best obtained from an intrapericardial location. Temporary shunting is a great help with IVC, SVC, and some smaller veins to decompress the field while a complete repair is done. Ultimate access to the injured vein may require division of overlying arteries. The right common iliac artery may be divided to allow access to the left common iliac vein and the distal inferior vena cava. Division of the internal iliac artery provides access to the internal iliac vein. When the surgeon is confronted with more complex maneuvers for hemorrhage control, the utility of endovascular control should be considered. If the injury can be identified, an intraluminal balloon can often be placed through it for control. If the injury cannot be clearly identified, remote access for intraluminal control can be very effective[22], provided that reasonable fluoroscopic imaging is available.

Once vascular control has been achieved, repair may then proceed using direct suture repair (venorrhaphy), venous patch angioplasty, or interposition venous grafting. Lateral venorrhaphy is suitable for limited injuries. Patch venoplasty with autogenous vein is useful for venous defects in which venorrhaphy would compromise the lumen by 50% or more. Internal jugular, internal iliac, saphenous, and superficial femoral veins have been used. Segmental defects may be managed with proximal and distal mobilization, debridement, and meticulous end-to-end anastomosis. Extensive loss of venous integrity can be managed with interposition vein graft. When replacement is needed for smaller veins, saphenous vein is the usual conduit. For innominate vein or superior or inferior vena cava replacement, the spiral vein technique may be suitable. Artificial substitutes have also been effective in these positions. Preservation of outflow is achieved when the correct repair is chosen for the appropriate defect magnitude, and can be enhanced with the adjuvant anticoagulation.

In some dire circumstances, the venous outflow must be sacrificed with ligation in order to save a patient's life.[19] In the setting of iatrogenic venous trauma, this tactic should be unusual due to the absence of other mitigating injuries. When necessary, extremity swelling can be anticipated and fasciotomy should be considered. When required centrally, in either the vena cava or portal system, massive third space fluid losses can also be expected and must be replaced. Transient reduction in arterial inflow may put involved extremities and organs at risk for ischemia. When this situation is encountered, consideration should be given to alternatives such as abdominal packing, resuscitation and warming, and subsequent planned endovascular solution or return to the operating room for a second attempt at open repair

ENDOVASCULAR SURGERY

Hemorrhage from venous injury occurring during endovascular interventions is initially arrested by appropriately-sized balloon inflation across the defect. Thereafter, the paradigm for vascular repair is distinctly different from open surgery. Instead of direct methods, the defect is indirectly sealed by first assuring normal venous outflow with the theoretic goal of achieving a balance between intra- and extra-vascular pressure. This may be accomplished by radially expanding the venous wall with prolonged angioplasty balloon inflation. If hematoma accumulation elevates extravascular pressures, this technique will be unsuccessful as venous collapse will lead to increased distal venous pressures and continued bleeding (Figure 17-1a). The addition of an intravascular stent can overcome venous collapse and allow extravascular forces to keep blood within the venous system. Once pressure balance is reached, the clotting system can effectively seal most perforations (Figure 17-1b). Very large venous injuries or those occurring within the low pressure environment of the thoracic cavity are not likely to respond to these therapeutic maneuvers. In these situations endovascular sealing becomes paramount and can be provided with a covered stent.

In the past the repair of venous injuries required open surgery. With the explosion in endovascular therapies, many venous injuries occur in the angiography suite. As such, hemorrhage control is initially endovascular. Once the injury is diagnosed, adequate intravenous access is critical for resuscitation. Establishing lower extremity access is important for thoracic venous injuries as upper extremity angiocatheters may simply deliver fluid and blood products through the injury into the chest. Subsequent strategies for therapy should be guided by the patient's hemodynamic stability, the type and location of the injury, and the availability of appropriate personnel and equipment. Hemodynamic stability allows for systematic injury delineation and treatment. As a rule, even though endovascular repair has been described,[37] iatrogenic thoracic venous injuries are best defined and managed in the operating room due to the propensity for rapid hemodynamic decompensation. In this setting, thoracotomy or median sternotomy can be easily accomplished for prompt control of either intrathoracic hemorrhage or decompression of cardiac tamponade. A hybrid endovascular operating room with full open surgical capacity and high quality fluoroscopic imaging is ideal for this situation. Intra-abdominal venous injury that occurs during endovascular treatment of chronic iliac venous occlusive disease is best managed with endovascular methods. Chronic perivenous scarring makes open surgical management treacherous, but promotes tamponade[3]once outflow has been facilitated with covered stents.[32] Consequently, remaining in the angiography suite with its high quality imaging is appropriate. Larger vena cava endovascular injuries will not generally allow such facile endovascular control and thus are best handled in an operating room environment that will allow for laparotomy. In contrast, peripheral venous endovascular injuries, because tamponade occurs into a small potential space, can be managed in the angiography suite. Venous injuries that occur during open surgery are almost always managed with open techniques. However, endovascular balloon occlusion can be useful for difficult hemorrhage control.[22] Occasionally, because of inability to safely access the venous injury, endovascular access and stent graft repair can salvage an untenable situation.[23-25,38] The vascular surgeon, of all vascular specialists, should not be trapped into one method of venous injury management. Recognition of the injury type, prompt assessment of hemodynamic status, and rapid inventory of equipment, both needed and available, for repair will allow the surgeon to pick the appropriate treatment modality.

REFERENCES

1. Meissner MH, Wakefield TW, Asher E, et al. Acute venous disease: Venous thrombosis and venous trauma. *J Vasc Surg*. 2007;46(6):S25–53.
2. Wright CB, Hobson RW. Hemodynamic effects of femoral venous occlusion in the subhuman primate. *Surgery*. 1974;75:453–60.

3. Neglen P, Hollis KC, Olivier J, et al. Stenting of the venous outflow in chronic venous disease: long-term stent-related outcome, clinical, and hemodynamic result. *J Vasc Surg.* 2007;46(5):979–90.

4. Kuter DJ. Thrombotic complications of central venous catheters in cancer patients. *Oncologist.* 2004;9(2):207–16.

5. Frizzelli R, Tortelli O, Di Comite V, et al. Deep venous thrombosis of the neck and pulmonary embolism in patients with a central cenous catheter admitted to cardiac rehabilitation after cardiac surgery: a prospective study of 815 patients. *Intern Emerg Med.* 2008;3:325–30.

6. Turcotte S, Dube S, Beauchamp G. Peripherally inserted central venous catheters are not superior to central venous catheters in the acute care of surgical patients on the ward. *World Journal of Surgery.* 2006;30(8):1605–19.

7. Liem TK, Yanit KE, Moseley SE, et al. Peripherally inserted central catheter usage patterns and associated symptomatic upper extremity venous thrombosis. *J Vasc Surg.* 2012;55(3):761–7.

8. Agarwal A. Central vein stenosis: Current concepts. *Adv Chronic Kidney Dis.* 2009;16:360–70.

9. Haskal ZJ, Trerotola S, Dolmatch B, et al. Stent graft versus balloon angioplasty for failing dialysis-access grafts. *N Engl J Med.* 2010;362(6):494–503.

10. Bittl JA. Venous rupture during percutaneous treatment of hemodialysis fistulas and grafts. *Cathet Cardiovasc Intervent.* 2009;74(7):1097–101.

11. Kornfield ZN, Kwak A, Soulen MC, et al. Incidence and management of percutaneous transluminal angioplast induced venous rupture in the "Fistula First" era. *J Vasc Interv Radiol.* 2009;20(6):744–51.

12. Da Ines D, Chabrot P, Motreff P, et al. Cardiac tamponade after malignant superior vena cava stenting: Two case reports and brief review of the literature. *Acta Radiologica.* 2010;51(3):256–9.

13. Nicholson AA, Ettles DF, Arnold A, et al. Treatment of malignant superior vena cava obstruction: metal stents or radiation therapy. *J Vasc Interv Radiol.* 1997;8(5):781–8.

14. Rizvi AZ, Kalra M, Bjarnason H, et al. Benign superior vena cava syndrome: Stenting is now the first line of treatment. *J Vasc Surg.* 2008;47(2):372–80.

15. Shah AS, Valdes J, Charlton-Ouw KM, et al. Endovascular treatment of hemodialysis access pseudoaneurysms. *J Vasc Surg.* 2012;55(4):1058–62.

16. Mattox K, Feliciano D, Burch J, et al. Five thousand seven hundred sixty cardiovascular injuries in 4459 patients. *Ann Surg.* 2012;209:698–705.

17. Timberlake G, Kerstein M. Venous injury: To repair or ligate, the dilemma revisited. *Am Surg.* 1995;61:139–45.

18. Youkey JR, Clagett GP, Rich NM, et al. Vascular trauma secondary to diagnostic and therapeutic procedures: 1974 through 1982. A comparative review. *Am J Surg.* 1983;146(6):788–91.

19. Oderich GS, Panneton JM, Hofer J, et al. Iatrogenic operative injuries of abdominal and pelvic veins: A potentially lethal complication. *J Vasc Surg.* 2004;39(5):931–6.

20. Rudstrom H, Bergqvist D, Ogren M, et al. Iatrogenic vascular injuries in Sweeden. A nationwide study 1987–2005. *Eur J Endovasc Surg.* 2008;35:131–8.

21. Wood K, DeVine J, Fischer D, et al. Vascular injury in elective anterior lumbosacral surgery. *Spine.* 2010;95:S66–75.

22. Tillman BW, Vaccaro PS, Starr JE, et al. Use of an endovascular occlusion balloon for control of unremitting venous hemorrhage. *J Vasc Surg.* 2006;43(2):399–400.

23. Schneider JR, Alonzo MJ, Hahn D. Successful endovascular management of an acute iliac venous injury during lumbar discectomy and anterior spinal fusion. *J Vasc Surg.* 2006;44(6):1353–6.

24. Zhou W, Bush RL, Terramani TT, et al. Treatment Options of Iatrogenic Pelvic Vein Injuries: Conventional Operative Versus Endovascular Approach. *Vasc and Endovasc Surg.* 2004;38(6):569–73.

25. Zahradnik V, Kashyap VS. Alternative management of iliac vein injury during anterior lumbar spine exposure. *Ann Vasc Surg.* 2012;26(2):277–8.

26. Nordestgaard AG, Bodily KC, Osborne R, et al. Major vascular injuries during laparoscopic procedures. *Am J Surg.* 1995;169(5):543–5.

27. Thiel R, Adams JB, Schulam PG, et al. Venous dissection injuries during laparoscopic urological surgery. *J Urol*. 1996;155(6):1874–6.
28. McAllister M, Bhayani SB, Ong A, et al. Vena caval transection during retroperitoneoscopic nephrectomy: Report of the complication and review of the literature. *J Urol*. 2004;172(1):183–5.
29. Cikrit DF, Dalsing MC, Sawchuk AP, et al. Vascular injuries during pancreatobiliary surgery. *Am Surg*. 1993;59(10):692–6.
30. Bartle EJ, Pearce WH, Sun JH, et al. Infrarenal venous anomalies and aortic surgery: Avoiding vascular injury. *J Vasc Surg*. 1987;6(6):590–3.
31. Titus JM, Moise MA, Bena J, et al. Iliofemoral stenting for venous occlusive disease. *J Vasc Surg*. 2011;53(3):706–12.
32. Adams MK, Anaya-Ayala JE, Davies MG, et al. Endovascular management of iliac vein rupture during percutaneous interventions for occlusive lesions. *Ann Vasc Surg*. 2012 May;26(4):575.e5–9. Epub 2012 Mar 19.
33. Kearon C, Akl EA, Comerota AJ, et al. Antithrombotic therapy for VTE disease. *Chest*. 2012;141(2 suppl):e419S–e494S.
34. Singh R, Mesh CL, Aryaie A, et al. Benefit of a single dose of preoperative antibiotic on surgical site infection in varicose vein surgery. *Ann Vasc Surg*. 2012;26:612–9.
35. De Martino RR, Nolan BW, Powell RJ, et al. Stent Graft repair of iatrogenic femoral arteriovenous fistula: A useful therapeutic approach in a hostile groin. *Vasc and Endovasc Surg*. 2010;44(1):40–3.
36. Kahn SR, Lim W, Dunn AS, et al. Prevention of VTE in nonsurgical patients. *Chest*. 2012;141(2 suppl):e195S–e226S.
37. Azizzadeh A, Pham MT, Estrera AL, et al. Endovascular repair of an iatrogenic superior vena caval injury: A case report. *J Vasc Surg*. 2007;46(3):569–71.
38. Erzurum VZ, Shoup M, Borge M, et al. Inferior vena cava endograft to control surgically inaccessible hemorrhage. *J Vasc Surg*. 2003;38(6):1437–9.

18

Common Femoral Endovenectomy for Postthrombotic Syndrome

Anthony J. Comerota, MD

INTRODUCTION

Natural history studies of anticoagulation for iliofemoral deep venous thrombosis (DVT) treated with anticoagulation alone have shown that, at 5 years, over 90% of patients have venous insufficiency, 15% have experienced venous ulceration, and up to 50% have venous claudication or restricted ambulation.[1,2] Moreover, many demonstrate impaired hemodynamics of venous return resulting in significantly and reduced quality of life.[1-3] A prospective observational study has shown that iliofemoral DVT patients have the most severe postthrombotic morbidity.[4] Unfortunately, most patients are treated with anticoagulation alone rather than a strategy of thrombus removal, as many physicians fail to appreciate the connection between iliofemoral venous obstruction and the subsequent severity of postthrombotic morbidity.

The pathophysiology of postthrombotic venous insufficiency is ambulatory venous hypertension, which is defined as elevated venous pressures during exercise[5,6] and is particularly severe when valvular incompetence and venous obstruction coexist. While valvular function can be quantified through ultrasonography, residual venous obstruction frequently goes undetected, even as it adversely affects venous hemodynamics. This inability to quantitate venous obstruction has led to a widespread under appreciation of its contribution to postthrombotic morbidity. Labropoulous et al.[7] measured venous pressure gradients in a spectrum of patients with postthrombotic venous disease and controls and found that chronic iliofemoral venous occlusion was associated with the highest resting and exercise venous pressure gradients.

Patients with postthrombotic iliac vein obstruction often can be successfully treated with angioplasty and stenting alone,[8,9] but if the chronic occlusive disease includes the common femoral vein (CFV), treatment is more challenging. Following percutaneous intervention, relative obstruction of the CFV can persist, leading to incomplete drainage of the femoral and profunda femoris venous systems and mitigating the benefit of iliac vein recanalization. Although stenting across the inguinal ligament can be performed, the risk of stent occlusion is increased in postthrombotic patients.[8] Moreover, personal observations have demonstrated that when a CFV stent compromises drainage from the profunda femoris veins, the patient's postthrombotic symptoms worsen. Based upon these observations, it seems appropriate to surgically eliminate the CFV obstruction and endoluminally recanalize the obstructed iliocaval segments.

The procedure described in this chapter is indicated for those patients with chronic postthrombotic iliofemoral venous obstruction causing severe postthrombotic syndrome and in whom the CFV is badly obstructed or occluded. The goal of the procedure is to provide unobstructed venous drainage from the profunda femoris vein to the vena cava. To date, we have treated 13 patients with severe postthrombotic iliofemoral/vena caval venous obstruction presenting with clinical class C3-C6 (CEAP classification). The duration of their obstruction ranged from 7 months to 25 years (mean 6.8 years).

OPERATIVE PROCEDURE

Preoperative preparation includes complete phlebography of the target leg, including the inferior vena cava, to document the extent of the patient's venous obstruction (Figure 18-1). A guidewire is maneuvered through the obstructed venous segments to ensure that passage through the occluded venous segments can be achieved and recanalization can be accomplished in the operating room. Two to three days prior to the procedure, patients are started on combined platelet inhibition with aspirin (81 mg/day)

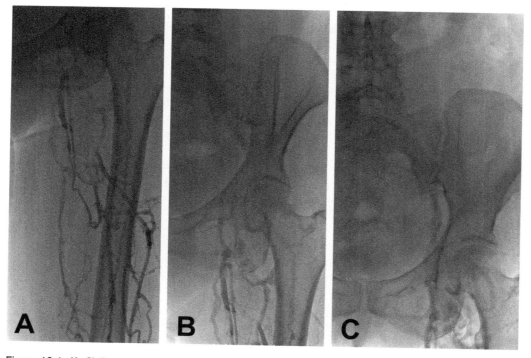

Figure 18-1. (A–C) Preoperative venogram demonstrates extensive venous of obstruction from the mid-thigh to the vena cava in a patient incapacitated following iliofemoral and femoropopliteal DVT seven months earlier. Reprinted from: *Vogel et al, J Vasc Surg. 55(1):129–35,* © *2012,* with permission from Elsevier.

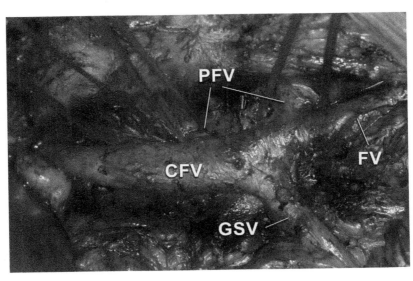

Figure 18-2. Operative exposure of the common femoral vein (CFV), femoral vein (FV), saphenofemoral junction (SFJ), and origins of the profunda femoris veins (PFV). Smaller tributaries are ligated or controlled with vessel loops. Dissection is extended cephalad to under the inguinal ligament exposing the distal external iliac vein (EIV). Reprinted from: *Vogel et al, J Vasc Surg. 55(1):129–35, © 2012*, with permission from Elsevier.

and clopidogrel (75 mg/day). Chlorhexidine showers twice daily are implemented and vitamin K antagonists (VKA) discontinued.

The CFV, common distal external iliac vein, cephalad portion of the femoral vein, and profunda femoris vein are exposed through a standard longitudinal inguinal incision. Control of all branches, especially posterior CFV branches, is obtained. Small tributaries are ligated or controlled with surgical clips (Figure 18-2). Patients are fully anticoagulated with 100 IU/kg of unfractionated heparin (UFH). A longitudinal venotomy is then performed which often incorporates the distal external iliac vein to the proximal femoral vein (Figures 18-3, 18-4). Dense fibrinous tissue and web-like synechiae are removed with sharp and blunt dissection well into the distal external iliac vein (Figure 18-5). Careful attention is given to the orifice of the profunda femoris vein(s) (Figure 18-5). In most patients, sharp excision is required, usually with small angled scissors, as the fibrous evolution of thrombus forms dense adherence to the vein wall. One can generally get an impression as to the proper plane, although the endovenectomy is unlike arterial endarterectomy, where the plaque cleanly peels away from the vessel wall, leaving a smooth arterial wall. Patch closure of the venotomy is performed using bovine pericardium or saphenous vein, leaving the distal centimeter open to introduce an 8 to 10 Fr sheath through which the endoluminal recanalization of the iliac venous segment is performed.

A separate stab incision is made below the inguinal wound through which the sheath is passed, traversing the subcutaneous tissue, and enters the CFV with minimal or no angle. A vascular tourniquet placed around the distal CFV secures the sheath (Figure 18-6). All clamps are left in place to limit the amount of stagnant blood in contact with the thrombogenic vein wall. The iliac venous system and, if necessary, vena cava are sequentially recanalized with guidewire passage, balloon dilation, and subsequent stenting. In general, Wallstents are preferred because of their high radial strength, with 14 to 18 mm stents used for the common iliac veins and 12 to 14 mm for the

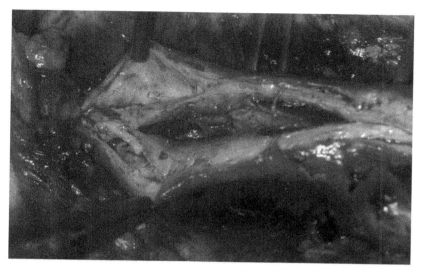

Figure 18-3. A longitudinal venotomy often incorporates the distal external iliac vein to the proximal femoral vein. Fibrotic transformation of occlusive thrombus is observed, with a remaining core of old thrombus. Reprinted from: *Vogel et al, J Vasc Surg. 55(1):129–35,* © *2012,* with permission from Elsevier.

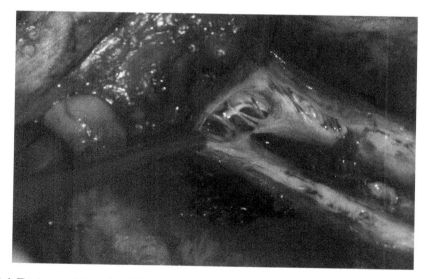

Figure 18-4. The lumen of the external iliac vein is noted to be diseased with the characteristic fibrous webs and synechiae. Reprinted from: *Vogel et al, J Vasc Surg. 55(1):129–35,* © *2012,* with permission from Elsevier.

external iliac veins. Stents are extended partially into the inferior vena cava (IVC), only to fully treat the iliac lesion. Occasionally, a stent may be brought below the inguinal ligament into endovenectomized CFV. It always terminates above the saphenofemoral junction. External iliac stents are placed initially, followed by stenting of the common iliac vein. If IVC stents are required, they will be placed first. Stents are post dilated to their target diameter. We have found intravascular ultrasound (IVUS) valuable in assessing the limits of the procedure and final result, and it is now used routinely.

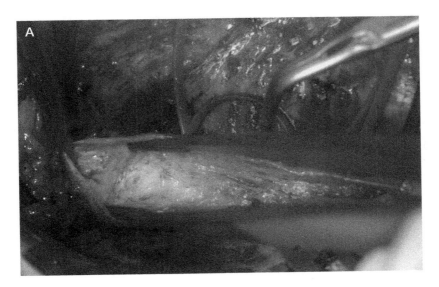

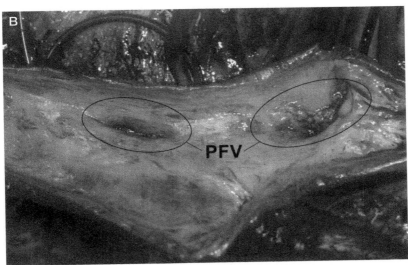

Figure 18-5. (A) Post endovenectomy, the distal external iliac and the common femoral vein is cleared of obstruction, **(B)** with the dissection extending into the orifice(s) of the profunda venous system. Reprinted from: *Vogel et al, J Vasc Surg. 55(1):129–35, © 2012*, with permission from Elsevier.

Following recanalization and venographic confirmation of unobstructed venous drainage from the CFV to the IVC (Figure 18-7), the sheath is removed and closure of the patch venoplasty is completed (Figure 18-8). A 7F silastic closed suction drain is brought through the stab wound used for the sheath and maintained on suction postoperatively until drainage volume is less than 20 cc/12 hrs. The incision is closed with several layers of running absorbable suture, obliterating dead space and ensuring lymphostatic and hemostatic closure of the subcutaneous tissue. Heparin is not reversed with protamine. In some patients, a silastic intravenous catheter was placed in a dorsal foot vein to infuse postoperative heparin; the intent was to achieve high concentrations of heparin in the treated veins while reducing the need for supratherapeutic

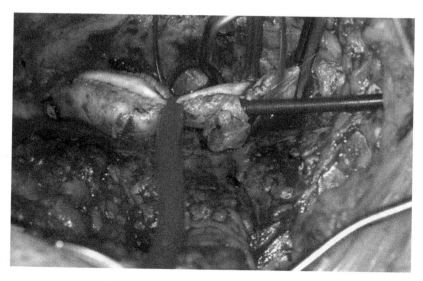

Figure 18-6. A sheath is inserted into the distal CFV and secured by placing a vascular tourniquet around the distal CFV. Clamps on all branch vessels remain in place. Reprinted from: *Vogel et al, J Vasc Surg. 55(1): 129–35*, © *2012*, with permission from Elsevier.

systemic anticoagulation. The remainder received standard intravenous therapeutic UFH infusion. The CFV is examined with a continuous wave Doppler after clamps are removed. If robust venous velocity signals are not present, a small arteriovenous fistula (AVF) is constructed.

Patients are anticoagulated postoperatively with unfractionated heparin converted to warfarin. Since most patients have had recurrent DVT, indefinite anticoagulation is planned. Clopidogrel is discontinued at 8 weeks postoperatively.

OPERATIVE COMPLICATIONS

In our series to date, one operative mortality has occurred: a patient died 9 days after discharge from an acute myocardial infarction. Three patients developed wound hematomas requiring operative evacuation and three developed early postoperative thrombosis. All recurrent thromboses were treated and all patients were discharged with patent reconstructions.

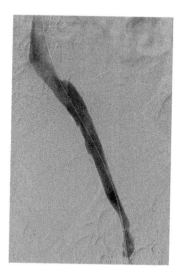

Figure 18-7. Intraoperative venogram following balloon dilation and stenting shows unobstructed drainage from the CFV to the IVC. Reprinted from: *Vogel et al, J Vasc Surg. 55(1):129–35*, © *2012*, with permission from Elsevier.

CLINICAL OUTCOMES

Both preoperative and postoperative evaluations are performed using the Venous Clinical Severity Score (VCSS), the Villalta scale, the clinical classification of CEAP, and completion of the validated VEINES-QOL/Sym questionnaire.

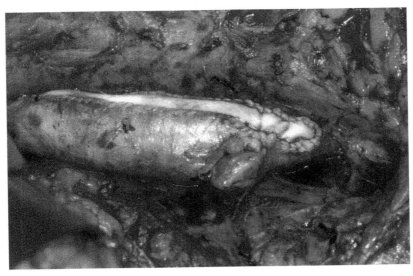

Figure 18-8. Following removal of the sheath, closure of the patch venoplasty is completed. The proximal femoral and saphenous veins were resected. Picture shows CFV patch extending onto the PFV. Reprinted from: *Vogel et al, J Vasc Surg. 55(1):129–35, © 2012*, with permission from Elsevier.

The VCSS identifies 9 clinical characteristics of chronic venous disease that are graded from 0 to 3 (absent, mild, moderate, severe) with specific criteria to avoid overlap or arbitrary scoring.[10] The Villalta scale consists of six clinician-rated physical signs and five patient-rated venous symptoms, of which each are rated on a four-point scale (0 = none, 1 = mild, 2 = moderate, 3 = severe). Points are summed to produce a total score (range 0–33). Subjects are classified as having PTS if the score is ≥5 or if a venous ulcer is present in a leg with previous DVT. The Villalta scale is a validated, reliable method of identifying patients with the postthrombotic syndrome.[11]

The CEAP clinical classification is based on a 7-point clinical assessment of venous disease.[12] The anatomical distribution of venous obstruction included the CFV and iliac venous segments in all patients. The VEINES-QOL/Sym questionnaire is a tool designed to assess quality of life (QOL) and symptoms of chronic venous insufficiency[13,14] and is modeled after the SF-36. All patients are followed at 3, 6, and 12 months and every 6 months thereafter.

In our cohort of patients, all clinical outcome measurements improved at 6 months and after following endovenectomy and iliac recanalization (mean follow-up 8.8 months). The mean preoperative VCSS of 17 dropped to 10 postoperatively (P = .02). Villalta scores improved from a mean of 14 preoperatively to 6 (P = .002). Overall QOL and symptoms improved as assessed by VEINES-QOL/Sym (P = .01 and .02, respectively). Preoperative CEAP scores in the study patients ranged from C4 (pigmentation changes, venous eczema, lipodermatosclerosis) to C5 (healed venous stasis ulceration) and C6 (active venous stasis ulceration).Two patients with preoperative ulcers had a CEAP classification change from 6 to 5 due to their ulcers healing post-endovenectomy. The remaining patients who had preoperative CEAP scores of 4 demonstrated improvement in all their symptoms.

Ultrasound evaluation at follow-up showed one segmental occlusion of the CFV; however, the patient was improved compared to preoperative status. The remaining patients continue to have patent veins.

DISCUSSION

Common femoral endovenectomy with endoluminal iliac vein recanalization is a promising treatment to eliminate proximal venous obstruction and reduce incapacitating postthrombotic morbidity. Since the iliofemoral venous segment is the single venous outflow channel from the leg, it is understandable that obstruction of this segment causes incapacitating morbidity.

As observed in our patient cohort, this procedure has the potential of substantially improving patient function and quality of life. Although the technical details have been previously reported,[15] several key elements are worth emphasizing. Complete control of all branches of the CFV is mandatory, as endovenectomy must be performed in a completely dry field. Ensuring unobstructed venous drainage from the profunda femoris vein into the patent vena cava is mandatory. Although IVUS was not used routinely early in our experience, we have found it to be a valuable adjunct and may have averted one of our early postoperative thromboses. Therefore, its use is now routine.

The construction of an adjunctive AVF was not performed in many cases because of the robust venous velocity signals obtained when the procedure was completed. However, aggressive anticoagulation with combined platelet inhibition led to a return to the operating room for evacuation of wound hematomas in 3 patients, which might have been avoided if AVFs had been constructed and less intense anticoagulation used.

Endovenectomy (or endophlebectomy) has been an infrequently reported procedure for venous obstruction. Early reports of removing obstruction from the superior vena cava[16–18] were followed by the case report of Breslau et al[19] who described successful treatment of an occluded saphenous vein functioning as a bypass graft. Gloviczki and Cho[20] suggested that CFV endovenectomy could be performed and Puggioni et al[21] reported that endovenectomy could be performed as part of a venous reconstructive procedure. More recently, Garg et al[22] described outcomes of 12 patients who underwent CFV endovenectomy, patch angioplasty, and stenting for chronic iliofemoral venous obstruction. They reported rather pessimistic results, which contrast with our observations thus far.

Iliac venous stenting has become the method of choice for correcting iliac venous obstruction.[23] Iliac stenting has for the most part been successful, with primary, assisted-primary, and secondary patency rates of 57%, 80%, and 86%, respectively, in postthrombotic patients, with low complication rates.[8] However, if the stent is extended below the inguinal ligament, there is at least a 3.8-fold risk of stent occlusion in postthrombotic limbs.[8,24] Despite the increased risk of occlusion, many postthrombotic patients require stenting into the CFV to adequately treat skip lesions and areas of residual stenosis which, if left untreated, might lead to recurrent thrombosis.[25,26] We believe that many of the failures in these patients are due to residual and underappreciated obstructive disease in the CFV.

As noted by Raju et al,[25,26] postthrombotic limbs are at a higher risk of recurrent occlusion and are the cause of the majority of failures (82% versus 100% 5-year patency in nonthrombotic iliac vein lesions [NIVL]).

Based upon personal experience, stenting into the distal CFV and potentially restricting drainage from the orifice of the profunda femoris vein in a postthrombotic CFV can lead to further compromise of venous outflow as a result of the stent compressing a fibrous flap across the profunda's orifice. When this occurs, there is notable progression of obstructive symptoms, with increasing edema, pain, and venous claudication.

Chronic central venous obstruction was the overriding pathology in our patients. Although all of our patients also had infrainguinal postthrombotic venous disease with damaged valves, their severe disability resulted from their iliofemoral/caval obstruction. Maleti and Lugli[27,28] reported constructing a neovalve in the femoral vein of patients with postthrombotic syndrome. The neovalve was constructed in patients without proximal obstruction, which is a different subset of patients than reported here. We did not perform any intervention below the common femoral vein.

By performing a hybrid procedure of open endovenectomy and endoluminal iliac recanalization, several important anatomical derangements can be corrected. First, the profunda femoris orifices can be disobliterated, thus allowing maximal drainage from the thigh and lower leg. Second, the multiple recanalization channels of outflow from dense fibrinous tissue with the synechiae in the CFV or CFV occlusions are cleared into the distal external iliac vein. Once completed, the iliac venous stenosis or occlusion can be stented into the endovenectomized portion of the external iliac vein or CFV, ensuring unobstructed flow to the inferior vena cava. This approach avoids skip lesions that might otherwise lead to reocclusion or continued functional compromise. While we attempted to keep stents above the inguinal ligament in the first several patients, we now believe it is reasonable to extend the stents below the inguinal ligament into the endovenectomized CFV if necessary; however, we believe it is imperative to keep the distal end of the stent above the saphenofemoral junction to ensure preservation of profunda femoris venous drainage. In several patients with severe disease of the femoral vein, it was ligated and the cephalad femoral vein resected. Occluded and incompetent saphenous veins are also ligated and the portion exposed within the incision resected.

This procedure has resulted in remarkable improvement in the clinical signs and symptoms of the postthrombotic syndrome in patients followed up to 24 months. No patients have clinically or physiologically deteriorated following their objective outcome assessment. Postoperative morbidity was acceptable, although with refinement of the technique as experience is gained, less operative morbidity should be expected. All patients returned to full daily activities, including employment for those not retired. Both patients with open venous ulcers healed without need for further surgical intervention.

CONCLUSION

Common femoral endovenectomy with iliocaval endoluminal recanalization is a safe and promising procedure for patients with chronic extensive postthrombotic iliofemoral/vena caval venous obstruction. It restores unobstructed venous drainage from the CFV to the vena cava, resulting in improved quality of life and reduced postthrombotic morbidity.

REFERENCES

1. Akesson H, Brudin L, Dahlstrom JA, et al. Venous function assessed during a 5 year period after acute ilio-femoral venous thrombosis treated with anticoagulation. *Eur J Vasc Surg.* 1990;4(1):43–8.
2. Delis KT, Bountouroglou D, Mansfield AO. Venous claudication in iliofemoral thrombosis: Long-term effects on venous hemodynamics, clinical status, and quality of life. *Ann Surg.* 2004;239(1):118–26.

3. Comerota AJ, Throm RC, Mathias SD, et al. Catheter-directed thrombolysis for iliofemoral deep venous thrombosis improves health-related quality of life. *J Vasc Surg.* 2000;32(1):130–7.

4. Kahn SR, Shrier I, Julian JA, et al. Determinants and time course of the postthrombotic syndrome after acute deep venous thrombosis. *Ann Intern Med.* 2008;149(10):698–707.

5. Shull KC, Nicolaides AN, Fernandes e Fernandes J, et al. Significance of popliteal reflux in relation to ambulatory venous pressure and ulceration. *Arch Surg.* 1979;114(11):1304–6.

6. Nicolaides AN, Schull K, Fernandes E. Ambulatory venous pressure: New information. In: Nicolaides AN, Yao JS, editors. *Investigation of Vascular Disorders.*New York: Churchill Livingstone; 1981. p. 488–94.

7. Labropoulos N, Volteas N, Leon M, et al. The role of venous outflow obstruction in patients with chronic venous dysfunction. *Arch Surg.* 1997;132(1):46–51.

8. Neglen P, Hollis KC, Olivier J, et al. Stenting of the venous outflow in chronic venous disease: Long-term stent-related outcome, clinical, and hemodynamic result. *J Vasc Surg.* 2007;46(5):979–90.

9. Kolbel T, Lindh M, Akesson M, et al. Chronic iliac vein occlusion: Midterm results of endovascular recanalization. *J Endovasc Ther.* 2009;16(4):483–91.

10. Meissner MH, Natiello C, Nicholls SC. Performance characteristics of the venous clinical severity score. *J Vasc Surg.* 2002;36(5):889–95.

11. Kahn SR. Measurement properties of the Villalta scale to define and classify the severity of the post-thrombotic syndrome. *J Thromb Haemost.* 2009;7(5):884–8.

12. Eklof B, Rutherford RB, Bergan JJ, et al. Revision of the CEAP classification for chronic venous disorders: Consensus statement. *J Vasc Surg.* 2004;40(6):1248–52.

13. Kahn SR, Lamping DL, Ducruet T, et al. VEINES-QOL/Sym questionnaire was a reliable and valid disease-specific quality of life measure for deep venous thrombosis. *J Clin Epidemiol.* 2006;59(10):1049–56.

14. Lamping DL, Schroter S, Kurz X, et al. Evaluation of outcomes in chronic venous disorders of the leg: Development of a scientifically rigorous, patient-reported measure of symptoms and quality of life. *J Vasc Surg.* 2003;37(2):410–9.

15. Comerota AJ, Grewal NK, Thakur S, et al. Endovenectomy of the common femoral vein and intraoperative iliac vein recanalization for chronic iliofemoral venous occlusion. *J Vasc Surg.* 2010;52(1):243–7.

16. Blondeau P, Wapler C, Piwnica A, et al. Deux cas de syndrome de la veine cava superierure trates chirurgicalement avec succes, l'un par desobstruction, l'autra par greffe. *Arch Mal Couer.* 1959;52:504.

17. O'Neill TH. In discussion of Scannel, J.C. and Shaw, R.S. Surgical reconstruction of the superior vena cava. *J Thor Surg.* 1954;28:163.

18. Templeton JY, III. Endvenectomy for the relief of obstruction of the superior vena cava. *Am J Surg.*1962;104:70–6.

19. Breslau RC, DeWeese JA. Successful endophlebectomy of autogenous venous bypass graft. *Ann Surg.* 1965;162:251–4.

20. Gloviczki P, Cho JS. Surgical treatment of chronic deep venous obstruction. In: Rutherford RB, editor. *Vascular Surgery.* 5th ed. New York: Elsevier; 2001. p. 2099–165.

21. Puggioni A, Kistner RL, Eklof B, et al. Surgical disobliteration of postthrombotic deep veins—endophlebectomy—is feasible. *J Vasc Surg.* 2004;39(5):1048–52.

22. Garg N, Gloviczki P, Karimi KM, et al. Factors affecting outcome of open and hybrid reconstructions for nonmalignant obstruction of iliofemoral veins and inferior vena cava. *J Vasc Surg.* 2011;53(2):383–93.

23. Meissner MH, Eklof B, Smith PC, et al. Secondary chronic venous disorders. *J Vasc Surg.* 2007;46 Suppl S:68S–83S.

24. Neglen P, Raju S. In-stent recurrent stenosis in stents placed in the lower extremity venous outflow tract. *J Vasc Surg.* 2004;39(1):181–7.

25. Raju S, Darcey R, Neglen P. Unexpected major role for venous stenting in deep reflux disease. *J Vasc Surg*. 2010;51(2):401–8.
26. Raju S, McAllister S, Neglen P. Recanalization of totally occluded iliac and adjacent venous segments. *J Vasc Surg*. 2002;36(5):903–11.
27. Lugli M, Guerzoni S, Garofalo M, et al. Neovalve construction in deep venous incompetence. *J Vasc Surg*. 2009;49(1):156–62, 162.
28. Maleti O, Lugli M. Neovalve construction in postthrombotic syndrome. *J Vasc Surg*. 2006;43(4):794–9.

19

Isolated Distal Deep Venous Thrombosis

Shipra Arya MD, SM and Peter K. Henke, MD

INTRODUCTION

Proximal lower extremity deep venous thrombosis (DVT) has been extensively studied in the last few decades and streamlined treatment guidelines have been well-established. However, management of distal lower extremity or *calf* DVT has been a matter of debate. The controversy stems from variable occurrence of proximal extension of the clot, risk of pulmonary embolism (PE) and risk of post-thrombotic syndrome.

ANATOMIC NOMENCLATURE

Distal lower extremity deep venous system is classified into two types: deep axial and muscular calf veins. The deep axial calf veins (DCV) include paired tibial (anterior and posterior tibial) and peroneal veins. They travel with the named arteries and each pair forms a confluent segment before draining into a trifurcation pattern to form the popliteal vein. Muscular calf veins (MCV) are the gastrocnemius and soleal veins. Gastrocnemius veins drain into the popliteal vein while the soleal veins drain into the posterior tibial or peroneal veins. There is debate whether muscular calf vein thrombosis should be classified as a DVT. Isolated distal (or *calf*) deep venous thrombosis (IDDVT), therefore, can be either deep calf vein thrombosis (DCVT) or muscular calf vein thrombosis (MCVT).

DIAGNOSIS OF IDDVT

The diagnosis of IDDVT is usually made on duplex ultrasound with compression. This has largely replaced venography that used to be gold standard for detection of DVT. The distal veins are difficult to image as compared to proximal veins and ultrasound is user dependent. The overall sensitivity and specificity of compression ultrasound is not

TABLE 19-1. EPIDEMIOLOGY AND NATURAL HISTORY OF ISOLATED DISTAL DVT (IDDVT) AND MUSCULAR CALF VENOUS THROMBOSIS (MCVT)

	IDDVT	MCVT only
Risk of clot propogation	3.8–32% [15]	3.7% [17]–16.3% [16]
Risk of clot propagation proximally	2.9–17.9% [15]	1.9% [17]–3% [16]
Presence of PE at diagnosis of IDDVT	5–56% [15]	7–50% [11, 19]
Risk of PE in follow up	0–6.2% [15]	0 [17]–4.6% [11]

PE: Pulmonary embolism

as good for distal veins as compared to proximal veins, but generally >90%.[1,2] The institutional protocols also vary in terms of compression ultrasonography limited to proximal veins instead of whole leg ultrasound or to include muscular calf veins as part of the DVT ultrasound scan. Recent studies have shown that recognition of lower extremity DVT using ultrasonography of the proximal veins (along with use of pretest probability and D-Dimer) or whole-leg ultrasonography, for symptomatic patients with suspected DVT, have equivalent results in terms of occurrence of symptomatic venous thromboembolic events at follow up.[3,4] These issues call into question whether diagnosis of IDDVT is clinically important. The latest American College of Chest Physicians Evidence-Based Clinical Practice Guidelines emphasize the use of pre-test clinical probability to diagnose distal DVT.[5] If isolated distal DVT is detected on whole-leg US, they suggest serial testing to rule out proximal extension over treatment (Grade 2C). In patients with high pretest probability, moderately or highly sensitive D-dimer assays should not be used as stand-alone tests to rule out DVT (Grade 1B).

Epidemiology and Natural History of IDDVT (Table 19-1)

The prevalence of IDDVT ranges from about 7 to 11% in suspected PE, and 4 to 15% in cases of suspected DVT. In patients with an established DVT by imaging, the proportion of IDDVTs varies between 23.4% and 59.7%.[6]

Some authors believe that DVT begins in calf veins, especially the soleal veins, and extends proximally.[7,8] Various studies describe the soleal[7–11] or the peroneal vein [12,13] as the most common site of thrombosis in the distal lower extremity. Thrombus in only a single or paired vein is found anywhere between 35–64% of the cases.[12,14] Multifocal origin of DVT, defined as thrombosis in at least two veins that do not anatomically communicate, is found in 22% of cases.[12]

Distal lower extremity thrombi propagate either proximally, distally or both. The most common area of propagation is the popliteal followed by femoral and common femoral veins. The risk of progression of thrombus to popliteal vein or higher is 2.9–17.9% in all IDDVTs[15] whereas only 2–3% of MCVTs propagate proximally.[16,17] Thombus can also propagate to adjacent tibial and soleal veins as well as contralateral thrombi develop in one fifth of the cases. Bilateral calf thrombi are present in 19% at presentation and 8% develop it during followup.[18] Muscular calf vein thrombosis (MCVT) is associated with PE with a prevalence of 7% to 50% at the time of diagnosis.[11,19]. Similarly IDDVT is associated with a 5–56% prevalence of PE.[15] It is impossible to say in these situations whether the calf vein or a proximal vein is the source of the pulmonary embolus. After diagnosis of IDDVT, the risk of future PE is much lower (0–6.2%).[15] Complete lysis of calf thrombi was found in 60–88% of the cases by

3 months without anticoagulation.[13,16,17] In those treated with anticoagulation, clot lysis was 96% at 6 months.[11]

Muscular calf vein thromboses usually present with pain while the deep axial calf vein thromboses are more often associated with swelling.[11,20] Up to one third of distal DVTs are asymptomatic at presentation.[21] During longer followup, persistent symptoms including pain, edema and pigmentation are found in 25–40% of patients. [21,22] Post thrombotic syndrome is of variable severity, with severe symptoms in 5% of patients.[23] Valvular reflux by duplex scanning of ipsilateral leg varies from 9–50%.[13,15] The rate of ulceration also varies from 0 to 11% after calf DVT.[13,21,22.]

Risk Factors for IDDVT (Table 19-2)

Patients with isolated calf DVT are usually younger, less likely to have a history of prior VTE, and tend to have fewer co-morbid conditions. They are more likely to have had a provoked event such as a recent surgery or a recent fracture, especially in the case of MCVT.[24] Galanaud et al compared risk factors for MCVT and DCVT and found recent surgery was significantly more associated with DCVT.[20] However, most studies to date on IDDVT have not included patients with hypercoagulable states and idiopathic VTE. A few studies, though, have shown a higher complication rate with idiopathic IDDVT.[25,26] Malignancy also seems to be a risk factor for bilateral IDDVT, as well as recurrence and complications of calf DVTs.[20,25]

TABLE 19-2. RISK FACTORS FOR ISOLATED DISTAL DEEP VEIN THROMBOSIS (IDDVT)[11,16,18,20,24]

IDDVT	DCVT only	MCVT only
Inpatient status	Hormone replacement therapy	Active cancer[a]
Younger age	Recent surgery (≤45 days)	Age >75 years[a]
Recent fracture	Recent plaster immobilization of lower limb(s)	Recent travel
Recent surgery		Recent surgery
		Recent trauma

[a]Bilateral MCVT
DCVT: Deep calf vein thrombosis; MCVT: Muscular calf vein thrombosis

Evidence for Treating IDDVT

The rationale for treating IDDVT lies in risk of thrombus propagation, pulmonary embolism, and post-thrombotic syndrome. Of these outcomes, numerous studies have now clearly shown prevention of thrombus propagation with anticoagulation.[10,13,18,27–29] Lagerstedt et al conducted a randomized control trial (RCT) on 51 patients comparing warfarin treatment of symptomatic IDDVT for 3 months versus no warfarin after a short course of intravenous heparin for 5 days in both groups. They showed no recurrences of VTE or proximal propagation of thrombus in the warfarin group at 3 months while the control group had 8 occurrences, including a pulmonary embolus.[27] Ferrara et al showed that the risk of progression of clot into femoral or popliteal veins with thromboses involving 2 or more distal veins is significantly higher than with thrombotic lesions confined to one distal vein.[14] Other risk factors associated with progression of thrombus include unprovoked or idiopathic DVT,[25,26,30] malignancy,[25] and initial clot burden.[11,19] Interestingly, an ultrasound finding of bilateral MCVT has a worse prognosis for all-cause mortality as compared to unilateral disease at 3-months (17.4% vs 6.1%).[20]

The risk of pulmonary embolism has not been as clearly established as thrombus propagation in the absence of anticoagulation. Lagerstedt et al had one PE event in the no anticoagulation arm of their RCT and no events in the warfarin arm.[27] Kakkar et al. showed clinically apparent pulmonary embolism in four of the nine patients in whom proximal propagation occurred with venographically documented postoperative DVT. [31] Asymptomatic deep axial vein DVT (DCVT) following total hip arthroplasty was studied in a prospective blinded trial by Pelligrini et al. No anticoagulation was associated with a significant risk of developing clinically evident pulmonary embolism within the first 8 weeks after operation.[29]

Post thrombotic syndrome (PTS) can develop after IDDVT with incidence rates similar to proximal vein DVT- mild PTS~ 21% and mod-severe PTS~5%.[23] Labropoulus et al showed that multiple calf vein segment involvement had more frequent and more significant PTS than thrombosis in a single calf vein. Calf vein involvement in the presence of proximal DVT was also found to increase the likelihood of PTS.[32]

Evidence Against Treating IDDVT

A recent randomized control trial comparing two point ultrasonography of proximal veins (common femoral and popliteal) to whole leg ultrasound for DVT showed higher initial prevalence of DVT in the whole-leg group compared with the 2-point group (absolute difference, 4.3%; 95% CI, 0.5%–8.1%), all of which was accounted for by 65 cases of IDDVT. However, the long-term outcome in terms of symptomatic venous thromboembolism was quite similar in the two groups. The authors speculated the need for recognition and anticoagulation of IDDVT cases and exposing them to increased risk of bleeding if there is no benefit in decreasing the future risk of VTE events.[3] Anticoagulation is associated with variable risk of bleeding in IDDVT patients, with major bleeding incidence around 0–4% [16,17,25,27] and overall bleeding risk upto 25%.[25] Longer duration of therapy is associated with increased risk of overall bleeding. [25]

Solis et al showed that IDDVT proximal propagation after total hip or knee arthroplasty was not influenced by anticoagulation. All thrombus propagations were detected within 2 weeks of the operative procedure. There were no pulmonary emboli or deaths, suggesting that postoperative IDDVT need not be routinely treated.[33] With regards to muscular calf vein thrombosis (MCVT), two studies[16,17] have shown a low risk of progression to proximal clot propagation (1.9–3%) and no occurrence of pulmonary embolism. Like Solis et al, they also showed that the risk of clot propagation was the highest within the first two weeks. Gillet et al did show a higher risk of pulmonary embolism in patients with untreated MCVT (~4.6%) but all except one case presented with extended MCVTs (several veins involved by the thrombosis), and all had a large venous thrombosis (diameter > 8 mm).[11] These findings suggest that IDDVT should be treated differently with regards to axial/muscular vein involvement, single/multiple calf vein thrombosis and extent of clot burden.

THERAPY AND CURRENT RECOMMENDATIONS

Various therapeutic strategies for anticoagulation have been proposed and studied in addition to lower extremity compression and ambulation for management of IDDVT.

Pinede et al showed that 6 weeks of anticoagulation is sufficient for IDDVT compared to a 12 week course while Lagerstedt et al used oral warfarin for 3 months in an RCT but did not compare it to a shorter duration of therapy.[25,27] In contrast, Ferrara et al have shown a 12 week course of warfarin to be superior to a 6 week duration therapy, at preventing thrombus propagation when 2 or more distal veins are involved.

According to the latest guidelines from ACCP, patients with severe symptoms and risk factors for extension are more likely to benefit from treatment over repeat US (Grade 2C). In patients with acute isolated distal DVT of the leg and without severe symptoms or risk factors for extension, serial imaging of the deep veins for 2 weeks is preferred over initial anticoagulation (Grade 2C). Patients at high risk for bleeding are more likely to benefit from serial imaging. Patients who place a high value on avoiding the inconvenience of repeat imaging and a low value on the inconvenience of treatment and on the potential for bleeding are likely to choose initial anticoagulation over serial imaging.

In patients with acute isolated distal DVT of the leg who are managed with initial anticoagulation, the therapy is the same as acute proximal DVT; i.e. 3 months of anticoagulation (Grade 1B). After 3 months of treatment, patients with unprovoked DVT of the leg should be evaluated for the risk-benefit ratio of extended therapy. In patients with acute isolated distal DVT of the leg who are managed with serial imaging, no anticoagulation is recommended if the thrombus does not extend (Grade 1B); anticoagulation if the thrombus extends but remains confined to the distal veins (Grade 2C); anticoagulation if the thrombus extends into the proximal veins (Grade 1B).

CONCLUSIONS

Management of isolated distal deep venous thrombosis is a controversial subject. While there is a definite risk of clot propagation in the absence of anticoagulation, the clinical importance and risk of further VTE events are poorly quantified. The consequences of treatment in terms of bleeding complications, mortality risk, and economic ramifications remain to be studied. A recent metaanalysis showed that anticoagulation therapy for IDDVT significantly reduces proximal thrombi propagation while no conclusions can be made regarding the effects of anticoagulation for clinically important outcomes such as PE, death, and bleeding.[34] A Cochrane review recently published also inferred that current data does not support a universal recommendation for treating IDDVT but the authors added "the option of no specific therapy other than support stockings and ignoring the calf is inappropriate given the established reality of clot propagation, clot recurrence, and small but not insignificant risk of PE".[15]

Based on the evidence summarized in this chapter, the following algorithm is proposed by us (Figure 19-1). We believe that IDDVT needs to be treated taking into account the risk factors, involvement of axial or muscular calf veins, risk of bleeding, and extent of clot burden. Adequately powered randomized clinical trials are needed in the future to answer the specific questions of clinical relevance of IDDVT, risk of VTE events, need for anticoagulation and duration of therapy.[35]

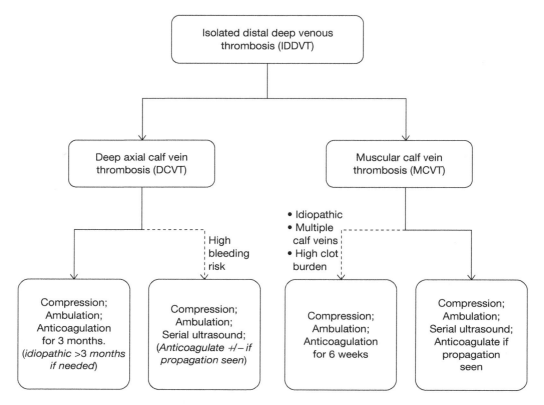

Figure 19-1. Treatment algorithm for Isolated Distal Deep Venous Thrombosis (IDDVT) (Solid arrows indicate preferred treatment strategy).

REFERENCES

1. Schellong, S.M., Complete compression ultrasonography of the leg veins as a single test for the diagnosis of deep vein thrombosis. *J Thromb Haemost*. 2003;89(2):228–34.
2. Goodacre, S., Systematic review and meta-analysis of the diagnostic accuracy of ultrasonography for deep vein thrombosis. *BMC Med Imaging*. 2005;5(1):6.
3. Bernardi, E., et al., Serial 2-Point Ultrasonography Plus D-Dimer vs Whole-Leg Color-Coded Doppler Ultrasonography for Diagnosing Suspected Symptomatic Deep Vein ThrombosisA Randomized Controlled Trial. *JAMA*. 2008;300(14):1653–1659.
4. Gibson, N.S., et al., Safety and sensitivity of two ultrasound strategies in patients with clinically suspected deep venous thrombosis: a prospective management study. *J Thromb Haemost*. 2009;7(12):2035–2041.
5. Bates, S.M., Diagnosis of DVT: Antithrombotic Therapy and Prevention of Thrombosis, 9th ed: American College of Chest Physicians Evidence-Based Clinical Practice Guidelines. *Chest*. 2012;141(2 suppl):e351S–418S.
6. Palareti, G. and S. Schellong, Isolated distal deep vein thrombosis: what we know and what we are doing. *J Thromb Haemost*. 2012;10(1):11–19.
7. Rollins, D.L., et al., Origin of deep vein thrombi in an ambulatory population. *AmJ Surg*. 1988;156(2):122–125.
8. Nicolaides, A.N., et al., The origin of deep vein thrombosis: a venographic study. *Br J Rad*. 1971;44(525):653–663.
9. Lohr, J.M., et al., Lower extremity calf thrombosis: To treat or not to treat? *J Vasc Surg*. 1991;14(5):618–623.

10. Schwarz, T., Therapy of isolated calf muscle vein thrombosis with low-molecular-weight heparin. *Blood Coagul Fibrinolysis*. 2001;12(7):597–9.
11. Gillet, J.-L., M.R. Perrin, and F.A. Allaert, Short-term and mid-term outcome of isolated symptomatic muscular calf vein thrombosis. *J Vasc Surg*. 2007;46(3):513–519.
12. Labropoulos, N., et al., Patterns and distribution of isolated calf deep vein thrombosis. *J Vasc Surg*. 1999;30(5):787–793.
13. Masuda, E.M., et al., The natural history of calf vein thrombosis: Lysis of thrombi and development of reflux. *J Vasc Surg*. 1998;28(1):67–74.
14. Ferrara, F., et al., Optimal Duration of Treatment in Surgical Patients With Calf Venous Thrombosis Involving One or More Veins. *Angiology*. 2006;57(4):418–423.
15. Masuda, E.M., et al., The controversy of managing calf vein thrombosis. *J Vasc Surg*. 2012;55(2):550–561.
16. MacDonald, P.S., et al., Short-term natural history of isolated gastrocnemius and soleal vein thrombosis. *J Vasc Surg*. 2003;37(3):523–527.
17. Schwarz, T., et al., Therapy of isolated calf muscle vein thrombosis: A randomized, controlled study. *J Vasc Surg*. 2010;52(5):1246–1250.
18. Lohr, J.M., et al., Calf vein thrombi are not a benign finding. *Am J Surg*. 1995;170(2):86–90.
19. Ohgi, S., Pulmonary embolism in patients with isolated soleal vein thrombosis. *Angiology*. 1998;49(9):759–64.
20. Galanaud, J.-P., et al., Comparison of the clinical history of symptomatic isolated muscular calf vein thrombosis versus deep calf vein thrombosis. *J Vasc Surg*. 2010;52(4): 932–938.e2.
21. Saarinen, J., Post-thrombotic symptoms after an isolated calf deep venous thrombosis. *J Cardiovasc Surg*. 2002;43(5):687–91.
22. Meissner, M.H., et al., Early outcome after isolated calf vein thrombosis. *J Vasc Surg*. 1997;26(5):749–756.
23. Prandoni, P., Symptomatic deep-vein thrombosis and the post-thrombotic syndrome. *Haematologica*. 1995;80(2 suppl):42–8.
24. Spencer, F.A., Isolated calf deep vein thrombosis in the community setting: the Worcester Venous Thromboembolism study. *J Thromb Thrombolysis*. 2012;33(3):211–7.
25. Pinede, L., et al., Comparison of 3 and 6 Months of Oral Anticoagulant Therapy After a First Episode of Proximal Deep Vein Thrombosis or Pulmonary Embolism and Comparison of 6 and 12 Weeks of Therapy After Isolated Calf Deep Vein Thrombosis. *Circulation*. 2001;103(20):2453–2460.
26. Parisi, R., Isolated distal deep vein thrombosis: efficacy and safety of a protocol of treatment. Treatment of Isolated Calf Thrombosis (TICT) Study. *Int Angiol*. 2009;28(1):68–72.
27. Lagerstedt, C.I., Need for long-term anticoagulant treatment in symptomatic calf-vein thrombosis. *Lancet*. 1985;2(8454):515–8.
28. Labropoulos, N., et al., Early Thrombus Remodelling of Isolated Calf Deep Vein Thrombosis. *Eur J Vasc Endovasc Surg*. 2002;23(4):344–348.
29. Pellegrini Jr, V.D., et al., Embolic complications of calf thrombosis following total hip arthroplasty. The Journal of Arthroplasty, 1993;8(5):449–457.
30. Astermark, J., et al., Low recurrence rate after deep calf-vein thrombosis with 6 weeks of oral anticoagulation. *J Intern Med*. 1998;244(1):79–82.
31. Kakkar, V.V., Natural history of postoperative deep-vein thrombosis. *Lancet*. 1969; 2(7614):230–2.
32. Labropoulos, N., et al., The effect of venous thrombus location and extent on the development of post-thrombotic signs and symptoms. *J Vasc Surg*. 2008;48(2):407–412.
33. Solis, M.M., et al., Is anticoagulation indicated for asymptomatic postoperative calf vein thrombosis? *J Vasc Surg*. 1992;16(3):414–419.
34. De Martino, R.R., et al., A meta-analysis of anticoagulation for calf deep venous thrombosis. *J Vasc Surg*. 2012.
35. Horner, D., The Anticoagulation of Calf Thrombosis (ACT) project: study protocol for a randomized controlled trial. *Trials*. 2012;13(1):31.

20

Algorithm for Bulging Varicose Veins

Marc A. Passman, MD

INTRODUCTION

Bulging varicose veins are dilated subcutaneous veins in the lower extremity that are >3 mm in diameter measured in the upright position, and may represent isolated primary varicosities or may be secondary to associated superficial, deep, and/or perforator insufficiency. The potential for primary varicose veins without associated axial or segmental reflux, dilated reticular veins, and venous telangiectases most commonly is from an intrinsic abnormality in the vein wall. On the other end of the spectrum, secondary varicose veins is associated with superficial venous insufficiency involving incompetence of the great saphenous vein (GSV), small saphenous vein (SSV) or saphenous branch systems, resulting in a branch pattern varicosities. Venous insufficiency can be isolated to the superficial venous system, or can include concomitant deep and perforator disease all of which can manifest as bulging varicose veins and can make decision making more complex.

Fortunately, bulging varicose veins especially when associated with superficial venous insufficiency are very amenable to surgical correction. Identification of superficial axial sources of reflux is important and when present treatment should include therapy directed at the source of superficial reflux in conjunction with varicose vein approaches, while secondary varicose veins in the absence of axial sources of refluxes can be treated directly. This chapter will review treatment of bulging varicose veins including evidence based guidelines, operative approaches, clinical decision making factors, and propose an algorithm for treatment.

EVIDENCE BASED GUIDELINES

Clinical practice guidelines of the Society for Vascular Surgery and the American Venous Forum published in 2011 provide a reasonable framework for clinical decision making based on current evidence. Recommendations are based on the Grading of Recommendations Assessment, Development, and Evaluation (GRADE) system, with the

TABLE 20-1. EVIDENCE BASED GUIDELINES FOR TREATMENT OF SUPERFICIAL VENOUS INSUFFICIENCY AND VARICOSE VEINS

Medical therapy

- Venoactive drugs (diosmin, hesperidin, rutosides, sulodexide, micronized purified flavonoid fraction, or horse chestnut seed extract [aescin]) in addition to compression for patients with pain and swelling due to chronic venous disease, in countries where these drugs are available. (Grade 2B)

- Pentoxifylline or micronized purified flavonoid fraction, if available, in combination with compression, to accelerate healing of venous ulcers is suggested. (Grade 2B)

Compression therapy

- Compression therapy using moderate pressure (20 to 30 mm Hg) for patients with symptomatic varicose veins. (Grade 2C)

- Against compression therapy as the primary treatment of symptomatic varicose veins in patients who are candidates for saphenous vein ablation. (Grade 1B)

- Compression as the primary therapeutic modality for healing venous ulcers. (Grade 1B)

- Compression as an adjuvant treatment to superficial vein ablation for the prevention of ulcer recurrence. (Grade 1A)

Endovenous thermal ablation

- Endovenous thermal ablations (laser and radiofrequency ablations) are safe and effective for treatment of saphenous incompetence. (Grade 1B)

- Because of reduced convalescence and less pain and morbidity, endovenous thermal ablation of the incompetent saphenous vein preferred over open surgery. (Grade 1B)

Open venous surgery

- For treatment of the incompetent great saphenous vein, high ligation and inversion stripping of the saphenous vein to the level of the knee. (Grade 2B)

- To reduce hematoma formation, pain, and swelling, postoperative compression in C2 patients for 1 week. (Grade 1B)

- For treatment of small saphenous vein incompetence, high ligation of the vein at the knee crease, about 3 to 5 cm distal to the saphenopopliteal junction, with selective invagination stripping of the incompetent portion of the vein. (Grade 1 B)

- To decrease recurrence of venous ulcers, ablation of the incompetent superficial veins in addition to compression therapy. (Grade 1A)

- Ambulatory phlebectomy for treatment of varicose veins, performed with saphenous vein ablation, either during the same procedure or at a later stage. If general anesthesia is required for phlebectomy, we suggest concomitant saphenous ablation. (Grade 1B)

- Transilluminated powered phlebectomy using lower oscillation speeds and extended tumescence as an alternative to traditional phlebectomy for extensive varicose veins. (Grade 2C)

- For treatment of recurrent varicose veins, ligation of the saphenous stump, ambulatory phlebectomy, sclerotherapy, or endovenous thermal ablation, depending on the etiology, source, location, and extent of varicosity. (Grade 2C)

Sclerotherapy

- Liquid or foam sclerotherapy recommended for telangiectasia, reticular veins, and varicose veins. (Grade 1B)

- For treatment of the incompetent saphenous vein, endovenous thermal ablation recommended over chemical ablation with foam. (Grade 1B)

Adapted from: Gloviczki P et al. The care of patients with varicose veins and associated chronic venous diseases: Clinical practice guidelines of the Society for Vascular Surgery and the American Venous Forum. J Vasc Surg. 2011;53:2S–48S.)

level of current evidence documented by A, B, C, and the strength of the recommendation rated as strong (1) or weak (2). The guidelines specific to treatment of superficial venous reflux including compression, endovenous thermal ablation, open superficial venous operations, and sclerotherapy proposed in this consensus statement are shown in Table 20-1, with supporting documents as listed in selected references [1–24].

OPERATIVE TECHNIQUES

Endovenous Thermal Ablation

Endovenous thermal ablation of the GSV or SSV systems with laser, radiofrequency or steam energy is usually performed as an outpatient procedure under local tumescent anesthesia. Using ultrasound guidance, percutaneous access is obtained in the target vein followed by wire, sheath and fiber position confirmed 1–2 cms from saphenofemoral junction for GSV and saphenopopliteal junction for SSV. Treatment is usually limited to the above the knee segment to avoid injury to the saphenous nerve which is in close proximity to the GSV in the calf, and limited to only a short segment of SSV to avoid injury to the sural nerve. Tumescence solution including lidocaine, epinephrine, and bicarbonate is infiltrated along the course of the saphenous vein to provide local anesthesia, localized vasoconstriction, extrinsic compression, and a heat sink barrier. Using a timed pullback of the laser or radiofrequency catheter, occlusion of saphenous vein is achieved by controlled heat delivered into the vein causing direct thermal injury to the vein wall causing endothelial destruction, collagen denaturation of the media, and thrombotic occlusion of the vein resulting in eventual fibrosis of the vein.

Complication rates are low including pain, bruising, hematoma, wound complications, and nerve injury. While there is occasional evidence of endovenous heat induced thrombosis extending into the deeper veins, deep venous thrombosis and pulmonary embolism is rare. Occlusion rates have ranged from 75% to 92% for radiofrequency, and 88%–100% for laser.

High Ligation, Division and Stripping

High ligation and division refers to detachment of the GSV through a small oblique groin incision at its confluence with the saphenofemoral junction and common femoral vein. Incision is usually located along the groin crease. Duplex ultrasound guidance can be used to limit incision size while still allowing appropriate visualization of the saphenofemoral junction and its tributaries. Through the groin incision, the subcutaneous plane over the GSV and saphenofemoral junction is developed. Understanding anatomic relationships and branch anatomy of the GSV at this location is important for most effective ligation technique. Most commonly, branch tributary veins at the saphenofemoral junction include inferior epigastric vein, superficial circumflex iliac vein, superficial external pudendal vein, deep external pudendal vein, lateral accessory saphenous vein, and medial accessory saphenous vein. It is important to identify and ligate all tributaries at the saphenofemoral junction to prevent persistent superficial venous flow directly into femoral vein and potential for recurrent reflux and varicosities. Flush ligation of the GSV at the saphenofemoral junction without narrowing of the femoral vein is performed to avoid a residual GSV stump as a potential source for thrombus formation and pulmonary embolism. Resection of the proximal 5–10 cm of GSV is performed through the exposed surgical field with distal ligation.

Stripping refers to removal of an extended segment of the GSV either with external stripper, intraluminal stripper (such as Codman or Myer) or perforation-invagination (PIN) stripper (such as Oesch). Most GSV reflux patterns will include thigh segment which is most routinely included in stripping. GSVstripping below the knee is rarely performed to avoid possible saphenous nerve injury, unless it is obviously incompetent with clinically significant reflux or in the setting of recurring calf varicosities. Through the groin exposure described for high ligation and division, and a distal counter incision at the level of intended stripping typically at the knee or ankle, using the intraluminal technique, the GSV is typically secured to the tip of the stripper with inversion of the vein as the stripper is pulled down through the distal incision. GSV stripping in the downward direction using the largest stripper head possible and use of a heavy silk suture attached to the GSV prior to stripping then allows recovery of the entire stripped GSV segment and tributaries back through the proximal groin incision thereby limiting the size of the distal incision. For PIN technique, a rod is used to puncture the vein and a small exit skin incision is used to retrieve the stripper and disconnected invaginated GSV. Expansion of PIN stripper techniques as well as additional techniques using ultrasound guidance for smaller incisions, tumescence anesthesia, leg elevation during stripping, and immediate compression wraps to decrease blood in the tunnel have led to less invasive options for stripping and more of shift into the outpatient setting than in the past.

For ligation, division, and stripping, reported complications include discomfort, bruising, bleeding, wound infection, deep venous thrombosis, and nerve injury which can range from temporary numb patches to neuropraxia along the sapheneous nerve distribution for GSV and sural nerve distribution for SSV based approaches. Potential for neoangiogensis at the saphenofemoral junction and recurrent varicosities has also been described.

Ambulatory Phlebectomy

Ambulatory phlebectomy techniques fall under various descriptors such as excisional phlebectomy, stab avulsion phlebectomy, hook phlebectomy, and micro-puncture phlebectomy. While the terminology can be confusing, the basic technique is the essentially the same. With advances in tumescence anesthesia, these phlebectomy techniques are able to be performed in the outpatient setting, are associated with low complications, high patient satisfaction, excellent cosmesis, and have become a safe and effective method for varicose vein removal. The positions of the varicosities are marked with the patient standing. For phlebectomy in the outpatient setting, tumescent anesthesia is infiltrated along the marked varicosities. Multiple tiny incisions are made with #11 blade, beaver blade, ophthalmic blade, or puncture hole using a large needle. With use of small profile phlebectomy hooks (such as Muller, Oesch, Tretbar, Ramelet, Varady or Dortu-Martimbeau), the targeted varicosity is brought up through the small incision and grasped with a hemostat or forcep for further mobilization and avulsion. Incisions are usually too small for suture and are brought together with steristrips.

There are some limitations with ambulatory phlebectomy, including need for multiple incisions, poor visualization, potential for incomplete resection, and technical challenges for patients with extensive varicosities. Potential complications associated with ambulatory phlebectomy are also low, mostly appearance related, and usually transient. Complaints can include allergic reaction to local anesthetic, skin blistering, subcutaneous dimpling, hypopigmentation, hyperpigmentation, induration, infection, contact dermatitis, skin necrosis, swelling, seroma, telangiectatic matting, numbness, nerve injury, traumatic neuroma, superficial venous thrombosis, and deep venous thrombosis.

Transilluminated Powered Phlebectomy

Transilluminated powered phlebectomy (TRIVEX™ system, InAVein, Lexington, MA, USA) combines visualization of varicosities using transillumination and directed resection using endoscopic technology. Instrumentation includes: *System Control Unit* as the central power unit with controls for xenon light source, irrigation pump, and resection oscillation speeds; *Illuminator Handpiece* connects to the control unit with a fiber optic cable and provides high intensity light for transillumination and tumescence irrigation control; *Resector Handpiece* has both 4.5 mm and 5.5 mm resector options, control of oscillation direction and rate, and connectors for suction tubing. General, epidural or spinal anesthesia is required. Through a tiny incision, the illuminator is placed a few millimeters deeper than the target varicosity and tumescence solution is infiltrated into the area along the course of the vein. Through a counter incision, the resector is positioned directly on the varicosity, and with powered oscillation, varicosities are mobilized free and then suctioned out of the leg. Addition of small dermal punch incisions allow for any blood or tissue debris that collects in the vein tract to be flushed out with further tumescence fluid. Overall, transilluminated powered phlebectomy is most effective for extensive varicose veins where the improved visualization allows for more complete resection with fewer incisions. However, for patients with fewer varicosities, the margin of benefit of transilluminated powered phlebectomy is less when compared to ambulatory phlebectomy.

Reported complications following transilluminated powered phlebectomy have varied considerably consisting primarily of ecchymosis and/or hematoma formation, paresthesias or nerve injury, skin perforation, superficial phlebitis, swelling, hyperpigmentation, and low potential for deep venous thrombosis. Although most studies reported fewer incisions for transilluminated powered phlebectomy compared to conventional surgery, differences in operating time have varied. With regard to cosmetic scores, outcomes were similar for both groups and overall patient satisfaction scores were not statistically different. Although there is no published data clearly showing any significant statistical advantage of transilluminated powered phlebectomy except for lower number of incisions, most of the published literature represents earlier generation system and techniques. With a newer generation system, smaller instrumentation, and modification of technique that allow for slower oscillation speed, higher suction, and extensive tumescence irrigation and drainage, most of these earlier problems have been eliminated with decreased potential for complications and improved outcomes over those previously reported.

Sclerotherapy

Sclerotherapy with liquid agents has been used primarily for treatment of telangiectasias and reticular veins <3 mm in diameter. Limitations for larger varicose veins include need for higher concentration of sclerosant, decreased effectiveness for larger veins based on less contact time of sclerosant with endothelial surface, and increased potential for leakage of sclerosant into normal superficial and deep venous system.

With foam reconstitution of detergent based sclerosants like sodium tetradecyl or polidocanol, options for treatment of larger varicose veins have increased. The most common technique uses a 3-way stopcock connected to two syringes to mix sclerosant with room air or carbon dioxide at predetermined ratios to create foam bubbled mixture which is injected directly into vein undergoing treatment. Leg elevation and ultrasound guidance are used to limit volume of foam spilling into systemic circulation, with treatment sessions usually limited to less than 20cc total volume.

Use of foam sclerotherapy has rapidly expanded for treatment of primary and recurrent varicose veins, great and small saphenous vein, and perforating veins. While several studies have suggested excellant results and low complications using foam sclerotherapy for these expanded uses, there is currently insufficient evidence to allow comparison of the effectiveness of foam sclerotherapy with other options. While used widely in Europe and other countries, foam reconstitution of sclerosant agents is not currently Food & Drug Administration (FDA) approved thereby limiting its use in the United States.

CLINICAL DECISION FACTORS FOR BULGING VARICOSE VEINS

Failure of Non-Operative Measures

Life style modifications including weight loss, leg elevation, elastic compression therapy and exercise are generally recommended for patients with venous insufficiency, but compliance and effectiveness is difficult. Venoactive medications have also been used for the treatment of chronic venous insufficiency. While many medications have been tried, most success has been noted with horse chestnut seed extract (aescin), micronized purified flavonoid fraction (rutosides, diosmin, hesperidin), pine bark extract, and pentoxifylline. While most of these medications have been shown to improve venous tone and decrease capillary permeability, leading to diminished symptoms from varicose veins, decreased inflammation and swelling and improved ulcer healing, overall effectiveness has been variable. However, a recent Cochrane meta-analysis failed to show sufficient evidence to support global use of the venoactive medications in the treatment of chronic venous insufficiency.

Compression is standard treatment for all patients with chronic venous insufficiency ranging from spider veins, varicose veins, venous edema, skin changes, and venous ulcerations, with most effectiveness seen in more advanced clinical venous classes. The goal of compression is to decrease venous reflux and improve calf muscle pump function, which has the net effect of decreasing ambulatory venous hypertension. Methods of compression include elastic graduated compression stockings for most patients with C1-3 disease, reserving paste gauze boots (Unnas boot), multilayered compression dressings, elastic and non elastic bandages, and pneumatic compression devices for advanced C4-6 venous disease that is not controlled with standard compression stockings. While implementation of these nonoperative measures prior to surgical intervention for superficial venous disease is important, the requirement of failure of these measures by third-party payers is not supported by scientific evidence. Unfortunately, most insurance plans require a trial of nonoperative measures, including compression therapy prior to providing coverage for superficial venous operations, and providers should work with patients and insurance carriers to most accurately represent medical justification for operative planning

Clinical Severity

Based on clinical severity, there are several considerations that should be factored into the decision to perform superficial venous operations: 1) Patients with more symptoms, higher clinical CEAP (C4/5/6) or higher venous clinical severity score (VCSS) will have a higher potential symptomatic benefit. 2) Larger varicose vein size and extensive varicose vein burden is less likely to resolve with isolated treatment of superficial axial venous reflux and may need additional therapy with either phlebectomy or sclerotherapy depending on the size, number, and distribution of residual varicosities. 3) Patients with recurrent varicose veins after prior venous intervention may represent a more severe group in which more extensive treatment is required. 4) Based on venous duplex ultrasound and additional plethysmography testing, patients who have more severe documented physiologic venous impairment would have expected higher margin of benefit and improvement in objective parameters. 5) Stratifying patients with isolated superficial venous reflux vs multilevel disease including deep and/or perforator venous insufficiency may have bearing on outcome, with extended venous treatment more often needed in the later group. 6) Patients with symptoms out of proportion to visualized infrainguinal reflux, or obstruction, varicosities in the inguinal or peroneal areas, presence of venous stasis ulcer or history of deep venous thrombosis extending to iliac veins may merit evaluation of the ilio-caval system.

Anatomic Varicose Vein Distribution and Pattern

An important factor in preoperative planning is anatomic distribution of varicose veins and their relationship to documented source of superficial venous reflux: great saphenous vein reflux with medial thigh and calf varicosities; anterior saphenous vein reflux with anterior lateral thigh varicosities; pudendal vein reflux with medial posterior thigh varicosities; small saphenous vein reflux with posterior calf varicosities; And reflux in posterior thigh circumflex vein (formerly the vein of Giacomini), the thigh extension of the SSV to the posterior accessory GSV, with posterior thigh varicosities. If a direct source of superficial reflux can be identified, then initial treatment of the axial source of reflux may result in increased potential for regression or complete resolution of associated varicosities. However, if noted pattern of varicose vein distribution does not match source reflux, then improvement of varicosities after treatment of superficial axial reflux is less likely, and further directed treatment of the varicosities will be required.

Staged vs Combined Approaches

Based on review of evidence supporting combined or staged approaches for treatment of superficial venous insufficiency and associated varicose veins, definitive recommendations are difficult. A fundamental principle for approaches to superficial venous insufficiency, whether using a combined or staged approach, is elimination of all sources of venous reflux. While saphenous vein based therapy is important in reducing venous hypertension, patient symptoms, and progression, proponents of combined approaches note that as a sole therapy, there is insufficient elimination of all varicose veins, incomplete reduction of all venous symptoms, higher potential for varicose vein recurrence, and additional frequent need for subsequent procedures. Proponents of a staged approach with saphenous based treatment first followed by selected phlebectomy only in those with persistent varicose vein problems argue that most varicose veins will improve or regress with direct isolated treatment of the underlying saphenous venous reflux and that unnecessary extra surgery is being performed on a significant number of patients undergoing combined approaches. Furthermore, by selectively reserving additional phlebectomy only for those with persistent varicose veins, less invasive techniques like sclerotherapy or microphlebectomy may be feasible at a later stage since prior varicosities may regress leaving less that may require subsequent treatment. While the global overview of evidence supports either approach as being acceptable, there are various factors that may make one approach preferred over the other in selected clinical scenarios based on clinical severity, risk profile, anatomic pattern, and patient preference, and providers should exercise best judgment in selection of either staged or combined approach on a case by case basis.

Operative Setting

While most endovenous thermal ablation and ambulatory phlebectomy procedures can be performed with local and tumescence anesthesia in an outpatient setting, saphenous division, traditional ligation & stripping and transilluminated powered phlebectomy approaches require general or regional anesthesia in a standard operating room setting. If closer hemodynamic monitoring, airway protection, or bleeding control is needed, the capacity of operating room to handle higher risk patients may also become a consideration. Furthermore, if general or regional anesthesia is required, then from an anesthetic risk standpoint, it may be better to perform a more extensive superficial venous operation to avoid need for multiple trips to the operating room. Ultimately, performing superficial venous operations in an outpatient ambulatory setting or operating room should be most importantly determined by the setting that is most appropriate and safest for the patient.

Patient Expectations

Patient preferences are important to factor into any decision to proceed with superficial venous operations. Engaging patients in a discussion regarding treatment alternatives, expected symptomatic improvement, postoperative recovery, compression, time off from work, potential complications, recurrence, cosmetic concerns, and potential financial burden should be done in an informed fashion and in an effort to realistically manage patient expectations. Helping patients make a balanced decision prior to superficial venous operations is critical to preventing dissatisfaction after operative intervention in what is sometimes considered a high maintenance patient group.

SUMMARY - ALGORITHM FOR BULGING VARICOSE VEINS

Coordinated treatment of bulging varicose veins involves comprehensive patient evaluation, appropriate venous testing usually with venous ultrasound as the cornerstone of diagnostic evaluation, and sound clinical decision making based on current evidence based guidelines. While non-operative measures focusing on compression are recommended as initial therapy, operative approaches offer additional opportunity for improved outcomes. A reasonable algorithm for treatment of bulging varicose veins should include:

- Determining severity of venous disease and response to nonoperative measures;
- Evaluating pattern of venous insufficiency and whether bulging varicosities are primary or are secondary from axial sources of reflux;

- Eliminating axial source reflux when present first, preferably with endovenous thermal ablation options, either as staged approach or combined with varicose vein directed approaches;
- For treatment of varicosities—ambulatory phlebectomy is preferred for most situations; Transilluminated powered phlebectomy may be most suitable for extensive varicose vein burden; Sclerotherapy is an option for smaller varicosities especially when persistent after staged approach.
- Using postoperative compression therapy protocol is recommended for optimal results.

REFERENCES

1. Barwell JR, Davies CE, Deacon J, et al. Comparison of surgery and compression with compression alone in chronic venous ulceration (ESCHAR study): Randomised controlled trial. *Lancet*. 2004;363(9424):1854–9.
2. Bergan J, Cheng V. Foam sclerotherapy for the treatment of varicose veins. *Vascular*. 2007;15(5):269–72.
3. Bountouroglou DG, Azzam M, Kakkos SK, et al. Ultrasound-guided foam sclerotherapy combined with sapheno-femoral ligation compared to surgical treatment of varicose veins: Early results of a randomised controlled trial. *Eur J Vasc Endovasc Surg*. 2006;31(1):93–100.
4. Campbell WB, Vijay Kumar A, Collin TW, et al. The outcome of varicose vein surgery at 10 years: Clinical findings symptoms and patient satisfaction. *Ann R Coll Surg Engl*. 2003; 85:52–7.
5. Carradice D, Mekako AI, Hatfield J, et al. Randomized clinical trial of concomitant or sequential phlebectomy after endovenous laser therapy for varicose veins. *Br J Surg*. 2009; 96: 369–75.
6. Disselhoff BC, der Kinderen DJ, Kelder JC, et al. Randomized clinical trial comparing endovenous laser with cryostripping for great saphenous varicose veins. *Br J Surg*. 2008;95(10):1232–8.
7. Dwerryhouse S, Davies B, Harradine K, et al. Stripping the long saphenous vein reduces the rate of reoperation for recurrent varicose veins: Five-year results of a randomized trial. *J Vasc Surg*. 1999; 29(4):589–92.
8. Eklöf B, Rutherford RB, Bergan JJ, et al; American Venous Forum International Ad Hoc Committee for revision of the CEAP classification. Revision of the CEAP classification for chronic venous disorders: Consensus statement. *J Vasc Surg*. 2004;40(6):1248–52.
9. Gloviczki P, Comerota AJ, Dalsing MC, et al. The care of patients with varicose veins and associated chronic venous diseases: Clinical practice guidelines of the Society for Vascular Surgery and the American Venous Forum. *J Vasc Surg*. 2011; 53:2S–48S.
10. Guyatt G, Gutterman D, Baumann MH, et al. Grading strength of recommendations and quality of evidence in clinical guidelines: Report from an American College of Chest Physicians task force. *Chest*. 2006;129:174–81.
11. Kakkos SK, Bountouroglou DG, Azzam M, et al. Effectiveness and safety of ultrasound-guided foam sclerotherapy for recurrent varicose veins: Immediate results. *J Endovasc Ther*. 2006;13(3):357–64.
12. Lurie F, Creton D, Eklof B, et al. Prospective randomized study of endovenous radiofrequency ablation (closure) versus ligation and vein stripping (EVOLVeS): Two-year follow-up. *Eur J Vasc Endovasc Surg*. 2005; 29(1):67–73.
13. Merchant RF, DePalma RG, Kabnick LS. Endovascular obliteration of saphenous reflux: A multicenter study. *J Vasc Surg*. 2002;35(6):1190–6.

14. Michaels JA, Campbell WB, Brazier JE, et al. Randomised clinical trial, observational study and assessment of cost-effectiveness of the treatment of varicose veins (REACTIV trial). *Health technology assessment (Winchester, England)*. 2006;10(13):1–196, iii-iv.

15. Mundy L, Merlin TL, Fitridge RA, et al. Systematic review of endovenous laser treatment for varicose veins. *Br J Surg*. 2005;92(10):1189–94.

16. Passman MA, Dattilo JB, Guzman RJ, Naslund TC. Combined endovenous ablation and transilluminated powered phlebectomy: Is less invasive better? *Vasc Endovascular Surg*. 2007; 41(1):41–7.

17. Perrin MR, Guex JJ, Ruckley CV, et al. Recurrent varices after surgery (REVAS), a consensus document. REVAS group. *Cardiovasc Surg*. 2000;8(4):233–45.

18. Porter JM, Moneta GL, International Consensus Committee on Chronic Venous Disease. Reporting standards in venous disease: An update. *J Vasc Surg*. 1995;21:635–45.

19. Puggioni A, Kaira M, Carmo M, et al. Endovenous laser therapy and radiofrequency ablation of the great saphenous vein: Analysis of early efficacy and complications. *J Vasc Surg*. 2005; 42(3): 488–93.

20. Rutherford RB, Padberg Jr FT, Comerota AJ, et al. Venous severity scoring: An adjunct to venous outcome assessment. *J Vasc Surg*. 2000;31:1307–12.

21. Scavee V. Transilluminated powered phlebectomy: Not enough advantages? Review of the literature. *Eur J Vasc Endovasc Surg*. 2006;31(3):316–9.

22. Tessari L, Cavezzi A, Frullini A. Preliminary experience with a new sclerosing foam in the treatment of varicose veins. *Dermatol Surg*. 2001;27(1):58–60.

23. Vasquez MA, Rabe E, McLaffertyt RB, Shortell CK, Marston WA, Gillespie D, et al. Revision of the venous clinical severity score: Venous outcomes consensus statement: Special communication of the American Venous Forum Ad Hoc Outcomes Working Group. *J Vasc Surg*.2010;52:1387–96.

24. Winterborn RJ, Foy C, Earnshaw JJ. Causes of varicose vein recurrence: Late results of a randomized controlled trial of stripping the long saphenous vein. *J Vasc Surg*.2004; 40:634–9.

SECTION V

Abdominal Aortic Disease

21

Practical Approaches to Type II Endoleaks After EVAR

James F. McKinsey, MD

INTRODUCTION

Since the initial inception of endovascular aneurysm repair (EVAR) by Parodi in 1991, there has been a concern for the effectiveness of this minimally invasive therapy.[1] Concerns include the short term peri-procedural risks as well as the long term risks of this procedure. Peri-procedural risks include acute risk of rupture, graft thrombosis and lack of exclusion of the aortic aneurysm by the endograft. Long term graft complications include graft migration, rupture, thrombosis and endoleak. An endoleak is defined as the persistent arterial perfusion of the aneurysm sac despite the presence of the endograft. Endoleaks are defined based on the location of the endoleak relative to the endograft. Type II endoleaks are defined by persistence of retrograde blood flow within the aneurysm sac via patent collaterals after endograft deployment. Flow into the aneurysm sac can come from inferior mesenteric, lumbar, internal iliac, sacral, gonadal and accessory renal arteries. Flow into the aneurysm sac can lead to continued sac pressurization and increased risk of rupture. Indications for intervention on type II endoleaks have changed over time. Initially, there was the thought that all type II endoleaks should be treated due to the uncertain long term impact of the endoleak.[2]

Currently, management of type II endoleaks has remained a somewhat individualized and controversial matter. The long-term history of type II endoleaks has still not been fully elucidated; this has contributed to the lack of consensus regarding the appropriate diagnostic and interventional management strategies to effectively deal with this problem.

Type II endoleaks can occur at anytime after endograft implantation, lifelong radiologic surveillance is required to periodically monitor for leaks. Type II endoleaks diagnosed within 30 days of the initial post-procedural imaging study are termed early or primary endoleaks. Late or delayed type II endoleaks are diagnosed after 30 days in a patient with a history of a negative initial diagnostic study after EVAR implantation. Persistent type II endoleaks are defined as those lasting longer than 6 months.

The reported incidence of type II endoleaks varies greatly in the literature with rates as high as 30% being reported. This is likely due to the fact that the development of type II endoleaks may be dependent on a wide array of factors including collateral vessel patency, aneurysmal thrombus burden, anticoagulation, endograft device construction, collateralization patterns and secondary interventions.[3] Simple type II endoleaks consist of a single artery that serves as an ingress and egress pathway for the leak. Whereas when multiple vessels are responsible for flow into and out of the aneurysm sac this is cateogorized as a complex type II endoleak.[4]

Based on observations that intrasac pressure in patients with type II endoleak can be equivalent to systemic pressure, some researchers have strongly advocated that immediate repair of type II endoleaks should be performed.[3] On the other hand, spontaneous regression of type II endoleaks may also occur in as many as 53% of patients within the first 6 months of EVAR implantation. Many other physicians support a policy of "watchful-waiting"and only intervene if there is a measureable increase in aneurysm sac size, or if no sac regression is noticed after a defined period of time.[5]

The appropriate interventional technique to employ to deal with type II endoleaks is also a matter of controversy amongst clinicians. Methods of intervention on type II endoleaks include minimally invasive and surgical interventions. Endovascular catheter-directed transarterial and translumbar embolization have been used to effectively obliterate retrograde flow into the aneursym sac. Laparoscopic and open surgical ligation of IMA and other sources of type II endoleaks have been reported but generally are not first line therapy.[6,7,8]

This chapter will begin with a brief review of the various imaging modalities used for surveillance of type II endoleaks. Risk factors for the development of type II endoleaks will be discussed, followed by endovascular and operative treatment strategies.

IMAGING

Quality imaging is essential for the diagnosis and surveillance of type II endoleaks. The incidence of type II endoleak may vary according to the sensitivity of the diagnostic method utilized. Type II endoleaks can be identified at the time of final angiogram during the time of EVAR implantation by identifying late retrograde flow into the aneurysm sac from native IMA or lumbar vessels or by the follow up imaging. Many centers will perform an initial imaging study one month after EVAR implantation, followed by a 6 month and then yearly study. Increased radiologic surveillance frequency may be indicated for patients with an endoleak or increase in aneurysm sac size. A number of different imaging tools have been used for postoperative detection of endoleaks including computed tomography angiography (CTA), ultrasonography (US), magnetic resonance imaging (MRI) and catheter-based angiography.

COMPUTED TOMOGRAPHY

Computed tomography angiography (CTA) is the most widely used imaging modality for the detection and study of type II endoleaks. CTA offers a non-invasive means to safely and rapidly acquire data that is accurate and reproducible. It allows for the assessment of numerous parameters including; changes in sac diameter, aortic remodeling and endograft positioning. The sensitivity of CTA has been shown to be superior to both ultrasound and angiography for the detection of endoleaks. Both the sensitivity and specificity of CTA for the detection of endoleaks has been shown to be greater than 90%.[9]

A multiphase study including precontrast, arterial, and delayed phase imaging should be performed to properly assess for endoleaks. Precontrast images are useful in order to differentiate calcification from contrast extravasation. Postcontrast images may identify low-flow type II endoleaks that are not well visualized in the arterial phase.[9,10] Golazarian et al. showed an 11% improvement in endoleak detection rate with biphasic helical CT compared to an arterial phase study alone. Direct comparison of noncontrast CT scans with the biphasic scan is also useful in distinguishing calcification and artifact from IV contrast in the setting of an endoleak.[11]

Limitations of CTA include cumulative radiation exposure and contrast-induced nephrotoxicity. Contrast-induced nephropathy is associated with increased morbidity and mortality. Affecting 7% to 12% of patient undergoing CT angiography.[12] In a recent study performed at Brigham and Women's Hospital to estimate cumulative radiation exposure in a cohort of 31,462 patients undergoing diagnostic CT, 33% of patients underwent 5 or more lifetime CT examinations. Fifteen percent of patients received estimated cumulative effective doses of more than 100mSv. Cumulative CT radiation exposure added incrementally to the baseline cancer risk in the cohort of patients.[13]

ULTRASOUND

Duplex ultrasound (US) is a readily available technology that can be used to detect the presence of Type II endoleaks and follow aneurysm sac progression. US is highly dependent on the operators experience, skill and technique. Patient factors including body habitus and bowel gas can limit the diagnostic utility of the study. The reported sensitivities for ultrasound detection of endoleaks ranges from 43% to 100%.[14] A prospective study comparing CTA and duplex ultrasound in 117 patients following EVAR showed ultrasound had an 86% sensitivity but had only a 45% positive predictive value for endoleak detection.[15] The detection of type II endoleaks was significantly less accurate than the detection of Type I endoleaks when studied by AbuRahma and colleagues (type I, 88% versus type II 50%, $p = 0.046$).[16] In comparison to CTA, ultrasound tends to underestimate aneurysm size. Improvements in ultrasound sensitivity for endoleak detection has been reported by authors using intravenous contrast infusion with perfluorocarbon microbubbles. McWilliams et al. demonstrated improved detection of endoleaks from a low of 12% with unenhanced color Doppler to 50% with enhanced Doppler.[17] Ultrasonography can be used to accurately identify specific branch vessel involvement in type II endoleaks and provides information on the direction of blood flow within the sac.

MAGNETIC RESONANCE IMAGING

Magnetic resonance imaging (MRI) is an alternative imaging method that has been found to be comparable to CTA and may indeed have a significantly higher sensitivity for identifying type II endoleaks. Haulon's group studied 52 patients that had undergone EVAR, MRI was more sensitive than CTA for detecting type II endoleaks, with a sensitivity of 100% and specificity of 82%.[18]

MRI is also particulary useful for patients with compromised renal function or known allergic reaction to intravenous contrast. Since life-long surveillance protocols are often required for patients that have undergone EVAR, MRI has the advantage over CTA by limiting repeated exposure to ionizing radiation.

Helical CTs and MRIs obtained in 31 patients following EVAR were compared to arteriography. MRA with gadolinium was found to have a 94% sensitivity for detecting type II leaks versus 50% sensitivity for helical CT ($p = 0.003$). It has been suggested that MRI might be useful for identifying endoleaks in patients with aneurysm sac changes that cannot be identified by CT.

Time-resolved magnetic resonance angiography (MRA) has been increasingly used to detect and classify endoleaks. Time-resolved MRA is able to detect the direction of blood flow within the aneurysm sac. Limitations of MRI include poor spatial resolution, small field of view and poor visualization of vascular calcifications. Image quality for patients that have stainless steel or elgiloy stent grafts may experience a significant degradation in imaging quality in comparison to patients with nitinol stent grafts.[9]

ANGIOGRAPHY

Catheter-based angiography is an invasive procedural method that can be used to accurately cateogorize endoleaks. Conventional angiography is limited as a screening test for detecting endoleak with a sensitivity of only 63%.[19] Gorich et al. have found aortography alone to be capable of detecting only 65% of endoleaks diagnosed by CT.[20]

Dynamic imaging via digital subtraction angiography, helps to more clearly distinguish endoleak subtypes in comparison to static CT imaging. Supraselective catheterization can aid in determining the direction of blood flow as well as therapeutic intervention. While CTA, MRA, and color duplex are all useful for screening, conventional arteriogram is still the considered the most accurate method to classify the type of endoleak.[2,3,4] Type II endoleak treatment via transcatheter embolization can also take place if arterial cannulation of the offending vessel can be achieved.

RISK FACTORS FOR THE DEVELOPMENT OF TYPE II ENDOLEAK

The etiology of type II endoleaks is multifactorial. Type II endoleaks have the highest prevalence of all endoleaks and the ability to determine which patients are at risk to develop a type II endoleak may eventually prove to be clinically useful. A number of authors have attempted to delineate what preoperative factors are responsible for the development of type II endoleak, with particular focus on the patency and size of lumbar and inferior mesenteric artery.

Marchiori et al. analyzed the data of 195 patients between 2003 and 2008, in an attempt to define predictive factors leading to the development of type II endoleaks.[21] Twenty-eight (13.4%) of patients were diagnosed with type II endoleaks. All the patients diagnosed with type II endoleaks had 4 or more patent lumbar arteries. In comparison to patients that developed transient type II endoleaks, the patients with persistent endoleaks had patent lumbar arteries with larger diameters (2.7 mm vs 1.5 mm). The presence of at least 4 patent lumbar arteries ($p < 0.001$), and at least 1 lumbar artery greater than 2 mm in diameter ($p < 0.001$) were positive predictive factors for the development of persistent endoleaks.

Warrier et al. identified specific variables associated with the development of type II endoleak after elective infrarenal aneurysm repair.[22] A retrospective analysis was conducted on 101 consecutive patients with a mean follow-up of 20 months. Postoperative imaging was obtained with CT and/or Duplex US at 1, 3, 6 months and yearly intervals thereafter. Type II endoleaks developed in 26 (25.7%) patients. Univariate and multivariate analysis was conducted to determine patient factors associated with the development of type II endoleaks. Fifty-four percent of the type II endoleaks were associated with an expanding aneurysmal sac. No aneurysms ruptured. The presence of a patent inferior mesenteric artery ($P < 0.001$) and sac enlargement ($P = 0.001$) were associated with development of endoleak after multivariate analysis ($P = 0.005$). Further assessment demonstrated that 70% of patients with an endoleak had a patent inferior mesenteric artery compared with only 26% of patients who did not develop an endoleak. In this study, the presence of four or more lumbar arteries ($P = 0.55$) was not associated with increased risk of type II endoleak.

Arko et al. reviewed the charts of 71 patients that were treated for infrarenal abdominal aortic aneurysm with an AneuRx bifurcated stent graft from 1996 to 1998. The presence or absence of type II endoleaks was determined from US and CTA for patients with greater than 1 year follow-up. Sixteen patients were identified with persistent type II endoleaks. In this study, a patent inferior mesenteric artery was present in 13 (81%) of patients with persistent endoleaks ($p < 0.01$). The number of patent lumbar arteries visualized preoperatively was 2.4 ± 0.6 in patients with persistent endoleaks ($p < 0.0001$). There were no ruptures related to the presence of a type II endoleak, but the aneurysm size did not decrease in patients with persistent type II endoleaks. A patent inferior mesenteric artery, or 2 or more lumbar arteries on preoperative CT angiography were independent preoperative risk factors for the development of persistent type-II endoleaks.[23]

Numerous studies have demonstrated the presence of patent inferior mesenteric and lumbar arteries are associated with an increased incidence of type II endoleak. Some authors have attempted preoperative embolization of large aortic side branches in an effort to reduce the incidence of type II endoleak. In one study twenty-three consecutive AAA patients had coil embolization of patent lumbar and inferior mesenteric arteries prior to endovascular repair.[24] Follow-up computed tomography, and duplex ultrasonography were obtained at 1, 30, 90, and 180 days after the stent-graft procedure and at 6-month intervals thereafter. Successful coil embolization was obtained in 65% of lumbar arteries and 100% of inferior mesenteric arteries. Over a mean 17-month follow-up period, 22 patients (1 intraoperative death), there was only 1 (4.5%) type II endoleak from a patent lumbar artery, with no sac expansion after 2 years.

Another study by Gould and his colleagues examined aortic side branch vessels with preoperative angiography and computed tomography. Embolization was performed prior to EVAR in 20 patients with patent lumbar and inferior mesenteric vessels. Follow-up CT was used to assess the presence of type II endoleak. Four (20%) patients developed type II endoleak during follow-up period. The onset of type II endoleak was later in patients that underwent preoperative embolization, however, these results suggest a lack of influence on preoperative embolization reducing the incidence of type II endoleak during the follow-up period.[25] This may be due to failure to ablate all aortic branches, collateralization or embolic vessel recanalization.

Despite a number of papers showing patent lumbar and inferior mesenteric artery can contribute to the development of type II endoleaks, routine preoperative embolization of patent side branches prior to EVAR is not uniformly practiced or recommended.[26]

Specific preoperative anatomic features related to aneurysm thrombus load may influence on the development of type II endoleaks. Maximum thickness of thrombus, percentage of sac circumference wall coverage, percentage of maximum sac area occupancy and thrombus thickness at each aortic branch ostium were all examined to investigate their relationship to the development of type II endoleaks. Postoperative CT, duplex US and angiography were reviewed to detect presence of type II endoleak. There were 38 (21.3%) patients with type II endoleaks. The median follow-up was 12 months (range 1–65 months). Results of univariate analysis showed significantly decreased risk of a type II endoleak in patients with a higher preoperative sac thrombus load.[27]

To determine whether specific endografts were related to the development of Type II endoleaks, Sheehan and colleagues retrospectively analyzed 1909 elective EVAR cases from 5 different aortic centers. Computer tomography was used to track and compare the rate of type II endoleaks among the different stent graft devices. Six different endografts were monitored (Talent, Lifepath, Excluder, Zenith, AneurRx, Ancure) for the development of type II endoleaks. Endoleak rates were examined at 1, 6, and 12 months, and yearly thereafter. 1909 patients underwent elective EVAR between 1996 and 2003. At 1 month, the overall rate of type II endoleak was 14.0% (range, 9.8% to 25.2%.) The Excluder had a significantly higher incidence of type II endoleaks at 1 month but was similar to most other grafts during longer term follow-up. No graft in this study had a long-term statistically significant difference in the rate of type II endoleak formation.[28]

Anticoagulation with warfarin has been shown to increase the overall endoleak rate. In a study spanning 7 years with 127 consecutive patients with infrarenal abdominal aortic aneurysms, computed tomography angiography follow-up showed the incidence of endoleak was significantly increased in patients undergoing warfarin therapy in comparison to patients undergoing antiplatelet therapy.[29] Type II endoleaks were also significantly more common in the warfarin group. The mean sac volume in the warfarin group had significantly increased compared to a mean sac volume decrease in the antiplatelet group. Fairman et al. also studied the effects of warfarin on type II endoleak rates. Warfarin treatment was not associated with a statistically significant increased rate of endoleak formation. However, delayed endoleaks tended to occur up to 5 times as often in the warfarin group as in the control group (p = NS). Furthermore, spontaneous resolution of type II endoleaks was not observed in the warfarin group, whereas it was observed in 31% of the control group (p = NS).[30]

TYPE II ENDOLEAK TREATMENT STRATEGIES

Deciding the appropriate timing for operative intervention in a patient with a type II endoleak can be challenging. The physician must determine what is the risk of adverse events occurring if the type II endoleak is not addressed. Intrasac pressures in patients with type II endoleaks can be equivalent to systemic pressure. Data from the EUROSTAR registry of 2463 patients from 87 European centers suggest an incidence of rupture after Type 2 endoleak of 0.52%.[31]

Some researchers advocate the immediate repair of type II endoleaks using transarterial or translumbar embolization to minimize the chance of rupture. While others base their timing to intervention on selective criteria relating to either aneurysm sac size change, or endoleak persistence over a defined time period. Many type II endoleaks will resolve spontaneously without any intervention at all. Most clinicians would agree to intervene on a type II endoleak if it is associated with any sign of aneurysm sac expansion, but the decision may not be so clear in patients with persistently stable sac size.

Silverberg et al. described an 8-year experience with type II endoleaks. Nine hundred sixty-five patients underwent EVAR at a single institution, 154 type II endoleaks were documented. Fifty-five patients (35.7%) type II endoleaks sealed spontaneously in a mean time of 14.5 months. Kaplan-Meier analysis, showed approximately 75% of type II endoleaks sealed spontaneously within five years.

80% of patients with type II endoleak remained free of sac enlargement, no patients experienced rupture or required conversion to open repair. Only 19 (12.3%) of patients with type II endoleak underwent intervention. The authors concluded type II endoleaks are relatively benign and a conservative approach with close follow-up is warranted in patients who have no evidence of aneurysm expansion.[32]

Rayt and colleagues reported a similar experience after examining 369 EVARs performed for infrarenal abdominal aortic aneurysms. Twenty-five isolated type II endoleaks were reported. Eighteen (72%) patients had no increase in sac size, 6 (24%) patients demonstrated sac enlargement. After a mean follow-up of 4 years 48% type II endoleaks spontaneously resolved, 48% remain under observation, only one patient underwent unsuccessful endovascular and laparoscopic intervention and remains under surveillance. No ruptures occurred and no patient required conversion to an open repair.[31]

A recent study performed by Karthikesalingam analyzed 10 series that reported the outcomes of isolated type II endoleaks in 231 patients. Meta-regression of the association between the threshold for intervention in patients with isolated type II endoleak after EVAR and the fate of the aneurysm sac was analyzed.[33] Articles were classified based on whether conservative, selective (intervention for 5-mm sac expansion or persistent type II endoleak greater than 6 months), or aggressive (any type II endoleak or persistent for 3 months) management strategies were employed. Type II endoleaks were managed conservatively in 71 patients (30.7%), selectively in 104 patients (45%) and aggressively in 56 patients (24.2%). Eight-four percent of patients had either stable or shrinking sacs during follow-up. No ruptures occurred. Meta-regression demonstrated no evidence that any strategy, compared to using a conservative approach, reduced sac expansion. The rarity of rupture and sac expansion confirmed the predominantly benign nature of isolated type II endoleak.

Persistent endoleaks have been associated with adverse late outcomes. Overall survival, aneurysm sac growth, reintervention rate, conversion to open repair, and abdominal aortic aneurysm rupture were examined in 873 patients undergoing EVAR.[34] Computed tomography scan assessment was performed <1 month after the operation and at least annually thereafter. Early type II endoleak was observed in 164 (18.9%) patients, with complete resolution occurring in 131 (79.9%) patients. Endoleaks persisted in 33 patients (3.8% of total patients; 20.1% of early type 2 endoleaks) for >6 months. Patients with persistent endoleak were at increased risk for aneurysm sac growth vs patients without endoleak (odds ratio [OR], 25.9; 95% confidence interval [CI] 11.8 to 57.4; $P < .001$). Patients with a persistent endoleak also had a significantly increased rate of reintervention (OR, 19.0; 95% CI, 8.0 to 44.7); $P < .001$). Four patients with type 2 endoleaks ruptured, with multivariate analysis showing persistent type II endoleak to be a significant predictor of aneurysm rupture ($P = 0.03$). Persistent type 2 endoleak was associated with an increased incidence of adverse outcomes, including aneurysm sac growth, the need for conversion to open repair, reintervention rate, and rupture. This data suggest that a conservative approach may not be prudent in all cases and continued close surveillance is warranted.

ENDOVASCULAR AND SURGICAL TREATMENT FOR TYPE II ENDOLEAK

A number of different treatment paradigms have been employed to treat type II endoleaks. Secondary procedures are required in up to 10% of patients per year to address type II endoleaks. Transarterial embolization involves direct intraluminal catheter access into the vessel perfusing the aneurysm sac. This is usually achieved from a transfemoral approach. Once supraselective catheterization of the ingress vessel is achieved embolization with coils, glue, thrombin or gelfoam is performed to obliterate retrograde flow into the aneurysm sac. Access to the sac may be quite circuitous; the inferior mesenteric vessel can be accessed by cannulating the superior mesenteric artery and directing the catheter through the middle colic artery or through the Arc of Riolan. (Figure 21-1a and b) Access to the lumbar arteries may require navigation through internal iliac artery branches. The presence of multiple vessels (complex type II) involved in an endoleak is associated with a higher failure rate for transarterial embolization.[35] Patients with complex type II endoleaks involving multiple vessels may benefit from a translumbar approach directly into the sac. With the patient in prone position, fluoroscopic or CT guidance can be used to directly puncture the sac. Rather than targeting individual vessels the nidus of the type II endoleak can be embolized.

Kasirajan et al. assessed the efficacy of transarterial coil embolization. 104 aortic stent grafts were deployed to exclude abdominal aortic aneursym over a 23-month period. CT follow-up was conducted at 6-month intervals. Eight patients with type II endoleak were identified during CT follow-up. Eight patients underwent superselective transarterial embolization. Access to the aortic sac was achieved in 6 of 8 patients. Aneurysm sac reduction occurred in 6 of 8 patients. One patient receiving warfarin anticoagulation therapy continued to have a small type II endoleak even after discontinuation of warfarin therapy.[36]

Another method of repairing a type II endoleak is a translumbar approach to the AAA sac and then embolization of coils or glue into the inflow and outflow sources as well as the sac itself. (Figure 21-2a and b) A retrospective study involving 84 patients

A

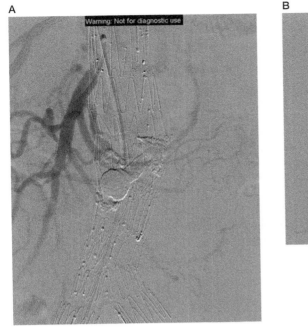

B

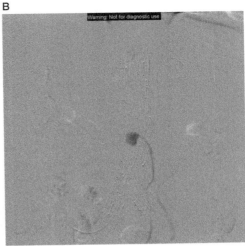

C

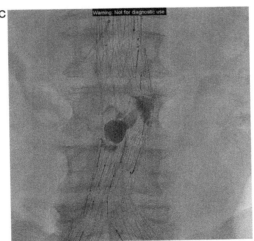

Figure 21–1. A. Type II endoleak involving retrograde flow in the IMA into aneurysm sac. **B.** Catheter placement from the SMA into the IMA and the aneurysm sac. **C.** Coil embolization with Glue of the AAA sac and origin of the IMA

with type II endoleaks, translumbar embolization was compared to a modifed transarterial embolization technique were the feeding artery and endoleak cavity were embolized.[33] Patients were followed for a mean period of 18.7 months. Sixty-two endoleaks were treated in the translumbar group and 23 endoleaks were treated in the transarterial group. Clinical success was achieved in 78% of the transarterial embolizations and 72% of the translumbar embolizations. Twenty-two percent of the transarterial embolizations had recurrent endoleaks. There was no significant difference between the two groups.

Another study comparing translumbar embolization and transarterial embolization techniques was conducted. Thirty-three angiographically proven type 2 endoleaks underwent treatment with either transarterial inferior mesenteric artery embolization (n = 20) or direct translumbar embolization (n = 13) during an 18-month period. Sixteen of twenty transarterial inferior mesenteric artery embolizations (80%) failed due to suspected recanalization of the endoleaks. All the translumbar endoleak procedures were successful with no procedural related complications. Twelve of 13 patients with translumbar embolization (92%) had a durable result, with a median follow-up period of 254 days. This study concluded that patients who underwent transarterial IMA embolization were significantly more likely to have recurrent endoleak than were the patients who underwent treatment with direct translumbar embolization.

Zanchetta performed a prospective nonrandomized study was between June 2003 and December 2005 to determine if fibrin glue embolization of the aneurysm sac at the time of EVAR was safe and beneficial. 84 consecutive patients were enrolled in the study. Selective catheterization of the AAA sac and fibrin glue injection into the aneurysm cavity were performed in the operating room during endografting. Selective sac catheterization and fibrin glue injection immediately after initial stent-graft deployment was successful in 83 (99%) of 84 case. In all these patients, aneurysm sac embolization and complete exclusion from retrograde perfusion was achieved, as confirmed by intraoperative angiography. The estimated primary and assisted primary clinical success rates at 2 years 91.3% and 98.8%, respectively. There were no early allergic-anaphylactic reactions or tissue reactions in the aneurysm sac or in the surrounding structures due to the fibrin glue.[37]

The major findings of this study were the low rate of delayed type II endoleak (2.4%, 2 patients) and the statistically significant decrease in the maximum transverse aneurysm diameter at follow-up

Open surgical approaches for the management of type II endoleaks should generally be reserved for percutaneous embolization failures in patients with rapidly enlarging sacs. Authors have described opening the aortic sac and over-sewing the holes of back-bleeding vessels, whilst leaving the endograft in place or ligation of the proximal IMA as it exits the AAA sac.[7]

Laparoscopic ligation of patent vessels feeding the aneurysm sac has been described by Richardson. One study conducted between 1995 and 2002, describes 213 patients had endografts placed for abdominal aortic aneurysm.[8] Four had enlarging aneurysms from type II endoleaks involving a patent IMA and underwent a secondary procedure. Two patients had endovascular embolizations through the superior mesenteric artery, and two patients underwent laparoscopic inferior mesenteric artery ligation.

One of the patients required a second laparoscopic procedure for a missed branch. Mean followup was 16 (range, 2–42) months. All patients have had complete resolution of endoleaks by CT scan. Laparoscopic ligation techniques to stop back bleeding from the IMA in expanding aneurysms after endovascular aortic aneurysm repair were successful with low morbidity and no mortality.[8]

Rarely stent graft explantation may be required for cases with failed endovascular or translumbar intervention or type II endoleaks or if the type II endoleak is associated with a concomitant type I and/or type III endoleak.

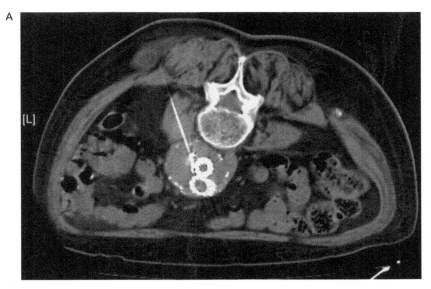

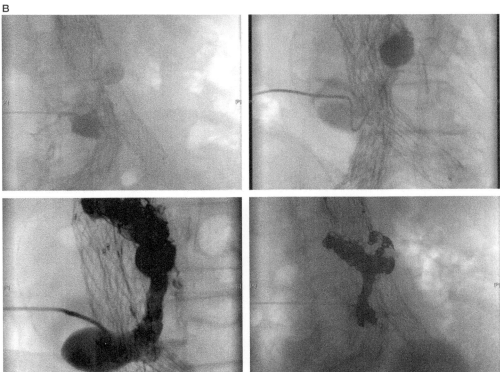

Figure 21–2. A. Type II endoleak into AAA sac with CT directed translumbar needle placement into AAA Sac Endoleak. **B.** Coil Embolization with Glue of sac and inflow vessels (Courtesy of Dr. Peter Schlossberg, Department of Interventional Radiology, Columbia University)

CONCLUSION

Type II endoleaks are not an uncommon occurrence after EVAR and most can be managed conservatively. The interventionalist must first confirm that the endoleak is in fact a type II endoleak and not a type I or III by objective evaluation by US, CT scan and if necessary angiography. Based on the review of the available data and our own clinical experience, we recommend the conservative management of type II endoleaks and reserve intervention for those patients that develop AAA sac expansion or AAA sac tenderness on physical examination. For those patients that re-intervention is indicated, we favor intra-arterial catheter directed intervention for confirmation of diagnosis and embolic occlusion of the inflow source. In those patients that we can not obliterate the inflow or outflow source then we will progress to a translumbar approach with both sac embolization and attempt to catheterize the inflow vessels and embolize those vessels also. It is a rare occurrence when one of these two treatment options are not successful. In these rare occasions graft explant has been performed.

REFERENCES

1. Parodi JC, Palmaz JC, Barone HD. Transfemoral intraluminal graft implantation for abdominal aortic aneurysms. *Ann Vasc Surg.* 1991 Nov: 491–499.
2. Maldonado TS, Gagne PJ. Controversies in the management of type "branch" endoleaks following endovascular abdominal aortic aneurysm repair. *Vasc Endovasc Surg.* 2003 Jan–Feb;37(1):1–12.
3. Gelfand DV, White GH, Willson SE. Clinical significance of type II endoleaks after endovascular repair of abdominal aortic aneurysm. *Ann Vasc Surg.* 2006 Jan;20(1):69–74.
4. Baum RA, Carpenter JP, Stavropoulous SW, et al. Diagnosis and management of type II endoleaks after endovascular aneurysm repair. *Tech Vasc Interv Radiol.* 2001 Dec;4(4):222–226.
5. Steinmetz E, Rubin BG, Sanchez LA, et al. Type II endoleak after endovascular abdominal aortic aneurysm repair: A conservative approach with selective intervention is safe and cost-effective. *J Vasc Surg.* 2004;39:306–313.
6. Zanchetta M, Faresin F, Pedon L, et al. Intraoperative Intrasac Thrombin Injection to Prevent Type II Endoleak After Endovascular Abdominal Aortic Aneurysm Repair. *J Endovasc Ther.* 2007 Apr;14(2):176–183.
7. Ferrari M, Sardella SG, Berchiolli R, et al. Surgical treatment of persistent Type 2 endoleaks, with increase of the aneurysm sac: Indications and technical notes. *Eur J Vasc Endovasc Surg.* 2005 Jan;29(1):43–46.
8. Richardson WS, Sternbergh C, Money SR. Laparoscopic Inferior Mesenteric Artery Ligation: An Alternative for the Treatment of Type II Endoleaks. *J Lap Adv Surg Tech.* 2004 July;1(13):355–358.
9. Shah A, Stavropoulos SW. Imaging surveillance following endovascular aneurysm repair. *Semin Interv Radiol.* 2009 Mar;26(1):10–16.
10. Maldonado TS, Gagne PH. Controversies in the mgmt. of type endoleak. *Vasc Endovasc Surg.* 2003 Jan–Feb;37(1):1–12.
11. Golzarian J, Murgo S, Dussaussois L, et al. Evaluation of abdominal aortic aneurysm after endoluminal treatment: Comparison of color Doppler sonography with biphasic helical CT. *AJR.* 2002 Mar;178(3):623–628.
12. Beeman BR, Doctor LM, Doerr K, et al. Duplex ultrasound imaging alone is sufficient for midterm endovascular aneurysm repair surveillance: A cost analysis study and prospective comparison with computed tomography scan. *J Vasc Surg.* 2009 Nov;50(5):1019–1024.

13. Sodickson A, Baeyens PF, Andriole KP, et al. Recurrent CT, cumulative radiation exposure, and associated radiation-induced cancer risk from CT of adults. *Radiology*. 2009 Apr;251:175–184.

14. Hiatt MD, Rubin GD. Surveillance of Endoleaks: How to detect them all. *Semin Vasc Surg*. 2004;17:268–278.

15. Manning BJ, O'Neill SM, Haider SN, et al. Duplex ultrasound in aneurysm surveillance following endovascular aneurysm repair: A comparison with computed tomography aortography. *J Vasc Surg*. 2009 Jan;49(1):60–65. Epub 2008 Oct 1.

16. AbuRahma AF, Welch CA, Mullins BB, et al. Computed tomography versus color duplex ultrasound for surveillance of abdominal aortic stent-grafts. *J Endovasc Ther*. Oct 2005;12(5):568–573.

17. McWilliams RG, Martin J, White D, et al. Detection of endoleak with enhanced ultrasound imaging: Comparison with biphasic CT. *J Endovasc Ther*. 2002 Apr;9(2):170–179.

18. Haulon S, Willoteaux S, Koussa M, et al. Diagnosis and treatment of type II endoleak after stent placement for exclusion of abdominal aortic aneurysm. *Ann Vasc Surg*. 2001 Mar;15(2):148–154. Epub 2001 Mar 1.

19. Armerding MD, Rubin GD, Beaulieu CF, et al. Aortic Aneurysmal disease: Assessment of stent-graft treatment-CT versus conventional angiography. *Radiology*. 2000 Apr;215(1):138–146.

20. Gorich J, Rilinger MN, Sokiranski R, et al. Leakages after endovascular repair of aortic aneurysms: Classification based or findings at CT, angiography, and radiography. *Radiology*. 1999 Dec;213(3):767–772.

21. Marchiori A, von Ristow A, Guimaraes M, et al. Predictive Factors for the development of Type II endoleaks. *J Endovasc Ther*. 2011 Jun;18(3):299–305.

22. Warrier R, Miller R, Bond R, et al. Risk factors for type II endoleaks after endovascular repair of abdominal aortic aneurysms. *ANZ J Surg*. 2008 Jan–Feb;78(1–2):61–63.

23. Arko FR, Rubin GD, Johnson BL, et al. Type-II endoleaks following Endovascular AAA Repair: Preoperative predictors and long-term effects. *J Endovasc Ther*. 2001 Oct;8(5):503–510.

24. Bonvini R, Alerci M, Antonucci F, et al. Preoperative Embolization of collateral side branches: A valid means to reduce type II endoleaks after endovascular AAA repair. *J Endovasc Ther*. 2003;10:227–232.

25. Gould DA, McWilliams R, Edwards RD, et al. Aortic side branch embolization before endovascular aneurysm repair: Incidence of type II endoleak. *J Vasc Interv Radiol*. 2001 Mar;12(3):337–341.

26. Rhee SJ, Ohki T, Veith FJ, et al. Current status of management of type 2 endoleaks after endovascular repair of abdominal aortic aneurysms sac thrombus load predicts type 2 endoleaks after endovascular aneurysm repair. *Ann Vasc Surg*. 2005;19(3):302–309.

27. Sampaio SM, Panneton JM, Mozes GI, et al. Aneurysm sac thrombus load predicts type 2 endoleaks after endovascular aneurysm repair. *Ann Vasc Surg*. 2005 May;19(3):302–309.

28. Sheehan MK, Ouriel K, Greenberg R, et al. Are type II endoleaks after endovascular aneurysm repair endograft dependent? *J Vasc Surg*. 2006 Apr;43(4):657–661.

29. Bobadilla JL, Hoch JR, Leverson GE, et al. The effect of warfarin therapy on endoleak development after endovascular aneurysm repair (EVAR) of the abdominal aorta. *J Vasc Surg*. 2010 Aug;52(2):267–271. Epub 2010 Jun 29.

30. Fairman RM, Carpenter JP, Baum RA, et al. Potential impact of therapeutic warfarin treatment on type II endoleaks and sac shrinkage rates on midterm follow-up examination. *J Vasc Surg*. 2002 Apr;35(4):679–685.

31. Rayt HS, Sandford RM, Salem M, et al. Conservative Management of Type 2 Endoleaks is not associated with increased risk of aneurysm rupture. *Eur J Vasc Endovasc Surg*. 2009 Dec;3(6):718–723. Epub 2009 Sep 19.

32. Silverberg D, Baril DT, Ellozy SH, et al. An 8-year experience with type II endoleaks: Natural history suggests selective intervention is a safe approach. *J Vasc Surg.* 2006 Sep;44(3):453–459.

33. Karthikesalingam A, Thrumurthy SG, Jackson D, et al. Current Evidence Is Insufficient to Define an Optimal Threshold for Intervention in Isolated Type II Endoleak After Endovascular Aneurysm Repair. *J Endovasc Ther.* 2012;19:200–208.

34. Jones JE, Atkins MD, Brewster DC, et al. Persistent type 2 endoleak after endovascular repair of abdominal aortic aneurysm is associated with adverse late outcomes. *J Vasc Surg.* 2007 Jul;46(1):1–8. Epub Jun 2007.

35. Baum RA, Carpenter JP, Golden MA, et al. Treatment of type 2 endoleaks after EVAR: Comparison of transarterial and translumbar techniques. *J Vasc Surg.* 2002 Jan;35(1):23–29.

36. Kasirajan K, Matteson B, Marek JM, et al. Technique and results of transfemoral superselective coil embolization of type II lumbar endoleak. *J Vasc Surg.* 2003 Jul;38(1):61–66.

37. Zanchetta M, Faresin F, Pedon L, et al. Intraoperative Intrasac Thrombin Injection to Prevent Type II Endoleak After Endovascular Abdominal Aortic Aneurysm Repair. *J Endovasc Ther.* 2007 Apr;14(2):176–183.

22

Next Generation Abdominal Endografts: Clinical Context and Devices

Andrew W. Hoel, MD

Endovascular aneurysm repair (EVAR) has rapidly expanded in its utilization in the treatment of abdominal aortic aneurysms (AAA) since first introduced in the early 1990s. This increase in utilization has been fostered by technological advancements over the last 20 years that have made EVAR safe and widely available. The objective of this chapter is to understand the current and future states of endograft technology and their implications for the management of AAA. We will first review studies comparing EVAR to open AAA repair (oAAA) to understand the minimal standards for EVAR outcomes. Because the advancement in technology is ongoing, we will also review current clinically available devices as they represent a substantial improvement from previous generation devices. We will next discuss the current status of endograft utilization including treatment of aneurysms outside of approved anatomic criteria. This finally leads to a discussion of emerging endograft technology that expands anatomic suitability for treatment with EVAR and heightens the potential for improved efficacy in the minimally invasive treatment of abdominal aortic aneurysms.

THE CURRENT STATE OF EVAR

It has been estimated that 2006 was the first year in which a greater proportion of AAA were treated annually with EVAR than oAAA.[1] Current estimates place EVAR at 60–80% of all infrarenal aneurysm repairs in the United States.[2-4] In the midst of this explosion in utilization in the last 10 years, the safety and efficacy of EVAR have been closely scrutinized in multiple clinical trials. The EVAR-1 trial,[5] the DREAM trial[6] and the OVER[7,8] trial have each ambitiously sought to compare EVAR with oAAA in a randomized, controlled fashion. Beyond their independent success, all three studies are made more remarkable by their similarity in results. Each study independently found a perioperative/30-day survival benefit for EVAR compared to oAAA. However, survival analysis demonstrated convergence of all-cause mortality such that in the EVAR-1 and DREAM trials, there was an equivalent survival between EVAR and oAAA at two years. Similarly, the OVER trial demonstrated an early survival advantage that disappeared by three years. Late aneurysm-related mortality appears to have a role in these results, particularly in the EVAR-1 and OVER trials. Reintervention and readmission following aneurysm repair is another important point of comparison between EVAR and oAAA. This secondary endpoint was examined in the DREAM and OVER trials where they demonstrated relative equivalence in intervention rates out to 5 years. In both of these studies, endograft related reinterventions in the EVAR group were balanced out by laparotomy-related admissions and interventions in the oAAA group.

The results of the randomized trials of EVAR versus oAAA were surprising, particularly considering that the participants in these studies are theoretically subject to improved outcomes as a result of the rigor in which they were treated and followed. However, these results are corroborated by a study of matched cohorts of Medicare beneficiaries undergoing EVAR or oAAA during a similar time interval (2001–2004) to the randomized trials. This study demonstrated similar findings of lower short-term morbidity and mortality, shorter hospital length of stay and higher likelihood of discharge home from the hospital for patients undergoing EVAR. However, like the randomized trials, this study demonstrated equivalent of all-cause mortality after 3 years. Importantly, there was a higher rate of laparotomy related complications following oAAA including incisional hernia and bowel obstruction, which at least partially offset the reintervention rate for patients that underwent EVAR.[9]

In spite of the consistency of the clinical trial data with results from administrative data, these results have been criticized, as many technology-based clinical trials are, for making conclusions based on outdated technology and limited clinical experience related to their use.[10] These concerns are supported by a more recent analysis of a Medicare analytic dataset, which also showed a perioperative reduction in morbidity and mortality for EVAR. However, this analysis demonstrated a persistent, albeit small, survival benefit for EVAR beyond three years. The many potential factors influencing these results include possible improved outcomes with new generation devices and better understanding by physicians of the long-term behavior of implanted devices. Similar to the OVER and DREAM trials, there was a higher rate of incisional hernia repair after oAAA, potentially balancing out late reinterventions for endograft related complications.[3]

In a broader sense, this decrease in morbidity and mortality over time is further supported by a meta-regression analysis of studies published between 1992 and 2002.[11] This analysis demonstrates a decrease in all-cause mortality, endoleak and post-EVAR aneurysm rupture rate in studies published during the evaluated interval. While a portion of this trend could be attributed to improved patient selection and technical expertise, it is also likely that advances in technology have contributed to better outcomes. Though it would be impossible to maintain a linear trend of improved outcomes into the present day, the contribution of technology to incrementally improved outcomes is apparent.

CURRENTLY AVAILABLE DEVICES

Nowhere is improvement of device technology more evident than when we look at the devices that are currently clinically available. There are 4 primary devices in widespread use clinically. Table 22-1 describes the pertinent anatomic criteria of each. Clinical data that

TABLE 22-1. CURRENT CLINICALLY AVAILABLE DEVICES IN THE UNITED STATES

Device	Anatomic indications	Delivery system
Cook Zenith	Proximal fixation: 15 mm infrarenal length, 18–32 mm diameter, angle ≤60 degrees.	Ipsi sheath: 18–22 F (7.1–8.5 mm OD)
	Distal fixation: 10 mm length, 7.5–20 mm diameter.	Contra sheath: 16–18 F
Endologix AFX	Proximal seal: 15 mm infrarenal length, 18–32 mm diameter, angle ≤60 degrees.	Ipsi sheath: 17 F (6.3 mm OD)
	Distal seal: 15 mm length, 10–23 mm diameter.	Contra sheath: 9 F
Gore Excluder	Proximal fixation: 15 mm infrarenal length, 19–29 mm diameter, angle ≤60 deg.	Ipsi sheath: 18–20 F (6.8 and 7.5 mm OD)
	Distal fixation: 10 mm length, 8–24 mm diameter.	Contra sheath: 16–18 F
Medtronic Endurant	Proximal fixation: 10 mm infrarenal length, 19–32 mm diameter (15 mm for neck angulation 60–75 degrees).	Ipsi sheath: 18–20 F (OD) (6.0–6.6 mm OD)
	Distal fixation: 15 mm length, 18–25 mm diameter.	Contra sheath: 16–18 F

*Ranges in sheath size depend on graft size, F = French

explicitly correlates currently available technology with improved patient outcomes is, and always will be, nearly impossible to demonstrate in real time. It is clear however that, generally speaking, devices have more robust stability and fixation and are delivered by lower profile systems compared to previous generation technology. With that in mind, it is worth commenting on each device individually.

Cook Zenith

Of currently available devices, the Zenith has been on the market in its current iteration the longest. It is a polyester graft with a stainless steel Z-strut framework. The bifurcated device has a suprarenal framework with active fixation. The bifurcated main body is deployed via an 18-French or 20-French integrated sheath system that maintains a constrained proximal end in a top cap while the contralateral gate is cannulated. This facilitates precise deployment in the proximal seal zone. Proximal fixation requires 15 mm of infrarenal seal and angulation ≤60 degrees. A new "Spiral-Z" iliac limb structure has been developed that is more flexible than the previous Z-strut structure. This configuration is designed to accommodate more tortuous iliac anatomy though no data of improved efficacy of this design change is yet available.

Endologix AFX

The AFX device expands on Endologix previous Powerlink device. Conceptually different in mechanism of function compared to other devices on the market, the bifurcated main body sits on the aortic bifurcation. Stability of the device is based largely on the columnar strength of the device's cobalt-chromium framework. This framework lies within a multilayer ePTFE barrier that is attached to the structure only at either end of the device. This is particularly important for the proximal aortic extensions, which achieves both proximal seal and stability against migration when the fabric billows out from the strut framework. The anatomic criteria for use includes 15 mm of proximal seal zone and angulation ≤60 degrees. The unique design of this device deserves careful consideration of the aortic anatomy prior to delivery.

Gore Excluder

The Excluder device has undergone multiple generations of innovation since it was first introduced. The most recent development is the C3 delivery system, which gives the physician an opportunity to reconstrain the proximal portion of the bifurcated device after it is partially deployed. This allows more precise positioning to maximized proximal seal. The device continues to use very low permeability PTFE bonded to a nitinol strut network and continues to be deployed by a rip-cord mechanism after delivery via an 18-French or 20-French sheath. Proximal fixation requires 15 mm of seal and neck angulation ≤60 degrees. Large "bell-bottom" iliac limbs are now available which expands the suitable common iliac diameter to 24 mm diameter. The Gore Dry Seal sheath is a useful adjunct component of the device because of an adjustable saline-filled valve, which facilitates improved hemostasis.

Medtronic Endurant

The Endurant device is the most recent offering from Medtronic. It builds on the technology developed in its previous generation of AneuRx and Talent infrarenal devices and features a high density polyester supported by variable width nitinol Z-struts. It employs suprarenal fixation that remains constrained until released by a top cap, which allows more accurate deployment in the infrarenal neck. Device delivery is achieved using a hydrophilic 18-French or 20-French system that does not require an additional sheath. Deployment is straightforward with a modified pin-and-pull delivery system. The use of a compliant balloon after device deployment does require exchange of the delivery system for a sheath. The device is FDA approved for aortic necks of 10 mm or greater with an infrarenal neck less than 60 degrees of angulation. Initial outcomes have been very good for the majority of parameters. However, it is worthy of note that a recent report described a nearly 5% rate of iliac limb occlusion at a mean follow-up of 12-months. This outcome is particularly important as lower profile, more flexible devices with hydrophilic sheaths are placed into more tortuous, smaller and diseased iliac anatomy.[12]

CONSIDERATIONS FOR DEVICE DELIVERY

The continued improvement in endograft technology has led to excellent outcomes in patients with suitable anatomy. However, there remains a substantial subset of patients with AAA who have suboptimal anatomy that does not meet strict anatomic criteria for an endograft. A growing body of literature is focusing on these patients.

A recent study of aortic anatomy in patients with infrarenal aneurysm of suitable diameter for repair demonstrated that only 25% of women and 46% of men had aortic neck anatomy suitable for EVAR by the most stringent IFU criteria (≥15 mm infrarenal neck, 18–32 mm diameter, ≤60 degree neck angulation). The most common reason for unsuitable anatomy was a short infrarenal neck followed by severe neck angulation. When you consider the additional factor of inadequate iliac access, the suitability for EVAR by the most stringent criteria (iliac diameter ≥6 mm but ≤20 mm) drops in women to 12% and in men to 32%.[13] These data are independent of eventual treatment strategy and demonstrate that current devices, if used within their anatomic thresholds, are suitable for only a portion of patients with infrarenal AAA.

The limited anatomic suitability for EVAR is particularly interesting in the clinical context of apparent higher rates of graft related complications in calcified and angulated aortic necks and in the setting of iliac artery calcifications and tortuosity.[14] Women, in particular, have been shown to have universally worse perioperative outcomes with higher mortality, more complications and a higher rate of type-1 endoleak compared to men.[15] These findings outline a clear opportunity, with technological innovation, to expand the pool of patients suitable for EVAR.

DEVICE DELIVERY OUTSIDE OF ANATOMIC CRITERIA

The long-term outcomes of EVAR are also likely affected by implantation of devices into patients that do not meet the anatomic criteria outlined in device instructions for use. A single center study of hostile neck anatomy (defined as length less than 10 mm, angulation greater than 60 degrees, diameter greater than 28 mm, or neck with calcifiation, thrombus or reverse taper) demonstrated significantly higher rates of Type I endoleak and perioperative complications.[16] In light of the association between late rupture risk and endoleak or graft migration,[17] it is reasonable to infer that device delivery outside of recommended anatomic criteria may increase the risk of late complications including rupture.

Adverse outcomes from EVAR outside of recommended anatomic criteria were also the focus of an observational study of post EVAR anatomy from a multicenter imaging database. This study demonstrated that aneurysms treated outside of recommend anatomic criteria had a high likelihood of continued expansion. Though potentially confounded by a selection bias, these findings do raise concern for continued aortic degeneration and increased rupture risk in aneurysms treated outside of the recommended anatomic criteria.[18]

THE FATE OF THE INFRARENAL AORTIC NECK POST EVAR

One of the important risks of treating aneurysms outside of recommended anatomic criteria is device implantation into diseased aorta. Because aneurysm formation is a biologically based phenomenon, it is likely that hostile aortic neck anatomy, in particular a conical or large diameter neck, is a manifestation of aorta at increased risk for late degeneration.

There is evidence for continued aortic neck dilation after EVAR in multiple studies and this is strongly associated with adverse midterm outcomes after EVAR including graft migration, the development of type 1 endoleak and continued aneurysm expansion. Aortic neck dilation after EVAR has been demonstrated in multiple studies with

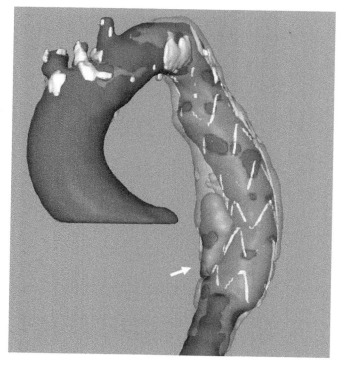

Figure 22-1. A Type 1B endoleak (white arrow) 6 month after treatment of a symptomatic penetrating aortic ulcer. This is an illustrative example of significant graft oversizing into a diseased segment of aorta with subsequent aortic degeneration. Radial force of the device on the aortic wall may have a role in this degeneration.

a prevalence of 35–59% of patients at 4-years. Additionally, there is evidence that this could be related to device oversizing, which is supported by the lower levels of aortic neck dilation seen with the use of balloon expandable devices in comparison to self expanding devices.[19] (Figure 22-1)

NEXT GENERATION EVAR DEVICES

As noted above, there have been significant advances in devices approved for EVAR in the United States. However, there remains a significant unmet clinical need to provide devices for a broader range of anatomy as well as an unrealized potential for better outcomes once those needs are met. There are multiple devices currently in clinical trials that have potential to address some of this need. Table 22-2 lists these devices and makes note of the clinical needs they address. The first group of devices are low profile devices that offer a endovascular option for small and diseased iliac anatomy. The second group of devices can treat hostile aortic neck anatomy including short and tortuous infrarenal necks. A third type of device worth discussing is a branched iliac device for the treatment of concurrent common iliac aneurysms.

TABLE 22-2. DEVICES IN CLINICAL TRIALS OR AWAITING FDA APPROVAL IN THE UNITED STATES

Device	Indication/Features	Expansion of anatomic criteria of current devices*	Main body (ipsi) delivery sheath
Incraft (Cordis)	Low profile for complex iliac anatomy.	Small iliac diameter.	13–15 F
Ovation (TriVascular)	Low profile for complex iliac anatomy. Proximal cuffs for short infrarenal neck.	Small iliac diameter. ≥7 mm infrarenal neck, minimum aortic diameter 15.5 mm.	14–15 F
Zenith LP (Cook)	Low profile for complex iliac anatomy.	Small iliac diameter.	16–17 F
Anaconda (Vascutek)	Repositionable proximal graft for maximal infrarenal fixation.		20–23 F (OD)
Aorfix (Lombard)	Flexible device for highly angulated infrarenal neck.	Infrarenal neck angulation up to 110 degrees.	22 F
Cook Fenestrated	Custom device. Juxtarenal AAA. Renal branches, SMA scallop.	≥4 mm infrarenal neck.	20 F
Nellix (Endologix)	"Sac anchoring endoprosthesis" for infrarenal and juxtarenal AAA.		17 F
Treovance (Bolton)	Low profile flexible device for complex anatomy.		18–19 F
Ventana (Endologix)	Off-the-shelf. Juxtarenal and pararenal AAA. Renal branches, SMA scallop.	Aortic neck below the SMA of ≥15 mm	17 F
Cook Branched Iliac	For common iliac artery aneurysm. Internal iliac branch graft.	Large common iliac diameter.	20 F

*Noting only features not present with currently available devices.

LOW-PROFILE DELIVERY SYSTEMS

Complex iliac anatomy including small diameter, significant tortuosity and calcification limits the access options for aortic devices without an adjunct procedure such as a retroperitoneal conduit or endoconduit. This is particularly relevant in women who, as we have noted, have a higher likelihood of small caliber iliac access. In addition to typical parameters of anatomic outcome, early results suggest that the patency of iliac limbs will be an important endpoint, likely due to small diameter graft outflow. This risk has potential to be offset by decreased risk of access complications due to the smaller delivery systems.

Incraft

Cordis Corportation has developed a new device platform that utilizes a nitinol and polyester graft with a bifurcated main body that fits into a 13–15 F (OD) delivery system. The main body is a modular bifurcated system with active suprarenal fixation. The three-piece device utilizes bilateral iliac limbs for distal seal. This device is currently in clinical trial and the inclusion criteria includes a broad range of aortic neck diameters which are likely broadly applicable to infrarenal anatomy.

Ovation

In similar fashion, TriVascular Corporation has developed a device that is based on a PTFE barrier with a nitinol framework. The bifurcated main body device is implanted via a 14 F or 15 F delivery system. The proximal device incorporates an active suprarenal fixation framework and is additionally supported by cuffs that are polymer injected at the time of deployment. This combination is designed for proximal fixation and seal into shorter necks (7 mm) than currently commercially available devices. This device has completed a phase III trial and has received FDA humanitarian use approval for use of its smallest diameter device in aortic necks with 15.5–17.4 mm diameter.

Zenith LP

Cook has built on their clinically approved technology to develop a low-profile device that replaces the stainless steel framework of its Zenith Flex device with a nitinol framework and utilizes a thinner polyester material. With these advances, the main body device fits into a 16-French or 17-French system. This is in contrast to the Zenith Flex device, which has an 18-French or 20-French delivery system, depending on graft size. This device is currently in a phase III trial. One-year outcomes were presented at the 2012 Vascular Annual Meeting and demonstrated generally excellent results though there was a 6.7% rate of graft limb occlusion. This rate of iliac limb occlusion underscores the need for continued close monitoring of this study outcome and careful patient selection.[20]

COMPLEX INFRARENAL NECK ANATOMY

The second major avenue of new device development is geared to complex aortic neck anatomy. As discussed above, there are three factors that make this endeavor worthwhile: (1) a small but significant prevalence of short and angulated necks in patients with infrarenal AAA—particularly women, (2) the existing need for adjunct procedures at the time of EVAR with currently available devices, particularly for Type Ia endoleak; and (3) an association between complex neck anatomy and continued aneurysm growth over time and degeneration of the proximal seal zone. There are a number of devices currently in clinical trials that seek to address these anatomic issues by a variety of means.

Anaconda

The Anaconda device was developed by Vascutek as a ringed nitinol system with active infrarenal fixation. The bifurcated aortic component is delivered through a 23-French (OD) sheath prior to the bilateral iliac limbs and is repositionable to allow greater precision in deployment. This allows utilization of the full extent of infrarenal fixation to minimize risk of Type Ia endoleak. Cannulation of the contralateral iliac limb is facilitated by a magnet system. The bilateral iliac limbs feature a ringed nitinol system to maximize flexibility in tortuous iliac anatomy. In the United States the Anaconda is currently undergoing phase II clinical evaluation of safety and effectiveness. A custom fenestrated device based on this platform is beginning clinical evaluation in the United Kingdom.

Aorfix

The Aorfix device utilizes a ringed nitinol support structure and a barbed "fish mouth" design for proximal fixation. The ringed nitinol construction provides additional flexibility allowing treatment of highly angulated infrarenal aortic necks. (Figure 22-2) The PYTHAGORUS trial is a Phase III evaluation of the device specifically evaluating the treatment of high-angle aortic necks (>60 degrees). Results presented at the 2012 Vascular Annual Meeting demonstrated an excellent safety and efficacy profile at 1-year in straightforward anatomy including no migration or endoleak in aortic necks less of less than 60 degrees of angulation. In highly angulated neck anatomy (60–110 degrees) for which this device is uniquely suitable, there was a 2.4% rate of type 1 endoleak and a 2.1% rate of device migration requiring reintervention—comparing favorably to a control group of open repair and to EVAR with other devices in highly angulated proximal neck anatomy.[21] Phase III clinical trials are ongoing.

Cook Fenestrated

The Cook Fenestrated device is designed for treatment of juxtarenal aortic aneurysms with an infrarenal neck ≥4 mm in length. Each device is made to a patient's precise anatomy and custom built to provide fenestrations to the bilateral renal arteries and a scallop or fenestration to the superior mesenteric artery. Use of this device requires relatively sophisticated measurement of the peri-renal and visceral aortic anatomy including angles of origin of the superior mesenteric and renal arteries. Implantation of this device involves cannulation of the bilateral renal arteries through graft fenestrations and deployment of renal stents or stent-grafts. This is key component of establishing a stable proximal seal zone. (Figure 22-3)

At this time, the Cook Fenestrated device has completed Plase III clinical trial and the results have been reported to the FDA. In 121 patients treated with the device, there was 100% technical success, no Type I or Type III endoleaks and no ruptures or conversions at 6-months. There was a 3.5% rate of branch stent occlusion and a

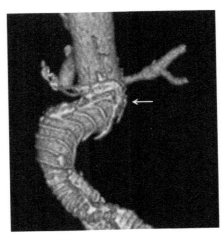

Figure 22-2. The Aorfix device is being evaluated in highly angulated aortic necks as part of a Phase III trial. Shown here is a bifurcated main body deployed in a 90 degree aortic neck. The "fish-mouth" proximal graft (white arrow) facilitates precise deployment in the peri-renal aorta.

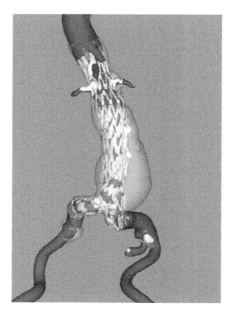

Figure 22-3. Three-dimensional reconstruction of a Cook Fenestrated device 1-month post implantation. Bilateral renal fenestrations are stented preserving renal perfusion.

6.9% rate of stenosis in a branch of which a small portion required reintervention. Based on these results, the FDA has granted regulatory approval for commercial distribution.[22]

Nellix

The Endologix Nellix system is a novel device consisting of two cobalt-chromium stents that are deployed in parallel from the infranrenal neck to the bilateral common iliac arteries via 17-French sheaths. Surrounding these stents are "endobags" which are subsequently filled with an inert polyethylene glycol. This results in anchoring of the system within the aneurysm sac to maintain endograft position. (Figure 22-4) The early published clinical experience has demonstrated efficacy in 34 patients. Of these 50% had anatomy considered unfavorable for currently available endografts. There were two patients with Type I endoleak in the study, the first a proximal endoleak that thrombosed spontaneously by 60-days, the second a distal endoleak for which the patient underwent extension of the iliac limb to correct. With mean 15-month follow-up there has been no instances of aneurysm expansion, no device migration and no new endoleaks.[23]

Treovance

The Treovance device from Bolton Medical is a modular bifurcated device with a Nitinol and polyester construction. Delivery system is 18–19 F OD depending on graft size. The proximal active fixation remains constrained until deployment of the bifurcated component is complete allowing increased precision proximally. The BENEFIT trial is a currently-enrolling US Phase I trial evaluating efficacy and safety of the device. The anatomic criteria for this trial includes neck angulation up to 75 degrees with an infrarenal neck length of 15 mm.

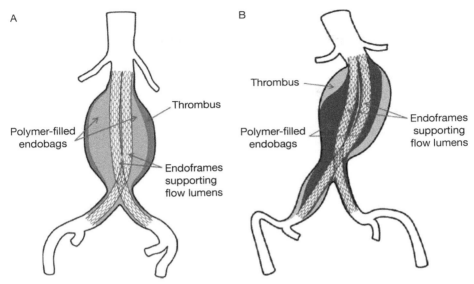

Figure 22-4. Schematic of the Nellix device in standard (a) and a short (b) infrarenal aortic neck. The unique device design has undergone human proof of concept study. Reprinted with permission from Krievins DK, et al. *Eur J Vasc Endovasc Surg.* 2011; 42(1):38–46.

Ventana

The Ventana device is an off-the-shelf branched device for the treatment of juxtarenal and pararenal aortic aneurysm. It is indicated for anatomy with ≥15 mm aortic neck below the origin of the superior mesenteric artery. It builds on, both literally and figuratively, the Endologix AFX unibody platform with the fenestrated device deployed as an aortic extension proximal to the bifurcated AFX device. The proximal extension features a large anterior scallop for the superior mesenteric artery and there are multiple configurations of renal branches available to treat a broad array of infrarenal and pararenal aneurysm anatomy. The design of the renal fenestrations allow for significant mobility along the lateral surface of the device facilitating cannulation of the bilateral renal arteries. Bilateral secondary sheaths integrated into the delivery system are used to cannulate the renal arteries prior to device deployment. It is through these sheaths that renal stent-grafts are deployed. (Figure 22-5) This device is currently undergoing Phase II evaluation for safety and effectiveness.

CONCURRENT ILIAC ANEURYSM

Multiple strategies have been developed to treat infrarenal aneurysms with concurrent iliac aneurysms including hypogastric coil embolization, hypogastric bypass and chimney grafts. The precise utility of hypogstric preservation is not determined, however there is a clear incidence of buttock claudication and even rare cases of necrosis in patients with hypogastric artery occlusion. In addition, risk of bowel and spinal cord ischemia is nominally increased with hypogastric occlusion, particularly in the setting additional adverse aortic anatomy. There is, therefore, a subpopulation that will likely benefit from internal iliac artery preservation at the time of EVAR.

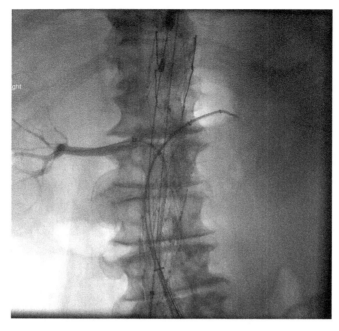

Figure 22-5. Angiogram of the Ventana device demonstrating concurrent cannulation of the bilateral renal arteries with the integrated sheath system. The aortic device is partially deployed in this image.

Cook Branched Iliac

The Cook Branched Iliac device was developed to preserve the hypogastric artery at the time of EVAR. This platform utilizes a 20-French ipsilateral and 12-French contralateral delivery system to place a branched device to preserve flow to the hypogastric artery. This is done prior to deployment of a standard Zenith bifurcated endograft. The branched hypogastric device is based on the stainless steel and polyester structure that is the same as the standard Zenith device. The internal iliac artery branch is a self-expanding nitinol and PTFE stent-graft. (Figure 22-6)

KEEPING TRACK OF ADVANCES

Learning about new developments in endovascular devices can occur via multiple parallel information streams including published literature, advertisements, presentations and word of mouth. Of course, the most important component of progress in device technology is the ability to deliver it to patients that need it. For that reason, keeping track of the progress of new devices through the regulatory pathways of the Food and Drug Administration is extremely useful. This is best achieved through on-line, searchable regulatory websites including www.clinicaltrials.gov and www.fda.gov. The Center for Device and Radiologic Health (CDRH) is the FDA branch responsible for the approval process of new endovascular technology. Their website (www.fda.gov/MedicalDevices) has a number of searchable databases that list details such as Premarket Approvals (PMA) and details of adverse events involving approved devices (Manufacturer and User Facility Device Experience/MAUDE).

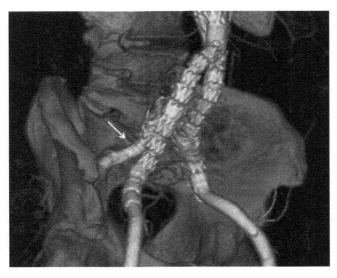

Figure 22-6. Post-operative CTA of a Cook Branched Iliac device demonstrating hypogastric preservation (white arrow) with a self-expanding stent graft in the setting of aortic and common iliac aneurysm.

SUMMARY

Endovascular treatment of abdominal aortic aneurysms is a mainstream and broadly applied technology in 2012. Favorable results of currently available technology ensure that this will continue. However, the lack of clear Level 1 evidence of a sustained benefit to EVAR beyond two years can be taken as a signal of the continued need for technological advancement in devices and better understanding of how these devices are optimally utilized. There remains a subset of the population with aneurysm anatomy that is not suitable for endovascular repair. The literature suggests that some of these are being treated with currently available endovascular devices. However, endovascular treatment of suboptimal anatomy that is outside of the defined anatomic criteria for EVAR represents an imperfect means of treating patients for which oAAA is not an appealing option. The coming years will see a more robust literature of this patient population as well as new devices with which to treat a broader spectrum of aortic aneurysms.

REFERENCES

1. Schwarze ML, Shen Y, Hemmerich J, Dale W. Age-related trends in utilization and outcome of open and endovascular repair for abdominal aortic aneurysm in the United States, 2001–2006. *J Vasc Surg.* Oct 2009;50(4):722–729.
2. Kent KC. Endovascular aneurysm repair--is it durable? *N Engl J Med.* May 20 2010; 362(20):1930–1931.
3. Jackson RS, Chang DC, Freischlag JA. Comparison of long-term survival after open vs endovascular repair of intact abdominal aortic aneurysm among Medicare beneficiaries. *JAMA.* Apr 18 2012;307(15):1621–1628.

4. Albuquerque Jr FC, Tonnessen BH, Noll Jr RE, et al. Paradigm shifts in the treatment of abdominal aortic aneurysm: Trends in 721 patients between 1996 and 2008. *J Vasc Surg.* Jun 2010;51(6):1348–1352; discussion 1352–1343.

5. Greenhalgh RM, Brown LC, Powell JT, et al. Endovascular versus open repair of abdominal aortic aneurysm. *N Engl J Med.* May 20 2010;362(20):1863–1871.

6. De Bruin JL, Baas AF, Buth J, et al. Long-term outcome of open or endovascular repair of abdominal aortic aneurysm. *N Engl J Med.* May 20 2010;362(20):1881–1889.

7. Lederle FA, Freischlag JA, Kyriakides TC, et al. Outcomes following endovascular vs open repair of abdominal aortic aneurysm: A randomized trial. *JAMA.* Oct 14 2009;302(14):1535–1542.

8. Lederle FA, Freischlag JA, Kyriakides TC. Long-term Comparison of Endovascular and Open Repair of Abdominal Aortic Aneurysm. *Vascular Annual Meeting.* National Harbor, MD2012.

9. Schermerhorn ML, O'Malley AJ, Jhaveri A, et al. Endovascular vs. open repair of abdominal aortic aneurysms in the Medicare population. *N Engl J Med.* Jan 31 2008;358(5):464–474.

10. Starnes BW, Kwolek CJ, Parodi JC, et al. Influence and critique of the EVAR 1 Trial. *Semin Vasc Surg.* Sep 2011;24(3):146–148.

11. Franks SC, Sutton AJ, Bown MJ, et al. Systematic review and meta-analysis of 12 years of endovascular abdominal aortic aneurysm repair. *Eur J Vasc Endovasc Surg.* Feb 2007;33(2):154–171.

12. van Zeggeren L, Van Herwaarden JA, Verhagen HJ, et al. Obstruction of the Endurant Endograft Post-EVAR; Incidence and Treatment Results. *Vascular Annual Meeting.* National Harbor, MD 2012.

13. Sweet MP, Fillinger MF, Morrison TM, et al. The influence of gender and aortic aneurysm size on eligibility for endovascular abdominal aortic aneurysm repair. *J Vasc Surg.* Oct 2011;54(4):931–937.

14. Wyss TR, Dick F, Brown LC, et al. The influence of thrombus, calcification, angulation, and tortuosity of attachment sites on the time to the first graft-related complication after endovascular aneurysm repair. *J Vasc Surg.* Oct 2011;54(4):965–971.

15. Mehta M, Byrne WJ, Robinson H, et al. Women derive less benefit from elective endovascular aneurysm repair than men. *J Vasc Surg.* Apr 2012;55(4):906–913.

16. Aburahma AF, Campbell JE, Mousa AY, et al. Clinical outcomes for hostile versus favorable aortic neck anatomy in endovascular aortic aneurysm repair using modular devices. *J Vasc Surg.* Jul 2011;54(1):13–21.

17. Wyss TR, Brown LC, Powell JT, et al. Rate and predictability of graft rupture after endovascular and open abdominal aortic aneurysm repair: Data from the EVAR Trials. *Ann Surg.* Nov 2010;252(5):805–812.

18. Schanzer A, Greenberg RK, Hevelone N, et al. Predictors of abdominal aortic aneurysm sac enlargement after endovascular repair. *Circulation.* Jun 21 2011;123(24):2848–2855.

19. Diehm N, Dick F, Katzen BT, et al. Aortic neck dilatation after endovascular abdominal aortic aneurysm repair: A word of caution. *J Vasc Surg.* Apr 2008;47(4):886–892.

20. Fairman R, Abraham C, Haulon S, et al. One year results from the Zenith low profile pivotal AAA Endovascular graft clinical study. *Vascular Annual Meeting.* National Harbor, MD 2012.

21. Fillinger MF. The Pythagoras U.S. Clinical trial of the Aorfix Endograft for Endovascular AAA repair (EVAR) with highly-angulated necks. *Vascular Annual Meeting.* National Harbor, MD 2012.

22. Zenith Fenestrated AAA Endovascular graft: Summary of safety and effectiveness data. Silver Springs, MD April 4, 2012 2012.

23. Krievins DK, Holden A, Savlovskis J, et al. EVAR using the Nellix Sac-anchoring endoprosthesis: Treatment of favourable and adverse anatomy. *Eur J Vasc Endovasc Surg.* Jul 2011;42(1):38–46.

23

EVAR Explants Definitive Remediation

Sean P. Lyden, MD

BACKGROUND

In the twenty years since the first endovascular abdominal aneurysm repair (EVAR) was reported,[1] hundreds of thousands of individuals have been treated with aortic stent grafts.[2,3] During this time we have also steadily seen the number of open aortic repairs decline.[4,5] Throughout these two decades we have seen the introduction of new devices and improvements to previously approved devices[6–8] as well as increasing physician experience and implantation skills.[5,9] Unfortunately no device has been uniformly successful and surveillance has identified endograft failures due to endoleak, migration, infection and rupture. Although some failures are salvageable by endovascular methods[10] many of these failures will require open conversion.[11,12]

The overall conversion rate is 0–9% based on published literature within various EVAR series. The true risk of conversion is difficult to ascertain as many patients are lost to follow-up or present to a different institution for removal. Devices that are placed outside of the instructions for use (IFU) have been found to have a higher risk of aneurysm growth and potential need for conversion.[13,14]

Early conversions are defined as occurring within 30 days of implantation and more commonly occur in patients that are treated with anatomy that is outside of the instructions for use for EVAR devices. A recent literature review found that the incidence of early conversion is 0.8–5.9% with a decrease in recent years.[15] Late conversions are defined as occurring later than 30 days after implantation and should not be due to poor planning or technical misadventures at the time of placement. However some patients may not have perioperative issues identified until after the first postoperative CT scan which is typically not done until 30 days after placement. A large review found a 1.7% incidence of late conversions, with the rate ranging from 0.4% to 22%.[15]

INDICATIONS

The reasons for early conversion are usually due to technical failures at placement and are outlined in Table 23-1.[16] Angulated and short necks are likely to lead to persistent type Ia endoleaks necessitating conversion.[14] Inexperience with devices or difficult anatomy can lead to inadvertent coverage of important visceral or renal vessels requiring conversion. Narrow distal aortic diameters and iliac tortuosity can lead to gate cannulation difficulties and inability to deliver the iliac limbs. Vessel rupture is another reason and may be due to small access vessel diameter or over aggressive balloon molding of seal zones. In most of these scenarios the reason for conversion is related to lack of technical skill, use of devices outside of the IFU or poor planning.

The indications for late explant of an aortic endograft are primarily related to device failure.[12,15,17–21] This may be related to endoleak, aneurysm sac enlargement, migration or any combination thereof. With the exception of a type IV endoleak, all types of endoleak (including endotension) have been reported as etiologies of post EVAR aneurysm rupture.[22–24] The need for explant may also be urgent or emergent due to graft infection, aortoduodenal fistulas, or rupture. Limb thrombosis may be a reason for removal if other endoluminal or surgical revascularization options fail.

Close monitoring of EVAR patients has helped identify and treat complications with secondary interventions.[25] Not all endoleaks are equal in terms of risk to the patient and literature supports early management of type I and III endoleaks to prevent aneurysm rupture.[26] While endovascular salvage of EVAR complications and even recurrent rupture is a viable and often successful option for many patients, conversion is required for those that fail.[10,20]

TABLE 23-1. REASONS FOR EARLY CONVERSION

Access Related:

Inability to deliver device

Rupture of the iliac vessels due to device being larger than access vessel or severely calcified

Device Placement:

Inability to cannulate the contralateral gate

Inability to retrieve delivery system

Rupture of aorta or iliac vessels from angioplasty

Coverage of renal or visceral vessels

Anatomy Issues:

Short proximal neck leading to proximal type Ia endoleak

Angulated neck >60 degrees leading to proximal type Ia endoleak

Narrow distal aortic neck leading to limb(s) thrombosis or inability to cannulate contralateral gate

Distal iliac angulation leading to limb thrombosis or type Ib endoleak

Small calcified iliac arteries more prone to rupture and inability to deliver the graft

Device Sizing:

Proximal graft undersized to native aorta leading to type Ia endoleak

Limb oversizing leading to compression in distal aorta

Large diameter limb brought into external iliac artery leading to thrombosis

PREOPERATIVE CONSIDERATIONS

The preoperative strategy should include identification of the type of endograft. This can be found in the patient's medical record or determined by plain abdominal x-ray or CT imaging. The presence of suprarenal fixation and type may impact the methods used to remove the device. Evaluation of contrast enhanced spiral CT imaging with thin (<1 mm) slices, delayed imaging and multiplanar reconstructions usually will allow identification of proximal or distal migration, component separation, endoleak type, or graft infection as the cause of endograft failure. The reason for failure may significantly alter the surgical approach, clamping positions and reconstruction options.

OPERATIVE TECHNIQUES

Case series documenting outcomes removing endografts have identified several technical challenges encountered during removal of endografts including: management of supra-renal components, endothelialization or incorporation of stents from endografts into the vessel wall, presence of external stents or barbs, and periaortic inflammation.[27–29]

In terms of exposure, both retroperitoneal and midline approaches have been used. There are advocates for each approach however devices with suprarenal fixa-tion have been more commonly approached by a retroperitoneal approach in most series. Both approaches are equally effective with the key being the anticipated proxi-mal clamp location. Cases without a suprarenal component and long aortic neck are suitable for infrarenal clamping. Early papers advocated infrarenal clamping with a temporary release to pull out proximal passive fixation devices. The ability to place a clamp above proximal active fixation can be of critical importance as removing the device from aorta can be made more difficult when the clamp is in the way.

In obtaining supra renal or visceral aortic control, the surgeon's preference and expertise should decide whether to use a transperitoneal versus retroperitoneal inci-sion. Periaortic inflammation can increase the difficulty of the exposure both proxi-mally and distally. The etiology for this inflammation is not well understood as it has been identified in grafts with both active and passive fixation and grafts with internal and external stents. This finding is unpredictable and not always present—even within similar graft types. In general, I believe endografts with proximal fixation or sealing problems are better approached from a retroperitoneal approach. This allows excellent exposure of the paravisceral aorta and the ability to choose the best location to place a clamp above the device. The retroperitoneal approach also allows proximal extension of the aortotomy above the renal or visceral arteries if necessary to facilitate removal. Once the graft has been removed, the clamp position should be moved a more distal location to limit the renal and visceral ischemic insult. Some have suggested the use of endoluminal proximal balloon occlusion supported by a large sheath however we find this approach to be cumbersome. To date there is no association between clamp positions (suprarenal vs. infrarenal) and peri-operative renal failure but just as with first time open aortic surgery clamping a diseased free portion of the aorta is critical. Distal exposure may require the ability to access the external and internal iliac arteries especially if the entire device is to be removed. An alternative distal control strategy is to clamp the endograft limbs once the aorta is opened then to use balloon occlusion of the endograft limbs once the graft is transected.

Once the proximal and distal control is obtained, opening the aortic sac in the midportion of the aneurysm without clamping (unless there is a proximal endoleak) allows evaluation and definitive identification of the source of failure. This confirms the type of endoleak and identifies secure areas of the graft in case complete removal is not possible. The iliac portion of endografts can be removed in segments when necessary or incorporated into a hybrid open repair when the limbs are adherent to the native vessel wall or extend far down into the external iliac artery. When distal limbs are left in place it is critical to make sure that they are not dislodged from their fixation points.

Some devices with uncovered proximal stents and devices that have had a giant balloon expandable stent placed across the proximal fixation into the native aorta can become covered with neointima, which will require endarterectomy of that portion of the aorta to allow removal. We sometimes use wire cutters to transect the uncovered stents allowing easier or partial or stepwise removal.

Treating the endoleaks without graft explantation is reasonable when patients will not tolerate complete removal. Transaortic graft sutures for fixation of type I endoleaks has been successfully performed as well as suturing through and through the proximal sealing stent and aortic wall with circumferential felt pledget reinforcement. Type II endoleaks have been treated with ligation of lumbar arteries or inferior mesenteric arteries.[11] Unfortunately, there are also reports of failures of these methods with proximal migration as well as development of new endoleaks. An open secondary intervention should not be performed if the patients' physiologic status would tolerate graft removal in my opinion. It is important to note, that if the procedure fails the risk of repeat open surgery is much higher. When possible we feel complete removal of the endograft should be the goal of the procedure.

The most commonly used maneuver to assist in successful removal of the aortic stent graft is a traditional 'clamp and pull' method. In stents with proximal barbs it is helpful to collapse the proximal stent. For Zenith devices (Cook Inc., Bloomington, IN), we have adopted the technique described by Koning which involves collapsing the device into a modified transected 20ml syringe (Figure 23-1).[29] By cutting off the closed end of a syringe, the syringe cylinder can be then used as a type of short sheath to recapture and separate the proximal stent safely from the aortic wall. The suprarenal portion is oftentimes covered with endothelium and gentle traction will perform a limited endarterectomy as the stents pull free from the aortic wall.

Metal wire cutters are a necessary instrument as they can help transect the device at any point with metal. They can be used to facilitate the removal of uncovered suprarenal fixation when it is not possible to collapse into a syringe. We have found the Endurant device (Medtronic, Santa Rosa, CA) proximal fixation impossible to remove by collapse into a syringe and have found wire cutters necessary to remove the uncovered proximal stent. When plans include leaving portions of well incorporated devices in situ, metal wire cutters are invaluable to create a place to safely suture to the remaining components. In patients who have large balloon expandable stainless steel stents within the aortic neck, these stents can be crushed with a clamp or divided with metal cutters to aid in atraumatic removal.

While removing the proximal device seems to concern most surgeons, removal of the distal limbs can be equally difficult. When a long length of the limb remains in a normal iliac artery it can be just as difficult to remove. Stent grafts with stents on the outside of the fabric can to be very adherent to the non-aneurysmal native distal vessel

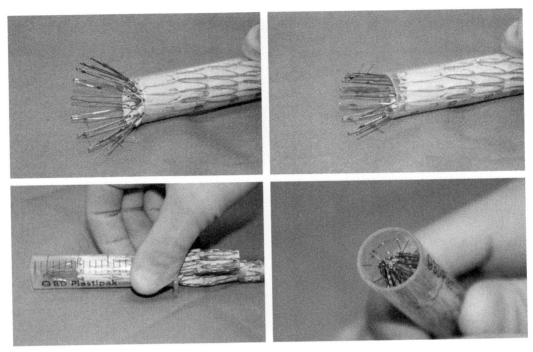

Figure 23-1. Using a 20cc syringe, the top stent is collapsed into the device, retracting the hooks from the wall of the aorta without damaging it. Copyright permission from Koning OH, Hinnen JW, van Baalen JM. Technique for safe removal of an aortic endograft with suprarenal fixation. *J Vasc Surg.* 2006; 43:855–857.

and thus more difficult to remove. Difficulty can also be encountered when a distal balloon expandable stent has been placed. When control is possible distal to the end of the endograft limbs, transection of the native artery and sewing at this level is many times the simplest solution. When the limbs are not removable or extend far down into the external iliac artery it is usually easier to do a hybrid reconstruction by suturing to the endograft limb and leaving it in place. Using sections of well-incorporated graft may potentially improve outcomes and reduce mortality by limiting the technical challenges of a more extensive operation. Late failure of hybrid repairs using transected endografts has not been reported. When portions of an endograft have been incorporated into the repair, closure of the aortic sac around the device may minimize potential device movement. In a series of 41 patients treated with conversion at our center, stent grafts were not completely removed due to 1) aneurysmal progression of the suprarenal segment with AAA exclusion and good distal fixation, 3) difficulty removing a well-incorporated endograft both proximally and distally, 3) isolated limb problem with good proximal fixation.[12] Hybrid reconstructions were performed in these patients (Figure 23-2A, B, C). Important factors when deciding when not to remove the entire endograft include: location of endograft problem (proximal or distal), extent of problem, and prevention of native tissue injury. Patients that have in-situ retention of a portion of the endograft still require lifelong CT surveillance as future complications of the remaining EVAR elements is possible. The last option is to bypass to an artery distal to the end of the device.

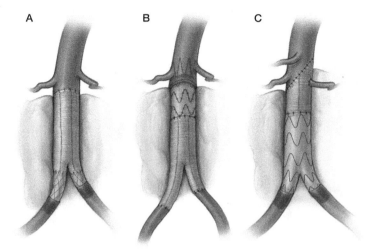

Figure 23-2. Hybrid reconstruction. Examples incorporating residual endografts into the aortic reconstruction. **A)** Incorporated proximal Zenith endograft into distal aortobiiliac repair. **B)** Proximal Dacron graft with distal AneuRx limbs. **C)** Beveled proximal Dacron graft with left renal implant anastomosed to distal Talent endograft. Copyright permission from Kelso RL, Lyden SP, Butler B et al. Late conversion of aortic stent grafts. *J Vasc Surg.* 2009; 49:589–595.

The rate of aortic graft infection has been estimated in a meta-analysis by Sharif et al to be 0.16% at 2 years after EVAR.[30] There have been reports of aortoduodenal fistulas even in cases without large aneurysm sacs.[31] The mechanism of the aortoduodenal fistula is unclear in EVAR as the graft is always covered by the aortic wall and may be related to the radial forces of the stent or primary or secondary infection. Further management of the infected graft is no different than primary management of infected aortic grafts or aortoduodenal fistulas.[32] The concepts of removing infected material, stump management, and debridement of infected tissue are unchanged.[33] A hybrid reconstruction is not an option as the presence of infection requires complete removal of all portions of the endograft.

POSTOPERATIVE CONSIDERATIONS

Compared to open primary aortic repair the postoperative management is similar. Cardiopulmonary and renal complications are the biggest risks. A large meta-analysis review also compared rates of conversion and mortality in both early and late explants. In 178 patients undergoing early conversion, the mortality rate was 12.4%.[15] The mortality in late conversion (279 patients) was similar at 10%. When further extrapolated to cases that underwent emergent late conversion for rupture the average mortality increased to 25.6%. This increase in mortality is a consistent finding amongst the various studies.[11,12,20] It is related not only to the emergent nature of the surgery but also to the increase cardiovascular risk of these patients, complexity of removal, and blood loss. Both the EUROSTAR registry and our own study found that patients presenting with rupture after EVAR had either type I or type III endoleaks and migration.[12,34] We suggest that these patients with these problems have higher risk and should be considered for expedited conversion if they fail endovascular options.

CONCLUSIONS

EVAR has revolutionized infrarenal aortic surgery. While the initial complication rate is lower than open repair, long-term follow-up data has confirmed the need to remove the device from some patients. With increased experience with conversion techniques elective late EVAR conversions can be performed with mortality risk similar to primary elective open aneurysm repair.

REFERENCES

1. Parodi JC, Palmaz JC, Barone HD. Transfemoral intraluminal graft implantation for abdominal aortic aneurysms. *Ann Vasc Surg.* Nov 1991;5(6):491–499.
2. Vogel TR, Symons R, Flum DR. The incidence and factors associated with graft infection after aortic aneurysm repair. *J Vasc Surg.* Feb 2008;47(2):264–269.
3. Landon BE, O'Malley AJ, Giles K, et al. Volume-outcome relationships and abdominal aortic aneurysm repair. *Circulation.* Sep 28 2010;122(13):1290–1297.
4. Chadi SA, Rowe BW, Vogt KN, et al. Trends in management of abdominal aortic aneurysms. *J Vasc Surg.* Apr 2012;55(4):924–928.
5. Sachs T, Schermerhorn M, Pomposelli F, et al. Resident and fellow experiences after the introduction of endovascular aneurysm repair for abdominal aortic aneurysm. *J Vasc Surg.* Sep 2011;54(3):881–888.
6. Makaroun MS, Tuchek M, Massop D, et al. One year outcomes of the United States regulatory trial of the Endurant Stent Graft System. *J Vasc Surg.* Sep 2011;54(3):601–608.
7. Hansen CJ, Aziz I, Kim BB, et al. Results from the Endologix PowerLink multicenter trial. *Semin Vasc Surg.* Jun 2003;16(2):166–170.
8. Ricotta JJ, 2nd, Oderich GS. The Cook Zenith AAA endovascular graft. *Perspect Vasc Surg and Endovasc Ther.* Jun 2008;20(2):167–173.
9. Traul D, Street D, Faught W, et al. Endoluminal stent-graft placement for repair of abdominal aortic aneurysms in the community setting. *J Endovasc Ther.* Dec 2008;15(6): 688–694.
10. Vourliotakis G, Bos WT, Beck AW, et al. Fenestrated stent-grafting after previous endovascular abdominal aortic aneurysm repair. *J Cardiovasc Surg. (Torino).* Jun 2010;51(3):383–389.
11. Chaar CI, Eid R, Park T, et al. Delayed open conversions after endovascular abdominal aortic aneurysm repair. *J Vasc Surg.* Jun 2012;55(6):1562–1569 e1561.
12. Kelso RL, Lyden SP, Butler B, et al. Late conversion of aortic stent grafts. *J Vasc Surg.* Mar 2009;49(3):589–595.
13. Schanzer A, Greenberg RK, Hevelone N, et al. Predictors of abdominal aortic aneurysm sac enlargement after endovascular repair. *Circulation.* Jun 21 2011;123(24):2848–2855.
14. Sternbergh WC, 3rd, Carter G, York JW, et al. Aortic neck angulation predicts adverse outcome with endovascular abdominal aortic aneurysm repair. *J Vasc Surg.* Mar 2002;35(3):482–486.
15. Moulakakis KG, Dalainas I, Mylonas S, et al. Conversion to open repair after endografting for abdominal aortic aneurysm: A review of causes, incidence, results, and surgical techniques of reconstruction. *J Endovasc Ther.* Dec 2010;17(6):694–702.
16. Pitoulias GA, Schulte S, Donas KP, et al. Secondary endovascular and conversion procedures for failed endovascular abdominal aortic aneurysm repair: Can we still be optimistic? *Vascular.* Jan–Feb 2009;17(1):15–22.
17. Forbes TL, Harrington DM, Harris JR, et al. Late conversion of endovascular to open repair of abdominal aortic aneurysms. *Can J Surg.* Jun 1 2012;55(3):038310.
18. Phade SV, Keldahl ML, Morasch MD, et al. Late abdominal aortic endograft explants: Indications and outcomes. *Surgery.* Oct 2011;150(4):788–795.

19. Brinster CJ, Fairman RM, Woo EY, et al. Late open conversion and explantation of abdominal aortic stent grafts. *J Vasc Surg.* Jul 2011;54(1):42–46.
20. Mehta M, Paty PS, Roddy SP, et al. Treatment options for delayed AAA rupture following endovascular repair. *J Vasc Surg.* Jan 2011;53(1):14–20.
21. Gambardella I, Blair PH, McKinley A, et al. Successful delayed secondary open conversion after endovascular repair using partial explantation technique: A single-center experience. *Ann Vasc Surg.* Jul 2010;24(5):646–654.
22. Koole D, Moll FL, Buth J, et al. Annual rupture risk of abdominal aortic aneurysm enlargement without detectable endoleak after endovascular abdominal aortic repair. *J Vasc Surg.* Dec 2011;54(6):1614–1622.
23. Vallabhaneni SR, Harris PL. Lessons learnt from the EUROSTAR registry on endovascular repair of abdominal aortic aneurysm repair. *Eur J Radiol.* Jul 2001;39(1):34–41.
24. Hinchliffe RJ, Singh-Ranger R, Davidson IR, et al. Rupture of an abdominal aortic aneurysm secondary to type II endoleak. *Eur J Vasc Endovasc Surg.* Dec 2001;22(6):563–565.
25. Resch T, Dias N. Treatment of endoleaks: Techniques and outcome. *J Cardiovasc Surg (Torino).* Feb 2012;53(1 Suppl 1):91–99.
26. van Marrewijk C, Buth J, Harris PL, et al. Significance of endoleaks after endovascular repair of abdominal aortic aneurysms: The EUROSTAR experience. *J Vasc Surg.* 2002;35(3):461–473.
27. Lyden SP, McNamara JM, Sternbach Y, et al. Technical considerations for late removal of aortic endografts. *J Vasc Surg.* 2002;36(4):674–678.
28. May J, White GH, Harris JP. Techniques for surgical conversion of aortic endoprosthesis. *Eur J Vasc Endovasc Surg.* 1999;18(4):284–289.
29. Koning OH, Hinnen JW, van Baalen JM. Technique for safe removal of an aortic endograft with suprarenal fixation. *J Vasc Surg.* Apr 2006;43(4):855–857.
30. Sharif MA, Lee B, Lau LL, et al. Prosthetic stent graft infection after endovascular abdominal aortic aneurysm repair. *J Vasc Surg.* Sep 2007;46(3):442–448.
31. Lyden SP, Tanquilut EM, Gavin TJ, et al. Aortoduodenal fistula after abdominal aortic stent graft presenting with extremity abscesses. *Vascular.* Sep-Oct 2005;13(5):305–308.
32. Laser A, Baker N, Rectenwald J, et al. Graft infection after endovascular abdominal aortic aneurysm repair. *J Vasc Surg.* Jul 2011;54(1):58–63.
33. Setacci C, De Donato G, Setacci F, et al. Management of abdominal endograft infection. *J Cardiovasc Surg (Torino).* Feb 2010;51(1):33–41.
34. Harris PL, Vallabhaneni SR, Desgranges P, et al. Incidence and risk factors of late rupture, conversion, and death after endovascular repair of infrarenal aortic aneurysms: The EUROSTAR experience. European Collaborators on Stent/graft techniques for aortic aneurysm repair. *J Vasc Surg.* 2000;32(4):739–749.

24

Perigraft Seromas Following Open Aortic Reconstruction

Joseph L. Karam, MD and Alexander D. Shepard, MD

INTRODUCTION

A perigraft seroma (PGS) is defined as a persistent, sometimes expanding, sterile fluid collection around a patent vascular graft. Such seromas are most commonly recognized following placement of a subcutaneously tunneled prosthetic graft, usually for dialysis access or axillofemoral bypass.[1,2] Perigraft seromas have been noted after open abdominal aortic reconstructions but are rare;[3–12] until very recently less than 15 cases had been reported with the largest series consisting of only five cases.[3] The increasing use of computed tomography (CT) scans and other cross-sectional imaging modalities has led to greater recognition of this pathology. Recent experience suggests an incidence significantly greater than reported in the older literature. Moreover, a variety of problems can result from such seromas, including persistent abdominal discomfort, sac rupture and acute limb-threatening ischemia from graft limb compression and thrombosis. This chapter reviews the literature as well as our institutional experience with PGS following open aortic reconstruction in an attempt to determine its true frequency, identify possible risk factors, and review management strategies.

DEFINITION

The earliest major reference to PGS is Blumenberg's classic 1985 paper wherein a PGS was defined as "a collection of clear, sterile fluid, confined within a nonsecretory fibrous pseudomembrane surrounding a vascular graft."[1] Some perigraft fluid accumulation is an expected component of the graft healing process and perigraft fluid up to six weeks following placement of an aortic prosthesis for occlusive disease is considered a normal CT finding; fluid present beyond six weeks is considered abnormal.[4] Fluid accumulation within the aneurysm sac following open AAA repair is the rule. However, over time, this fluid

253

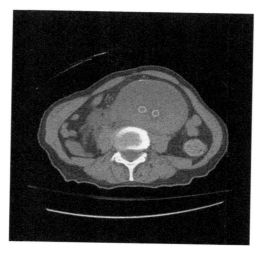

Figure 24-1. Computed tomographic image of a 10 cm perigraft seroma occurring six years after an open abdominal aortic aneurysm repair.

usually resolves and the aneurysm sac contracts around the aortic graft with a significant reduction in size. In most patients there is eventually complete or near-complete apposition of the native aneurysm sac to the aortic graft. Persistent expansion of the aneurysm sac with fluid is not normal.

Perigraft fluid can represent hematoma or seroma. The nature of the fluid can be determined by its radiodensity—simple body fluids such as cerebrospinal fluid and urine have a radiodensity of 0–10 Hounsfield units (HU) while blood is greater than 50 HU. Various reports in the literature describe PGS fluid as having a jelly-like consistency with a radiodensity usually less than 25 HU.[3,5,6] In analyzing our experience with PGS following open aortic surgery three criteria were used to define the presence of PGS. The fluid collection had to be present more than three months post graft implantation. The size of the collection had to be at least three centimeters in diameter. And finally the radiodensity of the fluid had to be ≤ 25 HU.[7] These criteria are relatively strict compared to others suggested in the literature but seem reasonable.[5] (Figure 24-1)

PATHOPHYSIOLOGY

Most cases of PGS involve prosthetic grafts, with only 1–2% reported to occur with vein grafts.[1] The cause of PGS remains unclear; abnormal transudation of fluid through graft pores and failure of normal graft healing/incorporation seem to be the common denominators in seroma formation.[2,8] All synthetic vascular prostheses have some degree of porosity to allow tissue ingrowth and normal graft healing. Anything that interferes with this incorporation process can potentially lead to a seroma. Immediately after implantation plasma proteins and formed blood elements infiltrate graft interstices from the luminal surface while extracellular fluids and proteins coat the outer surface. Over a period of weeks a compacted layer of fibrin coagulum lines the graft while fibroblasts in the perigraft tissue form collagen and induce tissue contraction around the graft. Graft incorporation produces a fluid tight seal. Factors that adversely affect this process can lead to continued graft porosity and slow leakage (ultrafiltration) of plasma fluid into the perigraft area.

Graft material and its properties appear to play an important role in PGS formation. While initial reports of PGS suggested that Dacron grafts were more commonly implicated than polytetrafluoroethylene (PTFE) grafts,[1] more recent experience have suggested just the opposite.[3,5,6,9,10] Almost all reported cases of PGS following open AAA repair have been done with PTFE grafts; there are only two cases in the literature of a PGS following Dacron graft repair of an AAA.[3–10] The increased prevalence of PGS following PTFE reconstructions may have to do with the increased porosity of PTFE (pores roughly 30 microns in size) compared to most currently available Dacron grafts. A similar problem has been noted with first generation PTFE endografts where PGS have been implicated as a cause of endotension following endovascular AAA repair.[11,12] Modification of these early grafts by adding an extra layer of PTFE has virtually eliminated this problem and highlights the potential problems associated with graft porosity.[11,13,14]

A variety of pathogenic mechanisms for increased graft porosity have been proposed including low-grade infection,[15] a fibrinolytic milieu retarding normal thrombotic sealing of graft pores,[9,16] and fibroblast inhibition leading to poor graft incorporation.[17] Some authorities have postulated that clinically and microbiologically silent infection by organisms such as "slime"-producing *staphylococcus epidermidis* may cause an exudative process resulting in a seroma.[3,9,18] Such an infectious process may also cause dissolution of the coagulum lining the graft leading to a transudation of serum. Microbiological testing, however, has never consistently proven an infectious etiology for PGS. Based on assays of coagulation and fibrinolytic factors in the plasma and aneurysm sac, Williams[16] hypothesized that local fibrinolysis may prevent sealing of the graft pores leading to continued transudation of serum. An association with long-term anticoagulation and PGS has only recently been documented.[7] Fibroblast inhibition by humoral fibroblast inhibitors has also been implicated in the genesis of PGS.[2] Investigators have observed that the histology of PGS tissue samples has demonstrated very sparse connective tissue around the graft in contrast to the mature connective tissue usually seen.[1]

It has also been suggested that various aspects of intra-operative graft handling can adversely affect graft integrity, particularly for PTFE. Anything that breaks the hydrophobic barrier of PTFE prior to establishing blood flow creates the potential for serous leakage through the graft wall. "Wetting" of the graft with serum, liquefied fat, blood, pressurized irrigating solutions,[15,19] or organic solvents[1] can have deleterious effects on graft porosity. Excessive graft handling with bloody gloves and localized graft manipulation have also been implicated.[8] Other possible predisposing factors highlighted in the literature include high blood pressure, low blood viscosity and low-grade patient allergy to the graft material.[1,2,16,20]

The fact that PGS has only been reported after open AAA repair as opposed to reconstructions for aortoiliac occlusive disease suggests that the aneurysm sac itself plays a significant role. The sac lining is devoid of fibroblasts and other connective tissue elements, which are important contributors to the graft incorporation/healing process.

HENRY FORD EXPERIENCE

To determine the frequency of PGS after open aortic reconstruction and possible associated risk factors we recently reviewed our experience.[7] All patients undergoing open AAA repair between 1995 and 2009 who had at least one post-operative cross-sectional imaging study were included. In this study PGS was defined as a perigraft fluid collection present > three months post-op, ≥3 cm in diameter, and with a radiodensity of ≤25 HU. Patient records were reviewed to determine possible risk factors for PGS. One hundred eleven study patients were identified of whom 20 (18%) had a PGS. All patients with a PGS had reconstruction with a PTFE graft and 20 of 98 (20.4%) patients with PTFE reconstructions developed a PGS. Average PGS size at the time of detection was 6.0 cm (range 3.0–11.0 cm) and in most patients the seroma involved the entire graft. The interval between graft implantation and PGS detection averaged 51 months (range 4–156 months).

To analyze possible risk factors for the development of PGS, patients who developed a seroma were compared to those who did not utilizing a number of demographic, comorbidity, operative, and post-operative variables. (Table 24-1) Univariate analysis identified smoking (P = 0.005), diabetes (P = 0.020), hyperlipidemia (P = 0.022), aneurysm extent (P = 0.031), left flank extraperitoneal operative approach (P = 0.003), reconstruction with a bifurcated graft (P = 0.002), and long-term anticoagulation (P = 0.010) as factors significantly associated with PGS formation. Reconstruction with a PTFE graft did not reach statistical significance (P = 0.069). On multivariate analysis, only four variables remained significant—reconstruction with a bifurcated graft, long-term anticoagulation, utilization of a left flank extraperitoneal approach, and smoking. (Table 24-2) Aneurysm extent approached but did not reach significance (P = 0.09). Of these factors, repair with a bifurcated graft (OR = 8.0) and anticoagulation (OR = 7.2) were the two variables that showed the strongest association with PGS development.

A similar review of patients with open aortic reconstructions for occlusive disease was also performed. The 213 patients undergoing aortofemoral bypass from 1995 to 2009 were reviewed. In the 96 patients who had an abdominal cross-sectional imaging study more than three months post-operatively, only two had a PGS fulfilling the same criteria as our AAA population for an incidence of 2%. Both these patients had PTFE reconstructions and had asymptomatic seromas, the largest of which was 4.7 cm in diameter. (Figure 24-2)

Review of this experience suggests several important findings. The incidence of PGS in this series was 18% (20/111 patients) for AAA patients, and 2% (2/96) for aortofemoral bypass patients is far higher than previously recognized. The true incidence of PGS after open AAA repair is probably even higher given the fact that the majority of CT scans performed, were obtained during the last half of the study interval. Most patients with PGS are asymptomatic and the deep location of these collections precludes detection by physical exam unless they are very large. Imaging studies are, therefore, necessary to make the diagnosis of PGS. With the widespread availability and extensive use of abdominal CT scanning, it seems likely that PGS following open AAA repair will be recognized with increasing frequency in the future.

Perigraft seroma after open aortic reconstruction appears to be largely a complication of PTFE grafts. This is congruent with the literature where PTFE is the implanted graft in the overwhelming majority of open aortic PGS cases. Only two cases of PGS following AAA repair with a Dacron graft have ever been reported.[9,10] The lower incidence of PGS following aortofemoral bypass suggests that the

TABLE 24-1. VARIABLES EXAMINED IN COMPARING PATIENTS WHO DEVELOPED A PERIGRAFT SEROMA WITH THOSE WHO DID NOT (ADAPTED FROM KADAKOL, ET AL., 2011)[7]

Demographics and co-morbidities

Age

Gender

Aneurysm size

Aneurysm extent—Limited:infrarenal, moderate:juxtarenal, extensive:suprarenal

Diabetes

Smoking

Hypertension

Dyslipidemia

Chronic obstructive pulmonary disease

Heart disease (Documented CAD and/or CHF)

Chronic kidney disease—Serum creatinine > 1.4 mg/dL

Poor nutritional status—Serum albumin < 3.6 mg/dL

Multiple allergies—Allergies to three or more allergens

Operative variables

Operative approach—Transperitoneal vs left flank extraperitoneal

Urgency—Ruptured vs intact aneurysm

Clamp level—Infrarenal vs suprarenal vs supraceliac

Polytetrafluoroethylene (PTFE) vs Dacron

Graft size

Tube vs bifurcated graft

Post-operative variables

Complicated vs uncomplicated post-operative course—Presence of one or more major post-op complications

Prolonged mechanical ventilation (>24 h)

Prolonged ICU stay (>3 days)

Post-operative infection—any culture-proven infection

Re-operation within 6 months (major operation related or unrelated to original repair)

Long-term anticoagulation

TABLE 24-2. FACTORS ASSOCIATED WITH DEVELOPMENT OF PERIGRAFT SEROMA BY MULTIVARIATE ANALYSIS (ADAPTED FROM KADAKOL, ET AL., 2011).[27]

Variable	Odds Ratio	P-value
Bifurcated vs tube graft reconstruction	8.0	.017
Anticoagulation	7.2	.003
Left flank extraperitoneal approach	7.1	.003
Smoking	5.6	.01
Aneurysm extent	4.2	.093
Diabetes	3.5	.010
Dyslipidemia	3.4	.531

aneurysm sac plays an important role in the formation of PGS. One could postulate that the sac wall is less conducive to complete graft incorporation/healing than the retroperitoneal tissues typically closed over an aortofemoral graft. This experience also suggests that coagulation abnormalities play a role in PGS formation. Anticoagulation was found to be the second most strongly associated factor in PGS

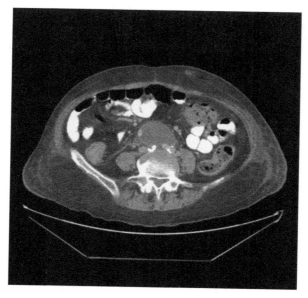

Figure 24-2. Computed tomographic image of a 4.1 cm perigraft seroma occurring 2 years after an aortobi-femoral bypass.

formation using multivariate analysis. In the single patient in our series in whom the seroma decreased in size over time, regression was temporally associated with discontinuation of chronic anticoagulation. The association between PGS and utilization of a left flank extraperitoneal approach or reconstruction with a bifurcated graft is unclear. Both of these factors may be markers for a more extensive aortic operation. This possibility is corroborated by the fact that aneurysm extent approached but did not reach statistical significance as a variable associated with PGS on multivariate analysis. Smoking as a risk factor for PGS makes sense given its well-recognized deleterious effects on wound healing.[21,22]

NATURAL HISTORY

The natural history of PGS following open AAA repair is unclear. The majority of patients in our series as well as those detailed in the literature remain asymptomatic. Most PGS are discovered incidentally on post-operative imaging studies obtained for other reasons. A small, but significant minority of patients (20% in our series), however, do develop symptoms. The most common symptom reported is persistent, vague abdominal discomfort presumed secondary to local compression associated with aneurysm sac expansion. The three patients in our series with abdominal symptoms all had PGS > 5 cm in diameter. Although the largest size encountered in our series was 11.0 cm, a gigantic, completely asymptomatic 28.0 cm in diameter PGS has been reported.[5] Presentation with chronic constipation or an abdominal mass have also been noted.[3,9]

Rarely a PGS can rupture leading to acute abdominal or back pain mimicking some of the symptomatology of a ruptured AAA. This picture can be very confusing to anyone who does not know about this entity. It is important to recognize the true nature of this condition and that its gravity is not the same as a ruptured AAA. We have encountered two cases of PGS rupture. Both patients had been followed with a known large (>9 cm) PGS and complaints of vague abdominal pain; one presented with the acute onset of worsened abdominal pain and the other with left flank pain. Both had undergone AAA repair with a bifurcated PTFE graft five years earlier. Both were hemodynamically stable, though the radiologic interpretation of both CT scans was "findings compatible with ruptured AAA." (Figure 24-3)

A final mode of presentation is bifurcated graft limb compression by the PGS. We have seen this in two patients. One patient presented with acute bilateral lower extremity ischemia from graft limb thrombosis resulting from compression of the limbs by the seroma. This patient had a suprarenal AAA repair in 2004 and presented in 2008 with sudden bilateral acute limb ischemia and was found to have occlusion of both graft limbs. He underwent successful catheter directed thrombolysis and a post-lysis CT angiogram showed evidence of a PGS causing compression of both graft limbs. (Figure 24-4) The decision was made to re-expand both graft limbs with stents. This patient has maintained continued patency with normal segmental pressures for four years. The degree of graft limb compression in the second patient is more modest and this patient is awaiting open intervention because of an associated suprarenal aneurysm. This complication is potentially preventable by monitoring for PGS with CT scans and timely intervention.

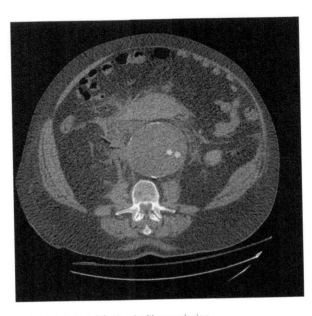

Figure 24-3. Adapted form Kadakol et al. [7]. Used with permission.

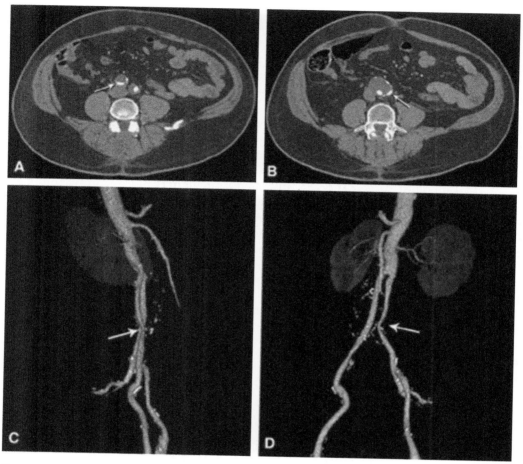

Figure 24-4. **A and B** CT scan slices showing right and left graft limbs respectively (*arrows*), **C and D** 3D reconstruction of CT-angiogram showing compressed right and left graft limbs, respectively (*arrows*).

MANAGEMENT

Asymptomatic seromas do not need intervention, however, it seems prudent to monitor them with periodic CT scans for stability and the rare case of graft limb compression. For symptomatic PGS, various treatment modalities have been attempted. Simple aspiration has been described in the literature but is frequently unsuccessful as it was in the one case in which we attempted it.[2,5] The seroma composition varies in consistency from a thin liquid to a frequently gelatinous collection, making reliable evacuation of a significant amount of material through even a large caliber catheter problematic. In addition, recurrence has been the rule. Injection of sclerosing agents, cryoprecipitate (fibrin glue), and topical thrombin have all been described as possible therapies but without documented outcomes.[1] Injection of microfibrillar collagen has been reported to result in the successful elimination of seromas complicating axillofemoral grafts,[2] but has not been documented with PGS following AAA repair. Techniques relying on catheter access to the seroma sac also run the risk of introducing infection, an obviously catastrophic complication.

Operative evacuation of the seroma with excision of the redundant sac wall and tight imbrication around the graft has also been described.[10] As might be expected, however, this approach has been associated with a high recurrence rate since it does not address the root cause(s) of seroma formation.[6,23] Williams reported a case of PGS treated with seroma evacuation and marsupialization of the aneurysm sac wall to the peritoneal cavity; at ten months follow-up the PGS had decreased in size.[16]

The most aggressive, and perhaps definitive method of treatment for PGS described in the early literature is evacuation of the seroma, excision of the associated "capsule," and replacement of the original graft with another type of graft material, usually Dacron for PTFE, routed through another tissue plane if possible.[1] This approach has been used with some success in treating PGS after axillofemoral bypass. A similar technique has been described for PGS after open AAA repair although in this situation it is not possible to route the graft through fresh tissue planes; instead redundant aneurysm sac wall is excised and then tightly closed around the new graft. Cuff and colleagues reported this approach as curative in one case.[23] We have used this approach in three patients—twice for PGS rupture and once for a patient with a large symptomatic (abdominal pain) PGS. The sac contents in all three cases were similar to that reported in the literature with thick gelatinous material. (Figure 24-5) Cultures were negative in all three cases. Both patients with PGS rupture had evidence of moderate bleeding from the ripped edges of the aneurysm sac wall. Early follow-up CT scans at four to six months post-operatively have shown some evidence of early PGS recurrence, but it is too early to comment definitively. In both cases juxta-anastomotic segments of the original PTFE bifurcation graft were retained raising the possibility that these short pieces of PTFE could be contributing to recurrent seroma formation.

An endoluminal solution has also been advocated. This approach involves re-lining the graft with covered stents similar to the solution described for treating type V endoleaks (so called endotension) that developed with some early generation aortic endografts, particularly the original Gore Excluder.[14] The first generation Excluder graft was constructed with a very thin, highly porous layer of PTFE which

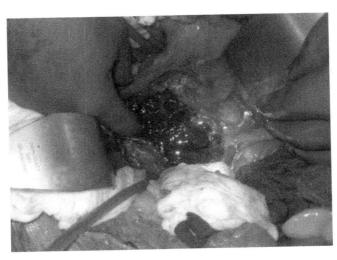

Figure 24-5. Operative photo of patient with ruptured perigraft seroma. Note blood-stained gelatinous contents.

was associated with a much higher than expected incidence of aneurysm sac enlargement—up to 32% as reported in original four year follow-up data.[24] Examining explanted Excluder devices for persistent aneurysm sac expansion, Goodney and colleagues described the presence of proteinaceous material deposition throughout the area where the graft was within the aneurysm, except the area where the docking limb overlapped with the contralateral limb, creating a double thickness graft surface.[14] This problem was eliminated in later models by adding another layer of PTFE to the graft. In patients with first generation Excluder grafts who experienced progressive aneurysm sac enlargement, re-lining the endograft with stent grafts led to seroma stabilization and/or resorption in a significant number of cases.[14,25] Salameh used this technique successfully in treating two patients with PGS.[13] While this approach does not allow evacuation of the seroma contents, a decrease in PGS size has been noted in the cases reported in the literature.[13] There may be theoretical concerns in small diameter limbs (≤8 mm in diameter) that such a re-lining procedure could narrow the lumen increasing the risk for limb thrombosis. Fortunately most open AAA repairs are performed with relatively large size grafts where graft limb narrowing would be unlikely. Patients with graft limb compression may be best treated with this endoluminal approach assuming they do not have symptoms from sac expansion. Even in this situation, it may be possible to wait for seroma resorption and aneurysm sac shrinkage or to evacuate the PGS cavity with a minimally invasive (laparoscopic) approach. Our first patient with graft limb compression has done well with stenting alone, and his PGS has remained stable in size despite continued use of warfarin anticoagulation. In retrospect use of covered stents may have been a better idea.

In view of the fact that PGS is far more common after open AAA repair than has been previously reported and that such seromas are not always benign, a strategy for surveillance seems appropriate. In our view, the best method for surveillance is abdominal CT scanning. Contrast enhancement is not necessary for seroma detection. Perigraft fluid with a radiodensity greater than 40 HU should raise suspicion that the collection may not be a simple PGS. Current guidelines suggest a surveillance CT scan five years after open AAA repair to look for new aneurysmal disease or a graft complication. In patients with a PTFE reconstruction, it may be prudent to obtain this first CT scan at two and one-half years. If no seroma is detected, resumption of a standard follow-up protocol seems appropriate. If a PGS is present, more frequent CT scans are necessary for follow up, especially if the PGS appears to be enlarging. In our experience, a PGS smaller than 5 cm rarely becomes symptomatic. Larger seromas need to be carefully evaluated for the possibility abdominal symptoms and graft-limb compression. If abdominal symptoms are thought to be secondary to the PGS, aspiration may be of benefit as a diagnostic test. Even partial decompression of the PGS may lead to symptom resolution/improvement, if only temporarily, confirming causation and strengthening indications for subsequent intervention. Graft limb compression of any significant degree needs to be addressed even if the patient is asymptomatic.

CONCLUSIONS

Perigraft seroma is an increasingly recognized complication after open aortic reconstruction with an incidence much higher than previously realized. It occurs much more frequently after AAA repair than after operations for aortoiliac occlusive disease and appears to be almost solely related to the use of PTFE grafts. Other risk factors identified in our analysis include use of anticoagulation post-operatively, tobacco use, reconstruction with a bifurcated graft, and utilization of a left flank extraperitoneal operative approach. Management of such PGS is variable and dependent on the size of the seroma and associated symptoms. Perigraft seromas <5 cm in diameter rarely cause problems and can be safely observed. Larger PGS are more frequently associated with symptoms and complications and should be followed more closely. Graft limb compression with thrombosis and PGS rupture are catastrophic complications requiring urgent interventions. A variety of treatment options exist for the management of PGS though as yet there are no definitive guidelines to suggest the best form of therapy. An endoluminal approach with graft re-lining with stent grafts seems reasonable for symptomatic PGS or those with significant graft limb compression involving non-small caliber limbs. Recognition of ruptured PGS as a diagnostic entity is important in order to avoid unnecessarily urgent celiotomy in an unprepared patient.

REFERENCES

1. Blumenberg RM, Gelfand MI, Dale WA. Perigraft seromas complicating arterial grafts. *Surgery*. 1985; 97:194–204.
2. Ahn SS, Machleder HI, Gupta R et al. Perigraft Seroma: Clinical, histologic, and Serologic Correlates. *Am J of Surg*. 1997;154:173–8.
3. Thoo CH, Bourke BM, May J. Symptomatic sac enlargement and rupture due to seroma after open abdominal aortic aneurysm repair with polytetrafluoroethylene graft: Implications for endovascular repair and endotension. *J Vasc Surg*. 2004;40:1089–94.
4. Auffermann W, Olofsson PA, Rabahie GN et al. Incorporation versus infection of retroperitoneal aortic grafts: MR imaging features. *Radiology*. 1989;172:359–62.
5. Lucas LA, Rodriguez JA, Oslen DM et al. Symptomatic seroma after open abdominal aortic aneurysm repair. *Ann Vasc Surg*. 2009;23:144–6.
6. Kat E, Jones DN, Burnett J et al. Perigraft seroma of open aortic reconstruction. *Am J Rad*. 2002;178:1462–4.
7. Kadakol AK, Nypaver TJ, Karam JL et al. Frequency, risk factors, and management of perigraft seroma after open abdominal aortic aneurysm repair. *J Vasc Surg*. 2011;54:637–43.
8. Bolton W, Cannon J. Seroma formation associated with PTFE vascular grafts used as arteriovenous fistulae. Dial Transplant 1981;10:60–3.
9. Risberg B, Delle M, Eriksson E et al. Aneurysm sac hygroma: a cause of endotension. *J Endovasc Ther*. 2001;8:447–53.
10. Arya N, O'Kane HF, Hannon RJ et al. Endoleak and endotension following open abdominal aortic aneurysm repair. *Ann Vasc Surg*. 2005;19:431–3.
11. Cho JS, Dillavou ED, Rhee RY et al. Late abdominal aortic aneurysm enlargement after endovascular repair with the Excluder device. *J Vasc Surg*. 2004;39:1236–42.
12. Ouriel K, Clair DG, Greenberg RK et al. Endovascular repair of abdominal aortic aneurysms: device specific outcomes. *J Vasc Surg*. 2003;37:991–8.
13. Salameh MK, Hoballah JJ. Successful endovascular treatment of aneurysm sac hygroma after open abdominal aortic aneurysm replacement: a report of two cases. *J Vasc Surg*. 2008;48:457–60.
14. Goodney PP, Fillinger MF. The effect of endograft relining on sac expansion after endovascular aneurysm repair with the original-permeability Gore Excluder abdominal aortic aneurysm endoprosthesis. *J Vasc Surg*. 2007;45:686–93.
15. LeBlanc J, Albus R, Williams WG et al. Serous fluid leakage: a complication following the modified Blalock-Taussig shunt. *J Thorac and Cardiovasc Surg*. 1984;88:259–62.

16. Williams GM. The management of massive ultrafiltration distending the aneurysm sac after abdominal aortic aneurysm repair with a polytetrafluoroethylene aortobiliac graft. *J Vasc Surg*. 1998;28:551–5.

17. Sladen JG, Mandl MA, Grossman L et al. Fibroblast inhibition: a new and treatable cause of prosthetic graft failure. *Am J of Surg*. 1985;149:587–90.

18. Bergamini TM, Bandyk DF, Govostis D et al. Infection of vascular prostheses caused by bacterial biofilms. *J Vasc Surg*. 1988;7:21–30.

19. Baker JD. Bleeding through PTFE grafts. *Eur J Vasc Surg*. 1987;1:41–3.

20. Kaupp HA, Matulewiecz TJ, Lattmier GL et al. Graft infection or graft rejection? *Arch Surg*. 1979;114:1419–22.

21. Kean J. The effects of smoking on wound healing process. *J wound care*. 2010; 19:5–8.

22. Silverstein P. Smoking and wound healing. *Am J of Med*. 1992;93:22S–24S.

23. Cuff RF, Thomas JH. Recurrent symptomatic aortic sac seroma after open abdominal aortic aneurysm repair. *J Vasc Surg*. 2005;41:1058–60.

24. W.L. Gore & Associates Inc. Gore Excluder bifurcated endoprosthesis. Annual Clinical Update, November 2004.

25. Ryu RK, Plaestrant S, Ryu J et al. Sac hygroma after endovascular abdominal aortic aneurysm repair: successful treatment with endograft relining. *Cardiovasc Intervent Radiol*. 2007;30:488–90.

25

Aortic Surgery and Interventions in Patients with Connective Tissue Disorders

James H. Black, III, MD

INTRODUCTION

Connective tissues serve as a framework or matrix to hold the cells and structures of our body together. The primary structural proteins of connective tissue are composed of collagen and elastin, which vary in type and amount within each of the body's tissues (see Table 25-1). A connective tissue disorder is a disease in which the primary target is either collagen or elastin proteins. While inflammation may affect these proteins and induce structural damage, such conditions often imply some element of autoimmunity, and are termed collagen vascular diseases or mixed connective tissue diseases. Such conditions and arteritides related to the vascular tree quite often have weaker genetic factors that predispose to their development. While clustering of aneurysms in multiply affected family members may indicate some element of an inheritance pattern, there are often greatly varying levels of expressivity and penetrance and no defined genetic test available to assist treatment. This chapter will discuss surgical and endovascular issues referable to the common connective tissue disorders affecting the arterial tree which have a

TABLE 25-1. STRUCTURAL ELEMENTS OF BLOOD VESSELS

Structural Proteins	Approximate Amount (% dry wt)	Function
Type I Collagen	20–40	Fibrillar network
Type III Collagen	20–40	Thin fibrils
Elastin, fibrillin	20–40	Elasticity
Type IV Collagen, Laminin	<5	Basal lamina
Type V and VI Collagen	<2	Function unclear
Proteoglycans (>30 types)	<3	Resiliency

studied natural history, a defined basis for genetic inheritance, and sufficiently understood pathophysiologic mechanisms to guide treatment paradigms. These "heritable disorders of connective tissue"[1] have severe vascular manifestations and include most commonly Marfan Syndrome (MFS), Vascular Type of Ehlers-Danlos Syndrome (EDS IV), Loeys-Dietz Syndrome (LDS), and Familial Thoracic Aortic Aneurysm and Dissection (TAAD).

MARFAN SYNDROME

Diagnosis and Surveillance

The incidence of Marfan Syndrome is about 2–3 per 10,000 individuals, although this estimate relies on proper recognition of all affected and genetically predisposed individuals.[2] A population based study in Scotland demonstrated the incidence at 1 in 9802 livebirths, although this number would underestimate the true incidence as features, particularly skeletal, of Marfan Syndrome become more apparent with growth. Furthermore, although the disorder is passed as a dominant Mendelian trait, about 25% of cases are due to sporadic de-novo mutations.[2] The disease has no gender predisposition, and the tall stature with long bone overgrowth (dolichostenomelia) leads to an increased incidence in athletes, particularly in basketball and volleyball.

The role of clinical genetic testing in establishing a diagnosis has assumed a new role in the *Revised Ghent* nosology published in 2010 (Table 25-2).[3] Over 500 mutations have been found, and 90% of the mutations are private within a pedigree. Even within families where the same mutation is shared, phenotypic variation is prominent. Thus, exacting a genotype-phenotype correlation is difficult. Once an individual is diagnosed with Marfan Syndrome, all first-degree relatives should be evaluated for the presence of the condition. In children, this may require repeated evaluations to avoid missing the disorder in evolution.

In this section, the focus will be placed on aortic and vascular pathology. For recommendations in regard to the other body systems, the readership may find useful information at the National Marfan Foundation Website (www.marfan.org). The clinical manifestations within the cardiovascular system which require attention are the atrioventricular valves, annuloaortic valve mechanism, the aortic root, ascending aorta, and the descending thoracic aorta.

Aortic aneurysm and dissection is the most life threatening manifestation of Marfan Syndrome. The threat is age dependent, and dilation at the sinuses of Valsalva can begin in-utero, thus life-long transthoracic echocardiography is needed. For patients with poor visualization of the aortic root and ascending aorta due to anterior chest deformity, CTA or MR-angiography (to avoid radiation exposure) is a viable substitute. In contrast to degenerative aneurysm, the dilation may be confined to only the aortic root and the not the ascending aorta. Normal aortic dimensions can vary widely with both age and size, and proper interpretation in patients affected by Marfan Syndrome requires age-dependent nomograms for those under 18 years of age. Lifestyle modifications are routinely recommended to patients once the diagnosis of Marfan Syndrome is established. A consensus document cited "burst" exertion such as sprinting, weight-lifting, basketball, and soccer should generally be avoided. Favored are recreational sports in which energy expenditure is stable and consistent over long periods of time, such as informal jogging, biking, and lap swimming.[4] Symptoms potentially referable to a cardiovascular cause, such as shortness of breath, presyncope, and chest

TABLE 25-2. 2010 GHENT CRITERIA FOR DIAGNOSIS OF MARFAN SYNDROME

Box 1: Revised Ghent criteria for diagnosis of Marafan Syndrome and related disorders.

In the absence of family history:

1. Ao (Z > 2) AND EL = MFS*
2. AO (Z > 2) and FBN1 = MFS
3. AO (Z > 2) and Systemic score (>7 pts) = MFS*
4. EL and FBN1 with known Ao = MFS

EL with or without Systemic AND with an FBN1 not known with Ao or no FBN1 = ELS
Ao (Z < 2) AND Systemic (>5 with at least one skeletal feature) without EL + MASS
MVP AND Ao (Z > 2) AND Systemic (<5) without EL = MVPS

In the presence of family history:

1. EL and FH of MFS (as defined above) = MFS
2. Systemic (>7) and FH of MFS (as defined above) = MFS*
3. Ao (Z > 2) above 20 years old, >3 below 20 years old) + FH of MFS (as defined above) = MFS

Box 2: Scoring of Systemic Features

- Wrist AND Thumb sign – 3 (wrist OR thumb sign – 1)
- Pectus carinatum deformity – 2 (pectus excavatum or chest asymmetry –1)
- Hindfoot deformity –2 (plain pes planus –1)
- Pneumothorax – 2
- Dural ectasia – 2
- Protrusio acetabuli – 2
- Reduced US/LS AND increased arm/height AND no severe scoliosis – 1
- Scoliosis or thoracolumbar kyphosis – 1
- Reduce elbow extension –1
- Facial features (3/5) –1 (dolichocephaly, enopthalmos, downsliding palpebral features, malar hypoplasia, retrognathia
- Skin striae – 1
- Myopia > 3 diopters – 1
- Mitral Vlave prolapse (all types) –1
- Maximum total: 20 points; score ≥7, indicates systemic involvement; US/LS, upper segment/lower segment ratio.

Box 3: Criteria for causal FBN1 mutation

- Mutation previously shown to segregate in Marfan family
- De Novo (with proven paternity and absence of disease in parents) mutation (one of the five following categories):
- Nonsense mutation
- Inframe and out of frame deletion/insertion
- Splice site mutations affecting canonical splice sequence or shown to alter splicing on mRNA/cDNA level
- Missense mutation affecting/creating cystein residues
- Missense affecting conserved residues of EGF consensus sequence
- Other missense mutations: segregation in family if possible + ansence in 400 ethnically matched control chromosomes, if no family history absence in 400 ethnically matched control chromosomes.
- Linkage of haplotype for n > 6 meiosies to the FBN1 locus.

*Caveat: without discriminating features of SGS, LDS, VEDS (as defined in Table 1) AND TGFBR1/2, collagen biochemistry, COL 3A1 testinting as indicated. Other conditions/genes will emerge over time.

Ao, aortic diameter at the sinuses of Valsalva above indicated Z-score or aortic root dissection; EL, ectopia lentis; ELS, ectopia lentis syndrome; FBN!, fibrillin-1 mutation (as defined in box 3); FBN1 not known with Ao, FBN1 mutation that has not previously been associated with aortic root aneurysm.dissection; FBN1 with known Ao, FBN1 mutation that has been identified in an individual with aortic aneurysm; MASS, myopia, mitral valve prolapsed, borderline Z-score (<2) aortic root dilation, striae, skeletal findings,; MFS, Marfan Syndrome; MVPS, mitral valve prolapsed syndrome; Systemic, systemic score (see Box 2); and Z, Z-score.

discomfort should prompt immediate withdrawal from activity and evaluation. Recent litigation suggests physician reliance on consensus statements to determine medically reasonable levels of activity in patients with cardiovascular abnormalities as appropriate.[5]

Surgical Treatment

The traditional threshold for surgical repair of the aortic root is 5 cm in patients with Marfan Syndrome. The association between aortic diameter and the risk of aortic catastrophe is clearly established, and aortic aneurysm size >6 cm predicts a 4-fold increase in risk for aortic rupture or dissection in patients with Marfan Syndrome.[6] While the aortic root is the site most often affected, once a dissection has occurred, degeneration of aneurysm may affect other segments of the aorta or its branches. Type A dissection during the initial aortic root surgery was the only independent predictor of distal aortic reoperation.[7] Long term survival is similarly reduced after Type A dissection in MFS despite successful root surgery, likely owing the unfavorable natural history afforded by these later aortic operations. This fact underlies the aggressive stance to consider arch repair in many acutely dissected MFS patients, including elephant trunk techniques. Indeed as the life expectancy of individuals affected by Marfan Syndrome has increased with prophylactic root replacement, it is plausible the remaining aorta, or other large arteries, may progress to require repair in the absence of antecedent dissection. The aging MFS patient this is at risk for multiple aortic segments, and after aortic root replacement, aortic operations in non-contiguous segments of the aorta are required in 50% of patients over a 26 year period.[7]

Surgery of the Descending Thoracic and Thoracoabdominal Aorta

The first successful replacement of the thoracoabdominal aorta in a patient with Marfan Syndrome was performed by Dr. Crawford in the 1980s. Prophylactic aortic replacement is indicated when the aortic diameter reaches 5.5–6.0 cm or if symptoms occur suspicious for aortic cause. Due to the frequent involvement of the descending aorta by extensive aortic dissections, surgery in these regions in Marfan Syndrome is often indicated for aortic diameter and chronic underlying dissection. As such, the extent of repairs in Marfan Syndrome tend to be greater, with 42–78% of all TAAAs being DeBakey Extent II.[8] As expected mean age of Marfan patients undergoing repair of TAAA is 34–48 years of age, younger than non-connective tissue disorder patients.[8,9] In comparison to patients with degenerative TAAA presenting for repairs, there was no higher rate of acute presentation with dissection or rupture in patients with Marfan Syndrome TAAA (6–8%, each).[9] Paraparesis and paraplegia rates after TAAA repair in Marfan Syndrome compare favorably with non-connective tissue disorder results, when matched for extent of repair required. Due to the very young mean age of the Marfan Syndrome patients undergoing TAAA repair versus the older mean age of degenerative TAAA patients, overall long-term survival was better in Marfan Syndrome patients.[9]

Juxtarenal and suprarenal aneurysms are not uncommon in the MFS patient after Type A dissection repairs. Thresholds for repair generally follow the non-syndromic patients at 5.5–6.0 cm. The repairs may be challenging as the dissection septum needs to be fully excised from the outer wall to uncover the many intercostals or lumbar arteries that require control. Failure to appreciate these many vessels under the dissection septum may lead to postoperative bleeding that usually mandate reexploration. For abdominal repairs, advanced techniques in hypothermia and perfusion are not necessary. By excising a wedge of the dissection septum above the collar of the anastomosis, the surgeon will leave a "fenestration" for the proximal true and false lumen to remain stable. (Figure 25-1A, B)

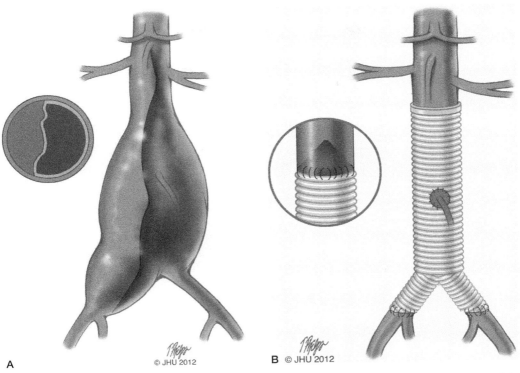

A   © JHU 2012   **B** © JHU 2012

Figure 25-1. **(A)** Abdominal aortic aneurysm secondary to chronic dissection is not uncommon as a later consequence of an index Type A dissection in Marfan syndrome patients. The extent of iliac involvement by the flap may incite asymmetric dilatation. **(B)** Graft reconstruction of dissected aortic segments is facilitated by removal of the dissection flap to the level of the proximal clamp, thus equilibrating flow in the proximal dissection areas.

Given the preponderance of Type II TAAA repairs in the available series, the freedom from further aortic repair is very low, owing to little aorta remaining to degenerate. As such, secondary aortic procedures in patients with Marfan Syndrome are often performed for pseudoaneurysm or aneurysm degeneration of the inclusion or Carrell patches. In a series of 107 patients who had TAAA repair including creation of visceral patches, 17 were know to have a connective tissue disorder.[10] With a mean time to diagnosis of 6.5 years, 3 of these 17 patients (17.6%) returned with aneurysmal degeneration of the visceral patch. By comparison, visceral patch aneurysms were noted in only 5.6% of atherosclerotic TAAA repairs.[10] All of these Marfan patients had inclusion patches that encompassed the celiac axis, superior mesenteric artery and both renal arteries, suggesting the visceral patch should be greatly reduced in all connective disorder patients to prevent late degeneration. Symptomatic presentation was noted in the series with a ruptured aneurysm appreciated in a patient (non-CTD) with a 6.1 cm patch aneurysm. Given the morbidity of the repair of the patch aneurysm (two intraoperative deaths among five patients taken to the operating room), the authors recommend maintaining an indication for repair of >6.0 cm.[10] Such a recommendation may be over- aggressive, so consideration of higher thresholds may be appropriate. In light of the appreciated morbidity of revision TAAA procedures, we have changed our reconstruction to include prefabricated dacron grafts with four branches for direct anastamosis to the origins of the renal and visceral vessels, thereby eliminating any retained aorta in the abdomen. For established visceral patch aneurysms, endovascular reconstruction with fenestrated grafts may provide a unique treatment paradigm and avoid revision procedures. (Figure 25-2 A, B, C)

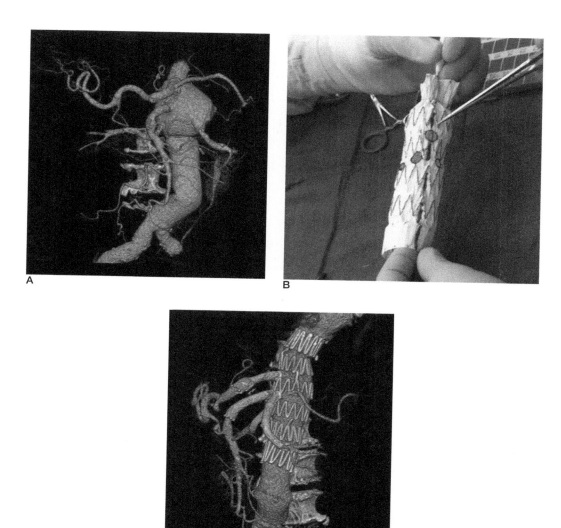

Figure 25–2. (A) Preoperative CTA of visceral patch aneurysm after TAAA reconstruction with standard inclusion patch of reno-visceral segment. **(B)** Standard TAA stent-graft can be modified to address the unique anatomy of the area—with all fenestrations anterior on the stent grafdt, given the anterior projection of the aneurysmal change. **(C)** Postoperative CTA demonstrating intact 4- branch endoluminal reconstruction of visceral patch aneurysm.

Endovascular Treatment

In general, aortic stent-grafts should not be used in the thoracic or abdominal aorta or for patients with other connective tissue diseases. The current approved devices have never been studied in the fragile milieu if the Marfan aorta (connective tissue disorder was an exclusion criteria during pivotal trials), and the question of physical damage to the aorta from the persistent radial force of the stent-graft remains (see Figure 25-3A, B) remains unanswered. A summary publication recommended endovascular repair *only* in instances of late localized pseudoaneurysm and stenting across native tissue aneurysm from "graft to graft."[11] A Society for Thoracic Surgery Consensus Statement recommended strongly against endovascular repair unless operative risk was deemed truly prohibitive by a center experienced in management of complex aortic disease, [12]but the stance was modified recently to support stent-graft therapy in cases of aortic rupture.[13] (Figure 25-3 A, B)

Series of MFS patients treated with endovascular therapy are now emerging with reasonable follow-up periods to determine clinical effectiveness. A report by Botta and colleagues,[14] examined 12 patients treated for dissection of the descending thoracic aorta after previous open aortic root/arch surgery. Five procedures were performed urgently and 7 were done in elective scenarios. In the immediate postoperative period, no paraplegia was encountered, However, in followup of a mean of 31 months, 25% of the patients required developed new dissection (retrograde into arch) or distally into the abdominal aorta. Waterman and colleagues[15] have recently published the largest series of MFS patients with stent-graft therapy, and the results are sobering. 44% of patients experienced primary failure of the stent-graft and many were converted to conventional surgical repairs. Among the primary treatment failures (7 of 16 patients), the mortality was 42%.

Indeed the issue of stent-graft induced new entry tears seems a persistent theme in patients with MFS.[16] A report of 650 patients treated for Type B dissection with stent-graft therapy revealed 22 events of SINE. The mortality of the new tears was substantial, with nearly 30% of patients dying from the event. The incidence of SINE in the patients with MFS was 33%, whereas, only 3% of patients with Type B dissection and no underlying MFS developed SINE. The authors conclude the stress-induced injury

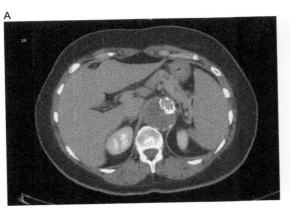
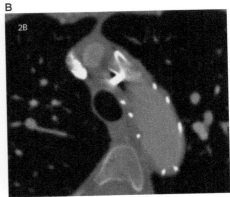

Figure 25–3. (A) Chronic aneurysmal change (5 cm) distal to stent-graft in Marfan syndrome patient one year after stent-graft placement for acute uncomplicated Type B dissection. (B) Axial CT scan asymptomatic showing bare-stent erosion through cephalad aspect of aortic arch.

of the stent-graft against the fragile aortic wall should be accounted for during design and placement of the endograft. While excessive oversizing should also be avoided, it is important to note the degree of oversizing was within IFU for the available devices to date. The same center has also elaborated their experience with stent-graft therapy in MFS to state "post-stent grafting RTAD (retrograde Type A dissection) represented the most common complication among Marfan patients."[17]

Conclusions

Marfan Syndrome has benefited from a century of progress in study of its pathogenesis and more recent refinements in surgical techniques to handle the cardinal manifestations within the cardiovascular system that plagued affected individuals. Proper genetic counseling, surveillance, and prudent application of modern surgical techniques have greatly modified the natural history of the disorder. Endovascular therapy of aortic disease has yet to have a defined long-term role, but may be of benefit in select instances of aortic rupture as a bridge to definitive therapy with open surgery and to address secondary aneurysms related to the initial conventional repairs.

VASCULAR TYPE EHLERS-DANLOS SYNDROME

Ehlers-Danlos Syndrome is a heterogeneous group of heritable disorders of connective tissue characterized by joint hypermobility, skin hyperextensibility, and tissue fragility affecting skin, ligaments, joints, blood vessels, and internal organs. There are many subtypes of the disorder (see Table 25-3), with the Classic Ehlers-Danlos Syndrome (Type I and II) being the most common, inherited as an autosomal dominant trait.[18] The importance of identifying the correct type cannot be underestimated because the natural history and modes of inheritance differ among the subtypes. Historically, the older literature did not clearly differentiate among the types, and the severe complications of the Vascular Type of Ehlers-Danlos Syndrome were cited as representative as the whole syndrome, thereby creating unnecessary anxiety. (Table 25-3)

TABLE 25-3. SUBTYPES OF EHLERS-DANLOS SYNDROME

Nomenclature		Skin(0-4+)	Joint Laxity(0-3+)	Features	Inheritance
New	Type	Elastic/Fragile			
Classical	I, II	+++/+++	+++	Vascular complications rarely	AD
Hypermobile	III	+/+	+++	Arthritis	AR
Vascular	IV	−/++++	+	Rupture of arteries, uterus, Intestine, thin skin	AD
Kyphoscoliotic	VIA, VIB	+++/++	+++	Hypotonia, osteoporosis kyphoscoliosis, rupture of Arteries, globe of eye	AR
Arthrochalasic	VIIC	++/+	+++	Hip luxations, osteoporosis	AD
Other	V	−/++++	+	Skin doughy and lax	AR X-linked
	VIII	++/++	++	Periodontal disease	AD
	IX	+/++	+	Lax skin, osteoporosis, bladder diverticula, retardation	X-linked
	X	+/+	++	Petechiae	?

Diagnosis and Surveillance

The prevalence of EDS IV is currently estimated to be 1:50,000 and is inherited in an autosomal dominant manner.[19] Approximately 50% cases represent new mutations, and as a rule, each patient or family carries a unique mutations in the COL3A1 gene which codes for type III procollagen. The overall life expectancy in EDS IV is dramatically shortened, largely as a result of vascular rupture, with median life span of 48 years (range 6–73 years).[20] In a study of 220 patients with EDS IV, confirmed by abnormal type III procollagen molecules, and 199 relatives with clinical diagnoses of EDS IV, major complications in childhood were rare, but 25% of the subjects suffered medical or surgical complications by age 20. By age 40, 80% had developed major complications.[20] Death occurred in 131 subjects, with vascular rupture of thoracic or abdominal vessels in 78(59%), 9 central nervous system hemorrhages (7%), and an unspecified bleeding source in 16 (12%). Organ rupture (heart, uterus, spleen, liver) caused death in 13 (10%) of the cases, and intestinal rupture led to demise in 10 (8%) subjects.[20]

EDS IV has the worst prognosis among the Ehlers-Danlos syndromes, and for this reason, examination of the patient is mandatory. Physical findings may mimic other EDS subtypes or other connective tissue disorders (see Table 25-4). The presence of any two or more of the major criteria is highly indicative of the diagnosis, and laboratory testing for abnormal collagen III or mutation analysis is strongly recommended. Such testing is both labor and time intensive, but should be considered strongly before any treatment course is chosen for the suspect affected individual.

Medical Therapy

Celiprolol has been advanced as a treatment of choice to reduce the incidence of vascular ruptures in EDS IV patients.[21] In a five year randomized study of 53 patients with suspected or proven EDS IV, celiprolol therapy reduced the incidence of vascular rupture to 20% versus 50% of control subjects. The trial has been criticized for the lack of uniform genetic

TABLE 25-4. DIAGNOSTIC CRITERIA OF EHLERS-DANLOS
SYNDROME, VASCULAR TYPE

Major diagnostic criteria

Thin, translucent skin

Arterial/intestinal/uterine fragility or rupture

Extensive bruising

Characteristic facial appearance (thin delicate nose, thin lips, hollow cheeks)

Minor diagnostic criteria

Acrogeria

Hypermobility of small joints

Tendon and muscle rupture

Talipdes equinovarus (clubfoot)

Early-onset varicose veins

Arteriovenous, carotid-cavernous sinus fistula

Pneumothorax/pneumohematothorax

Gingival recession

Positive family history, sudden death in (a) close relatives testing to prove all subjects had the disorder (only 33/53 had a COL3A1 mutation), and the fact that mean HR and blood pressure were actually higher than the control patients, This would suggest an alternate mechanism for the drug other than simple dP/dT effects. As such, prophylactic measures to control blood pressure and reduce atherosclerotic risk factors are recommended. Lifestyle modifications for EDS IV follow the general recommendations of other genetic disease as reviewed in the section within Marfan Syndrome earlier in this chapter. Daily doses of ascorbic acid (Vitamin C) have been offered on the theoretical basis of improving procollagen stability by conversion of proline residues the Y position within the Gly–X–Y sequences to hydroxyproline via prolyl hydroxylase. This enzyme requires ascorbic acid as a cofactor, and the resulting hydroxylation event allows the mature collagen molecule to fold into triple helix stably at body temperature.

Surgical Treatment

Surgical management of EDS IV is a formidable challenge.

Vascular catastrophe in EDS IV is not predictable, and vessel rupture can occur at any vessel diameter. Given the difficulty of handling the fragile tissues and vessels, management of spontaneous bleeding should be conservative as long as possible, especially in interstitial (muscular, retroperitoneal) spaces. Bleeding within the peritoneal cavity usually requires immediate transfusion; if surgery is required, vessel ligation with umbilical tapes appears to be the safest course versus direct repairs. Direct reconstructions must be tensionless, often pledgetted to reduce suture trauma, and reinforced circumferentially (Figure 25-4).

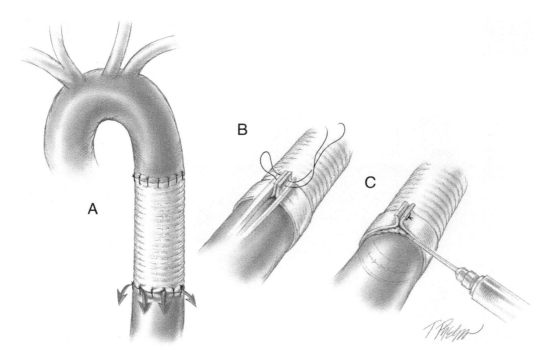

Figure 25-4. Step-wise depiction of rescue of deteriorating anastomosis with felt reinforcement and glue application. Constriction of the suture line area reduces pulse pressure stress across thin adventitial tissues.

The traditional risk assessment paradigm cites invasive procedures so fraught with complications that intervention should only be performed when faced with imminent risk of death. The presentation of patients with EDS IV can include arterial manifestations throughout the entire vascular tree. The outcomes of 31 patients over a 30 year period were studied retrospectively at tertiary referral center.[22] Among 24 patients, there were 132 vascular complications that prompted presentation for evaluation. While 85 of 132 complications were present before or during the first evaluation, 47 additional complications arose during a 6.3 year median follow-up. 15 of 31 patients underwent a vascular intervention with two operative deaths (one in an ascending aortic repair and one death, after a series of 8 operations, by anastamotic rupture of a carotid-subclavian graft). Overall procedure related morbidity was 46%, including a 37% incidence of postoperative bleeding and 20% re-exploration rate. Late graft-related complications occurred in 40% of arterial reconstructions, and included anastamotic aneurysm, anastamotic disruptions and graft thrombosis.

A report of EDS patients treated at the Johns Hopkins from 1994–2009 reveals some very important distinctions regarding the triage of patients with EDS IV.[23] In distinction to the Mayo Clinic series, where the preponderance of patients were treated emergently, most of the patients in the later contemporary series from Hopkins were treated electively. Overall perioperative bleeding and mortality was greatly reduced by comparison (see Table 25-5). Given success in the elective instance, it may be worthwhile to consider elective intervention in EDS IV patients before rupture and the ensuing stress compounds operative repair. Furthermore, it is also likely some improvement of the Hopkins series rests in its modernity. Undoubtedly, operative techniques have improved, and several methods are offered by the authors to explain their admirable results:

1. Liberal use of adjunctive techniques to reduce operative trauma in both the endovascular and operative setting.
2. Padded surgical clamps.
3. Permissive hypotension (SBP 70–80 mmHg) during vascular clamping and suture line testing.

EDS IV patients have been appreciated to have unique iliac aneurysms. The configuration usually spares the aortic bifurcation and the common iliac arteries "balloon" in a bell bottom fashion. (See Figure 25-5A & B). In such instances, repair should be

TABLE 25-5. OUTCOMES OF OPEN AND ENDOVASCULAR PROCEDURES IN EDS IV ENDOVASCULAR PROCEDURE (N = 9)

Procedure (N = 9)	
Operative death, no (%)	0(0)
In hospital death, no (%)	0(0)
LOS – median (IQR)	3 (1-6)
Any complication – no(%)	0(0)
Open Procedures (N = 9)	
Operative death, no (%)	1(11)
In hospital death, no (%)	1(13)
LOS, median (IQR)	7(6-8)
Any complication, no (%)	3(38)

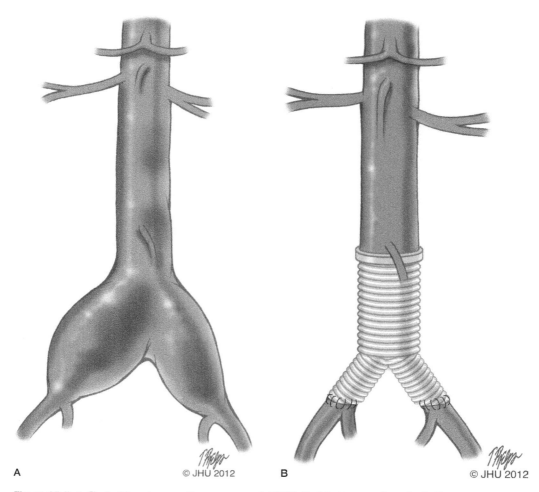

A   B

Figure 25-5. A: Typical iliac degenerative aneurysms in VEDS ("bell-bottom configuration"). The aorta is typically spared but the iliac bifurcations can be involved to varying degrees. **B:** Preserving the inferior mesenteric artery may be important if the tissue integrity off the internal iliac vessels requires bilateral ligations.

entertained in young patients electively, with emphasis on adjunctive measures to secure anastomoses as described earlier.

Ultimately, patient risk assessment and benefit compels any decision to proceed with a major surgical intervention. It is worthy to note that genetic analysis of specific mutations and collagen III biochemical assay does not predict clinical course.[23] But like most connective tissue disorders, clinical history can be informative. For patients with severe phenotypic features (such as very affected skin, facial morphology, etc.), those with early age onset, and those with prior complicated courses, complications can be expected. Furthermore, as median survival is 48–54 years, older patients may develop intolerance to procedural manipulations versus prior uncomplicated medical or surgical events, and assume a higher risk profile as vessel fragility worsens over a lifetime in EDS IV.

Endovascular Treatment

Endovascular approaches to coil embolize aortic branch vessels and other medium sized arteries has been successful in presentations of hemorrhage.[22] Indeed, a recent report of endovascular interventions in a spectrum of EDS patients revealed a very favorable safety profile.[24] (See Table 25-5) Arterial access can precipitate femoral rupture and pseudoaneurysm formation, especially when large devices are necessary. Solely diagnostic angiography should be avoided because of severe morbidity and the risk of vessel dissection and/or perforation during selective catheterization or from the puncture site itself. In one study, the major complication rate from arteriography was 67% with a 12% mortality[25], although the benefit of more contemporary lower-profile catheter and endovascular devices may favorably impact this historically high percentage. Consideration should be given to open repair of any access puncture, especially when larger French size is introduced, given the rate of complications reported (Figure 25-6). Accordingly, stent-graft therapy for aortic aneurysm has not been reported in significant sample, and long term durability and threat to the fixation zones in the setting of chronic outward radial force may increase secondary interventions. As such, there is general agreement that stent-graft therapy in EDS IV (and other connective tissue disorders) should be avoided.

Conclusions

There are no specific therapies for EDS IV, and life expectancy is shortened most often by vascular catastrophe. Proper identification of patients presenting with major diagnostic criteria should prompt biochemical investigation of type III procollagen production. Patient self-education in this disorder, often to inform treating physicians, may influence management of specific vascular complications, as well as pregnancy and reproductive counseling. With the advent of newer scientific methodologies using genetically defined animal models to discover new pathophysiologic pathways, it is hoped novel medical paradigms may evolve to favorably impact patients affected by EDS IV.

Loeys-Dietz syndrome is a multisystem disorder with a classic triad of craniofacial abnormality (90%), hypertelorism (wide set eyes, 90%), and arterial tortuousity/aneurysm (98%).[26] The disease is caused by heterozygous mutations in the genes encoding transforming growth factor β receptors 1 and 2 (TGFBR1 and TGFBR2, respectively). Cardiovascular involvement is a hallmark of Loeys-Dietz Syndrome, but aneurysms are not limited to the aortic root but can occur throughout the vascular tree. Arterial tortuousity, particular of the supra aortic vessels should prompt consideration of the disease.[27] Due to the early age of presentation of dramatic pathology, Vascular Type Ehlers-Danlos Syndrome is often considered along with the LDS disease. It could not be more critical to differentiate the two, either on clinical exam to determine the LDS triad or biochemical testing to confirm EDS IV, as surgical management and tissue fragility is dramatically more challenging in EDS IV than LDS patients.

The new diagnosis of a patient as affected by Loeys-Dietz Syndrome should prompt a head to toe CT or MR imaging study to determine the presence of arterial pathology outside the aortic root. Since involvement of supraaortic trunks and vertebral vessels is not uncommon, surgical exposure may be difficult, and embolization approaches considered. Given the widespread involvement of the arterial pathology in this disorder, multiple operations or interventions on a single patient is not uncommon.

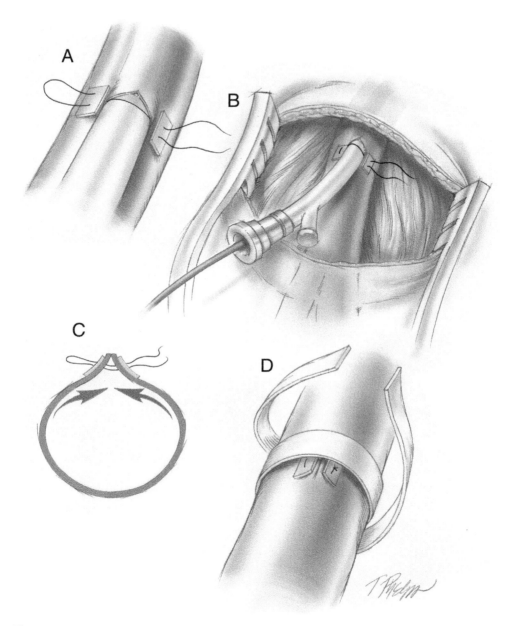

Figure 25-6. Technique for buttressed repair of femoral insertion site if large diameter sheaths are required or if femoral catheterization has previously resulted in hemorrhage. (A, B) "U stitch" placement is performed before needle insertion. (C-D) Inversion of puncture site with tying may obviate need for vascular clamping. 360-degree felt buttress to reduce delayed rupture of puncture site.

Surgical Treatment

Early results after surgical treatment of aneurysm in Loeys-Dietz are now emerging due to the very recent characterization of clinical and genetic features specific to the disease. Tissue handling and aortic anastamoses is favorable, and a small series of aortic root replacement patients in adults and children demonstrated no operative mortality, but 3 of 21 patients died in follow-up of thoracic aorta (N = 2) and abdominal aorta (N = 1) rupture.[28] In the authors institution, there have 5 patients who returned for descending thoracic aortic replacement after prior ascending/VSRR repairs. In distinction to the experience with MFS that Type A dissection usually incites the later operations of the descending aorta, in LDS these aneurysms seem more likely to form de-novo. Three of these patients returned thereafter with patch aneurysms after prior thoracoabdominal repairs, and were confirmed as LDS on subsequent TGFBR testing. As in Marfan Syndrome, this experience suggests patch size should be limited, or preferably avoided by direct anastamosis with multiple branched dacron graft (See Figure 25-7). Based upon the experience in the aortic root with premature rupture at small diameters, a general recommendation for repair of any aortic segment in adults would be 5 cm, or growth of aneurysm more than 0.5 cm in one year.[28] Recommendations for repair of peripheral aneurysms in LDS have not been determined, but rate of growth and absolute size both factor into the decision, making regular surveillance with high quality imaging critical. (Figure 25-7)

Conclusions

Loeys-Dietz Syndrome is unique among connective tissue disorders in the aggressive nature of aneurysms to rupture and/or dissect at very young age, the widespread involvement of the arterial tree, and characteristic craniofacial features. Since age at presentation and subtle cutaneous changes may first raise EDS IV as a lead diagnosis in the differential, *separating the diagnosis of LDS from VEDS is critical*, as management paradigms move aggressively toward prophylactic repairs in LDS, while EDS IV paradigms are conservative.

FAMILIAL THORACIC AORTIC ANEURYSM AND DISSECTION SYNDROME

Familial studies suggest 11–19% of all non-syndromic TAAD patients have a first degree relative with TAAD.[29] Pedigree analysis suggests Familial TAAD is inherited as a predominantly autosomal dominant disorder with decreased penetrance and variable expression yielding considerable clinical heterogeneity.[29] Genetic mapping of loci in familial TAAD had provided new insights into the pathogenesis of aneurysms throughout the aorta.

α-actin mutations have recently been discovered to cause 14% of Familial TAAD.[30] The actin proteins are highly conserved and are critical cytoskeletal elements. Aortic tissue demonstrates cystic medial degeneration with focal areas of marked vascular smooth muscle proliferation. Interestingly, Familial TAAD patients with ACTA2 mutations also are noted to have significant livedo reticularis, a physical finding not encountered in the other connective tissue disorders. As age at presentation is older than the other CTDs, it may be increasingly attractive to consider stent-graft therapy for the majority of these FTAAD patients. As in other CTDs, such patients should be counseled that stent-graft therapy may not have the admirable results seen in atherosclerotic aneurysm patients and mandates close serial follow-up.

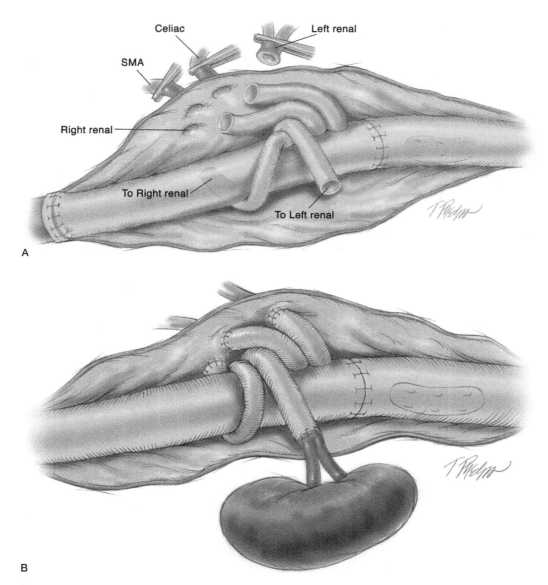

Figure 25-7. Technique for total aortic exclusion for repair of visceral-renal abdominal segment. **(A)** Graft is connected to proximal dacron graft and to the aortic bifurcation and exposed to pulsatile flow. **(B)** With full aortic graft, proper length sizing and orientation of individual graft can be achieved. Grafts will assume circumference of graft and thus reduces the risk of kinking.

SUMMARY

As these CTD patients age, portions of the vascular tree other than the ascending aorta may become affected, placing vascular surgeons in the management paradigm of these challenging patients. Patients with connective tissue disorder currently should maintain regular surveillance, seek expert opinion when intervention is contemplated, and receive genetic counseling to maintain reproductive health. When intervention is chosen, proper operative preparation and use of adjunctive techniques may foster a more successful outcome. Endovascular interventions in patients with connective tissue disorders will require further study, but in select instances may be preferred and life-saving.

REFERENCES

1. McKusick V: *Heritable Disorders of Connective Tissue*. St. Louis, CV Mosby, 1956.
2. Judge DP, Dietz HC: Marfan's Syndrome. *Lancet*. 2005;366:1965–1976.
3. Loeys BL, Dietz HC, Braverman AC, et al. The revised Ghent Nosology for the Marfan Syndrome. *J Med Genet*. Jul 2010; 47 (7):476–85.
4. Maron BJ, Chaitman BR, Ackerman MJ, et al. Recommendations for physical activity and recreational sports participation for young patients with genetic cardiovascular diseases. Circulation. 2004;109:2807–2816.
5. Maron BJ, Mitten MJ, Quandt EF, et al. Competitive athletes with cardiovascular disease: the case of Nicholas Knapp. *N Engl J Med*. 1998;339:632–1635.
6. Davies RR, Goldstein LJ, Coady MA, et al. Yearly rupture or dissection rates for thoracic aortic aneurysm: simple prediction based on size. *Ann Thor Surg*. 2003;73:17–27.
7. Girdauskas E, Kuntz T, Borger MA, et al. Distal aortic reinterventions after root surgery in Marfan patients. *Ann Thor Surg*. 2008; 86: 1815–20.
8. Lemaire SA, Carter SA, Volguina IV, et al. Spectrum of aortic operations in 300 patients with confirmed or suspected Marfan Syndrome. *Ann Thor Surg*. 2006;81:2063–78.
9. Dardik A, Krosnick T, Perler BA, et al. Durability of thoracoabdominal aortic aneurysm repair in patients with connective tissue disorders, *J Vasc Surg*. 2002;36:696–703.
10. Dardik A, Perler BA, Roseborough GS, et al. Aneurysmal expansion of the visceral patch after thoracoabdominal aortic replacement: an argument for limiting patch size? *J Vasc Surg*. 2001;34:405–10.
11. Milewicz DM, Dietz HC, Miller C. Treatment of aortic disease in patients with Marfan Syndrome. *Circulation*. 2005;111:e150–e157.
12. Expert consensus document on the treatment of descending thoracic aortic disease using endovascular grafts. *Ann Thor Surg*. 2008;85:S1–41.
13. Writing Group Members. 2010 ACCF/AHA/AATS/ACR/ASA/SCA/SCAI/SIR/STS/SVM Guidelines for the diagnosis and management of patients with thoracic aortic disease. *Circulation*. 2010; 121: e266-369.
14. Botta L, Russo V, Palombara CL, et al. Stent graft repair of descending thoracic aortic dissection in patients with Marfan Syndrome: An effective alternative to open reoperation? *J Thorac Cardiovasc Surg*. 2009; 138:1108–14.
15. Waterman AL, Feezor RJ, Lee WA, et al. Endovascular treatment of acute and chronic aortic pathology in patients with Marfan Syndrome. *J Vasc Surg*. 2012; 55:1234–41.
16. Dong ZH, Fu W, Wang Y, et al. Stent-graft induced new entry tear after endovascular repair for Stanford type B aortic dissection. *J Vasc Surg*. 2010;52: 1450–8.
17. Dong ZH, Fu WG, Wang YQ, et al. Retrograde Type A aortic dissection after endovascular stent graft placement for treatment of Type B dissection. *Circulation*. 2009;119:735–741.
18. Steinman B, Royce PM, Superti-Furga. Ehlers-Danlos Syndrome. In: *Connective Tissue and its Heritable Disorders*. Wiley-Liss, 431–523, 2002.
19. Superti-Furga A, Steinman B, Byers PH. Type III collagen deficiency. *Lancet*. 1989;1:903–904.
20. Pepin M, Schwarze U, Superti-Furga A, Byers PH. Clinical and genetic features of Ehlers-Danlos Type IV, the vascular type. *N Engl J Med*. 2000;342:673–80.
21. Ong KT, Perdu J, DeBacker J, et al. Effect of celiprolol on prevention of cardiovascular events in vascular Ehlers-Danlos syndrome: a prospective, open, blinded endpoints trial. *Lancet*. 2010 Oct; (30) 376(9751): 1476–84.
22. Oderich GS, Panneton JM, Bower TC. The spectrum, management and clinical outcome of Ehlers-Danlos Syndrome Type IV: A 30 year experience. *J Vasc Surg*. 2005;42:98–106.

23. Brooke BS, Arnaoutakis G, McDonell N, et al. Contemporary management of vascular complications associated with Ehlers-Danlos Syndromes. *J Vasc Surg*. 2010 Jan;51(1):131–8.

24. Lum YW, Brooke BS, Arnoutakis G, et al. Endovascular procedures in patients with Ehlers-Danlos syndrome: a review of clinical outcomes and iatrogenic complications. *Ann Vasc Surg*. 2012 Jan;26 (1): 25–33.

25. Cikrit DF, Miles JH, Silver D. Spontaneous arterial perforation: the Ehlers-Danlos specter. *J Vasc Surg*. 1987;5:248–255.

26. Loeys BL, Schwarze U, Holm T. Aneurysm syndromes caused by mutations in the TGF-receptor. *N Engl J Med*. 2006;355:788–798.

27. Loeys B, Chen J, Neptune E, et al. A syndrome of altered cardiovascular, craniofacial, neurocognitive, and skeletal development caused by mutations in TGFBR1 and TGFBR2. *Nat Genet*. 2005;37:275–281.

28. Williams JA, Loeys BL, Nwakanma LU, et al. Early surgical experience with Loeys-Dietz: A new syndrome of aggressive thoracic aortic aneurysm disease. *Ann Thorac Surg*. 2007;83:s757–763.

29. Albornoz G, Coady MA, Roberts M, et al. Familial thoracic aortic aneurysms and dissections—incidence, modes of inheritance, and phenotypic patterns. *Ann Thorac Surg*. 2006;82:1400–1406.

30. Pannu H, Avidian N, Tran-Fadulu V, et al. Genetic basis of thoracic aortic aneurysms and dissections, potential relevance to abdominal aortic aneurysms. *Ann NY Acad Sci*. 2006;1085:242–255.

Visceral and Renal Artery Disease

26

Visceral Artery Reconstruction

Thomas D. Willson, MD and Heron E. Rodriguez, MD

INTRODUCTION

Visceral artery reconstruction is indicated in the context of multiple clinical conditions. More often, revascularization is needed for the treatment of atherosclerotic occlusive disease. Less commonly, visceral reconstruction is performed after aortic and visceral artery dissection, trauma or during treatment of visceral artery aneurysms. In this chapter, we will review the indications, and surgical techniques used for reconstruction of the celiac axis, superior mesenteric and renal arteries.

INDICATIONS FOR VISCERAL RECONSTRUCTION OTHER THAN OCCLUSIVE DISEASE:

Trauma

Major abdominal vascular injury is common in civilian trauma, accounting for up to 30% of traumatic vascular injuries.[1,2] Gunshot wounds have a higher rate of vascular injury, about 25%, than do stab wounds, 5–10%.[2,3] Blunt mechanisms such as rapid deceleration (shearing) and crushing are responsible for only 3–10% of all traumatic vascular injuries.[2-4]

Veins and arteries are injured with the same frequency; large vessels such as the inferior vena cava (IVC) and the aorta are the most frequently involved. In terms of intraabdominal arteries, the superior mesenteric artery accounts for about 10% of abdominal vascular injuries.[1] Mortality, typically due to exsanguination, is high and actual or suspected major vessel injury is a hard indication for laparotomy. Management of SMA trauma depends upon the location of the injury. Proximal injuries, above the level of the middle colic artery typically require revascularization due to total gut ischemia. Injuries distal to that point can frequently be managed by branch ligation and small segmental bowel resection.[2,3]

Injuries to the celiac artery are extremely rare and almost always penetrating. They can frequently be managed by ligation due to the rich collateral supply from the SMA system.[1-3]

Trauma to the renal vasculature accounts for up to 14% of abdominal vascular injuries with the left renal artery about 1.5 times more likely to be injured than the right.[5] Blunt trauma to the renal arteries is rare, but rapid deceleration can cause intimal tears, thrombosis, or avulsion. Hemodynamic stability in these patients is dependent upon retroperitoneal tamponade; once this is lost, decompensation is nearly immediate. As a rule, zone 2 retroperitoneal hematomas with a penetrating mechanism demand exploration. If discovered within six hours of presentation, renal revascularization should be attempted.[1,2,5]

Dissection

Isolated dissection of any of the visceral arteries is a rare occurrence. More commonly, dissection of the SMA, celiac trunk, or renal arteries is a consequence of aortic dissection. When the aorta is not involved, dissections can be spontaneous, mycotic, traumatic, inflammatory, or iatrogenic in nature.[6] The existing literature regarding superior mesenteric and celiac artery dissection is sparse. Case series are typically small and no randomized trials of conservative versus operative management have been performed. In the reported cases, the SMA is the most commonly involved, followed by the celiac artery, the hepatic artery, and finally the splenic artery.[6,7] Takayama and colleagues reported a series of 19 patients over 10 years with an average of 20.9 month follow-up and put the relative prevalence of these dissections at 57.9% for the SMA, 36.8% celiac, 10.5% hepatic, and 5.3% splenic. Signs of ischemia are indications for operation, but otherwise the rich collateral blood supply between the celiac and SMA systems means that involvement of only one vessel is, for the most part, well tolerated and can be managed conservatively. In Takayama's study, only one patient underwent surgical correction of the dissection; there were no mortalities.[6] Others have reported the same experience with most patients being managed expectantly or with anticoagulation. Endovascular or open revascularization is rarely needed.

Renal artery dissections are commonly associated with dissection of the abdominal aorta. Surgical intervention is undertaken with two goals: first, to prevent or mitigate end-organ damage, and second, to improve renovascular hypertension.[8]

The available literature consists mostly of small case series. Work by Muller and colleagues described 39 patients over 13 years who underwent renal artery reconstruction following dissection. Of these lesions, 25 were spontaneous, 10 were associated with aortic dissection, and 4 were iatrogenic. Over the same time period, 655 patients underwent renal artery reconstruction for occlusive disease. Flank, lumbar, and abdominal pain are the most common presenting symptoms. Hypertension is present in over 90%; signs of renal compromise are present in 9–13% of patients.[8]

Aneurysm

Aneurysms are relatively uncommon within the splanchnic vessels, occurring in less than 1% of the general population. Generally speaking, rapid enlargement or symptomatic aneurysms warrant urgent surgical intervention. In general, a size threshold of 2 cm has been proposed for treatment of splanchnic aneurysms regardless of the presence of absence of symptoms.[9-14] These recommendations are generally based on small, retrospective studies due to the rarity of these lesions. Table 26-1 details the relative frequency of splanchnic

TABLE 26-1. VISCERAL ANEURYSM FREQUENCIES AND INDICATIONS FOR REPAIR

Vessel	% of visceral aneurysms	Indications for Repair
Celiac	5%	*General Criteria:* Symptomatic or rapidly enlarging
		Size Criteria: >2 cm recommended
Hepatic	20%	*General Criteria:* Symptomatic; rapidly enlarging; polyarteritis nodosa; fibromuscular dysplasia
		Size Criteria: >2 cm recommended
Splenic	60%	*General Criteria:* Symptomatic; rapidly enlarging; pregnancy; women of childbearing age; portal hypertension; liver transplant candidates
		Size Criteria: >2 cm recommended
Gastric/Gastroepiploic	4%	*General Criteria:* diagnosis of aneurysm; 70% mortality with rupture; rupture is presenting symptom in up to 90%
		Size Criteria: any size
Pancreaticoduodenal/ Gastroduodenal	PDA: 2% GDA: 1.5%	*General Criteria:* diagnosis of aneurysm; no correlation between size and rupture rate
		Size Criteria: any size
Superior Mesenteric	5%	*General Criteria:* diagnosis of aneurysm; high mortality with rupture; most are symptomatic on presentation
		Size Criteria: any size
Terminal Branches	2%	*General Criteria:* diagnosis of aneurysm; most reported ruptures are <1 cm diameter
		Size Criteria: any size
Renal	Prevalence: 0.1% (autopsy) 1% (angio)	*General Criteria:* Symptomatic or rapidly enlarging; hypertension; acute dissection; pregnancy
		Size Criteria: 2 cm traditional; unclear relationship between size and rupture risk

aneurysms as well as the indications for treatment. Renal artery aneurysms are traditionally not included in the count of splanchnic aneurysms, so overall, rather than relative prevalence is noted.

As endovascular techniques have improved, open surgery has become a less common method of correcting visceral aneurysms.[13] Additionally, some visceral aneurysms, such as splenic artery lesions, can be dealt with by removal of the end organ rather than arterial reconstruction.[12]

CELIAC AXIS

Exposure of the Celiac Axis and Its Branches

The celiac trunk arises from the aorta at a nearly right angle at the level of the first lumbar vertebra, just below the aortic hiatus. It is generally approached via an upper midline laparotomy. Unlike the retroperitoneal approach, this allows for access to the hepatic artery and for evaluation of end organ perfusion. Alternatively, a thoracoabdominal approach with exposure of the intraperiotneal organs is also feasible.

Upon entry into the peritoneal cavity, the triangular ligament of the liver is divided and the left lobe is retracted to the right. With the aid of a nasogastric tube that is easily palpated, the esophagus and the stomach are retracted laterally. The gastrohepatic ligament is divided, allowing access to the lesser sac. By dividing the left crus of the diaphragm, the supraceliac aorta and the origin of the celiac artery are exposed. Exposure of the celiac artery can be extended distally by transecting the posterior peritoneal layer just above the superior border of the pancreas. The left coronary vein typically passes across the celiac trunk from the lesser curvature before draining into the portal vein.

Trifurcation into common hepatic to the right, splenic to the left, and left gastric in the cranial direction is typical and is seen in up to 89% of patients.[15,16] A gastrosplenic trunk with a separate hepatic origin is the most common variation, accounting for another 5-8% of patients. Uncommon aberrant arrangements include hepatogastric and hepatosplenic trunks while a common origin of the celiac axis and superior mesenteric artery is exceedingly rare.[15] Opening the hepatoduodenal ligament just above the pylorus allows for exposure of the proximal portion of the hepatic artery. From there it courses along the left edge of the common bile duct into the hilum of the liver. Careful dissection of the soft tissue encapsulating the common bile duct will reveal this portion of the hepatic artery. The terminal branches are highly variable, so it is imperative to fully identify any branches encountered at this point to prevent devascularization of portions of the liver, stomach, or gallbladder. If hepatorenal bypass is planned, the hepatic artery can also be approached via a right subcostal incision to facilitate simultaneous exposure of the kidney.

The splenic artery runs leftward along the superior border of the pancreas giving off a dorsal pancreatic branch and other, smaller branches. Meticulous dissection along the pancreatic edge is required as the artery is frequently tortuous and takes a winding course before giving off the short gastric arteries and left gastroepiploic arteries and finally entering the splenic hilum. Frequently, the splenic artery divides into multiple branches prior to entering the hilum; these should be individually skeletonized for work around the splenic hilum. The short gastric and left gastroepiploic arteries may arise from the main branch or from these smaller branches. If splenorenal bypass is planned, the splenic artery can also be approached via a left subcostal incision to facilitate simultaneous exposure of the kidney.

The left gastric artery is relatively short and can be found ascending in the retroperitoneum to the lesser curvature at the level of the gastroesophageal junction.

REVASCULARIZATION OF THE CELIAC AXIS AND ITS BRANCHES

Aortoceliac Bypass

Isolated revascularization of the celiac artery alone is relatively uncommon. More commonly, this operation is performed as part of an aorto-celiac-mesenteric bypass for chronic mesenteric ischemia. The most common indication for stand-alone celiac revascularization is aneurysm. In many cases, the celiac artery can be ligated and the diseased section resected with minimal consequence to the patient. Due to extensive collateralization through the SMA system, the rate of hepatic necrosis with this approach is low.[10,17]

Aortoceliac bypass has been described for the treatment of aneurysm, dissection, mesenteric ischemia, and median arcuate ligament syndrome. Once the celiac axis is exposed as previously described, each branch must be individually isolated and controlled. An aortotomy is made twice the diameter of the chosen conduit and an end-to-side anastomosis is performed using running monofilament suture. Attention is then turned to the diseased segment of the celiac axis. The artery is ligated proximally and the segment excised. The conduit and artery are spatulated and anastomosed end-to-end, again using running monofilament suture.

Polytetrafluoroethylene (PTFE), polyethylene tetraphthalate, and autologous vein conduits have been used successfully for this bypass. There is no randomized controlled data comparing autologous vein to synthetic graft material for this application as there are simply too few cases performed. Small series and case reports demonstrate good long-term patency with either vein or synthetic conduit, though some authors believe PTFE to be more durable.[11] We consider either acceptable for this application.

Aortohepatic Bypass

Like the celiac trunk, the hepatic artery has excellent collateralization from the SMA system. In many cases, isolated hepatic artery lesions can be treated with simple ligation or embolization.[12] Sometimes, however, the collateral circulation is insufficient or the patient's condition mandates reconstruction of the hepatic artery. In particular, it is imperative that the hepatic circulation remain intact in patients with cirrhosis or any sign of liver dysfunction.

The hepatic artery is exposed as previously described and proximal and distal control are obtained. The supraceliac aorta is then exposed. A longitudinal arteriotomy is made on the anterolateral wall of the aorta, approximately twice the diameter of the conduit. An end-to-side anastomosis is performed using monofilament suture. The diseased segment of the hepatic artery can then be ligated proximally and excised. The distal end of the hepatic artery is spatulated as is the conduit and the two are anastomosed end-to-end using monofilament suture.

Proximal Splenic Artery Reconstruction

Isolated splenic artery revascularization is rarely needed. It can be approached through the omental bursa, as previously described, or through the retroperitoneum once the pancreas has been mobilized.

Due to its tortuosity, splenic artery reconstruction is frequently accomplished by simply excising the diseased segment, releasing the proximal and distal portions of the artery, and performing a primary anastomosis.[13,14] This is possible even when the lesion in question can only be excluded, not excised, such as an intrapancreatic splenic artery aneurysm. If, for whatever reason, neither ligation of the artery nor primary reanastomosis is possible, reversed saphenous vein is used as a conduit for bypass. The proximal and distal anastomoses are both performed in an end-to-end fashion after spatulating the artery and vein graft.

Hilar Splenic Artery Reconstruction

The hilar portion of the splenic artery is rarely, if ever, reconstructed. Splenectomy is the most commonly performed operation for lesions of the distal and hilar splenic artery.[12,13]

When the lesion in question involves not only the hilar portion of the artery, but intrasplenic branches as well, this approach is mandatory.[12] In some cases, the distal pancreas must also be sacrificed due to inadequate blood supply following splenic artery ligation and splenectomy. When lesions, such as aneurysms, involve single branches of the splenic artery as they enter the hilum and do not involve the intrasplenic vessels, simple ligation without splenectomy is an adequate treatment. This will usually result in segmental infarction of the spleen, but the majority of the organ will be adequately perfused.

SUPERIOR MESENTERIC ARTERY

Exposure of the Superior Mesenteric Artery

The origin of the superior mesenteric artery lies behind the pancreatic neck at the level of the first or second lumbar vertebra.

The SMA courses caudally at an acute angle from its origin, crossing over the uncinate process and third portion of the duodenum before entering the root of the small intestine mesentery. Multiple structures are crowded around the SMA origin and the surgeon must be cognizant of their location both to avoid bleeding and preserve the vasculature. The left renal vein is lodged in the angle between the aorta and the SMA. The splenic vein runs across the origin while the superior mesenteric vein runs parallel and just to the right of the SMA before merging to form the portal vein.

Exposure of the SMA origin is accomplished through a midline laparotomy or a retroperitoneal approach. Upon entry into the abdominal cavity, a left-to-right medial visceral rotation (the Mattox maneuver) is performed. The peritoneal reflection anchoring the left colon, spleen, and splenic flexure is divided, allowing the left colon, gastric fundus, spleen, and pancreatic tail to be rotated medially. The left kidney need not be rotated in order to access the SMA origin. If rapid exposure is required, such as in trauma, stapler division of the pancreatic neck permits immediate direct exposure.

Exposure of the more distal SMA, beyond the first five centimeters or so, is typically less complicated. A Kocher maneuver permits access through the root of the mesentery while direct dissection onto the artery is also possible. The omentum and the transverse colon are reflected cephalad while the small bowel is packed to the right side of the abdomen and the sigmoid colon into the left lower quadrant. The ligament of Treitz and the superior duodenal attachments are released to allow full rightward mobilization of the fourth portion of the duodenum. At this point, the SMA is palpated at the level of the transverse colonic mesentery. Layer-by-layer dissection of the overlying soft tissue with ligation of small crossing vessels and lymphatics completes the exposure.

REVASCULARIZATION OF THE SUPERIOR MESENTERIC ARTERY

Antegrade (Supraceliac) Aortomesenteric Bypass

Antegrade aortomesenteric bypass has long demonstrated both efficacy and durability for reconstruction in the context of chronic mesenteric ischemia.[18–20] This procedure can also be used in cases of aneurysm, dissection, or trauma involving the SMA or its branches.

Jimenez et al. demonstrated 100% secondary patency and 94% primary assisted patency at five years for this type of bypass.[18] Quoted mortalities are 11–29% with high morbidity and long hospital stays, but these data are based on studies of CMI patients.[18,19]

Because of the requirement for supraceliac aortic clamping, decompensated patients, patients with renal insufficiency, and other marginal candidates may be better served by retrograde bypass. The advantage of antegrade bypass is that the supraceliac aorta is typically less involved with atherosclerotic disease than the infrarenal aorta, which is an important consideration even when the procedure is not performed for occlusive disease.[19]

The procedure begins with an upper midline incision carried from just below the umbilicus up to the level of the xiphoid process. It is important to reach the level of the diaphragm with the skin incision so as to facilitate later exposure of the aorta. Just as with celiac artery exposure, a nasogastric tube is placed to allow easy palpation of the esophagus. The triangular ligament of the liver is divided, allowing its retraction to the right; the esophagus is retracted to the left. Division of the diaphragm exposes the supraceliac aorta. The dissection is carried onto the celiac axis for complete exposure. Lateral dissection is performed to permit cross-clamping.

Attention is then turned to the superior mesenteric artery. When the pathology is located close to the origin, the superior border of the pancreas can be released and the organ retracted caudad to expose the artery. When the pathology is more extensive or distal, the artery is exposed within the mesentery.

A retropancreatic tunnel is created by blunt, fingertip dissection along the left edge of the aorta connecting the SMA dissection to the supraceliac. A Penrose drain is passed through this tunnel. At this point, heparin, mannitol, and furosemide are administered. The estimated time for aortic cross-clamping is approximately fifteen minutes. If the surgeon cannot accomplish the anastomosis in that time or if the patient is unable to tolerate a brief test-clamp, partial occlusion clamping should be considered instead.

Synthetic graft is used in the face of a non-contaminated field as it has been found to be more durable in this location than saphenous vein graft. The graft is placed through the tunnel, cross-clamp is initiated, and the proximal anastomosis is performed using running monofilament in an end-to-side fashion. Once the proximal anastomosis is complete, the aortic clamp is released and the conduit is clamped in its place. The diseased segment of SMA is then ligated proximally and divided distally. An end-to-side anastomosis is performed using running monofilament after spatulation.

When antegrade bypass is performed for occlusive disease, a hepatic or celiac limb is frequently added in addition to the aorto-mesenteric bypass. In this case, a bifurcted type graft is used with the shorter, superior limb being anastomosed to the celiac and the inferior limb being tunneled through the retropancreatic space to the SMA.

Retrograde (Infrarenal) Aortomesenteric or Iliomesenteric Bypass

Retrograde aortomesenteric bypass is typically less technically challenging for the surgeon and less physiologically challenging for the patient, making it an excellent operation for higher risk patients who cannot tolerate supraceliac clamping. Primary and assisted patency rates for retrograde bypass, when properly performed, are equivalent to antegrade bypass.[18–20] The drawback, of course, is that the infrarenal aorta tends to be more atherosclerotic and it can be difficult to find an appropriate site for grafting. Originating the bypass from the common iliac artery is frequently easier and provides a more direct route for the conduit, reducing the risk of kinking.[20] Usually, it is sufficient to reconstruct only the superior mesenteric artery using the retrograde approach.

The SMA is exposed through the mesentery near the takeoff of the middle colic artery as described previously. The retroperitoneum is opened and the inferior aorta and common iliac arteries are exposed. Once a suitable landing site is chosen, attention is returned to the SMA. An end-to-side anastomosis is performed between the conduit and the SMA. Whether the heel or the toe of the graft is positioned on the proximal portion of the artery depends upon how the graft will lie within the closed abdomen. It is imperative that the surgeon visualizes the final position to avoid post-operative kinking and acute bowel ischemia. Once the proximal anastomosis is complete, the viscera are returned as much as possible to their native position while still allowing exposure of landing site. The bypass is evaluated for kinking and then the distal anastomosis is performed in an end-to-side fashion. The retroperitoneum is closed to prevent the graft from coming into contact with the bowels. Omental coverage may be needed in thin patients to completely exclude the graft.

Either synthetic graft or autologous vein can be used to create this bypass.[18–20] The advantage of autologous vein is that it can be used in contaminated fields or when bowel resection is performed. Reinforced synthetic graft, on the other hand, has less tendency to kink. In either case, the principle is to form a "lazy C," gently curving the bypass into position rather than a short straight shot, which is more prone to kinking when the viscera are returned to their normal position.

RENAL ARTERY

The renal arteries arise from the abdominal aorta at the level of the top of second lumbar vertebra. The left is typically situated slightly higher than the right. On the right side, the artery passes behind the IVC. Before entering the renal hilum, each artery divides into anterior and posterior trunks. Anywhere from two to five branches can be found entering the hilum. Branch points behind the IVC are common. Frequently, the renal artery will also send a branch to the adrenal gland; this can be ligated without consequence.

In terms of variation, only about 72% of patients will have classic, single-vessel anatomy. The next most common variations are a single artery with an early upper pole branch in 13% and duplicated renal arteries entering the hilum in 11%. Less common variations include completely separate upper (6%) or lower (3%) pole arteries. A patient may have different anatomy on each side.[15]

EXPOSURE OF THE RENAL ARTERIES

Correct choice of renal artery exposure depends upon the indication for surgery and the planned operation. The arteries can be approached individually via subcostal, flank, midline, or transverse incisions depending upon what other vasculature needs to be exposed. Simultaneous bilateral exposure is possible by midline or transverse supraumbilical celiotomy.[21]

For simultaneous exposure of both renal arteries, we recommend midline laparotomy, although a transverse supraumbilical incision will provide similar exposure.

Once the peritoneal cavity is entered, the omentum and transverse colon are reflected cephalad. The small bowel is eviscerated and mobilization of the duodenum proceeds by incision of the ligament of Treitz and release of other attachments. Once the duodenum is free, it is reflected to the right side. The posterior peritoneum overlying the aorta can then be incised and the dissection plane carried up to the level of the left renal vein and then across to the renal hilum. The left renal vein almost always lies over the origin of the renal arteries; its mobilization is necessary to properly expose the origins. The pancreas it should be retracted gently cephalad and the vein dissected free all the way to the hilum. An umbilical tape can then be used to provide retraction and exposure of the left renal artery. At this point, the medial edge of the IVC should be mobilized and retracted laterally; this will expose the origin of the right renal artery.

The right renal artery may be exposed through any of the incisions previously mentioned and proper choice will depend upon the planned operation. Once the peritoneum has been entered, the lateral peritoneal attachments of the ascending colon and hepatic flexure are released, allowing the right colon to be medialized. A Kocher maneuver permits medialization of the duodenum and pancreas to expose the IVC. The right renal vein should now be identified and isolated. Mobilization of the lateral edge of the IVC combined with medial retraction will expose the origin of the right renal artery. We recommend complete dissection of the renal artery from origin to hilum to ensure that all branches are accounted for and controlled.

Exposure of the left renal artery proceeds in similar fashion to the right. Once the peritoneum has been entered, the lateral attachments of the left colon and splenic flexure are released. The spleen is then released from its diaphragmatic and renal attachments. Finally, the retroperitoneal attachments of the distal pancreas are released and the viscera are medialized. The left renal vein is isolated and encircled with umbilical tape. Lumbar, gonadal, and adrenal veins are ligated as needed to provide adequate retraction and exposure of the artery. Again, we recommend dissection of the renal artery from its origin to the renal hilum to ensure that all branches have been isolated.

REVASCULARIZATION OF THE RENAL ARTERIES

Renal Artery Reimplantation

Like the splenic artery, the renal arteries tend to have a significant amount of redundancy. This means that when the diseased segment is relatively short and close to the origin, enough mobilization can often be gained to allow the artery to be reanastomosed to itself or reimplanted into the aorta, eliminating the need for vein graft or synthetic conduit.[22] The origin of the vessel is ligated, the artery is transected and an aortotomy is made slighty below the level of the renal artery stump. The distal vessel is spatulated and anastomosed to the aorta using monofilament suture.

Aortorenal Bypass

Aortorenal bypass proceeds in much the same fashion as reimplantation of a redundant renal artery. The preferred conduit is saphenous vein although hypogastric artery and synthetic grafts are viable alternatives, particularly in the face of a hypoplastic or sclerotic saphenous vein.[21]

The renal artery is exposed as previously described and, once the conduit has been harvested, the artery is ligated and transected. An aortotomy is made at least three times the diameter of the graft using two or three passes of an aortic punch. An end-to-side anastomosis if created between the conduit and the aorta. The aortic clamp is then released while the graft is clamped. The distal renal artery is spatulated as is the graft and the two are anastomosed end-to-end. When polar branches are present in the diseased segment of renal artery, they can be incorporated into the bypass via end-to-side anastomoses. This is typically done after the aortic anastomosis and before the distal anastomosis to ensure a tension free result.

Hepatorenal Bypass

Hepatorenal bypass is usually performed through a right subcostal incision.[22,23] The hepatic artery is isolated within the hepatoduodenal ligament as described in the celiac exposure section. The gastroduodenal artery should be identified and preserved during dissection, as it can provide important collateral flow to the bowel. If necessary to gain greater exposure, however, the artery can be ligated and transected.[22] The right renal artery is exposed via Kocher maneuver as previously described. Saphenous vein is carefully procured from the patient's leg, though synthetic graft can also be used.

If the gastroduodenal artery has been ligated, the stump is removed and the arteriotomy is continued onto the common hepatic artery, allowing for a wide anastomosis. If the gastroduodenal has been preserved, the arteriotomy is performed more proximally on the common hepatic artery. The vein is spatulated and sutured in place end-to-side using running monofilament. At this point, the distance to the target site on the renal artery should be measured. Accurate measurement is important to avoid both kinking of and tension on the bypass. Once an appropriate site has been selected, the renal artery is ligated and transected. The distal end is then anastomosed end-to-end to the vein graft, the viscera returned to their native positions, and the abdomen closed.

Splenorenal Bypass

Splenorenal bypass is performed through a left subcostal incision.[22,23] Unlike other bypasses, in this case the splenic artery serves as both the inflow source and the conduit. The splenic artery is exposed as previously described by dissecting free the inferior edge of the pancreas. The left renal artery is then exposed via a Mattox maneuver as detailed previously. Once both arteries have been exposed and mobilized, the splenic artery is transected distally and tunneled though the retropancreatic plane. The renal artery can then be ligated and transected. The arteries are spatulated and anastomosed end-to-end. The viscera are rotated back to their anatomic positions and the abdomen is closed. Routine splenectomy is not performed.[22]

Ex-Vivo Renal Artery Reconstruction

Reconstruction of the main renal artery can normally be accomplished rapidly and the kidneys are relatively tolerant to ischemia. Pathology affecting the hilar branches of the artery, however, is typically much more time consuming to reconstruct. Many pharmacologic therapies have been promoted for renal protection, but hypothermia remains the gold standard. Once the vasculature of the renal hilum is reconstructed, the kidney is returned to the renal fossa. Altenratively, autotransplantation in to the iliac fossa can also be performed.[22]

An extended subcostal incision is used to enter the abdomen unless autotransplantation is planned, in which case a midline laparotomy is performed. To perform this operation, the renal artery is exposed just as before. Next, Gerota's fascia is opened and the kidney is released from its attachments. The ureter is dissected free and controlled with umbilical tape. A side-biting clamp is used to control the renal vein, which is then transected with a section of IVC wall. The renal artery is then ligated and transected. The kidney is flushed with cold renal preservative solution, wrapped in cold, moist laparotomy pads, and placed in a bowel bag filled with ice and chilled saline.

Reconstruction of the hilar branch vessels requires either a branched conduit, such as branched saphenous vein or hypogastric artery, or numerous end-to-side anastomoses. Once the arterial reconstructions are complete, the kidney is replaced into its fossa. The renal vein and excised patch of IVC are reanastomosed to the IVC defect in a method analogous to a patch angioplasty. The viscera are replaced into their natural positions and the abdomen is closed.

REFERENCES

1. Asensio JA, Chahwan S, Hanpeter D, et al. Operative management and outcome of 302 abdominal vascular injuries. *Am J Surg*. 2000 Dec; 180(6): 528–33.
2. Asensio JA, Forno W, Roldan G, et al. Abdominal vascular injuries: injuries to the aorta. *Surg Clin N Am*. 2001 Dec; 81(6): 1395–1416.
3. Asensio JA, Forno W, Roldan G, et al. Visceral vascular injuries. *Surg Clin N Am*. 2002 Feb; 82(1): 1–20.
4. Cox EF. Blunt abdominal trauma: A 5-year analysis of 870 patients requiring celiotomy. *Ann Surg*. 1984 Apr; 199(4): 467–74.
5. Tillou A, Romero J, Asensio JA, et al. Renal vascular injuries. *Surg Clin N Am*. 2001 Dec; 81(6): 1417–30.
6. Takayama T, Miyata T, Shirakawa M, et al. Isolated spontaneous dissection of the splanchnic arteries. *J Vasc Surg*. 2008 Aug; 48(2): 329–33.
7. Goueffic Y, Costargent A, Dupas B, et al. Superior mesenteric artery dissection: Case report. *J Vasc Surg*. 2002 May; 35(5): 1003–5.
8. Muller BT, Reiher L, Pfeiffer T, et al. Surgical treatment of renal artery dissection in 25 patients: Indications and results. *J Vasc Surg*. 2003 Apr; 37(4): 761–8.
9. Carr SC, Mahvi DM, Hoch JR, et al. Visceral artery aneurysm rupture. *J Vasc Surg*. 2001 Apr; 33(4): 806–11.
10. Messina LM, Shanley CJ. Visceral artery aneurysms. *Surg Clin N Am*. 1997 Apr; 77(2): 425–42.
11. Stone WM, Abbas MA, Gloviczki P, et al. Celiac artery aneurysms: A critical reappraisal of a rare entity. *Arch Surg*. 2002 Jun; 137: 670–4.
12. Pulli R, Dorigo W, Troisi N, et al. Surgical treatment of visceral artery aneurysms: A 25-year experience. *J Vasc Surg*. 2008 Aug; 48(2): 334–42.
13. Sachdev-Ost U. Visceral artery aneurysms: Review of current management options. *Mt Sinai J Med*. 2010; 77:296–303.
14. Chiesa R, Astore D, Guzzo G, et al. *Ann Vasc Surg*. 2005; 19(1): 42–8.
15. Valentine RJ, Wind GG. Anatomic Exposures in *Vascular Surgery*. 2nd ed. New York, NY: Lippincott, Williams, & Wilkins; 2003.
16. Koops A, Wojciechowski B, Broering DC, et al. Anatomic variations in the hepatic arteries in 604 selective celiac and superior mesenteric angiographies. *Surg Radiol Anat*. 2004; 26: 239–44.

17. Graham LM, Stanley JC, Whitehouse WM, et al. Celiac artery aneurysms: Historic (1745–1949) and contemporary (1950–1984) differences in etiology and clinical importance. *J Vasc Surg*. 1985 Sep; 2(5): 757–64.

18. Jimenez JG, Huber TS, Ozaki CK, et al. Durability of antegrade synthetic aortomesenteric bypass for chronic mesenteric ischemia. *J Vasc Surg*. 2002 Jun; 35(6): 1078–84.

19. English WP, Pearce JD, Craven TE, et al. Chronic visceral ischemia: Symptom-free survival after open surgical repair. *Vasc Endovasc Surg*. 2004; 38(6): 493–503.

20. McMillan WD, McCarthy WJ, Bresticker MR, et al. Mesenteric artery bypass: Objective patency determination. *J Vasc Surg*. 1995 May; 21(5): 729–41.

21. Benjamin ME, Dean RH. Techniques in renal artery reconstruction: Part I. *Ann Vasc Surg*. 1996 May; 10(3): 306–14.

22. Benjamin ME, Dean RH. Techniques in renal artery reconstruction: Part II. *Ann Vasc Surg*. 1996 Jul; 10(4): 409–14.

23. Moncure AC, Brewster DC, Darling RC, et al. Use of the splenic and hepatic arteries for renal revascularization. *J Vasc Surg*. 1986 Feb; 3(2): 196–203.

27

In Situ Renal Artery Aneurysm Repair

William P. Robinson III, MD

INTRODUCTION

Renal Artery Aneurysms (RAAs) are a rare entity with the preponderance of evidence regarding their treatment coming from a limited number of referral centers. While few vascular surgeons have extensive experience with RAAs, moat vascular surgeons will encounter RAAs during their career. The goals of this chapter are twofold. The first is to review the incidence and natural history, pathophysiology, diagnosis, and operative indications related to RAA. The second is to review *in situ* RAA repair including patient selection, operative techniques, and outcomes.

INCIDENCE

Renal Artery Aneurysms are a rare entity with an incidence of approximately 0.1% in the general population, .7–1.3% of patients undergoing abdominal and renal arteriograms, and .7% undergoing computed tomographic angiography.[1-4] RAAs account for 22% of visceral artery aneurysms.[5] Most RAAs are discovered in relatively young patients, with a peak incidence between 40 and 60 years of age, which points the association of RAAs with underlying arterial pathology. In multiple series of RAA repair, the mean age is between 46 and 51 years of age.[6-11] Aneurysms secondary to fibrodysplasia are more common in younger women, but there is equal incidence in males and females if this etiology is excluded.[9] Even if asymtomoatic, they are incidentally detected with increased use of computed tomography and angiography.[12,13]

PATHOPHYSIOLOGY AND RISK FACTORS

Types of renal artery aneurysms include true aneurysms, which are either sacular or fusiform, dissecting aneurysms, intra-renal aneurysms, or false aneurysms most often secondary to trauma. More than 90% of renal artery aneurysms are extra parenchymal.[1,14]

Approximately 75% of true renal artery aneurysms are sacular and are generally less than 5 cm in diameter. These occur predominantly at the main renal artery bifurcation.[15] Most are thought to be secondary to either atherosclerosis or a congenital defect in the arterial wall. The internal elastic lamina is particularly weak at arterial bifurcations which explains the propensity for RAA formation at first and second order renal artery branch points.[1] Atherosclerosis is considered risk factor for RAAs as in many cases it is the only potential risk factor identified. However, the role of atherosclerosis in RAA pathophysiology is unclear and atherosclerosis may be secondary to aneurysm formation rather than the cause of aneurysm development.

Fusiform aneurysms are generally the result of a post stenotic dilatation distal to significant renal artery stenosis which results from either atherosclerosis or arterial fibrodysplasia.[1,14,15] Major risk factors include fibromuscular dysplasia (FMD), which is seen in 25–50% of RAAs.[7,11,16] RAAs are most often associated with the medial fibrodisplasia variant of FMD, tend to be smaller than 2 cm, more often affect the main renal artery, and have the typical angiographic appearance of a "string of beads."[1] Larger RAAs can occur with FMD however, as in one study macroaneurysms of the renal artery were found in 9.2% of adults with FMD.[1]

Spontaneous dissections of the renal artery are rare but can lead to pseudo-aneurysms. Stanley, et al. reported a series in which 14 of 57 cases were due to spontaneous dissection.[1] An intimal defect associated with atherosclerosis or dysplastic arterial disease is probably the underlying etiology. Blunt trauma and iatrogenic injury caused by wires and catheters can also lead to renal artery dissection and subsequent psuedonaeurysm.[1,14]

Approximately 80% of patients with RAA have HTN.[1,9,11] Hypertension is believed to be a risk factor for RAA formation and growth as it is with aneurysms in other arterial beds. Hypertension may also be the result of RAAs, though the mechanism by which RAA elicits renovascular hypertension remains poorly defined. Among patients undergoing renal arteriography for evaluation of hypertension, the incidence of RA is 2.5%.[1]

A variety of other arteriopathies have also been implicated in RAA formation including polyarteritis nodosa and Behcet's arteritis, as well as mycotic and inflammatory RAAs. Neurofibromatosis is a documented risk factor for development of RAAs in children and young adults. RAAs have also been reported in association with renal cell cancer, renal transplantation, Williams syndrome, and tuberous sclerosis.

CLINICAL PRESENTATION AND DIAGNOSIS

The majority of renal artery aneurysms are asymptomatic and incidentally discovered on abdominal imaging to investigate other pathology.[12,13] However, in one series, 34% of renal artery aneurysms repaired had presented with symptoms.[6] The most dreaded complication of renal artery aneurysms is rupture. Less than 5% of RAAs repaired present with rupture.[1,13] Ruptured RAAs present with abdominal or flank distension and pain and signs and symptoms of acute hemorrhage. Abdominal or flank pain or fullness with an intact RAA but no other intrabdominal pathology must be presumed to be secondary to aneurysm expansion with pending rupture.

RAAs are frequently associated with severe renovascular hypertension. The aneurysm may be associated with a significant renal artery stenosis which is the source of hypertension.[1,9,13,17] Large series, however, have documented severe hypertension in the absence of associated stenosis in the majority of patients.[8,10] Potential mechanisms include distal microembolization with parenchymal hypoperfusion and resultant renin-mediated vasoconstriction, flow reduction from extensive intra-aneurysmal thrombus, or compression or kinking of adjacent renal artery branches by the aneurysm.[1,8,9,18] The most plausible phenomenon is the Windkessel phenomenon, in which the aneurysm alters flow and dissipates downstream arterial pressure in distal segmental braches and the afferent arteriole, thereby initiating the rennin-mediated hypertension.

Renal infarction from embolization has been described, and loss of kidney function is a concern, particularly in a solitary kidney.[10,16] In addition, renal artery dissection and associated aneurysms is often asymptomatic, but can cause acute flank or back pain, hematuria, and hypertension.

Given the relatively small size of most RAAs and location, physical exam is unreliable in detection of RAAAs. The diagnosis is made via imaging. First-line noninvasive imaging often includes duplex ultrasound and conventional computed tomographic scanning, particularly when pathology other than RAA is suspected.[13] If RAA is suspected, however, spiral computed tomographic angiography (CTA), magnetic resonance imaging (MRI), or conventional angiography is recommended (Figure 27-1).[4,19] Subtraction angiography via selective renal artery catheterization remains the gold standard modality and multiple imaging angles is recommended order to delineate RAA anatomy and branch vessel involvement to plan elective repair (Figure 27-2).

INDICATIONS FOR REPAIR OF RENAL ARTERY ANEURYSM

Rupture

Rupture of a RAA is an obvious indication for repair. The mortality of ruptured renal artery aneurysms in males and non-pregnant females is reported that 10–25%.[13] Most

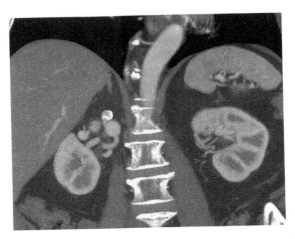

Figure 27-1. Computed tomographic (CT) scan with intravenous contrast demonstrating two right renal artery aneurysms measuring 1.8 and 1.3 cm in diameter in a 71-year-old male patient who presented with right flank pain, hematuria, and severe hypertension.

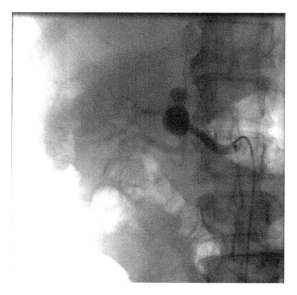

Figure 27-2. Selective digital subtraction right, renal artery angiogram demonstrating the arterial anatomy in the same patient. Note that the larger aneurysm involves the main renal artery bifurcation and a second aneurysm involves the main bifurcation and the upper pole segmental artery.

often, a ruptured RAA necessitates nephrectomy due to hemodynamic instability, a large perinephric hematoma, and the extended renal ischemic time. In certain instances of a contained rupture in a stable patient, *in situ* repair the aneurysm with salvage of the kidney may be advisable, particularly in the instance of a solitary kidney.

Dissection

RAAs associated with dissections that are either symptomatic in the form of flank pain or threaten the viability of the kidney require emergent repair. Nephrectomy is often required because dissections often extend into small renal branch vessels, which makes repair difficult to perform in the time available to salvage an ischemic kidney.

Hypertension

Renal artery aneurysms can cause hypertension, though the exact mechanism is not clearly defined.[8,9] The reported blood pressure response in hypertensive patients after renal artery aneurysm repair has been uniformly beneficial with improved blood pressure control and reduction of antihypertensive medications in properly selected patients.[1,7–11,20] Some authors recommend a conservative approach with criteria for surgical repair identical to that for intervention for renal artery stenosis, namely diastolic blood pressure greater than 90 mmHg despite three antihypertensive medications.[21] Others recommend a more liberal approach with repair of any RAA associated with significant hypertension or any RAA greater than 1 cm with difficult to control hypertension.[8,10] The decision to repair a renal artery aneurysm associated with hypertension should be tailored to individual patient based on their comorbidities, response to antihypertensive medications, and anticipated difficulty of repair based on the aneurysm anatomy. Renal artery aneurysm repair should be undertaken in patients of acceptable operative risk with difficult -to -control hypertension and anatomy amenable to repair with low risk of nephrectomy. Coexistent stenoses should be repaired along with the aneurysm. Mild post-stenotic dilatations associated with hemodynamically significant stenoses resulting from fibromuscular disease are treated with balloon angioplasty. The indication is the stenotic lesion and not the aneurysm.

Elective Repair for the Prevention of Rupture

Indication for repair of an asymptomatic renal artery aneurysm for prevention of rupture is controversial because the natural history of RAAs is not clearly defined. Traditionally, repair has been recommended for RAAs greater than 2 cm in diameter.[14] However, the expected rate of growth has not been delineated and definitive evidence for rupture risk based on RAA size is lacking. While rupture of RAAs smaller than 2 cm has been reported, small RAAs less than 1.5–2.0 cm have a generally benign course with extremely low rates of rupture on mid-term to long-term follow-up.[1,2,8,12,16,22] Henke et al followed 86 aneurysms (mean size 1.3 cm) in 61 patents for 72 months without evidence of symptoms or rupture.[8] In another series, there were no ruptures in a group of 18 patients with RAAAs Less than 2.6 cm who were followed for 1 to 16 years.[9] However, there is selection bias in reports of RAAs followed conservatively, as many larger aneurysms were repaired. Few series report follow-up on any aneurysms greater than 3 cm.

Given the lack of definitive data, recommendations for elective repair vary considerably. Some authors recommend repair for RAAs that are 1.5 to 2 cm or greater.[8,10] Others have recommended a expectant management for any RAA <2.5 cm, and still others expectant management for any RAA less than 3.0 cm.[16,21] The most common recommendation and our recommendation is to consider 2.0 cm diameter as the threshold for elective repair assuming there is a low risk of nephrectomy and acceptable operative risk.[5,21,22,8] Weighing all evidence, this remains a reliable approach in this young patient population with good life expectancy. Aside from RAAA size, some have suggested that calcification may be protective against RAA rupture. Because there is also evidence that the degree of calcification of a RAA does not impact rupture risk, others believe that calcification of an RAA should not be a factor in consideration for repair.[13]

As with other splanchnic aneurysms, pregnancy greatly increases the risk of rupture.[1,6,13] Rupture during pregnancy has been reported in RAAs as small as 1 cm diameter.[9] Rupture during pregnancy maternal and fetal mortality of 55% and 85% respectively.[23] While the exact risk of rupture during pregnancy remains uncertain, repair is recommended in any women of child bearing age regardless of aneurysm size.[6,8,9,21,23]

In summary, indications for renal artery aneurysm repair are tailored to individual patient presentation with elective surgical repair of RAAs greater than 2 cm in size in good candidates and repair of any RAA in women of child-bearing age. Aneurysms between 1.5 and 2 cm should be considered for repair based upon severity of HTN, comorbidities, and RAA anatomy impacting surgical risk.

OVERVIEW OF REPAIR OF RENAL ARTERY ANEURYSMS

Repair of RAA is a challenging operation because most aneurysms extend into first and second order branches of the renal artery. In general, RAA repair is more challenging than revascularization for renal artery stenosis. In addition, the repair must be performed expeditiously in order to limit renal warm ischemic time to less than 45 minutes.[8,11,21]

The optimal method of repair of renal artery aneurysms are controversial. Many recent series espouse the use of *ex vivo* techniques for open repair of complex renal artery aneurysms involving renal branch vessels.[7,17] There have also been increasing number of reports of both *ex vivo* and *in situ* laparoscopic repair of renal artery aneurysms.[24] In addition, the use of a variety of endovascular techniques for RAA repair, including stent grafting and coil embolization, have been described.[25] The lack of consensus regarding the optimal method of repair is due in part to the lack of data on the outcomes of open repair of RAA, with the majority of data coming from a few select high volume centers with particular interest in renal reconstruction.[7,8,10] Analysis of any particular surgical approach is difficult because of the wide variety techniques employed by surgeons at different centers and even within centers with a particular interest in RAA repair.

PATIENT SELECTION FOR IN SITU REPAIR

In many contemporary series, an *in situ* technique can be utilized in greater than 70% of all renal artery aneurysm repairs (Table 27-1).[8,11,16,20] Pfeiffer et al. report that *in situ* techniques were utilized in 132 of 136 repairs over a 20 year period.[10] Series from other institutions report use of *in situ* techniques in 20% to 60% of cases, with a corresponding increased preference for *ex vivo* techniques.[6,7,17] In our institution, an *in situ* technique is utilized in all cases when anatomically feasible which is approximately three-fourths of cases. An *ex vivo* approach is reserved for cases when very distal subsegmental branch or intrahilar location of the RAA prevents adequate distal vascular control for reconstruction. *Ex vivo* repair includes division of the renal vessels and ureteral mobilization and/or division to allow aneurysm resection and vascular reconstruction either on the anterior abdominal wall or on a back table. And orthotopic or iliac fossa replantation follows.

TECHNIQUE OF *IN SITU* REPAIR

Exposure

Wide exposure is achieved with either a subcostal or 10th interspace flank incision which allows a retroperitoneal approach and full mobilization of the kidney from both the anterior and posterior aspects (Figures 27-3 and 27-4). In our experience, both incisions are generally well tolerated. Approximately 70% of unilateral repairs can be performed via a retroperitoneal approach on both the right and left. Retroperitoneal mobilization of the kidney is particularly important when the RAA involves a posterior branch of the renal artery, as it is necessary to approach the renal arteries posteriorly. The left renal artery usually lies directly beneath the cephalad border of the left renal vein. The vein must be mobilized in order to fully expose the main renal artery and its branches, which may require ligation

TABLE 27-1. MAJOR CONTEMPORARY SERIES OF RENAL ARTERY ANEURYSM REPAIR WITH *IN SITU* TECHNIQUES

First Author, Year	Study Years	RAAs repaired *In Situu*/Total RAAs Repaired	Mean Size (cm)	RAA Location[μ] N (%)	Approach	Techniques Utilized (n)
Chandra, 2010	2003–2008	7/10	2.1 ± 0.4*	Main Bifurcation: 7 (70%) Proximal Branch: 2 (20%) Distal Branch: 1 (10%)	Transperitoneal: 2 Retroperitoneal: 5	Aneurysmectomy w/ vein patch: 4 prosthetic patch: 2 primary repair: 1
Dzsinich, 1993	1978–1990	16/35	1.7	nr	nr	Aneurysmectomy w/ primary repair: 3 vein patch: 1 prosthetic patch: 2 Ligation/resection with aortorenal bypass: 17 (Dacron 3, saphenous vein 13, composite 1) Ligation:5
English, 2004	1987–2003	44/72	2.6 (1.3–5.5)	Branch: 56 (78%)	Subcostal Incision/ transperitoneal†	Bypass‡ Aneurysmorraphy w/ exclusion patch angioplasty Bypass with Aneurysmorraphy
Henke, 2001	1965–2000	168 RAAs in 96 patients/121 patients	1.5	Main RA: 27 (15%) Main Bifurcation: 80 (43%) Proximal and distal segmental branches: 97 (52%)	Transverse umbilical, TP approach with medial visceral rotation	Aneurysmectomy w/ Primary closure or artery replantation: 63 Aneurysmectomy w/ bypass graft: 33

(Continued)

TABLE 27-1. *(Continued)*

First Author, Year	Study Years	RAAs repaired In Situ/Total RAAs Repaired	Mean Size (cm)	RAA Location[b] N (%)	Approach	Techniques Utilized (n)
Lumsden, 1996	1972–1992	7/10	2.1 ±1.5*	Main RA: 15 (52%) Proximal and distal segmental Branches: 12 (44%) Intraparenchymal: 1 (4%)	nr	Aneurysmectomy w/ vein patch: 1 primary repair: 2 Ligation with aortorenal bypass: 3 (Dacron 3, vein 1)
Martin, 1989	1973–1987	13/19	2.03	Main RA: 5/43 (12%) Main bifurcation: 22/43 (51%) Distal Branch: 14/43 (33%) Intraparenchymal 3/43 (7%)	nr	Aneurysmectomy w/ primary repair or vein patch: 6 Resection with interposition or aortorenal bypass graft: 7
Murray, 1994	1971–1993	23/84	nr	In situ repair used only for RAAs at main renal bifurcation	Midline Transperitoneal	Aortorenal bypass with branched internal iliac autograft
Pfeiffer, 2003	1980–2001	132/136	1–2 cm in 45 patients w/risk factor; >2 cm in 49 patients	Main RA: 83 (61%) Branch arteries: 49 (36%)	Midline transperitoneal for proximal RAAs Lumbar retroperitoneal for peripheral RAAs	Aneurysmectomy w/ tailoring: 37 saphenous vein graft: 40 tailoring and vein graft: 7 Resection and reanastomosis: 14 resection, reanastomosis, vein graft: 3 PTFE bypass: 5 Homologous vein graft: 1

First Author, Year	Study Years	RAAs repaired *In Situ*/Total RAAs Repaired	Mean Size (cm)	RAA Location[υ] N (%)	Approach	Techniques Utilized (n)
Robinson, 2011	1984–2009	22/26	2.3 ± 0.7	Main RA: 1 (3%) Bifurcation and first-order branches: 18 (70%) Second order branches: 7 (27%)	Midline transperitoneal for coexistent AAA or bilateral RAA repair: 5 Subcostal: 12 Flank/10th interspace: 8 Thoracoretroperitoneal: 1	Resection w/ Autogenous bypass/interposition: 11 Primary anastomosis to conjoined branches: 3 Aortic reimplantation: 2 Aneurysmorraphy w/ Vein patch angioplasty: 6 Tailored primary closure: 1 Autogenous bypass: 1 Exclusion: 2

* of entire cohort , including those observed or repaired without in situ repair
† stated by authors to be preferred approach
‡ techniques includes those for both *in situ* and *ex vivo* repairs
υ designate location of all RAAs, including those managed with observation or *ex vivo* repair

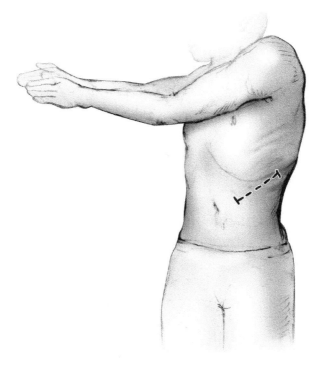

Figure 27-3. Tenth Interspace Flank Incision. Patient is positioned in 60 degree lateral decubitus position with hips rotated and the bed flexed to "open up" the space just below the costal margin. A "kidney rest" or towel roll under the contralateral flank is used. Incision extends from Tip of 10th rib toward umbilicus.

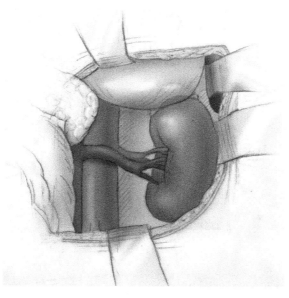

Figure 27-4. Exposure of Kidney. Flank exposure with retroperitoneal mobilization to the midline provides ready exposure of the anterior kidney to the level of the hilum and also allows posterior mobilization of the kidney if necessary.

of adrenal, gonadal, or lumbar branches to permit retraction. The right renal artery more often lies beneath the caudal aspect of the right renal vein. A midline or transverse abdominal transperitoneal approach is reserved for bilateral renal artery repairs and repairs performed simultaneously with aortic reconstruction.[11] In this instance, the left renal vessels are exposed via a meal visceral rotation and the right, renal vessels are exposed via an extended Kocher maneuver.

Techniques of Resection and Renal Artery Reconstruction

A variety of techniques for *in situ* repair have been described. Because there may be multiple RAAs which occur both at first and second-order branch points and thus involved multiple segmental branches, the surgeon must be both creative and flexible in adapting techniques of reconstruction to the renal artery anatomy (Figure 27-5). Occasionally, redundancy in both the inflow and outflow renal arteries may allow a tailored primary repair with end-to-end anastomosis after aneurysm resection (Figure 27-6). Most commonly, resection of the involved segment of artery followed by interposition grafting or bypass grafting from the aorta to the distal renal artery is required. Surgeons employ this technique in approximately 50 to 70% of *in situ* repairs in most series.[10, 11, 16]

Because renal artery aneurysms frequently involve renal artery branch points, it is not possible fully resects the aneurysm and maintain a common outflow that would perfuse all renal parenchyma. Resection and interposition or bypass grafting thus frequently require adjunctive techniques in order to maintain perfusion to all or the majority of renal parenchyma. A common reconstruction is to re-implant a segmental renal artery in an end- to-side fashion to the main renal artery or interposition vein graft (Figure 27-7). Alternatively, a segment of harvested internal iliac artery with

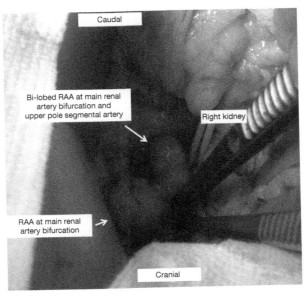

Figure 27-5. Exposure of RAAs. Intraoperative photographs of two right renal artery aneurysms in the same patient. The larger RAA obscures the proximal main renal artery which is deep to it and the lower pole segmental branch. The smaller aneurysm is bi-lobed and involves the main bifurcation and the segmental branch to the upper pole.

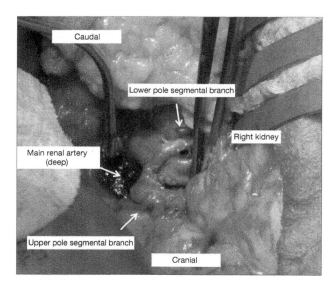

Figure 27-6. Repair of RAAs. Intraoperative photograph of *in situ* repair of the two renal artery aneurysms. Both aneurysms were resected, and the common orifice of the distal main renal artery and lower pole segmental branch was anastomosed in an end-to-end fashion to the upper pole segmental branch.

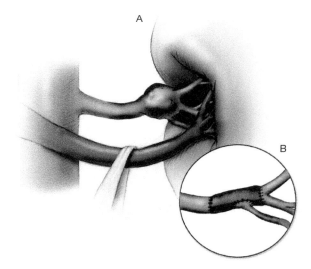

Figure 27-7. Aneurysm Resection and Interposition Graft. Circumferential aneurysm involvement necessitated segmental renal artery resection and vein interposition grafting. Note that segmental branches are too widely splayed to allow anastomosis to a single conjoined outflow target so a lower pole segmental artery has been re-implanted on the graft.

multiple branches provides an excellent autologous conduit as the artery branches can be anastomosed to small branches of the main renal artery. Yet another technique involves "conjoining" of adjacent segmental branches with a side-to-side anastomoses in order to create a common outflow channel to the renal parenchyma into which the renal artery or graft can be sewn in an end-to-end configuration. Saphenous vein is the preferred conduit due to its conformability and excellent size match with the renal artery. In cases where aortorenal grafting or renal artery interposition grafting is not possible, splenorenal bypass and hepatorenal bypass can be utilized for left and right RAAs respectively.

Aneurysmectomy with primary closure or patch angioplasty (Figure 27-8) can be performed for saccular aneurysms or aneurysms which do not involve the majority of the circumference of the renal artery wall. This is a relatively straightforward technique and the preferred method when aneurysm anatomy allows. In this technique, we excise all grossly aneurismal tissue but will spare uninvolved portions of the renal artery wall in order to allow reconstruction. Saphenous vein is preferred for patch angioplasty but both PTFE and Dacron patches have been utilized. In most series, this method constitutes approximately 1/3 of *in situ* repairs.[6,10,11,16]

In situ repair requires meticulous dissection and identification of aneurysm anatomy to allow for a direct repair with less than 45 minutes warm renal ischemic time to prevent acute tubular necrosis. Intravenous heparin (100 units per kilogram) is administered before renal artery clamping in reconstruction. When greater than 40 minutes warm ischemic time would be required, we flush the kidney with 500 to 1000 ml of manitol-infused heparinized Ringers solution (2500 u/L) at 4°C. The perfusate is drained with a small angiocatheter in the renal vein after it is flushed through the kidney.

In situ repair can be utilized for a ruptured renal artery aneurysm if the patient is stable and bleeding is easily controlled. Aneurysm anatomy must be amenable to a relatively straightforward reconstruction. Often, however, juxtarenal hematoma does not allow safe control of the proximal renal arteries and aortic clamping is required. Patient instability and pro-longed ischemia of the kidney may require nephrectomy.

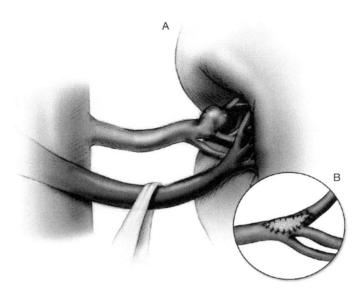

Figure 27-8. Aneurysmectomy and Vein Patch Angioplasty. Note the resection of grossly aneurismal arterial wall and reconstruction with vein patch to maintain perfusion to segmental branches.

OUTCOMES OF *IN SITU* REPAIR

Short-Term Outcomes

Elective *in situ* RAA repair by well-trained surgeons can be performed with excellent success and low early morbidity and mortality (Table 27-2). Most recent contemporary series of in situ repair reported mortality of less than 2%.[6–11,17,20] Technical success in reconstruction is reported in greater than 90% of patients in recent series with a rate of nephrectomy after a failed repair of 8% or less.[6–11,16,17,20] Rates of significant postoperative morbidity have been reported between 0 and 28%.[6–11,16,17,20] Median length of stay averages 5 to 7 days.[11,20]

  Comparisons of short-term outcomes with *in situ* and *ex vivo* techniques are limited and difficult to make. Chandra et al. report that in a series of 14 patients, there was higher blood loss with *ex vivo* in comparison to *in situ* repair, but no difference in transfusion requirements and overall operative time. There was a trend toward shorter time to oral intake when *in situ* aneurysmectomy with arterial reconstruction was performed via a retroperitoneal approach.[20]

Long-Term Outcomes

Data regarding long-term follow-up of renal artery reconstructions for RAA remains limited to that provided by a few select centers (Table 27-3). Data on long-term outcome is particularly important for two reasons. First, RAAs occur in relatively young patients with good life expectancy. Second, it is necessary to establish standards to which emerging therapies will be compared.

Patency of Reconstruction

In modern series with follow-up beyond one year, a primary patency of 81% and 100% with *in situ* reconstruction is reported (Table 27-3).[7,8,10,11,17,20] Though direct comparison of *in situ* and *ex vivo* repair is very difficult to make due to selection bias, there appears

TABLE 27-2. SHORT-TERM OUTCOMES OF *IN SITU* RENAL ARTERY ANEURYSM REPAIR

First Author, Year	RAAs repaired in situ/Total RAAs Repaired	Technical Success	Nephrectomy s/p repair	Major Morbidity	Mortality
Chandra, 2010	7/10	100%	0	28%	0%
Dzsinich,1993	16/35	94%	0	6%	0%
English, 2004[†]	44/72	98.6%	0%	12%	1.6%
Henke, 2001	96/121	91%	8.3%	8.3%	0%
Lumsden,1996	7/10	100%	0%	0%	10%[x]
Martin, 1989	13/19	100%	0%	nr	0%
Murray, 1994	23/84	100%	nr	nr	0%
Pfeiffer, 2003	132/136	96.8%	2.6%	17%	<1%
Robinson, 2011	22/26	96%	4%	12%	0%

nr = not reported in study
[†] includes combined outcomes of *in situ* and *ex vivo* repairs
[x] 1 death in patient who underwent concomitant repair of suprarenal AAA

TABLE 27-3. LONG-TERM OUTCOMES OF *IN SITU* RENAL ARTERY ANEURYSM REPAIR

First Author, Year	Follow-Up, n	Primary Patency	Impact on HTN	Renal Function	Recurrent RAA/ Rupture	Survival
Chandra, 2010	12 mo in 10 pts	100%	Significantly reduced # of meds (2.3 vs. 3.8)	nr	0%/0%	100%
Dzsinich, 1993	nr	nr	Improved: 50%	nr	nr/nr	nr
English, 2004[†]	47 mo in 72 pts	96% (100% in situ, 93% ex vivo)	Improved: 54% Cured: 21% Unchanged: 25%	Improved:60%[μ] Unchanged:20%[μ] Decline:20%[μ]	0%/0%	91% estimated at 120 months
Henke, 2001	91 mo in 145 pts	93%	Significantly Improved BP and reduced # of meds (1 vs. 2)	nr	nr/0%	>80%
Lumsden, 1996	37 mo[∞]	nr	Improved or cured: 100%[γ]	nr	nr/0%	nr
Martin, 1989	97 mo in 18 pts	nr	Cured: 12% Improved: 65% No change: 23%	nr	nr/0%	89%
Murray, 1994	90 mo in 53 pts	92%	Cured: 87% Improved: 13%	No change: 83% Worse: 13%	0%	nr/nr
Pfeiffer, 2003	46 mo in 83 pts	81% (100% tailored vs. 73% graft[*])	Cured: 25% Improved: 22%	Mean post-op Cr 1.1 (no pre-op Cr reported)	0%/0%	97%
Robinson, 2011	99 mo in 18 pts	94%	82% improved with reduced # of meds (1.1 vs. 2.6)[Ω]	post-op Cr: 1.1vs. pre-op 1.2 1.3 p = NS	0%/0%	100%

nr = not reported in study
[*] p < .05
[μ] among patients with pre-operative renal insufficiency
[∞] including patients followed expectantly
[Ω] In 11 patients with severe HTN
[γ] in 4 patients who preoperative lateralizing renins

to be no difference in patency between these 2 methods of repair. English et al reported a primary patency of 100% in 44 patients after *in situ* repair and 93% in 28 patients undergoing *ex vivo* repair at an average of 47 months follow-up. Due to the wide variety of reconstruction techniques employed in published reports, it is difficult to make comparisons between the various types of in situ reconstructions such as bypass grafting, interposition grafting, and aneurysmorrhaphy with patch angioplasty. Pfeiffer et al. did report a patency of 100% with aneurysmectomy with "tailoring" which was significantly better than the 73% patency with aneurysmectomy and bypass grafting.[10] No other groups have reported differences in patency based on reconstruction technique employed.

Impact on Hypertension

Renal artery aneurysm repair has been shown to have a beneficial effect on blood pressure control in properly selected patients (Table 27-3). Though there is little uniformity in the manner in which the impact of RAA repair on blood pressure response has been reported, contemporary series have almost uniformly reported significant improvement or cure of hypertension in 75 to 100% of cases.[7–9,11,16,17,20]. A few studies have reported a 50% reduction in antihypertensive medication requirements confirmed at long-term follow-up out to 99 months.[8,11,20] Martin et al. reported the most consistent blood pressure response in patients with documented renovascular hypertension whose renal vein renin measurements and/or split function studies lateralized to the side of the renal artery aneurysm.[9] However, studies to identify the kidney responsible for renin-mediated hypertension can be falsely negative and excellent blood pressure response has been consistently observed after RAA repair in patients with medically-refractory hypertension without a lateralizing study.[8–11] Most authors do not think that a lateralizing study is necessary before repair of in RAA for severe hypertension.[9–11] The excellent long-term outcomes for control of hypertension have led to the recommendations for repair of renal artery aneurysms as small as 1 cm, which are associated with refractory hypertension regardless of whether there is a coexistent renal artery stenosis.[8, 10] It is not unreasonable to assume that the lifelong benefit of improved blood pressure control and cost savings on antihypertensive medications could be substantial.

Preservation of Renal Function

Studies show that *in situ* RAA repair can be performed with good preservation of renal function, even in complex reconstructions of 1st and 2nd order segmental branches. In studies which report postoperative renal function, no significant postoperative renal insufficiency has been observed. English et al. reported that among patients with preoperative renal insufficiency, 60% had improvement, 20% saw no change, and 20% had declined in renal function after RAA repair. These positive outcomes with *in situ* RAA reconstruction highlights the benefit of expeditious repair with limited renal ischemic time, as well as the need for meticulous technique for durable long-term renal perfusion.

Freedom from RAA Rupture and Recurrence

In situ repair provides durable cure of RAA. Although the frequency and type imaging studies which have been utilized for surveillance after RAA repair varies considerably in major contemporary series, there have been no reported cases of RAA recurrence or late RAA—related deaths (Table 27-3). There has been theoretic concerns that repair of an RAA with aneurysmectomy with either primary or patch closure may predispose to aneurysm recurrence and RAA—related morbidity because aneurysmal tissue may be left behind. This concern does not appear to be borne out in the literature. There was no evidence of RAA recurrence and 77 aneurysms repaired by this technique that had imaging studies at long-term follow-up.[11] Other authors have endorsed the durability of in situ aneurysmectomy and patching or primary closure. As with any aneurysm repair, all aneurysmal tissue must be resected, leaving behind only normal arterial wall for reconstruction.

Long-Term Survival

Long-term survival has been reported to be between 80% and 100% at a mean follow-up ranging from 46 to 99 month (Table 27-3).[7–11] This is indicative of the fact that renal artery aneurysms occur in a relatively young patient population, primarily in the 5th and 6th decades of life, with good expected longevity. Excellent long-term survival also provides evidence for the durability of RAA repair via *in situ* techniques.

SURVEILLANCE

Little data exists to guide recommendations for surveillance of RAA repairs or RAAs followed conservatively. Given the extended life expectancy in these patients, surveillance of *in situ* recommendation is warranted. CTA provides excellent anatomic detail to evaluate for recurrence or lesions which threaten the patency of the renal artery reconstruction (Figure 27-9). English et al. have demonstrated that in the hands of expert sonographers duplex ultrasonography provide accurate routine surveillance of RAA repair.[7] A reasonable surveillance protocol is to obtain a CTA at 1 month and 1 year after repair and, if no concerns exist, to follow intermittently with bilateral renal artery duplex thereafter.

SUMMARY

Indications for repair of RAA include ruptured or otherwise symptomatic RAAs, recalcitrant hypertension believed to be secondary to a RAA, and RAAs associated with kidney-threatening dissection. Although the size threshold at which repair of asymptomatic

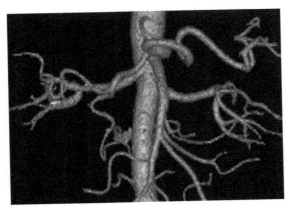

Figure 27-9. Surveillance Imaging after In Situ Repair. Postoperative CTA in the same patient demonstrating the elimination of both RAAs and patent segmental arteries to both the upper and lower pole with good perfusion of the kidney.

RAAs is recommended remains controversial, most recommend repair at a diameter between 2 and 3 centimeters in males and women beyond child-bearing age. RAAs in women of child-bearing age should be repaired irrespective of size. Though surgeon and institution preference of techniques varies considerably in the published literature, approximately 70% or greater of RAAs have been repaired via an *in situ* method in many series. The array of techniques utilized include resection and bypass or interposition grafting, aneurysmectomy and primary closure or patching, and adjunctive techniques such as "conjoining" of adjacent renal artery branch vessels. The goal of all *in situ* RAA repairs is to resect all aneurysmal tissue and provide durable reconstruction of renal perfusion while limiting kidney warm ischemic time. *In situ* repair of RAA is associated with low morbidity and mortality, beneficial blood pressure response, and good preservation of renal function. *In situ* RAA repair has shown good long–term outcomes including patency of reconstruction, freedom from aneurysm recurrence and rupture, and excellent long-term survival which is important in this young patient population. The outcomes of *in situ* repair of RAA establish the standards by which emerging therapies such as endovascular treatment should be measured.

REFERENCES

1. Stanley JC, Rhodes EL, Gewertz BL, et al. Renal artery aneurysms. Significance of macroaneurysms exclusive of dissections and fibrodysplastic mural dilations. *Arch Surg.* 1975;110(11):1327–33.
2. Tham G, Ekelund L, Herrlin K, et al. Renal artery aneurysms. Natural history and prognosis. *Ann Surg.* 1983;197(3):348–52.
3. Ersdman G. *Acta Radiol.* 1957(155(suppl)):104.
4. Zhang LJ, Yang GF, Qi J, et al. Renal artery aneurysm: Diagnosis and surveillance with multidetector-row computed tomography. *Acta Radiol.* 2007;48(3):274–9.
5. Deterling RA, Jr. Aneurysm of the visceral arteries. *J Cardiovasc Surg.* (Torino) 1971; 12(4):309–22.
6. Dzsinich C, Gloviczki P, McKusick MA, et al. Surgical management of renal artery aneurysm. *Cardiovasc Surg.* 1993;1(3):243–7.
7. English WP, Pearce JD, Craven TE, et al. Surgical management of renal artery aneurysms. *J Vasc Surg.* 2004;40(1):53–60.
8. Henke PK, Cardneau JD, Welling TH 3rd, et al. Renal artery aneurysms: a 35-year clinical experience with 252 aneurysms in 168 patients. *Ann Surg.* 2001;234(4):454–62; discussion 62–3.
9. Martin RS 3rd, Meacham PW, Ditesheim JA, et al. Renal artery aneurysm: selective treatment for hypertension and prevention of rupture. *J Vasc Surg.* 1989;9(1):26–34.
10. Pfeiffer T, Reiher L, Grabitz K, et al. Reconstruction for renal artery aneurysm: Operative techniques and long-term results. *J Vasc Surg.* 2003;37(2):293–300.
11. Robinson WP 3rd, Bafford R, Belkin M, et al. Favorable outcomes with in situ techniques for surgical repair of complex renal artery aneurysms. *J Vasc Surg.* 53(3):684–91.
12. Henriksson C, Bjorkerud S, Nilson AE, et al. Natural history of renal artery aneurysm elucidated by repeated angiography and pathoanatomical studies. *Eur Urol.* 1985;11(4):244–8.
13. Stanley J. Natural History of Renal Artery Stenosis and Aneurysms. *In* Calligaro KD and Dean RH, eds. Modern Management of Renovascular Hypertension and Renal Salvage. Baltimore: William and Wilkins, 1996. pp. 15.
14. Fry W. Renal artery aneurysm. *In* Ernst CB, Stanley JC, eds. *Current Therapy in Vascular Surgery*: Philadelphia: BC Decker, 1987. pp. 363.

15. Poutasse, EF. Renal artery aneurysms: Their natural history and surgery. *J Urol.* 1966; 95(3):297–306.

16. Lumsden AB, Salam TA, Walton KG. Renal artery aneurysm: A report of 28 cases. *Cardiovasc Surg.* 1996;4(2):185–9.

17. Murray SP, Kent C, Salvatierra O, et al. Complex branch renovascular disease: management options and late results. *J Vasc Surg.* 1994;20(3):338-45; discussion 46.

18. Youkey JR, Collins GJ Jr., Orecchia PM, et al. Saccular renal artery aneurysm as a cause of hypertension. *Surgery.* 1985;97(4):498–501.

19. Takebayashi S, Ohno T, Tanaka K, et al. MR angiography of renal vascular malformations. *J Comput Assist Tomogr.* 1994;18(4):596–600.

20. Chandra A, O'Connell JB, Quinones-Baldrich WJ, et al. Aneurysmectomy With Arterial Reconstruction of Renal Artery Aneurysms in the Endovascular Era: A Safe, Effective Treatment for Both Aneurysm and Associated Hypertension. *Ann Vasc Surg.* 2009.

21. Calligaro KD. Renovascular Disease: Aneurysms and Arteriovenous Fistula. *In* Cronenwett JL, Johnson KW, eds. Rutherford's Vascular Surgery, Vol. 2. Philadephia: Saunders, 2010. pp. 2243–47.

22. Hidai H, Kinoshita Y, Murayama T, et al. Rupture of renal artery aneurysm. *Eur Urol.* 1985; 11(4):249–53.

23. Cohen JR, Shamash FS. Ruptured renal artery aneurysms during pregnancy. *J Vasc Surg.* 1987;6(1):51–9.

24. Giulianotti PC, Bianco FM, Addeo P, et al. Robot-assisted laparoscopic repair of renal artery aneurysms. *J Vasc Surg.* 51(4):842–9.

25. Bruce M, Kuan YM. Endoluminal stent-graft repair of a renal artery aneurysm. *J Endovasc Ther.* 2002;9(3):359–62.

28

Open Surgical Treatment of Mesenteric Occlusive Disease

Margaret C. Tracci, MD, JD and Kenneth J. Cherry, MD

INTRODUCTION

Mesenteric ischemia, in both its chronic and acute forms, remains among the most challenging clinical situations in vascular surgery and continues to be associated with significant morbidity and mortality. Chronic mesenteric ischemia (CMI) and the acute-on-chronic form of acute mesenteric ischemia (AMI) are typically associated with atherosclerotic lesions of the vessel origin and proximal arterial segments. The mesenteric circulation is characterized by rich collateralization. These collaterals include the gastroduodenal and pancreaticoduodenal communications between the celiac axis and SMA; the marginal artery of Drummond and arc of Riolan that, along with the numerous vasa recta, link the SMA and IMA circulation; and the superior rectal and other essential pelvic collaterals arising from the hypogastric artery. This anatomic redundancy is consistent with the typical clinical finding of involvement of two, if not all three, of the mesenteric vessels at the time symptoms emerge. It is widely presumed that factors resulting in compromise of collaterals, such as prior intestinal surgery or ligation of the inferior mesenteric artery in conjunction with aortic reconstruction, render a patient more susceptible to clinical ischemia. The presentation of acute mesenteric ischemia (AMI) may represent either the acute-on-chronic pattern of thrombosis of a diseased vessel (most frequently in the setting of multivessel disease) or sudden embolic occlusion of a nondiseased vessel. The latter generally involves a single vessel, the superior mesenteric artery, and its dramatic presentation and often devastating clinical course are thought to be attributable to the lack of opportunity to develop robust collaterals in the absence of chronic ischemic pressures.

EPIDEMIOLOGY

Patients treated with revascularization for CMI in a review of National Inpatient Sample (NIS) data were, on average, 65.5 years old and predominantly female (76.2%) and Caucasian (90.7%).[1] Nonatherosclerotic etiologies account for a much smaller (10%) proportion of patients presenting with CMI. This population is typically younger with gender ratios reflective of underlying associated conditions such as vasculitis.[2]

Acute mesenteric ischemia may arise in the setting of either in situ thrombosis of preexisting CMI or acute occlusion by emboli of cardiac or aortic origin. A recent review of American College of Surgeons National Surgical Quality Improvement Program (ACS-NSQIP) data found that the average age of revascularized AMI patients was 66.4 years. 54 percent were female and 84% Caucasian. In this sample, patients were evenly divided between thrombotic (acute-on-chronic) and embolic etiologies.[3] The distribution of these underlying etiologies does not appear to have changed significantly over the past two decades.[4]

Unsurprisingly, in a systematic review of the literature, associated factors included tobacco use (30–88%), hypertension (28–56%), chronic renal insufficiency (4–25%) and diabetes mellitus (2–12%) and other atherosclerotic disease was commonly present. In the series reviewed, 34–58% of patients had concurrent coronary artery disease, 20–73% peripheral arterial disease, and 11–50% cerebrovascular disease.[5]

CLINICAL PRESENTATION

Virtually all patients treated for CMI relate a history of abdominal pain, which is often described as cramping in nature and located in the epigastrium or midabdomen. A significant proportion describe the classic symptoms of postprandial pain, with onset 30–60 minutes following a meal, followed by gradual resolution. This is frequently accompanied by significant involuntary weight loss and deliberate avoidance of foods associated with these symptoms or of normal meals, entirely. Less commonly, patients may describe persistent diarrhea, constipation, nausea, or vomiting.[5] Endoscopy, while typically nondiagnostic, may in some cases demonstrate ischemic ulceration of the stomach or colon or atrophic mucosal changes.

While the hallmark of AMI is sudden onset of severe abdominal pain, up to two thirds of these patients have underlying chronic mesenteric atherosclerotic disease and more than half may give a history of CMI symptoms. In one large series, the mean duration of these symptoms was 5.5 months prior to presentation with AMI.[4] (Ryer) In patients with the embolic form of AMI, a history of atrial fibrillation is common (43–50%) and may suggest the diagnosis.[4,6]

DIAGNOSIS

Though the clinical presentation and history may suggest a diagnosis of chronic or acute mesenteric ischemia, diagnostic imaging is generally essential to confirm the diagnosis and plan appropriate treatment.

Duplex ultrasound provides a rapid, noninvasive screening tool that is both sensitive and specific for hemodynamically significant stenosis of the mesenteric arteries. Moneta et al. have established a widely used set of velocity criteria for findings predictive of greater than 70% stenosis of the mesenteric vessels, including a peak systolic velocity of greater than 275 cm/sec in the SMA and 200 cm/sec in the celiac artery. Other characteristics such as elevated end-diastolic flow velocity in the SMA and flow reversal in the celiac collaterals suggestive of retrograde filling are also consistent with hemodynamically significant stenosis.[7]

True anatomic imaging is crucial prior to surgical intervention to establish the etiology and anatomic extent of disease. Both CT and MR angiographic imaging permit three-dimensional reconstruction. CT angiography permits accurate assessment of anatomy, lesion extent, calcification, and vessel caliber. Exceptionally high resolution images may be acquired on contemporary 32- or 64-channel multidetector CT scanners within a matter of seconds, rendering this a favored diagnostic modality. Renal insufficiency may limit the administration of both the iodinated contrast required for CTA and, since the reporting of several cases of nephrogenic systemic fibrosis, gadolinium used for MR angiography.

Contrast arteriography can provide additional diagnostic information about patency when vessels are so heavily calcified as to compromise CT assessment of the lumen. It also provides information about physiological characteristics such as the speed and direction of flow. Typically, anteroposterior and lateral views are obtained, with the latter acquired in both inspiratory and expiratory phases. If intervention is anticipated, thought should be given to whether brachial or femoral access is preferable to provide optimal vessel access and system "pushability." In cases of renal insufficiency, it may be possible to substitute CO_2 in part or in total for iodinated contrast, although image quality is typically compromised.

SURGICAL TECHNIQUES

Supraceliac Graft Reconstruction

An upper midline incision carried as far cephalad as possible along the course of the xyphoid is made. Distally, the incision is made down to, or slightly past, the umbilicus. A nasogastric tube should be in place so that the esophagus is easily palpable. The left lobe of the liver is mobilized by division of the triangular ligament. Care is taken not to injure the hepatic veins. The lesser omentum is entered. The liver is folded on itself; padded retraction is used to retract the liver to the patient's right and the esophagus to the left.

The exposed diaphragmatic fibers and crura are incised on the anterior surface of the aorta, and carried circumferentially about the celiac artery and the origins of the common hepatic and splenic arteries. The lateral surfaces of the aorta are dissected sufficient to allow secure and comfortable clamp placement. The phrenic arteries are usually encountered and are divided and ligated during this exposure. We usually divide and ligate the left gastric artery also, as it is most commonly very small. This latter maneuver facilitates creation of the retropancreatic tunnel for the limb to the superior mesenteric artery (SMA).

If the SMA lesion is very proximal and localized, the recipient site on the SMA may be dissected free here. Incision of the areolar tissue on the upper border of the pancreas coupled with gentle caudad retraction of the pancreas will allow for exposure and reconstruction at this site. More usually, however, the SMA lesion is extensive and exposure of the SMA in an infracolic location is required. The usual infracolic approach is used. The ligament of Treitz is incised and the SMA is palpated and exposed distal to the atherosclerotic lesion. Care is taken to avoid injury to posterior branches of the artery or to the surrounding small veins. Repair of such injuries may be time consuming.

A retropancreatic tunnel is created bluntly with the fingers. Proximally, the blunt dissention is started in the space created by division of the left gastric artery. The finger is passed to the left side of the aorta behind the pancreas. Distally, the tunnel should end just to the left of the SMA, allowing the graft to be in the correct plane with the recipient portion of the SMA. A rubber tubing or umbilical tape is placed in the tunnel.

The patient is heparinized. In addition, Lasix and mannitol are given. It is our preference also to give fenoldopam or low dose dopamine. Control is obtained of the supraceliac aorta with a stout, angled clamp such as a Supraceliac Clamp (Figure 28-1) which allows posterior angulation of the clamp to occlude intercostal or lumbar arteries, and also keeps the clamp handles out of the surgeon's way. Distally, a Hypogastric Clamp (Figure 28-2) is placed, its angulation allowing clamping of the lumbar vessels posteriorly. The tips of the clamp are in close apposition, thereby preventing annoying back bleeding. (Figure 28-3) We prefer aortic cross clamping as opposed to partial clamping, as the former provides excellent anterior aortic access, allowing creation of a secure and comfortable anastomosis, especially at the two apices of the suture line. Aortic ischemia time should be between 10 and 15 minutes, and certainly less than 20 minutes.

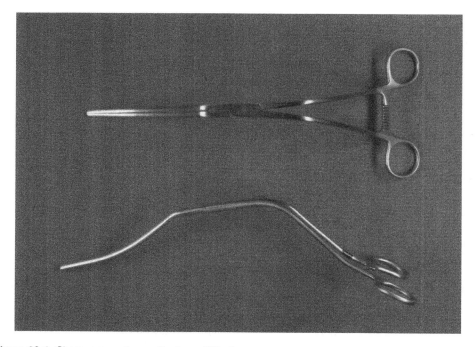

Figure 28-1. Cherry supraceliac aortic clamp (Pilling)

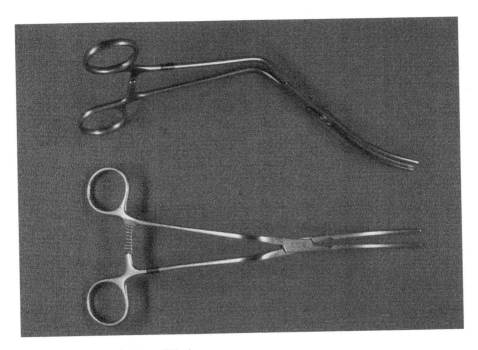

Figure 28-2. Wylie hypogastric clamp (Pilling)

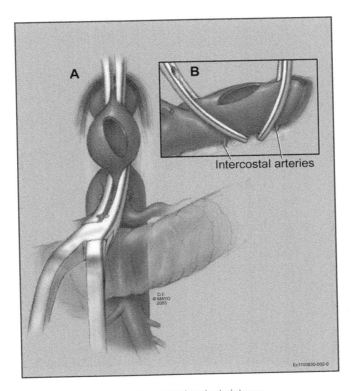

Figure 28-3. Two clamp technique for supraceliac control and arteriotomy.

The aortotomy is made on an oblique angle, from 11 o'clock to 5 o'clock, rather than vertically. Usually, a 12 × 7 knitted Polyester graft is chosen, fashioned to fit, and sutured end-to-side with 4-0 or 5-0 permanent suture is used. The upper limb at 11 o'clock will go to the celiac artery, and the lower, at 5 o'clock, to the SMA. This orientation allows for reduced protrusion of the graft trunk into the lesser sac and a pleasing course for both the celiac artery and the SMA limbs, without kinking.

The celiac artery anastomosis may be end-to-end or end-to-side, depending on anatomic features and the extent of the lesion. The arteriotomy is usually extended along the axis of the common hepatic artery, or indeed may be to either of the two major branch arteries of the celiac. 4-0 permanent suture is used. After appropriate forward and back bleeding, flow is established to the celiac artery. If necessary, the native celiac artery stump is oversewn.

The limb to the SMA is brought through the retropancreatic tunnel. Control is obtained of the SMA, and a vertical arteriotomy made. This anastomosis is most commonly done in an end-to-side manner with 5-0 or 6-0 permanent suture. (Figure 28-4) Flow is established after appropriate bleeding and irrigation of the graft. The lesser sac is closed and the mesentery overlying the distal SMA graft reapproximated. The abdomen is closed in standard manner.

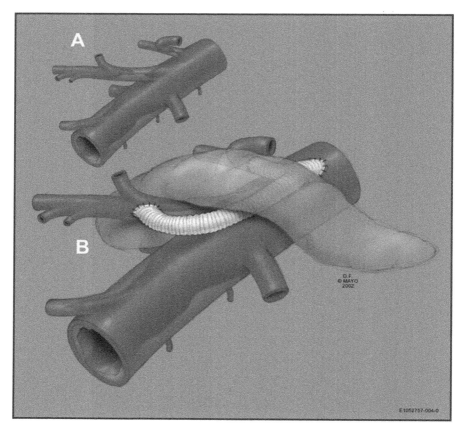

Figure 28-4. Anatomic representation of antegrade bifurcated reconstruction of the celiac and superior mesenteric arteries. Note retropancreatic course of superior mesenteric artery graft.

Infrarenal Graft Reconstruction

Although both the celiac artery and the SMA may be reconstructed from an infrarenal route, it is our practice to reconstruct the SMA only. Patency has been shown to be very good to excellent. It is preferable to originate these grafts from the common iliac arteries rather than the infrarenal aorta. These iliac-origin grafts assume a more pleasing conformation, lying in the same axial (vertical) plane as the aorta, rather than in a plane perpendicular to the aorta, as is seen with grafts arising from the infrarenal aorta itself. (Figures 28-5, 28-6) That perpendicular orientation, coupled with the return of the viscera to their anatomic position following reconstruction, make these aortic-origin grafts prone to kinking.

The SMA is exposed in an infracolic location by division of the Ligament of Treitz as described above. The chosen common iliac artery is exposed in standard manner.

The patient is heparinized. We perform the SMA anastomosis first. A 7- or 8-mm knitted polyester or ringed PTFE graft is used. In the face of infection, saphenous vein may be used. Anecdotally, its patency is quite good when used in this ilio-SMA location. The heel of the graft may be at the proximal or distal end of the vertical SMA arteriotomy, depending on the patient's anatomy, the site of the arteriotomy, and the surgeon's judgment of the conformation of the graft in the closed abdomen. The heel is usually at the distal end of the arteriotomy as one would generally anticipate.

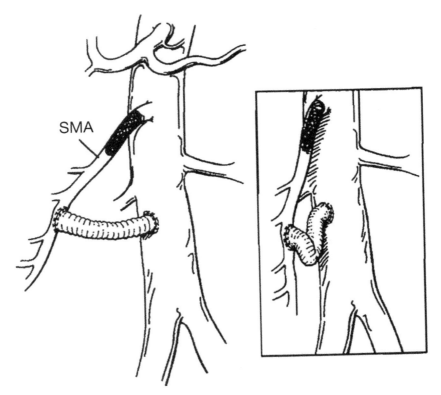

Figure 28-5. Retrograde graft from the distal aorta to superior mesenteric artery demonstrates a tendency to kink when the mesentery is returned to normal anatomic position.

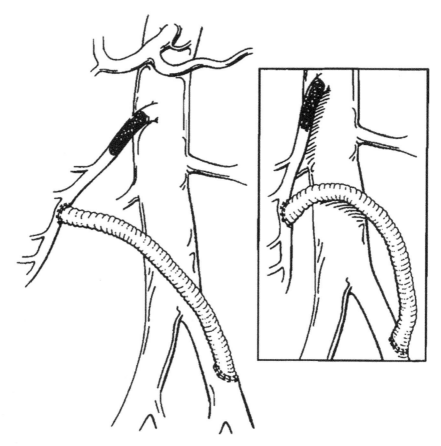

Figure 28-6. C-configured retrograde graft from the common iliac artery to the superior mesenteric artery is more resistant to kink formation with a range of positioning.

When perfoming the iliac artery anastomosis, we relax the retraction as much as possible to permit the graft to approximate the anatomic position anticipated for it in the closed abdomen, without undue length. This anastomosis is usually performed with running 4-0 or 5-0 permanent suture in an end-to-side manner. Appropriate forward and back bleeding is permitted, and flow established to the SMA. (Figure 28-7)

The mesentery and the retroperitoneum are closed over the graft. If necessary in these very thin patients, an omental flap is placed to exclude the graft from the gastrointestinal tract. Closure is performed in standard manner.

Transaortic Visceral Endarterectomy

Endarterectomy of the mesenteric arteries (and the renal arteries if necessary) may be indicated if the patient has extensive and/or densely calcific atherosclerosis of the abdominal aorta precluding either supraceliac or infrarenal reconstruction. It may also be chosen in the face of gross contamination to avoid synthetic graft placement. Done electively, transaortic visceral endarterectomy may be combined with infrarenal aortic graft reconstruction.

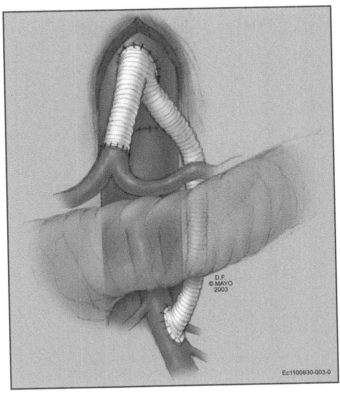

Figure 28-7. Completed antegrade bifurcated reconstruction of the celiac and superior mesenteric arteries. Note slightly oblique orientation of limbs, which minimizes kinking of the graft.

Either a low-lying thoraco-retroperitoneal incision or a midline incision with medial visceral rotation may be employed. The distal thoracic aorta is dissected free as are the visceral vessels. The left kidney is left in its bed, to allow full exposure of the SMA as far along its course as necessary. The infrarenal aorta is dissected free.

The patient is given heparin, Lasix and mannitol. Again, it is our preference to give fenoldopam or low-dose dopamine prior to clamp placement. Control is obtained of the thoracic and abdominal aorta. A trap door aortic incision, or a lateral vertical aortotomy, is made, based on the pattern of atherosclerosis and the particular goals of the operation. This incision is angled between the SMA and the left renal artery. The endarterectomy is begun in the proximal aorta in the correct plane and extended into the involved visceral vessels. (Figure 28-8) The lesion in the celiac artery most frequently ends at the major bifurcation of that artery. The lesion in the SMA may, and usually does, extend for several inches. In that case, the endarterectomy of the SMA is carried out for an inch or so, and the plaque transected and removed. (Figure 28-9) This will permit safe clamping of the SMA origin subsequently. The distal infrarenal aortic site is tacked down if necessary, or readied for infrarenal grafting if that is planned. The aortotomy is closed with running 4-0 permanent suture. (Figure 28-10) Just prior to completion, appropriate forward and back bleeding is allowed and flow restored sequentially to the visceral arteries and the lower extremities.

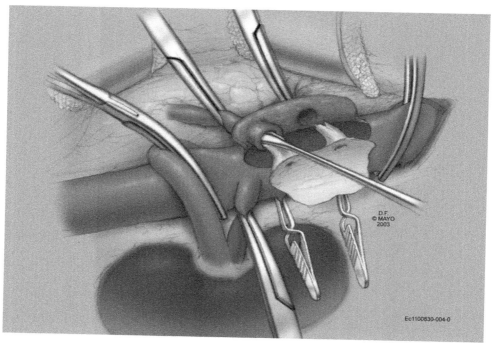

Figure 28-8. "Trapdoor" incision permits endarterectomy of the celiac and superior mesenteric arteries. This may be oriented more posteriorly to permit treatment of the renal arteries, if necessary.

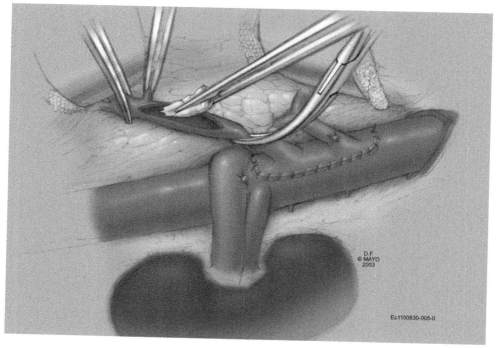

Figure 28-9. A longitudinal counterincision on the superior mesenteric artery permits extended endarterectomy, if necessary.

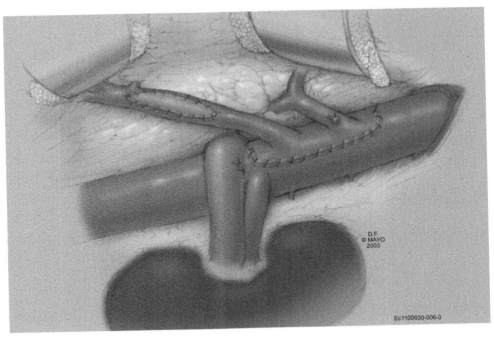

Figure 28-10. Completed transaortic endarterectomy of the celiac and superior mesenteric arteries. Note patch closure of superior mesenteric artery counterincision.

A clamp is placed across the origin of the SMA where it has undergone endarterectomy. A completion endarterectomy of the SMA is performed, through either a horizontal or vertical incision dependent on the pattern of disease. This is done without the burden of prolonged aortic, celiac, and renal artery ischemia time. The incision is closed in an appropriate manner for the arteriotomy employed. A longitudinal incision may require patch repair, while primary closure is generally appropriate for a transverse arteriotomy.

Surgical Embolectomy

A midline laparotomy is performed. The transverse colon is retracted cephalad and the small intestine to the patient's right side, as for infrarenal aortic exposure. The proximal SMA is located at the root of the mesentery. The proximal SMA is circumferentially dissected with great care taken to preserve the accompanying vein and small proximal SMA branches. Systemic heparin is administered. The SMA may be controlled proximally and distally with silastic loops or vascular clamps. If a purely embolic phenomenon is suspected, a transverse arteriotomy may be performed and a 3 French Fogarty balloon catheter passed proximally to ensure brisk inflow and then distally. Great care must be taken not to overinflate the balloon or otherwise traumatize the distal SMA, which may be prone to dissection. The arteriotomy may then be closed with interrupted 6-0 permanent sutures.

If there is any suspicion of coexistent occlusive disease or of embolic debris extending into branch arteries, a longitudinal arteriotomy is preferred, as this facilitates thromboendarterectomy, described above, or retrieval of embolus from these secondary vessels. The longitudinal incision may be closed using an appropriate patch fashioned of saphenous vein or bovine pericardium.

Other Approaches

Exotic sources of inflow such as the axillary artery and the ascending aorta have been described recently.[8,9] The hybrid approach of laparotomy with retrograde placement of mesenteric stents has been most thoroughly reported by the Dartmouth group.[10] This approach appears to hold significant promise, particularly in the acute setting, where laparotomy is obligatory and the retrograde access facilitates rapid crossing of often difficult flush SMA occlusions. In at least one instance, the authors have combined endovascular stent placement with a limited retrograde endarterectomy to address a densely calcified flush occlusion of the proximal SMA.

OUTCOMES

Review of recent series of open interventions for chronic mesenteric ischemia suggests that revascularization of these patients may be accomplished with relatively low morbidity and mortality and with durable results. (Table 28-1) Several groups report early mortality rates of only 2–3 percent.[11,12,13] In these series, bypass, either antegrade or retrograde, was the primary method of revascularization for CMI. However, Mell et al. reported excellent results in a series of 80 patients, more than half of whom were treated with endarterectomy, either alone or in combination. Early mortality in this report was 3.8% with complication and 5 year survival rates comparable to other large contemporary series.[14]

Some investigators relied on clinical assessments of patency, but where consistently evaluated with imaging, primary patency rates of 80–90 percent at a year were widely reported, with 5 year rates ranging from 59 to over 90 percent.[11,12,13,15,16] A multicenter comparison of clinical outcomes following antegrade and retrograde grafts for CMI suggested similarly excellent symptom-free survival at one year (95.2% vs 88.2%).[17]

Data regarding outcomes following open surgical treatment of acute mesenteric ischemia reflect the fact that the two leading etiologies, embolic and thrombotic disease, suggest different underlying disease processes as well as different surgical approaches. The mortality rate of patients presenting with embolic disease likely reflects, in part, the comorbidities of this population, which consistently demonstrates a higher prevalence of cardiac disease, atrial fibrillation, and CHF than those presenting with thrombosis.[18,19] Early mortality for all etiologies ranges from 22–47% in recent large series and exceeds 90% in many historical reports.[18] (Table 28-2) Data are mixed with regard to whether embolic or thrombotic AMI is associated with a higher mortality rate.[4,18,19] However, mortality is consistently associated with advanced age, need for bowel resection, delay in diagnosis, and severity of presentation.[4,18,19,20]

It appears that mortality rates following revascularization for both AMI and CMI have trended down over the past several decades. Schermerhorn et al. reviewed data from the National Inpatient Sample (NIS) from 1988–2006 and found that the post-revascularization mortality rate decreased from 15% to 8% in CMI and 49% to 30% in AMI before and after 2000, respectively.[19] While this trend may be attributable to factors ranging from a growing surgical experience to improved perioperative care, it has also been noted that the prevalence of endovascular therapies has increased over this time period, surpassing that of open surgery in both this series and the Mayo Clinic

TABLE 28-1 OUTCOMES FOLLOWING OPEN RECONSTRUCTION FOR CHRONIC MESENTERIC ISCHEMIA

Author (Year)	# Patients/vessels	# Vessels involved	Type of repair	Early mortality	5 year survival	Morbidity	Recurrent symptoms	Patency	Followup
Oderich (2009)[11]	146/265	1v 3 (2%) 2v 63 (43%) 3v 80 (55%)	Bypass 136 (93%) Endarterectomy 10 (7%)	2.7%	72 ± 5%	36%	8 (6%)	1° 88 ± 2 2° 97 ± 2 (5 years)	36 mos (4-179)
Mell (2008)[14]	80/134	1v 8 (10%) 2v 29 (36%) 3v 43 (54%)	Bypass 29 (36%) Endarterectomy 37 (46%) Combined 14 (18%)	3.8%	64.5%	26.3%	9 (11%)	NR	46 mos (1-206)
Kruger (2007)[22]	39/67	1v 7 (18%) 2v 9 (22%) 3v 24 (59%)	Bypass 39 (100%)	2.5%	75%	12%	2 (5%)	1° 92.4% (5 years)	39 mos (4-161)
Biebl (2007)[23]	26/NR	1v 0 (0%) 2v 8 (31%) 3v 18 (69%)	Bypass 22 (85%) Endarterectomy 4 (15%)	13%	NR	42%	11% mild-moderate	NR	25 mos
Atkins (2007)[13]	49/88	1v 2 (4%) 2v 19 (39%) 3v 28 (57%)	Bypass 31 (63%) Endarterectomy 7 (14%) Patch 4 (8%)	2%	65%	39%	11 (22%)	1° 90% ± 4 (1 year) 2° 87% =/-5 (2 years)	15 mos (0-32)
Park (2002)[24]	98/179	NR	Bypass 79 (81%) Endarterectomy 5 (5%) Reimplantation 1 (1%) Patch angioplasty 1 (1%) Combination 12 (12%)	5.1%	62%	21.4%	6 (6%)	NR	1.9 yrs (0-9.6)
Jiminez (2002)[15]	47/100	1v 1 (2%) 2v 10 (21%) 3v 36 (77%)	Bypass 47 (100%)	10.6%	74%	66%	3 (6%)	1° 69% ± 17 2° 100%	31 mos (1-119)
Kansal (2002)[17]	37/60	NR	Bypass Antegrade 21 (54%) Retrograde 18 (46%)	8%	72.2% (4 yr)	84%	NR	NR	25 mos (0-95)
Cho (2002)[16]	25/41	1v 0 (0%) 2v 5 (20%) 3v 20 (80%)	Bypass 24 (59%) Endarterectomy Local 7 (17%) Transaortic 10 (24%)	4%	77%	NR	NR	1° 59% (5 years)	5.3 yrs (30d-36.3 yrs)
Kasirajan (2001)[25]	85/130	1v 4 (5%) 2v 32 (38%) 3v 49 (58%)	Bypass 60 (71%) Endarterectomy 19 (22%) Patch angioplasty 6 (7%)	8.2%	64%	32.9%	10 (13%)	NR	5 yrs

* included 10% treated for acute presentation

TABLE 28-2. OUTCOMES FOLLOWING OPEN SURGICAL TREATMENT FOR ACUTE MESENTERIC ISCHEMIA

Author (Year)	# Patients	Etiology	Revascularization method	Bypass conduit	Bowel resection	Second look	Resection at second look	Morbidity	Early mortality	Survival	Followup
Ryer (2012)[26]	82	Thrombosis 49 Embolus 29 Dissection 2	Bypass 39 Antegrade 20 Retrograde 19 Embolectomy 37 Endarterectomy 6	Prosthetic 33 Vein 6	33 (40%)	42 (51%)	20 (48%)	68%	22%	53.7% 1 yr	2.6 =/- 3.4 yrs
Newton (2011)[3]	142	Thrombosis 71 Embolus 71	Bypass 55 Embolectomy 71 Endarterectomy 16	Prosthetic 38 Vein 17	48 (34%)	NR	NR	69%	30%	NR	NR
Kougias (2007)[6]	72	Thrombosis 48 Embolus 24	Bypass 33 (46%) Embolectomy 22 (31%) Patch angioplasty 9 (12%) Reimplantation 5 (7%) Endartectomy 3 (4%)	Prosthetic 11 Vein 22	22 (31%)	38 (53%)	15 (39%)	39%	31%	58% 5 yrs 28% 10 yrs	NR
Edwards (2003)[20]	76	Thrombosis 44 Embolism 32	Bypass 16 Embolectomy 18 Patch angioplasty 3 Endarterectomy 2 Other/Combination 4	Prosthetic 9 Vein 7	28*	34 (44%)	17 (50%)	55%	47%	18% 5 yrs	NR
Endean (2001)[18]											

* Of 43 patients revascularized. Of the total study group, 16 received exploration alone and 18 bowel resection alone.

series in 2002.[19,21] The review of NIS data did carefully compare the characteristics of patients treated with open versus endovascular therapy between 2000 and 2006 and noted decreased mortality in both CMI and AMI groups treated with angioplasty with or without stenting.[19] Commentary on this study has noted that not all lesions are amenable to endovascular therapy, that lesions not suitable for this approach may require more complex revascularization, and that the endovascular treatment population in this study required fewer bowel resections, perhaps suggesting a subacute or overall milder manifestation of disease.[4]

DISCUSSION

Ample data demonstrate that with careful technique and excellent perioperative management, chronic mesenteric arterial occlusive disease may be surgically reconstructed with excellent results. The current era brings both beneficial advances in critical care and endovascular technique and persistent concern over the diminished exposure of trainees to complex open reconstructions. Schermerhorn et al. have reviewed nearly 20 years of NIS data and found that, although the number and proportion of cases treated with endovascular means has increased over time, the number of patients requiring open surgery for CMI has remained relatively stable. Occluded stents and other failures of prior endovascular and open therapy will also continue to require surgical reconstruction.

The importance of identifying and addressing chronic mesenteric ischemia prior to an acute presentation cannot be overemphasized. Between 40–54% of patients with AMI attributed to mesenteric thrombosis give a history of prior CMI symptoms.[4,6] Crucially, the early mortality rate increases radically, from 2–13% in the chronic stage of disease to 62%–70% when the patient progresses to an acute presentation, suggesting that the critical opportunity for intervention is prior to this transition.[18,20]

While endovascular therapy for acute mesenteric ischemia may confer some benefit, where the underlying lesion is amenable, the authors maintain that laparotomy is virtually mandatory and that a second look operation 24–48 hours later should be considered similarly mandatory where any bowel initially appeared to be at risk. One need look no farther than the fact that approximately half of the second look operations in the reviewed series resulted in initial or additional resection of intestine to justify an aggressive approach in this regard.[4,6,20] Furthermore, the presence or possibility of threatened bowel and abdominal contamination significantly complicates reconstruction, as it necessitates the avoidance, if possible, of synthetic graft. Endarterectomy in this territory is infrequently performed and poses a significant challenge for most operators. Autologous grafts are more prone to technical issues related to graft length and configuration in the retrograde position and to long term patency issues. Endovascular techniques and innovative hybrid approaches such as retrograde endarterectomy and stent placement may ameliorate some of these concerns, but do not eliminate the mortality differential between chronic mesenteric occlusive disease treated in the chronic and acute settings.[19]

REFERENCES

1. Derrow AE, Seeger JM, Dame DA, et al. The outcome in the United States after thoracoabdominal aortic aneurysm repair, renal artery bypass, and mesenteric revascularization. *J Vasc Surg*. 2001;34:54–61.
2. Oderich GS. Current concepts in the management of chronic mesenteric ischemia. *Curr Treat Options Cardiovasc Med*. 2010;12:117–130.
3. Newton WB III, Sagransky MJ, Andrews JS, et al. Outcomes of revascularized acute mesenteric ischemia in the American college of surgeons national surgical quality improvement program database. *Am Surg*. 2011;7:832–838.
4. Ryer EJ, Oderich GS, Bower TC, et al. Differences in anatomy and outcomes in patients treated with open mesenteric revascularization before and after the endovascular era. *J Vasc Surg*. 2011;53:1611–1618.
5. Moawad J, Gewertz BL. Chronic mesenteric ischemia: clinical presentation and diagnosis. *Surg Clin N Amer*. 1997;77(2): 357–369.
6. Kougias P, Lau D, El Sayed HF, et al. Determinants of mortality and treatment outcome following surgical interventions for acute mesenteric ischemia. *J Vasc Surg*. 2007;46:467–474.
7. Moneta GL, Lee RW, Yeager RA, et al. Mesenteric duplex scanning: a blinded prospective study. *J Vasc Surg*. 1993;17(1):79–84.
8. Karkos CD, McMahon GS, Markose G, et al. Axillomesenteric bypass: an unusual solution to a difficult problem. *J Vasc Surg*. 2007;45:404–407.
9. Chiche L, Kieffer E. Use of the ascending aorta as bypass inflow for treatment of chronic intestinal ischemia. *J Vasc Surg*. 2005;41:457–461.
10. Wyers MC, Powell RJ, Nolan BW, et al. Retrograde mesenteric stenting during laparotomy for acute occlusive mesenteric ischemia. *J Vasc Surg*. 2007;45:269–275.
11. Oderich GS, Bower TC, Sullivan TM, et al. Open versus endovascular revascularization for chronic mesenteric ischemia: risk-stratified outcomes. *J Vasc Surg*. 2009;49:1472–1479.
12. Kruger AJ, Walker PJ, Foster WJ, et al., Open surgery for atherosclerotic chronic mesenteric ischemia. *J Vasc Surg*. 2007;46:941–945.
13. Atkins MD, Kwolek CJ, LaMuraglia GM, et al. Surgical revascularization versus endovascular therapy for chronic mesenteric ischemia: a comparative experience. *J Vasc Surg*. 2007;45:1162–1171.
14. Mell MW, Acher CW, Hoch JR, et al. Outcomes after endarterectomy for chronic mesenteric ischemia. *J Vasc Surg*. 2008;48:1132–1138.
15. Jiminez JG, Huber TS, Ozaki CK, et al. Durability of antegrade synthetic aortomesenteric bypass for chronic mesenteric ischemia. *J Vasc Surg*. 2002;35:1078–1084.
16. Cho J-S, Carr JA, Jacobsen G, et al. Long-term outcome after mesenteric artery reconstruction: a 37-year experience. *J Vasc Surg*. 2002;35:453–460.
17. Kansal N, LoGerfo FW, Belfield AK, et al. A comparison of antegrade and retrograde mesenteric bypass. *Ann Vasc Surg*. 2002;16:591–596.
18. Endean ED, Barnes SL, Kwolek CJ, et al. Surgical management of thrombotic acute intestinal ischemia. *Ann Surg*. 2001;233(6):801–808.
19. Schermerhorn ML, Giles KA, Hamdan AD, et al. Mesenteric revascularization: management and outcomes in the United States, 1988–2006. *J Vasc Surg*. 2009;50:341–348.
20. Edward MS, Cherr GS, Craven TE, et al. Acute occlusive mesenteric ischemia: surgical management and outcome. *Ann Vasc Surg*. 2003;17:72–79.
21. Oderich GS, Gloviczki P, Bower TC. Open surgical treatment of chronic mesenteric ischemia in the endovascular era: when is it necessary and what is the preferred technique? *Semin Vasc Surg*. 2010;23:36–46.
22. Kruger AJ, Walker PJ, Foster WJ, et al. Open surgery for atherosclerotic chronic mesenteric ischemia. *J Vasc Surg* 2007;46:941–945.

23. Biebl M, Oldenburg WA, Paz-Fumagalli R, et al. Surgical and interventional visceral revascularization for the treatment of chronic mesenteric ischemia—when to prefer which? *World J Surg.* 2007;31:562–568.
24. Park WM, Cherry KJ Jr, Chua HK, et al. Current results of open revascularization for chronic mesenteric ischemia: a standard for comparison. *J Vasc Surg.* 2001;35:853–859.
25. Kasirajan K, O'Hara PJ, Gray BH, et al. Chronic mesenteric ischemia: open surgery versus percutaneous angioplasty and stenting. *J Vasc Surg.* 2001;33:63–71.
26. Ryer EJ, Kalra M, Oderich GS, et al. Revascularization for acute mesenteric ischemia. *J Vasc Surg.* 2012;55:1682–1689.

Contemporary Management of Acute Type B Aortic Dissection

Colin P. Ryan, MS and Timur P. Sarac, MD

BACKGROUND

Aortic dissection is a rare but devastating disease that occurs in 5–10 people per million each year and is the most common life-threatening aortic disease.[1,2] While surgical repair is the standard treatment for acute <u>ascending</u> aortic dissection, treatment of acute <u>descending</u> aortic dissection is a contentious point. Uncomplicated acute Stanford type B dissection (ABAD) has been shown to be manageable with optimal and aggressive anti-hypertensive and anti-impulse therapies as well as vigilant follow-up by the 2009 INSTEAD trial.[3] However, complications related to ABAD occur in 25–50% of patients with a variety of treatments advocated based on presentation status.[4] Complications related to ABAD include intractable pain, refractory hypertension, impending or frank rupture, anterograde or retrograde dissection extension, localized pseudoaneurysm, and malperfusion of aortic branch vessels leading to ischemia.[5] Our focus is on one of the most serious complications of ABAD: malperfusion.

Ischemia caused by acute type B aortic dissection (ABAD) is a life-threatening medical emergency and occurs in approximately 15–42% of all ABAD patients. Malperfusion has been associated with significantly higher morbidity and mortality rates in ABAD patients.[1,6–9] Recently, thoracic endovascular aortic repair (TEVAR) has been utilized in the treatment of ischemia-complicated ABAD (icABAD). This procedure seeks to seal the entry tear, stent open the true lumen, and, if possible, completely occlude the false lumen in a proximal to distal fashion. A growing body of knowledge has advocated TEVAR as the preferred treatment method for emergency ABAD treatment, though no clear consensus has yet been made.[8,10,11]

Data concerning the outcomes of TEVAR for icABAD is limited to small subsets of most study populations or by short-term follow-up.[1,12] Therefore, in addition to providing an overview concerning the clinical features, imaging modalities, and treatment options pertaining to descending aortic dissection, this review focuses on progress made in treating icABAD using endovascular stent grafting.

PATHOPHYSIOLOGY OF DISSECTION-RELATED MALPERFUSION

Aortic dissection, regardless whether in the ascending or descending aorta, begins with a transverse tear in the tunica intima that allows blood to flow between the intimal and adventitial vessel layers. This tear does not normally involve the entire circumference of the aorta but proceeds in a longitudinal and circumferential manner.[13] As both the native aortic lumen and the intima-adventitial space fill, a false lumen is created. Both lumens run parallel to one another. Pulsatile blood flow into this newly formed false lumen primarily causes propagation in a proximal-to-distal fashion. In rare instances however, retrograde extension has been observed.[2] An intimal flap is formed that begins to compress the true lumen of the aorta due to pressure buildup in the false lumen. This compression can cause partial or complete obstruction of the true lumen resulting in distal malperfusion.

Two distinct mechanisms of aortic branch vessel occlusion have been reported. Dynamic obstruction occurs when a proximal entry tear forms without a large distal reentry tear to allow outflow from the false lumen. The resulting intimal flap balloons outward and can compress the true lumen to a point where it either causes a functional collapses the thoracic aorta's true lumen or prolapses into branch vessel ostia.[14] Static obstruction involves extension of the dissection into the branch vessel lumen itself, which thereby compresses the true branch vessel lumen; this can lead to thrombosis of the branch vessel false lumen.[14] Two perfusion patterns complicated by static obstruction have been recognized. First, the dissection extends into a branch vessel with a dominant and patent true lumen with a small false lumen that may or may not be perfused. Second, the dissection may affect the patency of the true lumen in a branch vessel due to false lumen compression with malperfusion as an endpoint. This false lumen may or may not have detectable blood flow.[15]

Blood pressure in the false lumen can rise to a significantly higher level when distal communication with the aortic true lumen is limited. This increase in pressure in combination with stagnant blood that is in contact with thrombogenic adventitial tissue promotes thrombogenesis in the distal false lumen. Presentation with partial false lumen thrombosis is an independent mortality risk factor due to higher diastolic and mean arterial pressure within the false lumen when no distal reentry tear forms.[16]

A combination of dynamic and static obstruction may result in partial or complete avulsion of a branch vessel ostium from the true lumen. When avulsion occurs, the torn flap of the branch vessel true lumen can prolapse into the branch vessel and completely obstruct blood flow. Likewise, a patent false lumen can continue perfusing the branch vessel. Regardless of primary treatment type chosen, ostial avulsion almost always requires branch vessel stenting to the true lumen for reperfusion because of branch vessel intimal flap obstruction.[4]

CLINICAL PRESENTATION OF ICABAD

Distal aortic dissection most often presents in men in their fifth to seventh decade of life who have a history of hypertension and tobacco use.[13,17] Men are more likely to suffer from essential hypertension than women and also comprise a larger percentage of adult smokers in the US.[18,19] Hypertension increases hemodynamic forces that are constantly stressing aortic wall, and this anatomical stress is due to the mobility of the aortic arch versus the immobility of the descending thoracic aorta.[2] Use of stimulants like cocaine, MDMA, and others are associated with an increased risk of dissection. Pregnancy is the greatest risk factor for women under 40 years of age due to the changes in hemodynamics and hormone concentrations during gestation.[20] Additional risk factors include congenital connective tissue disorders such as Marfan, Ehlers-Danlos, and Loeys-Dietz syndromes, a family history of aortic disease, concurrent cardiovascular disease, and a bicuspid aortic valve.[17,21]

Female gender and prior aortic disease have been previously identified as independent predictors of short-term mortality.[7] Women are reported to present at later times following ABAD and be diagnosed at a later time than men due to atypical clinical presentation. Women often do not report abrupt sharp pain instead experiencing gradual onset of pain. This also delays IV beta-blocker infusion, as it takes longer to diagnose without typical clinical symptoms. When malperfusion and ischemia are involved, this increase in time correlates to an increase in short-term mortality. Women are also more likely to be hypertensive and suffer ABAD at an older age.[22] Indeed, in recent publication from the Cleveland Clinic, female gender had a significant association with increased 30-day mortality (Men HR: 0.42; CI [0.18–0.96]; p = 0.04).[23]

ABAD patients report a ripping or tearing pain in the back or abdomen in up to 92% of patients reporting pain as severe or their worst ever.[8] However, 4.5–7% of patients report no pain at all.[13,21] Mesenteric ischemia should be definitively considered when abdominal pain is reported because mesenteric reperfusion prior to central aortic repair is very important for reducing early mortality.[24] Refractory pain following optimization of blood pressure, while long considered a complication warranting further intervention, commonly can safely be treated with conservative therapy in the absence of clinical or radiographic signs of worsening symptoms; however, there is still controversy as to whether this group represents a subcategory at high risk for further complications.[25]

Hemodynamic abnormalities are another clinical sign of ABAD. Hypertension is present in 50–82% of patients.[7] Many ABAD patients present with blood pressures indicative of hypertensive crises, and systolic blood pressures as high as 250 mmHg were observed in the Cleveland Clinic series.[23] In an attempt to overcome true lumen compression, a massive catecholamine release drives blood pressure to very high levels. Additionally, renal malperfusion stimulates renin release, increasing blood pressure even further. While hypotension and shock have been associated with high risk of early death, ABAD rarely presents with these symptoms.[13] Fifty-seven of the 61 patients (93.4%) in the Cleveland Clinic cohort had a history of hypertension prior to dissection, reemphasizing the association of high blood pressure and dissection.[23]

Malperfusion-specific clinical signs and symptoms should be examined at initial presentation and again following blood pressure optimization. Lower extremity ischemia may present with a variety of symptoms including ischemic rest pain, off-pallor, paresthesia not associated with a neurological source, and pulse deficits. Malperfusion of intercostal vessels or collateral vessels of the left subclavian artery (LSA) may lead to spinal cord ischemia that present as paraparesis or paraplegia. Rising creatinine levels and oliguria following medical optimization both suggest renal ischemia. Absence of bowel sounds, an acute abdomen, and rising lactate levels are all signals of mesenteric ischemia.[1] Renal and mesenteric ischemic complications have been associated with high perioperative morbidity and mortality in the greater context of all ABAD patients[26], though we recently reported a large cohort of cases complicated by malperfusion, and did not identify one specific type of ischemia as a predictor of early death.[23]

ABAD is diagnosed properly in a variable range of 15–43% of patients, mainly due to the low prevalence of aortic dissection in patients presenting with chest or back pain. Molecular blood assays have been proposed for diagnosing aortic dissection. Both smooth muscle myosin and plasma D-dimer assays have been studied as inexpensive and rapid tests that have high specificity and sensitivity for judging a patient's dissection status.[21] Further adoption of these tests could help to decrease missed ABAD diagnoses by emergency room physicians, but until such time as they are substantiated, imaging studies will remain the standard for confirming or ruling out aortic dissection.

IMAGING TECHNIQUES FOR TEVAR TREATMENT OF ICABAD

Understanding the extent of dissection propagation and locating the site of the primary entry tear are two of the main goals for deciding a patient's clinical course. Two classification systems have been devised for differentiating between ascending aortic arch and descending aortic dissections. Michael DeBakey, M.D. was the first to organize a dissection classification system in 1965.[27] This system classified dissections into three types: Type I has a primary entry tear in the ascending aortic arch with propagation through both the arch and distal thoracic aorta, type II dissection has a primary entry tear in the ascending aorta but is confined to Criado zones 0 and 1, and type III dissection places the primary entry tear in the distal aorta. Type III dissections were further broken down into type IIIa dissection and type IIIb dissections by Larson and Edwards.[28] Type IIIa are those with a primary entry tear distal to the LSA with both proximal and distal propagation. Type IIIb dissections also have the primary entry tear at a site distal to the LSA but only have distal propagation and may involve the abdominal aorta.

Stanford classification of dissection was proposed in 1970 by Daily et al and simplified dissections into type A and type B. Type A dissections include Debakey types I and II and can include Debakey type III when retrograde dissection beyond the LSA occurs. Type B dissections involve Criado zones 2, 3, and 4 in the descending aortic arch and aorta without dissection propagation beyond the LSA.[29]

The imaging standard for suspected aortic dissection is thin-cut computed tomography angiography (CTA) from the neck to femoral heads. This scan allows for a rapid assessment of patient status, though advanced TEE or arterial-weighted magnetic resonance angiography (MRA) are alternative modalities.[20] Multiplanar 3D reconstruction is critical for sizing and understanding the optimal deployment angle for endovascular stent graft placement as well as determining the degree of atherosclerosis to assess embolism risk.[5] Chest radiography is rarely used as a diagnostic method for dissection as mediastinal widening is routinely the only visible abnormality occurring in 45–90% of patients.[8,21]

Regardless of which treatment method is utilized, proximal landing zone assessment and access determination must be established. Adequate proximal landing zone varies by stent design, but a diameter ≥20mm but ≤40 mm is recommended due to currently available devices, with a proximal landing length of ≥20 mm.[5,30] Coverage of the left subclavian artery is the primary concern for icABAD as this requires CTA or MRA scanning of the head to check for non-dominant left vertebral artery and a patent Circle of Willis.[5] Revascularization by extra-anatomic subclavian artery bypass is a topic of debate, particularly in the case of patient extremis. Intentional occlusion of the LSA to create an appropriate proximal landing zone is well tolerated in most cases. However, excessive manipulation of endovascular implements such as guidewires, catheters, and grafts at or proximal to the level of the LSA has been associated with stroke due to emboli. Two of 3 patients who suffered stroke in the CCF cohort had complete occlusion of the LSA, which gives us reason to recommend a minimalistic approach to endovascular manipulations within the descending aortic arch.[23]

Imaging is vital for assessing percutaneous access vessels to be used in endovascular interventions. Tortuosity, atherosclerotic and calcified buildup, and access vessel caliber all need to be examined. Most surgeons recommend using the access vessel with larger caliber and less atherosclerosis and tortuosity as the primary access vessel.[5] Iliac conduits may be used for highly tortuous and plaque-laden or small caliber arteries that are not amenable to use of a TEVAR delivery system.[2] Proper identification of challenging access vessels can dictate the proper access method for endovascular therapy and prevent complications such as femoral and iliac dissection or pseudoaneurysm.

Assessment for spinal protective measures completes the gamut of preoperative assessment required to submit a patient to TEVAR for icABAD. If time and clinical circumstances are favorable, we recommend spinal cord drainage.

TREATMENT METHODS FOR ABAD-INDUCED MALPERFUSION

Medical Management

Aggressive antihypertensive and anti-impulse therapy should be administered when ABAD is suspected. Medical management for aortic dissection aims to reduce the mobility of the intimal flap and decrease false lumen pressure to relieve dynamic obstruction of the true lumen. A target heart rate of less than 60 BPM, a systolic blood pressure less than 100–120 mmHg, and/ a mean arterial pressure of less than 60–70 mmHg should be the clinical goals of medical therapy, and unlike the management of most hypertensive crises, the blood pressure needs to be lowered as quickly as possible.[17,31] Beta-adrenergic blockers should be the first-line therapies for ABAD hypertensive crises with esmolol as the recommended agent.[31,32] Sodium nitroprusside or hydralazine can be used to rapidly lower blood pressure so long as beta-blockers are first administered to prevent aortic pulse wave increase caused by baroreceptor stimulation.[32] For patients suffering from heart failure, calcium channel blockers can be used alternatively to prevent exacerbation of this comorbidity. Combining beta blockers with hydralazine or nitroprusside is almost always effective for establishing blood pressure control, reducing shear forces on the aortic wall, and decreasing the impulse force of pulsatile blood flow.[33] Additionally, angiotensin-converting enzyme (ACE) inhibitors can be useful for countering the effects of renin secreted by the kidneys in response to malperfusion. All patients presenting to our institution are treated with some combination of the above-listed therapies to achieve the described goals. The need for large doses of antihypertensive and anti-impulse medications is an independent sign of possible true lumen collapse caused by an overwhelming dynamic obstruction,[17] and this should warrant evaluation for endovascular treatment to avoid complications.

While the majority of ABAD patients are treated and discharged following medical optimization, those showing clinical signs or laboratory values consistent with complications require further intervention. Treatment modalities for complicated ABAD differ based on time to presentation. Acute and chronic dissection are described throughout the literature with 14 days after the initial event set as the determining factor for one classification or the other. Though this is an arbitrary determination, important implications for treatment and outcomes exist between the two groups.[2]

Open Surgical Aortic Graft Replacement

Treatment options for ischemia-complicated ABAD (icABAD) are numerous and include open surgical aortic graft replacement, thoracic endovascular aortic repair (TEVAR) with endovascular stent-grafting, open or endovascular fenestration of the intimal flap, or extra-anatomic surgical bypass.[34,35] Surgical graft repair was previously the standard treatment for icABAD. A recent large series presented results of open surgical treatment without cardiopulmonary bypass in the majority of patients via a left posterolateral thoracotomy. Their only reported indications were rupture or emergent rupture. Impending rupture characteristics were defined as aortic diameter ≥5 cm, hemorrhagic pleural effusion, acute dissection in a previously aneurysmal descending aorta, and unrelenting pain despite medical optimization. In-hospital mortality was 22.4% with cardiac dysrhythmia, renal failure, and left vocal cord paralysis as the tope 3 reported complications.[36]

Open surgical graft repair in emergent cases has been associated with high morbidity and mortality.[1,37] Perioperative mortality rates range from 22.4% for the above-reported cohort[36] to 29% in the most recent analysis of the International Registry of Aortic Dissection (IRAD).[38] For cases complicated by ischemia, the surgical mortality rate exceeds 50%[39] with a perioperative mortality rate for cases complicated by mesenteric ischemia being reported at 88%.[22] Furthermore, serious complications have been reported to occur in up to 78% of patients undergoing open surgical repair.[40] Because patients are usually elderly and present in serious condition, the physical trauma of such extensive surgery has lead to the search for alternative less invasive therapies. Finally, central aortic grafting may not alleviate distal malperfusion due to dynamic vs. static obstruction, dissection complexity, and lack of false lumen flow obliteration.[13] Better treatment options for these patients have been proposed to achieve more favorable morbidity and mortality rates.

Endovascular Fenestration

Endovascular fenestration is one proposed treatment method for icABAD caused by dynamic obstruction. This procedure is performed either with a balloon or via a 'percutaneous scissor' technique and aims to relieve malperfusion caused by dynamic obstruction. For both surgical procedures, access to bilateral femoral arteries and also the left brachial artery is obtained. Balloon fenestration is carried out by first puncturing the intimal flap with a flexible endovascular stylet using intravascular ultrasound (IVUS) guidance. This puncture is typically made at or beyond the level of T12. A 15–20 mm balloon is then advanced over the transluminal guidewire and inflated to create a large distal reentry tear.[41] Percutaneous scissoring starts by advancing two stiff guidewires through the same introducer sheath with one guidewire being directed into each lumen. The introducer sheath is then advanced over both guidewires, achieving the same end as balloon fenestration.[42] Patel et al from the Michigan group reported a technical success rate defined as flow restoration to malperfused renal arteries in 96% of patients with short-term mortality of 17.4% (12 patients) in a cohort of icABAD patients. The celiac and superior mesenteric arteries were not included in their report. The sole univariate risk factor for early mortality was advanced age with trends seen for decreased survival in patients with historical peripheral vascular disease and dialysis requirement post-operatively. Complications including stroke in 3 patients (4.3%), dialysis for acute renal failure in 10 patients (14.5%), and paraplegia in 2.9% were noted. While fenestration is effective at relieving malperfusion, false lumen rupture was the cause of death in 5 of the 12 short-term mortality cohort patients. Additionally, 68% of patients required adjunctive branch vessel or true lumen stenting to achieve reperfusion of ischemic vascular beds.[43] Fenestration is useful for relieving the effects of dynamic obstruction but does so in a way that essentially downgrades icABAD to an uncomplicated dissection. This prevents aortic remodeling from occurring as is common in patients treated with endografts.[43] Also, the unpredictability of flow dynamics and intimal flap action following fenestration of the visceral aorta limits its effective use to the distal aorta.[13] By eliminating the serious risks inherent with ischemia, fenestration is effective as a therapy for icABAD. However, the adventitia of the false lumen remains the only barrier to aortic rupture. Further investigation of whether fenestration should serve as a primary treatment or a bridge therapy to false lumen exclusion via stent-grafting or open repair is strongly suggested.

Thoracic Endovascular Aortic Repair (TEVAR)

Michael Dake first reported on the use of TEVAR for acute aortic dissection in 1999.[6] His team placed stent grafts in 19 patients, 15 of whom had type B dissection. All branch vessels that were occluded by dynamic obstruction were reperfused while 6 of 15 branch vessels occluded by static obstruction had flow restoration. Their report of a 16% perioperative mortality rate was superior to open surgery (31.4% 30-day mortality) at the time.[44] TEVAR has since been popularized for treatment of complicated ABAD by a large number of retrospective studies and meta-analyses. Improvements made in stent-graft design and operative technique as well as accumulation of experience treating ABAD with TEVAR have reduced the in-hospital mortality rate to 10.1% in the latest IRAD analysis of TEVAR treatment for complicated ABAD.[38]

The TEVAR procedure at our institution involves three-vessel access with right common femoral artery open cut-down, and left common femoral and left brachial percutaneous access. Open access is important in our opinion due to the frailty of the peripheral vessels observed in icABAD patients and frequent extension of the dissection flap distally. In most cases, intravascular ultrasound is used in conjunction with conventional angiography throughout the procedure to assist and confirm access in the true lumen. For patients with preoperative acute renal insufficiency or failure, care should be taken to use minimal as little iodinated contrast as necessary.

Goals of TEVAR for icABAD patients are to seal the proximal entry tear, expand the true lumen, and restore flow to malperfused aortic branch vessels. The length of vessel treated is at the discretion of the surgeon with these goals taken into consideration. However, recognition of the risk of spinal cord ischemia with extensive descending aortic or LSA coverage needs to be considered while doing so. However, is not unusual for simple coverage of the entry to not be enough to restore perfusion. In addition, the aortic wall remains diseased, and therefore, we now routinely cover as much aorta as possible to provide adequate restoration of flow in addition to sealing as much tear as possible. Five to ten percent oversizing of the graft is recommended to ensure a proximal seal, and we do not routinely post dilate. Adjunctive branch vessel stenting is occasionally performed to assist true lumen expansion in the face of compromised flow due to static obstruction of branch vessels. TEVAR serves to rapidly relieve symptoms associated with dynamic obstruction while also sharply reducing the risk of false lumen rupture due to primary entry tear occlusion.

OUTCOMES OF TEVAR FOR ICABAD

No randomized control studies have been performed with TEVAR for complicated ABAD cases due to ethical issues and the emergent nature of the disease. However, recent series have reported favorable rates of short-term mortality and morbidity among icABAD patients. Trimarchi et al presented results from a recent IRAD review that compared complicated to uncomplicated ABAD. Short-term mortality was 10.1% for patients receiving endovascular treatment versus 28.6% for open surgical patients with complicated ABAD. Independent predictors of mortality were age >70 years, female gender, preoperative acute renal failure, preoperative limb ischemia, and signs of a periaortic hematoma.[38] This compares favorably to a 2006 review of the IRAD data for long-term survival in complicated ABAD patients in which the in-hospital mortality for endovascular and surgical patients was 11% and 29% respectively. The 2006 review had prior aortic aneurysm, history of atherosclerosis, pleural effusion on chest radiograph, and in-hospital hypotension/shock as additional independent predictors of mortality.[7] Subsequent studies have confirmed these results as well as the predictors of mortality.

A study sanctioned by the SVS Outcomes Committee in order to establish 30-day performance goals for TEVAR stent manufacturers investigated results of TEVAR for complicated ABAD at 5 IDE sites. Thirty-day mortality for patients with malperfusion in their acute cohort was 8.6% while actuarial 1-year mortality of 11.3%. Interestingly, the authors proposed that the high hazard phase for complicated ABAD persists to 90 days or greater. Major adverse events experienced within 30 days of treatment including early mortality, stroke, MI, acute renal failure, respiratory failure, paraparesis/paraplegia, and bowel ischemia were reported to occur in 34.5% of the 61 patients presenting with malperfusion.[1]

Recently, two series using a hybrid of covered proximal stent grafts with bare metal stents in the descending aorta for complicated ABAD have been published. The so-called PETTICOAT (Provisional ExTension To Induce COmplete ATtachment) trial and the STABLE (Study of Thoracic Aortic type B dissection using endoLuminal rEpair) trial place a covered thoracic stent graft over the proximal entry tear and then continue to place overlapping bare metal stents along the length of the dissection flap until complete occlusion is achieved. Results of these trials were promising with 30-day mortality reported at 5% (2 of 40) for the STABLE trial and none (0 of 25) in the PETTICOAT trial. However, the number of patients in these series with visceral ischemia was low. Mesenteric and renal ischemia in the STABLE trial were reported at 18.5% and 62% and in the PETTICOAT trial at 8% and 20% respectively.[3,30] It must be stated that both acute and chronic ABAD patients were included in both trials so further studies examining this methodology are recommended.

A recent Cleveland Clinic report reviewed 61 patients with icABAD who were treated with TEVAR between November 1999 and March 2011.[23] Signs of malperfusion for inclusion were any of the aforementioned clinical signs or laboratory values indicative of malperfusion and/or imaging results showing evidence of malperfusion to one or more vascular beds. Visceral ischemia was present in 54 patients (88.5%). Multiple vascular beds were affected in 70.5% of patients with 26.2% showing signs of ischemia in 3 or more vascular beds. Thirteen patients (21%) died within 30 days. Seven of these patients (54%) had irreparable ischemic damage despite technical success of TEVAR and died due to multiple organ failure or reperfusion injury. No patient during short or long-term follow-up died due to aortic rupture. Actuarial survival at 6, 12, 36, and 60 months was 75%, 71%, 60%, and 50% respectively. Univariate factors associated with increased survival were male gender (HR: 0.42, p = 0.042) and non-smoking status (HR: 0.031, p = 0.047). In the surviving cohort, partial or complete thrombosis of the false lumen was achieved in 72% of patients with remaining flow into the false lumen originating through distal reentry tears.

In this series, freedom from reintervention for patients at 6, 12, 36, and 60 months, were 84%, 76%, 68%, and 42% respectively. Branch vessel stenting was negatively associated with freedom from reintervention (HR: 4.33, p=0.012) as this signified a more complex static obstruction of the aortic branch vessels that could not be fully relived by central aortic grafting.[23] Based on this experience, we believe that further advances in endograft technology are needed to serve the needs of patients. Recognition of this need has been previously addressed in the literature. Nienaber et al performed meta-analysis of both survival and freedom from reintervention on studies published up until December 2010. They reported reintervention rates of around 20% at 1 year postoperatively with a trend toward increasing rates after this time point.[45] Until new devices or new procedures are presented and tested, routine follow-up every 3 months for the first year following TEVAR for icABAD and yearly thereafter must be stressed for both patients and providers.

Our study highlighted the importance of rapid diagnosis and treatment of icABAD. More than half of the short-term mortality cohort died due to complications of their ischemia despite technical success in restoring blood flow to their ischemic vascular beds. Harris et al examined the relationship between treatment outcomes and delayed recognition and treatment of type A dissection. They found a mortality rate of 1% per hour from presentation to treatment suggesting that time is of the essence for these patients.[46] We suggest that complicated type B dissection be aggressively treated based on the results of our study and further recommend that outcomes of treatment for icABAD be compared to time to treatment in the near future.

COMPLICATIONS OF TEVAR FOR ICABAD

Arguably the most devastating complication of TEVAR is retrograde type A dissection. Reported in 1.33–5% of patients, this complication routinely requires aortic valve resuspension and complete ascending arch replacement (Akin et al, Lombardi et al 2012). Retrograde dissection is associated with a mortality rate of 42% in the European Registry on Endovascular Aortic Repair Complications (Eggebrecht et al 2009). Aortic insufficiency can rapidly develop as a result of the dissection extending to the aortic root. We reported a rate of dissection extension in 14 patients with 10 of these being distal extension and 4 of them being retrograde extensions. Four of these patients underwent a second TEVAR operation and four underwent open surgery as reintervention.

Risk factors for retrograde dissection have been proposed using clinical observation. Authors of the STABLE trial recommend ensuring a proximal landing zone of ≥20 mm of healthy aorta in an attempt to land the graft as far proximal of the entry tear as possible. (Lombardi et al). Oversizing of the stent graft is another proposed risk factor as the radial outward force of the graft itself can cause further intimal tearing, though this was not the conclusion of European Registry group who observed median oversizing of 6%. They proposed over-ballooning of the stent graft following deployment, bare metal springs on the proximal end of the stent graft, and iatrogenic intimal injury as the three main mechanisms of retrograde type A dissection.[12] We do not recommend routinely ballooning. Great care needs to be taken to avoid hard contact with the diseased aortic wall during graft deployment and guidewire manipulation as the patients presenting with dissections are prone to further damage. Stent grafts with a proximally covered end may also be of use. Continued observation of this rare but critical complication is needed.

Central nervous system catastrophes including stroke and paraplegia have been routinely expressed as troubling complications of TEVAR throughout the literature.[3,9,12,47] Stroke was witnessed in 3 of 61 patients examined in the CCF study (4.9%).[23] It is interesting to note that 2 of the 3 had intentional LSA occlusion by the stent graft. The authors also identified coverage of the left subclavian artery as an independent risk factor of follow-up mortality.[23] Recent research has shown trends in higher rates of CVA in patients with LSA occlusion.[48] This finding is substantiated by the STABLE trial in which all patients who suffered strokes had LSA coverage. They concluded that emboli due to guidewire manipulation at the level of or proximal to the left subclavian artery could be a contributing factor to strokes in these patients.[3] The need to cover the LSA with a thoracic stent graft in order to occlude the primary entry tear indicates the severity of aortic disease present, which could also contribute to the early mortality of the patient. Further research into coverage of the LSA with a TEVAR graft for the treatment of ischemia is warranted. If necessary and if the patient clinical condition allows, we recommend concomitant carotid subclavian bypass.

Paraparesis and paraplegia are a devastating complication of TEVAR for icABAD as well. Spinal cord ischemia on presentation is most often caused by dynamic obstruction of the aortic collateral vessels supplying the spinal column and carries similar risk factors to stroke. Proposed risk factors include >20 cm of descending aortic stent graft coverage, coverage of the T8-L2 region, previous infra-renal aortic surgery, LSA coverage, and.[5,9,49] Again, while flow may be reestablished via TEVAR, excessive time to treatment can cause permanent nerve damage for patients. Patients who are at risk for or present with spinal cord ischemia should receive a preoperative spinal drain. By reducing the CSF fluid pressure surrounding the cord, the blunt force of complete spinal column reperfusion will be less damaging. This can be accomplished with a lumbar puncture at the L3 interspace with maintenance of 10 cm water pressure.[50] Postoperative paraparesis and paraplegia are disconcerting complications that require aggressive treatment. Spinal cord ischemia was an independent risk factor for decreased freedom from reintervention in the Cleveland Clinic study (HR: 5.39, p = 0.017).[23] Maintenance of mean arterial pressure ≥70 mmHg as well as previously described spinal drain placement can be effective in preventing many cases of potential paraplegia.

SUMMARY

ABAD patients with suspected symptoms of malperfusion require prompt treatment to attempt reversal of ischemic conditions. Prompt and accurate diagnosis combined with effective, rapid imaging techniques can substantially limit morbidity and mortality of icABAD patients. We presented promising data on the use of TEVAR to treat icABAD in which we demonstrated complete resolution of ischemia in 57 of 61 patients treated with no cases of aortic rupture witnessed. Improvements in clinical recognition, rapid imaging modalities, stent design, and treatment methods will continue to improve the outlook for ABAD patients. Furthermore, we recommend further investigation into the promising results of both the PETTICOAT and STABLE trials for treatment of type B dissection. TEVAR for icABAD, despite a lack of Level I evidence, shows promising results on the way to future treatments for this devastating disease.

REFERENCES

1. White RA, Miller DC, Criado FJ, et al. Report on the results of thoracic endovascular aortic repair for acute, complicated, type B aortic dissection at 30 days and 1 year from a multidisciplinary subcommittee of the Society for Vascular Surgery Outcomes Committee. *J Vasc Surg*. 2011;53(4):1082–90.
2. Hinchliffe RJ, Halawa M, Holt PJ, et al. Aortic dissection and its endovascular management. *J Cardiovasc Surg* (Torino). 2008;49(4):449–60.
3. Lombardi JV, Cambria RP, Nienaber CA, et al. Prospective multicenter clinical trial (STABLE) on the endovascular treatment of complicated type B aortic dissection using a composite device design. *J Vasc Surg*. 2012;55(3):629–40.e2.
4. Midulla M, Fattori R, Beregi JP, et al. Aortic dissection and malperfusion syndrome: a when, what and how-to guide. *Radiol Med*. 2012;2012 Apr 1. [Epub ahead of print]
5. Adams JD, Garcia LM, Kern JA. Endovascular repair of the thoracic aorta. *Surg Clin North Am*. 2009;89(4):895–912, ix.
6. Dake MD, Kato N, Mitchell RS, et al. Endovascular stent-graft placement for the treatment of acute aortic dissection. *N Engl J Med*. 1999;340(20):1546–52.
7. Tsai TT, Fattori R, Trimarchi S, et al. Long-term survival in patients presenting with type B acute aortic dissection: insights from the International Registry of Acute Aortic Dissection. *Circulation*. 2006;114(21):2226–31.
8. Fattori R, Tsai TT, Myrmel T, et al. Complicated acute type B dissection: is surgery still the best option?: A report from the International Registry of Acute Aortic Dissection. *JACC Cardiovasc Interv*. 2008;1(4):395–402.
9. Fattori R, Mineo G, Di Eusanio M. Acute type B aortic dissection: current management strategies. *Curr Opin Cardiol*. 2011;26(6):488–93.
10. Verhoye JP, Miller DC, Sze D, Dake MD, Mitchell RS. Complicated acute type B aortic dissection: midterm results of emergency endovascular stent-grafting. *J Thorac Cardiovasc Surg*. 2008;136(2):424–30.
11. Dake MD. Endovascular stent-graft management of thoracic aortic diseases. *Eur J Radiol*. 2001;39(1):42–9.
12. Eggebrecht H, Nienaber CA, Neuhäuser M, et al. Endovascular stent-graft placement in aortic dissection: a meta-analysis. *Eur Heart J*. 2006;27(4):489–98.
13. Atkins MD, Black JH, Cambria RP. Aortic dissection: perspectives in the era of stent-graft repair. *J Vasc Surg*. 2006;43 Suppl A(2):30A–43A.
14. Williams DM, Lee DY, Hamilton BH, et al. The dissected aorta: percutaneous treatment of ischemic complications--principles and results. *J Vasc Interv Radiol*. 8(4):605–25.

15. Orihashi K, Sueda T, Okada K, Imai K. Perioperative diagnosis of mesenteric ischemia in acute aortic dissection by transesophageal echocardiography. *Eur J Cardiothorac Surg.* 2005;28(6):871–6.

16. Tsai TT, Evangelista A, Nienaber CA, et al. Partial thrombosis of the false lumen in patients with acute type B aortic dissection. *N Engl J Med.* 2007;357(4):349–59.

17. Bogdan Y, Hines GL. Management of acute complicated and uncomplicated type B dissection of the aorta: focus on endovascular stent grafting. *Cardiol Rev.* 2010;18(5):234–9.

18. Carretero OA, Oparil S. Essential Hypertension : Part I: Definition and Etiology. *Circulation.* 101(3):329–35.

19. Centers for Disease Control and Prevention. Vital Signs: Current Cigarette Smoking Among Adults Aged ≥ 18 Years—United States, 2005–2010. *Morbidity and Mortality Weekly Report* 2011;60(33):1207–12 [accessed 2012 Jan 24].

20. Upadhye S, Schiff K. Acute aortic dissection in the emergency department: diagnostic challenges and evidence-based management. *Emerg Med Clin North Am.* 2012;30(2):307–27, viii.

21. Khoynezhad A, Rao R, Trento A, Gewertz B. Management of acute type B aortic dissections and acute limb ischemia. *J Cardiovasc Surg* (Torino). 2011;52(4):507–17.

22. Nienaber CA, Fattori R, Mehta RH, et al. Gender-related differences in acute aortic dissection. *Circulation.* 2004;109(24):3014–21

23. Ryan CP, Mastracci T, Vargas L, Srivastava S, Eagleton M, Kelso R, Lyden S, Clair D, Sarac TP. Progress in management of visceral Ischemia from type B dissections. *J Vasc Surg.* 2012 (in press).

24. Deeb GM, Williams DM, Bolling SF, et al. Surgical delay for acute type A dissection with malperfusion. *Ann Thorac Surg.* 1997;64(6):1669–75.

25. Januzzi JL, Movsowitz HD, Choi J, Abernethy WB, Isselbacher EM. Significance of recurrent pain in acute type B aortic dissection. *Am J Cardiol.* 2001;87(7):930–3.

26. Nienaber CA. Influence and critique of the INSTEAD Trial (TEVAR versus medical treatment for uncomplicated type B aortic dissection). *Semin Vasc Surg.* 2011;24(3):167–71.

27. Debakey ME, Henly WS, Cooley DA, Morris GC, Crawford ES, Beall AC. Surgical management of dissecting aneurysms of the aorta. *J Thorac Cardiovasc Surg.* 1965;49:130–49.

28. Larson EW, Edwards WD. Risk factors for aortic dissection: a necropsy study of 161 cases. *Am J Cardiol.* 1984;53(6):849–55.

29. Daily PO, Trueblood HW, Stinson EB, Wuerflein RD, Shumway NE. Management of acute aortic dissections. *Ann Thorac Surg.* 1970;10(3):237–47.

30. Melissano G, Bertoglio L, Rinaldi E, et al. Volume changes in aortic true and false lumen after the "PETTICOAT" procedure for type B aortic dissection. *J Vasc Surg.* 2012;55(3):641–51.

31. Feldstein C. Management of hypertensive crises. *Am J Ther.* 14(2):135–9.

32. Blumenfeld J. Management of hypertensive crises: the scientific basis for treatment decisions. *Am J Hypertens.* 14(11):1154–67.

33. Estrera AL, Miller CC, Safi HJ, et al. Outcomes of medical management of acute type B aortic dissection. *Circulation.* 2006;114(1 Suppl):I384–9.

34. Apostolakis E, Baikoussis NG, Georgiopoulos M. Acute type-B aortic dissection: the treatment strategy. *Hellenic J Cardiol.* 51(4):338–47.

35. Barnes DM, Williams DM, Dasika NL, et al. A single-center experience treating renal malperfusion after aortic dissection with central aortic fenestration and renal artery stenting. *J Vasc Surg.* 2008;47(5):903–910.

36. Bozinovski J, Coselli JS. Outcomes and survival in surgical treatment of descending thoracic aorta with acute dissection. *Ann Thorac Surg.* 2008;85(3):965–70.

37. Svensson LG, Kouchoukos NT, Miller DC, et al. Expert consensus document on the treatment of descending thoracic aortic disease using endovascular stent-grafts. *Ann Thorac Surg.* 2008;85(1 Suppl):S1–41.

38. Trimarchi S, Tolenaar JL, Tsai TT, et al. Influence of clinical presentation on the outcome of acute B aortic dissection: evidences from IRAD. *J Cardiovasc Surg* (Torino). 2012;53(2):161–8.

39. Cambria RP, Brewster DC, Gertler J, et al. Vascular complications associated with spontaneous aortic dissection. *J Vasc Surg*. 1988;7(2):199–209.
40. Roseborough G, Burke J, Sperry J, Perler B, Parra J, Williams GM. Twenty-year experience with acute distal thoracic aortic dissections. *J Vasc Surg*. 2004;40(2):235–46.
41. Chavan A, Rosenthal H, Luthe L, et al. Percutaneous interventions for treating ischemic complications of aortic dissection. *Eur Radiol*. 2009;19(2):488–94.
42. Midulla M, Renaud A, Martinelli T, et al. Endovascular fenestration in aortic dissection with acute malperfusion syndrome: immediate and late follow-up. *J Thorac Cardiovasc Surg*. 2011;142(1):66–72
43. Patel HJ, Williams DM, Meerkov M, et al. Long-term results of percutaneous management of malperfusion in acute type B aortic dissection: implications for thoracic aortic endovascular repair. *J Thorac Cardiovasc Surg*. 2009;138(2):300–8.
44. Hagan PG, Nienaber CA, Isselbacher EM, et al. The International Registry of Acute Aortic Dissection (IRAD): new insights into an old disease. *JAMA*. 2000;283(7):897–903.
45. Nienaber CA, Kische S, Ince H, Fattori R. Thoracic endovascular aneurysm repair for complicated type B aortic dissection. *J Vasc Surg*. 2011;54(5):1529–33.
46. Harris KM, Strauss CE, Eagle KA, et al. Correlates of delayed recognition and treatment of acute type A aortic dissection: the International Registry of Acute Aortic Dissection (IRAD). *Circulation*. 2011;124(18):1911–8.
47. Jazaeri O, Gupta R, Rochon PJ, Reece TB. Endovascular approaches and perioperative considerations in acute aortic dissection. *Semin Cardiothorac Vasc Anesth*. 2011;15(4):141–62.
48. Zipfel B, Buz S, Hammerschmidt R, Hetzer R. Occlusion of the left subclavian artery with stent grafts is safer with protective reconstruction. *Ann Thorac Surg*. 2009;88(2):498–504.
49. Riesenman PJ, Farber MA, Mendes RR, Marston WA, Fulton JJ, Keagy BA. Coverage of the left subclavian artery during thoracic endovascular aortic repair. *J Vasc Surg*. 2007;45(1):90–95.
50. Gravereaux EC, Faries PL, Burks JA, et al. Risk of spinal cord ischemia after endograft repair of thoracic aortic aneurysms. *J Vasc Surg*. 2001;34(6):997–1003.

SECTION **VII**

Thoracic Aortic
Disease

30

Acute Type B Dissections: Open Surgical Options

Joseph S. Coselli, MD and Scott A. LeMaire, MD

ACUTE TYPE B AORTIC DISSECTION

The Stanford classification of aortic dissection categorizes dissection according to whether the ascending aorta is involved: type A dissection involves the ascending aorta, and type B dissection does not. Type B dissection generally begins with an intimal tear in the proximal descending thoracic aorta. This tear initiates separation of the vessel's medial layer, resulting in a new channel—the false lumen—that progresses down the length of the descending thoracic aorta and often extends into the abdominal aorta.

The acute period of aortic dissection is defined as the first 14 days after the inciting intimal tear and separation of the aortic wall, which is generally heralded by the sudden onset of severe pain. Most patients with acute type B dissection stabilize upon receiving aggressive medical treatment consisting primarily of anti-impulse therapy and serial imaging. However, approximately 39% of patients with acute type B dissection present with or develop life-threatening sequelae and are categorized as having "complicated dissection."[1] The most feared complication is aortic rupture, which is caused by dilatation and disruption of the fragile, torn outer wall of the false lumen. Another major complication is malperfusion of organs—particularly the abdominal viscera and spinal cord—or the lower extremities. The true lumen and false lumen are separated by the dissecting membrane, a fragile boundary that oscillates within the aorta and can interfere with blood flow within the aorta and any of the branch arteries in either a static or a dynamic fashion. Impaired branch-vessel blood flow leads to organ ischemia—manifesting as paraplegia, bowel infarction, liver failure, or acute renal failure—or severe limb ischemia.[2]

INDICATIONS FOR OPEN SURGICAL REPAIR

Open surgical repair of the aorta in patients with acute type B dissection has traditionally been reserved for patients with complicated dissection; thus, it has been employed in a relatively small proportion of patients with type B dissection.[3] As endovascular options—including fenestration, branch vessel stenting, and thoracic aortic stent-graft placement[1*]—for treating complicated acute type B dissection have expanded, open surgery is used even less frequently. (Because algorithms regarding the choice between an endovascular procedure and an open operation for a given patient depend on many factors, are highly institution dependent, and are rapidly evolving, such decisions will not be discussed in this chapter.) In the near future, open surgery may be reserved for patients with complicated dissection in whom endovascular repair is not feasible, and for those in whom endovascular repair has not alleviated the life-threatening complication. Nevertheless, given the gravity of these two scenarios, open surgery will remain a critical component of the surgeon's armamentarium when treating patients with acute type B dissection.

Approximately 22% of patients with acute type B dissection present with aortic rupture, which may be contained by adjacent tissues (usually manifesting as localized periaortic hematoma on imaging studies) or may be complete (often termed "free rupture" and usually manifesting as shock with hemothorax, hemoperitoneum, or massive retroperitoneal hematoma).[4] Patients with aortic rupture (Figure 30-1) undergo immediate surgery to stop bleeding and replace the ruptured segment with a prosthetic graft. Additionally, patients with symptoms and signs that signal a high risk of impending rupture—such as refractory pain, refractory hypertension, and rapid aortic expansion— also undergo open surgery to prevent a catastrophic event. Similarly, patients whose acute dissection is superimposed upon a preexisting aneurysm (Figure 30-2) are at high risk for rupture and warrant urgent open surgical repair.

Malperfusion of vital organs or the limbs occurs in approximately 20% of patients with acute type B aortic dissection and is associated with an increased risk of death.[5,6] In many cases, an endovascular procedure can be performed to restore flow in compromised branch arteries.[3,7] When endovascular procedures are not feasible or are unsuccessful, open surgical procedures are often indicated. Patients with malperfusion of the organs supplied by the celiac and superior mesenteric arteries undergo emergent intervention to prevent liver failure and bowel necrosis. Although unilateral renal malperfusion is generally not considered an indication for operative intervention, open surgical repair might be warranted in patients with bilateral renal ischemia. Patients with lower-extremity ischemia can undergo extraanatomic bypass procedures to restore limb perfusion. Spinal cord malperfusion resulting in paraplegia has not traditionally been considered an indication for open surgical repair of the aorta.[8]

STRATEGIC CONSIDERATIONS

There are several strategic considerations specifically related to the open surgical treatment of complicated acute type B aortic dissection. The first is selecting the type of open procedure to use in a given case. Patients with rupture, impending rupture, or acute dissection superimposed upon a preexisting aneurysm generally require graft replacement of the descending thoracic aorta or, less commonly, the thoracoabdominal aorta. In selected cases of malperfusion, bypass to the affected branch artery may suffice. For example, patients with lower-extremity ischemia can undergo femoral artery–to–femoral artery bypass to correct unilateral malperfusion. A right axillary artery–to–right femoral artery bypass can

---

* The use of stent-grafts in patients with aortic dissection is currently an off-label application of these devices in the United States.

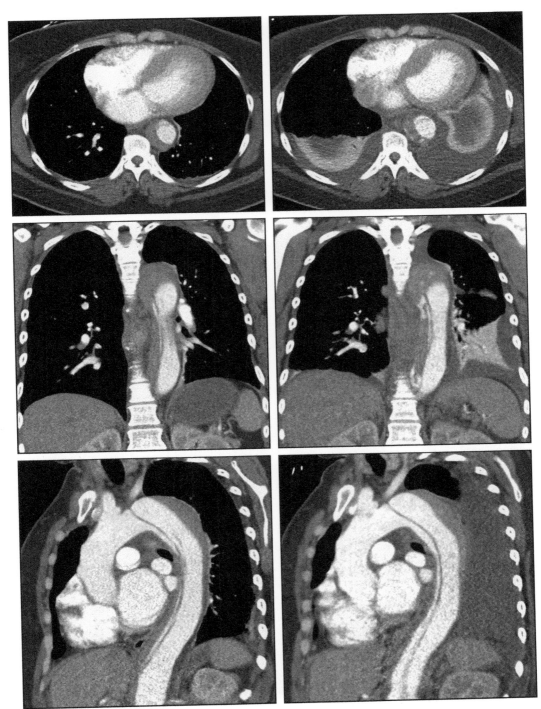

Figure 30-1. Computed tomography images from a patient who had a moderately dilated thoracoabdominal aortic aneurysm secondary to chronic dissection. The patient subsequently developed a superimposed acute dissection (left panels) that progressed to rupture 4 days later (right panels). The patient was transferred to our institution and underwent successful emergency graft replacement of the thoracoabdominal aorta. Used with permission from Baylor College of Medicine.

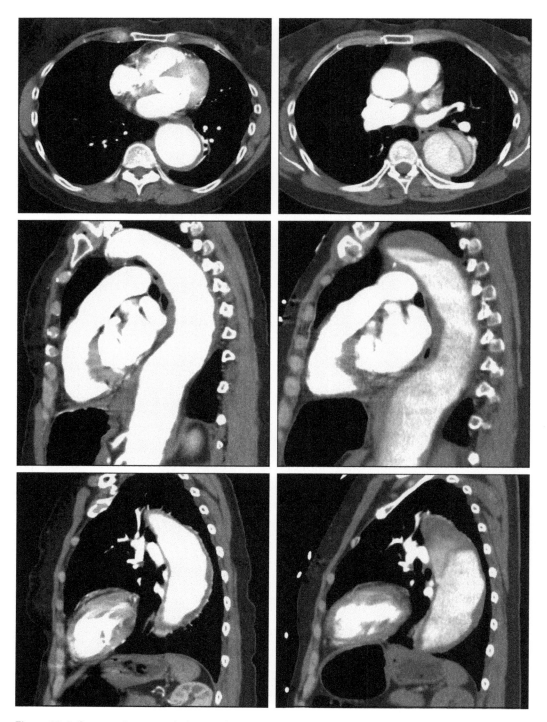

Figure 30-2. Computed tomography images from a patient who had a large thoracoabdominal aortic aneurysm (left panels). Four weeks later, the patient developed a superimposed acute type B dissection (right panels), prompting transfer to our institution for surgical treatment. The patient underwent successful urgent graft replacement of the thoracoabdominal aorta. Used with permission from Baylor College of Medicine.

be added to the femoral-femoral bypass procedure in patients with bilateral lower-limb ischemia. When adequate inflow arteries are available, bypass grafts to malperfused visceral branches can alleviate ischemia.[9,10] When malperfusion cannot be corrected by bypass grafting, open aortic fenestration procedures—in which a segment of the dissecting membrane is excised through an aortotomy—are an excellent option for restoring blood flow to ischemic viscera.[7,11,12] Because fenestration procedures enable the correction of malperfusion without the need to replace aorta, they are generally associated with better outcomes than aortic replacement operations in these patients.

The second strategic consideration relates to the use of adjuncts to provide spinal cord protection during aortic repair. Patients undergoing open repair of the descending thoracic or thoracoabdominal aorta in the presence of acute dissection are at high risk of developing postoperative paraplegia.[13] In fact, acute dissection is a major factor in two models that were developed to calculate the risk of spinal cord complications after surgical repair of descending thoracic aortic aneurysms and thoracoabdominal aortic aneurysms.[14,15] In an attempt to mitigate the increased risk of spinal cord ischemia, surgical teams often use spinal-cord–protective adjuncts more liberally during open repairs for acute type B dissection than they would during elective repairs. For example, in patients with acute dissection, we strongly consider using cerebrospinal fluid drainage and left heart bypass regardless of the planned extent of repair.[15–17]

The third issue to consider is the extent of aortic replacement. A tenet of open surgical repair of acute type B dissection is focusing on addressing the life-threatening problem while minimizing the overall extent of aortic replacement, thereby reducing the risk of perioperative complications. It is therefore common to replace relatively short segments of the aorta in these patients, targeting the area that has ruptured, undergone rapid expansion, or precipitated malperfusion. This strategy of limited repair is not feasible in some patients, particularly those with acute dissection superimposed upon a large preexisting thoracoabdominal aortic aneurysm; such patients are at an extremely high risk of developing paraplegia.[13,18]

The final strategic consideration relates to the extreme fragility of the aortic tissue encountered in patients with aortic dissection. The friable aortic wall is prone to tearing during suturing, making it difficult to ensure hemostatic anastomoses; this problem is compounded in patients with connective tissue disorders. It is common to use smaller needles and finer suture material when sewing the acutely dissected aorta than when sewing an aorta without dissection or with chronic dissection. In some cases, the fragility of the aortic wall may preclude using the standard island technique to reattach a set of visceral or intercostal arteries; alternative reattachment techniques, such as using branch grafts, can be useful in this situation. Extra reinforcement with felt strips or pledgets, as well as surgical adhesives or sealants, may help secure a tenuous anastomosis.

SURGICAL TECHNIQUES FOR OPEN AORTIC REPAIR

Intraoperative Preparation

Many aspects of preparing the patient with acute type B dissection for operation are similar to those related to elective repair of descending thoracic and thoracoabdominal aortic aneurysms.[16,19–23] The endotracheal intubation strategy needs to enable single right-lung ventilation. Placement of a right radial arterial catheter ensures uninterrupted blood pressure monitoring should the aortic arch need to be clamped proximal to the left subclavian artery. Avoiding hypertension—an important aspect of management in any patient with an aneurysm—is essential in patients with acute aortic dissection. In hemodynamically stable patients, placement of a cerebrospinal fluid drain should be considered. The patient is secured in a modified right lateral decubitus position, with the shoulders rotated to about 60 degrees from horizontal and the hips rotated to about 30 degrees from horizontal, thereby enabling access to both groins. Cell-saving and rapid-infusion devices are routinely set up to enable shed blood salvage and rapid volume replacement, respectively.

Aortic Exposure

When the aortic repair will only involve the descending thoracic aorta, a left thoracotomy is made after single right-lung ventilation is initiated. The left thorax is usually entered through the sixth intercostal space, although the fifth interspace is preferable when the repair will primarily involve the proximal descending thoracic aorta, especially when there is a rupture or large aneurysm in this region. When the repair will involve the thoracoabdominal aorta, the thoracotomy incision is curved inferiorly and extended across the costal margin and toward the umbilicus. The thoracoabdominal aorta is exposed by performing medial visceral rotation through a transperitoneal approach and dividing the diaphragm circumferentially, leaving a 3- to 4-cm rim of diaphragm attached to the lateral and posterior chest wall. During the opening and aortic exposure phases of the operation, the patient's temperature is allowed to slowly drift downward toward 32 to 33°C (nasopharyngeal) to capitalize on the protective effects of mild hypothermia.

Graft Replacement Procedures

An aortic clamp site is then prepared a few centimeters proximal to the area being repaired. Whenever possible, the clamp site is prepared distal to the left subclavian artery. Frequently, however, the clamp needs to be placed between the left common carotid artery and the left subclavian artery; this necessitates placing another clamp (eg, a bulldog clamp) across the proximal left subclavian artery. In either case, when exposing the distal aortic arch, the surgeon attempts to preserve the left recurrent laryngeal nerve. However, preserving the nerve can be challenging in acute dissection cases, particularly when there is periaortic hematoma in the region, and in many cases is simply not possible. In patients with free rupture, blood and hematoma are rapidly evacuated from the region adjacent to the desired aortic clamp site; the area of rupture is manually compressed while a proximal clamp site is quickly prepared. In patients with contained rupture, the area containing the periaortic hematoma is avoided whenever possible until a proximal clamp site is secured. Heparin (1 mg/kg) is routinely administered intravenously before the aorta is clamped.

When feasible from hemodynamic and anatomic standpoints, left heart bypass can be a valuable adjunct when repairing acute type B aortic dissection, especially when a substantial length of aorta needs to be replaced. Cannulation is performed after heparin administration and before aortic clamping. The tip of an angled drainage cannula is placed in the left atrium through an opening in the left superior pulmonary vein. The inflow cannula can be placed in either the left femoral artery or the distal descending thoracic aorta; when this cannula is placed, care is taken to ensure that flow will pass through the true lumen, not the false one. To avoid retrograde extension of the dissection, the proximal aortic clamp can be placed before pump flow is initiated. Left heart bypass flow is then started and increased to a target rate of 1.5 to 2.5 L/min.

A second clamp is placed across a more distal aspect of the aorta, thereby isolating the site of the proximal extent of repair between the clamps.

The aorta is opened distal to the proximal aortic clamp. This opening is usually made into the false lumen. The dissecting membrane is identified and excised. Patent intercostal arteries are oversewn with 2-0 silk sutures. The site of the proximal anastomosis is prepared by transecting the aorta, taking care to leave a cuff of intact aorta that is approximately 3 cm in length, and separating the medial wall from the underlying esophagus. Preparing the aorta in this manner ensures that the entire aortic circumference will be included in the proximal anastomosis and reduces the chance of incorporating the esophagus into the suture line. A coated polyester graft—usually between 20 and 24 mm in diameter—is then sewn to the proximal aortic cuff, often with a 4-0 polypropylene suture. Individual polypropylene mattress sutures with felt pledgets can be used to reinforce the anastomosis. Alternatively, a second polypropylene suture can be sewn in a running fashion along the entire initial suture line.

If the proximal clamp was placed distal to the left subclavian artery, it is left in place during the next phase of the repair. However, if the proximal aortic clamp was placed between the left common carotid and left subclavian arteries, it is ideal to reposition the clamps so that perfusion of the left common carotid artery can be restored. After the patient is placed in head-down position, the clamp on the left subclavian artery is removed, the proximal portion of the graft is deaired, and the proximal clamp is moved from the arch to the proximal aspect of the graft.

In many patients with acute type B dissection, graft repairs can be limited to the descending thoracic aorta. If left heart bypass is being used, pump flow can be either continued (which is facilitated by moving the distal aortic clamp to the aorta near the diaphragm) or stopped (followed by removal of the distal aortic clamp). The remainder of the aortic segment being replaced is then opened longitudinally, and the dissecting membrane is excised from this section. As discussed above, the goal of the operation is to correct the immediate life-threatening problem (eg, rupture, large aneurysm), and not to replace the entire dissected aorta; the extent of the aortic replacement should be limited accordingly. Patent intercostal arteries are generally oversewn with 2-0 silk suture. The site of the distal anastomosis is inspected, and the true lumen is identified. Although it is helpful to make a transverse cut in the aorta here, it is not necessary to fully transect the aorta at this level. When the graft is cut to its final length, leaving it 1 or 2 cm longer than necessary helps reduce the amount of tension at the fragile anastomoses. The distal anastomosis is created with 4-0 polypropylene suture and is sewn in a manner that obliterates the entry into the false lumen; this ensures that all of the flow is directed into the true lumen and often alleviates distal malperfusion.

When graft replacement extends into the thoracoabdominal segment, left heart bypass is stopped after the proximal anastomosis is completed. The distal aortic clamp is removed. If the inflow cannula had been placed in the aorta, this cannula is also removed. The aorta is then opened longitudinally along the length being replaced, and care is taken to incise the aorta posterior to the origin of the left renal artery.

The dissecting membrane is then excised, and the origins of the celiac axis, superior mesenteric artery, and both renal arteries are identified. When dissection extends into a visceral branch, this can be dealt with in several ways. First, the dissecting membrane within the artery can be simply excised or fenestrated, especially when the dissection only extends a short distance into the vessel. When the arterial dissection is more extensive, it may be possible to use interrupted fine polypropylene sutures to tack the artery's dissecting membrane to the outer vessel wall, thereby obliterating the false channel; this approach facilitates standard reattachment of the vessel as part of an island of aortic tissue that is sewn to an opening in the side of the graft. Alternatively, the artery can be reattached by using a branch graft (generally an 8- or 10-mm polyester graft), and the false channel can be obliterated within the end-to-end suture line. It is also possible to ensure the patency of the artery's true lumen by deploying a balloon-expandable stent (6- or 7-mm in diameter) into the vessel under direct vision; however, although this technique works well in patients with atherosclerotic stenosis or chronic dissection, it should be used with caution when one is dealing with fragile, acutely dissected arteries.[24]

If left heart bypass has been used, a Y-limb from the inflow line of the circuit can be used to deliver selective perfusion to the celiac and superior mesenteric arteries through 9-Fr balloon perfusion catheters. Another set of balloon perfusion catheters is inserted into the renal arteries to enable intermittent delivery of cold crystalloid solution to the kidneys, thereby enhancing renal protection.[25] Placing these catheters and inflating their balloons within acutely dissected arteries requires great care to ensure perfusion of the true lumen and to avoid exacerbating vessel dissection or causing arterial rupture.

After perfusion to the abdominal viscera is initiated, attention is turned to any exposed intercostal arteries. During elective thoracoabdominal aortic aneurysm repair, large, patent intercostal arteries that are located below the T7 level and exhibit marginal backbleeding are considered excellent candidates for reattachment. However, in patients with acute dissection, the adjacent aortic tissue may be too fragile to create a secure island-type anastomosis. As an alternative approach, an 8- or 10-mm branch graft can be used to connect 1 or 2 intercostal ostia to the aortic graft after the other portions of the repair have been completed. This technique reduces the length of the anastomosis and provides the bailout option of graft ligation in the event that bleeding cannot be controlled. Although it is tempting to sequentially move the aortic clamp below each newly created anastomosis (thereby restoring perfusion of the attached vessels), this can lead to troublesome bleeding, dealing with which delays completion of the distal anastomoses and prolongs aortic clamp time.

In extent I thoracoabdominal aortic repairs, the distal anastomosis is performed at the level of the visceral branches, generally in a beveled fashion. As described above for repairs limited to the descending thoracic aorta, the distal anastomosis is fashioned to obliterate the false lumen and direct all flow into the true lumen. As with the other anastomoses, techniques to improve hemostasis at the distal suture line include using 4-0 polypropylene suture for the anastomosis, placing interrupted polypropylene mattress sutures with felt pledgets to provide reinforcement, using a second polypropylene suture to oversew the initial suture line, and judiciously applying topical hemostats or sealants.

In extent II repairs (as well as many extent III and IV repairs), the distal anastomosis is performed in the infrarenal aorta, often just proximal to the aorto-iliac bifurcation. Therefore, before this anastomosis is begun, the visceral branches need to be reattached to the graft. This is often done by attaching the island of aortic tissue surrounding the 4 visceral ostia to an opening cut in the side of the graft. In some patients—particularly those with preexisting aneurysms in this region—the left renal artery is substantially displaced away from the other 3 vessels. In this situation, it is best to incorporate only the celiac, superior mesenteric, and right renal arteries in the island reattachment, and later (ie, after the distal anastomosis is completed) reattach the left renal artery separately by using an 8-mm branch graft. As with the intercostal artery island reattachment technique, creating a hemostatic visceral artery island anastomosis can be extremely challenging in patients with acute dissection. When the surrounding aortic tissue appears unsuitable for suturing, individual branch grafts can be anastomosed to each of the visceral vessels, usually after the distal aortic anastomosis is completed.

Before the distal anastomosis is performed, the infrarenal aorta is inspected. The inferior mesenteric artery origin is identified and ligated, and lumbar arteries are evaluated for potential reattachment. The distal anastomosis is then created with 4-0 polypropylene suture. If the dissection extends beyond the anastomosis site, the false lumen is obliterated within the suture line. When the anastomosis is nearly completed, the impending clamp removal is communicated to the anesthesiology team so that they can prepare for the associated hemodynamic changes.

After the distal anastomosis is completed, the patient is placed in a head-down position, the graft is deaired, and the aortic clamp is removed. Intravenous protamine is administered to reverse the effects of heparin. Intravenous indigo carmine dye is also administered to ensure renal perfusion; the appearance of blue dye in the urine signifies arterial flow to at least one of the kidneys. All suture lines are carefully inspected to ensure hemostasis. After surgical hemostasis has been adequately secured, blood products are administered as needed to correct coagulopathy. The abdominal cavity is inspected to ensure adequate perfusion of the viscera. The presence of pulses is also confirmed in the iliac and femoral arteries.

Occasionally, aortic clamping is not feasible because of rupture or an extremely large aneurysm involving the proximal descending thoracic aorta. In these situations, cardiopulmonary bypass and hypothermic circulatory arrest are used.[26] This is generally established by placing a long atriocaval drainage cannula through the left femoral vein, an arterial inflow cannula in the left femoral artery, and a drainage cannula in the left superior pulmonary vein. Once the patient has been adequately cooled (target nasopharyngeal temperature <18°C), circulatory arrest is established. In some cases, a clamp can be placed across the mid- or lower descending thoracic aorta and distal aortic perfusion can be delivered through the femoral cannula. The aorta is opened, and the proximal anastomosis site is prepared as described above. A graft with a side-branch near the proximal end is selected and sewn to the proximal aortic cuff. After the proximal anastomosis is completed, a Y-limb from the arterial line of the cardiopulmonary bypass circuit is connected to the side graft. Pump flow is established though the side graft to deair the aortic arch and the graft. The main graft is then clamped distal to the side branch, which restores perfusion to the heart and brachiocephalic branches. The remainder of the aortic repair proceeds as described previously except that selective visceral perfusion and cold crystalloid renal perfusion are not used. After the repair has been completed and the patient has been adequately rewarmed, the patient is weaned from cardiopulmonary bypass.

Fenestration Procedures

In patients who are undergoing surgery specifically to correct visceral malperfusion, an aortic fenestration procedure can be performed. This approach restores blood flow to ischemic organs while minimizing the extent of the aortic repair. Consequently, these procedures are generally associated with a lower risk of morbidity and mortality than graft replacement operations in patients with acute dissection and visceral ischemia.[7,12] Aortic exposure and clamping are performed as described for graft replacement operations. In one approach to the fenestration procedure, a longitudinal, posterolateral opening is made in the visceral segment of the aorta, and the dissecting membrane is fully excised from this segment. The aortotomy is then closed with polypropylene suture; felt strips can be incorporated in the closure to provide reinforcement. Another approach involves transecting the aorta and excising the dissecting membrane from the proximal stump. Then, when the ends of the aorta are sewn back together, the suture line is constructed to obliterate the distal false lumen.

CONTEMPORARY CLINICAL EXPERIENCE

Between January 2002 and April 2012, we performed open surgical repair of the aorta in 32 patients with acute type B dissection. The mean age of this group, which comprised 20 men (63%) and 12 women (38%), was 60 ± 15 years (range, 24 to 83 years). Seven patients had genetically-triggered aortic disease, such as Marfan syndrome (6 patients) and Loeys-Dietz syndrome (1 patient).

The dissection was confined to the descending thoracic aorta in 13 patients (41%) and extended into the abdominal aorta in 19 (59%). Seven patients (22%) had rupture. One patient (3%) underwent surgery to treat malperfusion; flow was compromised in the superior mesenteric artery in this patient. Two patients underwent surgery because of refractory pain. The remaining patients presented with a dangerously large aneurysm, indicating either rapid expansion of the false lumen before presentation or a dissection superimposed on a preexisting aneurysm. The mean maximum diameter of the descending thoracic aorta for the overall group was 6.2±0.8 cm (range, 4.8 to 7.5 cm).

Graft replacement of the descending thoracic aorta was performed in 9 patients (28%). Twenty-one patients (66%) underwent graft replacement of the thoracoabdominal aorta; Crawford extents of repair were extent I in 14 patients, extent II in 5, and extent III in 2. One patient underwent open fenestration of the thoracoabdominal aorta, and 1 patient underwent graft replacement of the juxtarenal aorta.

Clamping proximal to the left subclavian artery was necessary in 12 patients (38%). Cardiopulmonary bypass and hypothermic circulatory arrest were used in 3 patients. Left heart bypass was used in 20 patients (63%), selective visceral perfusion was used in 4 (13%), and cold renal perfusion was used in 10 (31%). Cerebrospinal fluid drainage was used in 23 patients (72%). Intercostal or lumbar arteries were reattached in 13 patients (41%); in 2 patients, branch grafts were used for this purpose in lieu of the traditional island technique. In 7 patients, one or more branch grafts were used to reattach the visceral branches; the left renal artery was the most common visceral branch reattached in this manner (5 patients). Bypass grafts to the iliac or femoral arteries were performed in 2 patients.

The overall operative mortality rate was 6%. The 2 operative deaths occurred during the initial hospitalization; 1 occurred within 30 days of the procedure. One patient had postoperative bleeding that necessitated reoperation. Spinal cord complications occurred in 6 patients (19%); deficits were transient in 3 patients and permanent in 3. One patient suffered a stroke. Acute renal failure necessitating dialysis developed in 4 patients (13%); dialysis dependency was transient in 2 and permanent in 2. Respiratory failure occurred in 13 patients (41%), and 13 patients (41%) had left vocal cord paralysis. The median postoperative intensive care unit length of stay was 7 days (range, 2 to 64 days), and the median postoperative hospital length of stay was 15 days (range, 5 to 100 days).

Acknowledgments

The authors thank Matt D. Price, MS, RHIA, Samantha Zarda, RHIA, Michael S. Hughes, and Jeffrey Whorton, RHIA, for clinical data management; Stephen N. Palmer, PhD, ELS, and Susan Y. Green, MPH, for editorial support; and Scott A. Weldon, MA, CMI, for assistance with figure preparation.

REFERENCES

1. Trimarchi S, Jonker FH, Froehlich JB, et al. Acute type B aortic dissection in the absence of aortic dilatation. *J Vasc Surg*. 2012 [E-pub ahead of print].
2. Williams DM, Lee DY, Hamilton BH, et al. The dissected aorta: part III. Anatomy and radiologic diagnosis of branch-vessel compromise. *Radiology*. 1997;203:37–44.
3. Slonim SM, Miller DC, Mitchell RS, et al. Percutaneous balloon fenestration and stenting for life-threatening ischemic complications in patients with acute aortic dissection. *J Thorac Cardiovasc Surg*. 1999;117:1118–1126.
4. Garbade J, Jenniches M, Borger MA, et al. Outcome of patients suffering from acute type B aortic dissection: A retrospective single-centre analysis of 135 consecutive patients. *Eur J Cardiothorac Surg*. 2010;38:285–292.
5. Fattori R, Tsai TT, Myrmel T, et al. Complicated acute type B dissection: Is surgery still the best option? A report from the International Registry of Acute Aortic Dissection. *JACC Cardiovasc Interv*. 2008;1:395–402.
6. Hiratzka LF, Bakris GL, Beckman JA, et al. 2010 ACCF/AHA/AATS/ACR/ASA/SCA/ SCAI/SIR/STS/SVM guidelines for the diagnosis and management of patients with thoracic aortic disease: a report of the American College of Cardiology Foundation/ American Heart Association Task Force on Practice Guidelines, American Association for Thoracic Surgery, American College of Radiology, American Stroke Association, Society of Cardiovascular Anesthesiologists, Society for Cardiovascular Angiography and Interventions, Society of Interventional Radiology, Society of Thoracic Surgeons, and Society for Vascular Medicine. *Circulation*. 2010;121:e266–369.
7. Pradhan S, Elefteriades JA, Sumpio BE. Utility of the aortic fenestration technique in the management of acute aortic dissections. *Ann Thorac Cardiovasc Surg*. 2007;13:296–300.
8. Nagano N, Kikuchi K, Amano A, et al. Should we consider surgical intervention for spinal cord ischemia due to acute type B aortic dissection? *Eur J Cardiothorac Surg*. 2009;35:547–549.
9. Holfeld J, Gottardi R, Zimpfer D, et al. Bail-out visceral bypass grafting for acute intestinal ischemia after endovascular stent-graft placement in a complicated type B dissection. *Thorac Cardiovasc Surg*. 2009;57:110–111.
10. Uchida N, Shibamura H, Katayama A, et al. Surgical strategies for organ malperfusions in acute type B aortic dissection. *Interact Cardiovasc Thorac Surg*. 2009;8:75–78.
11. Howell JF, LeMaire SA, Kirby RP. Thoracoabdominal fenestration for aortic dissection with ischemic colonic perforation. *Ann Thorac Surg*. 1997;64:242–244.
12. Trimarchi S, Jonker FH, Muhs BE, et al. Long-term outcomes of surgical aortic fenestration for complicated acute type B aortic dissections. *J Vasc Surg*. 2010;52:261–266.
13. Coselli JS, LeMaire SA, de Figueiredo LP, et al. Paraplegia after thoracoabdominal aortic aneurysm repair: Is dissection a risk factor? *Ann Thorac Surg*. 1997;63:28–35; discussion 35-36.
14. Acher CW, Wynn MM, Hoch JR, et al. Combined use of cerebral spinal fluid drainage and naloxone reduces the risk of paraplegia in thoracoabdominal aneurysm repair. *J Vasc Surg*. 1994;19:236–246; discussion 247–248.
15. Coselli JS. The use of left heart bypass in the repair of thoracoabdominal aortic aneurysms: current techniques and results. *Semin Thorac Cardiovasc Surg*. 2003;15:326–332.

16. Coselli JS, LeMaire SA. Tips for successful outcomes for descending thoracic and thoracoabdominal aortic aneurysm procedures. *Semin Vasc Surg.* 2008;21:13–20.

17. Coselli JS, LeMaire SA, Köksoy C, et al. Cerebrospinal fluid drainage reduces paraplegia after thoracoabdominal aortic aneurysm repair: Results of a randomized clinical trial. *J Vasc Surg.* 2002;35:631–639.

18. Bozinovski J, Coselli JS. Outcomes and survival in surgical treatment of descending thoracic aorta with acute dissection. *Ann Thorac Surg.* 2008;85:965–970; discussion 970–971.

19. Huh J, LeMaire SA, Weldon SA, et al. Thoracoabdominal aortic aneurysm repair: Open technique. *Op Tech Thorac Cardiovasc Surg.* 2010;15:70–85.

20. LeMaire SA, Rice DC, Schmittling ZC, et al. Emergency surgery for thoracoabdominal aortic aneurysms with acute presentation. *J Vasc Surg.* 2002;35:1171–1178.

21. Vaughn SB, LeMaire SA, Collard CD. Case scenario: Anesthetic considerations for thoracoabdominal aortic aneurysm repair. *Anesthesiology.* 2011;115:1093–1102.

22. Wong DR, LeMaire SA, Coselli JS. Managing dissections of the thoracic aorta. *Am Surg.* 2008;74:364–380.

23. Wong DR, Parenti JL, Green SY, et al. Open repair of thoracoabdominal aortic aneurysm in the modern surgical era: Contemporary outcomes in 509 patients. *J Am Coll Surg.* 2011;212:569–579; discussion 579–581.

24. LeMaire SA, Jamison AL, Carter SA, et al. Deployment of balloon expandable stents during open repair of thoracoabdominal aortic aneurysms: A new strategy for managing renal and mesenteric artery lesions. *Eur J Cardiothorac Surg.* 2004;26:599–607.

25. Köksoy C, LeMaire SA, Curling PE, et al. Renal perfusion during thoracoabdominal aortic operations: Cold crystalloid is superior to normothermic blood. *Ann Thorac Surg.* 2002;73:730–738.

26. Coselli JS, Bozinovski J, Cheung C. Hypothermic circulatory arrest: Safety and efficacy in the operative treatment of descending and thoracoabdominal aortic aneurysms. *Ann Thorac Surg.* 2008;85:956–963; discussion 964.

31

Endovascular Management of Type B Aortic Dissections

Paul D. DiMusto, MD and Gilbert R. Upchurch Jr., MD

INTRODUCTION

There are approximately 9,000 new cases of aortic dissection in the United States each year. Uncomplicated type B aortic dissections are traditionally managed with medical therapy, controlling blood pressure and heart rate, with 30-day mortality rates between 4% and 10%. However, there is no consensus regarding the management of complicated type B dissections presenting with malperfusion or refractory pain. Open surgical management of these patients carries an excessive mortality rate. Therefore, endovascular aortic fenestration and branch vessel stenting to relieve malperfusion was developed as an alternative to open surgical repair. While endovascular fenestration and stenting relieves malperfusion, it does not prevent late aneurysm degeneration of the aorta, which can occur in up to 30% of patients. More recently, the use of endovascular stent grafts to cover the primary and proximal entry tear has been examined, with the belief that this approach treats most cases of malperfusion and in theory prevents late aneurysm formation. The objective of this chapter is to examine the literature surrounding the endovascular management of type B aortic dissections.

BACKGROUND

Aortic dissection involves a tear in the intima of the aorta, allowing blood to flow within layers of the media. This creates a false lumen for blood flow in the intramural space, which may compress the true lumen or extend into branch arteries creating malperfusion. Additionally, the dissected aorta can chronically become aneurysmal, leading to eventual rupture. It is estimated that dissections of the descending thoracic aorta occur with an incidence of 2 to 3.5 cases per 100,000 person-years.[1,2] Common causes of aortic dissection include long standing hypertension, connective tissue disorders, and trauma.[3,4]

Dissections involving the thoracic aorta can be classified according to the Stanford or DeBakey systems. In the Stanford classification, a type A dissection involves the ascending aorta, while a type B does not. Under the DeBakey classification, a type I dissection begins in the proximal aorta and extends distally, involving both the ascending and descending thoracic aorta. A type II dissection is confined to the ascending aorta, while a type III dissection is confined to the descending aorta (similar to Stanford type B). Dissections can also be classified temporally into acute, sub-acute, and chronic phases. The acute phase is defined as less than 14 days from the onset of symptoms, sub-acute 15–30 days, and a chronic dissection is defined as more than 31 days from the onset of symptoms. Finally, dissections are typically classified as complicated or uncomplicated, with complicated dissections involving malperfusion, rupture or impending rupture, refractory hypertension, or continued pain.[5] Approximately 30% of type B dissections are complicated at initial presentation.[6]

The management of an aortic dissection is based typically on the type, time course, and associated symptoms, such as malperfusion. Type B dissections require tight blood pressure control to attempt to minimize the extent of dissection, to decrease false lumen distention, and to reduce the risk of aortic rupture. This is commonly done with beta blockade, as these agents reduce the heart rate and contractile force of the heart, while also decreasing systemic blood pressure.[4] Additional anti-hypertensives are often required.

SURGICAL MANAGEMENT OF TYPE B DISSECTIONS

The management of a type B dissection classically depends on whether the dissection is considered complicated or not. For uncomplicated type B dissections, medical management is advocated as it has been shown to have a lower mortality than surgical intervention, particularly in the acute phase. Surgical intervention for uncomplicated type B dissections is classically reserved for those patients who develop complications in the chronic phase. Aneurysmal dilation of the false lumen will develop in 20% to 50% of patients with type B dissections within 1 to 5 years, eventually leading to the need for repair to prevent aortic rupture.[7,8]

Complicated type B dissections, in contrast, require intervention in the acute phase to alleviate malperfusion or refractory hypertension. Mortality rates for surgical intervention are extremely high in this setting. The IRAD investigators reported on 82 patients undergoing open surgical intervention for type B dissection and described an overall in-hospital mortality rate of 29%.[9] The in-hospital mortality rate was 39% for patients undergoing surgery within the first 48 hours and 18% for those having surgery more than 48 hours after the onset of symptoms. Independent predictors of surgical mortality for a type B dissection were an age greater than 70 years and pre-operative shock or hypotension. New neurological deficits were seen in 23% of patients, with 9% suffering a stroke, and approximately 5% developing paraplegia. In 2008, the same investigators reported an in-hospital mortality rate of 34% in 59 patients undergoing open surgical intervention for complicated type B dissections.[6] These patients had a 40% in-hospital complication rate with 3 (5%) developing paraplegia.

ENDOVASCULAR FENESTRATION AND STENTING FOR COMPLICATED TYPE B DISSECTIONS

Given the high morbidity and mortality rates associated with open surgical intervention, less invasive alternatives were sought to treat malperfusion associated with a complicated type B dissection. In the 1990s, as endovascular techniques continued to evolve, the concept of endovascular fenestration and stenting to treat malperfusion became popular.[10] Endovascular fenestration and stenting requires extensive endovascular skill and experience, but can relieve the symptoms of malperfusion with a lower risk of morbidity and mortality than open surgery. The theoretical disadvantage of this technique is that it promotes blood flow through the false lumen, which potentially can lead to progressive dilation and aneurysm development, with the possibility of eventual rupture.[11]

Williams et al. classified branch vessel compromise secondary to aortic dissections as either static or dynamic.[12] Static obstruction occurs when the course of dissection intersects the origin of a branch vessel and the aortic hematoma propagates into that vessel wall, thereby constricting the lumen. Dynamic obstruction results from prolapse of the dissection flap across the branch vessel origin. Additionally, dynamic narrowing of the aorta proximal to a branch vessel ostium may compromise a vessel otherwise spared by the dissection flap. Finally, a combination of any of these mechanisms may also be present.

The technique of endovascular fenestration and stenting begins with an angiographic evaluation of malperfusion directed at finding and treating ongoing branch artery obstructions. Intravascular ultrasound (IVUS) is performed from the ascending aorta to the iliac arteries to define the relationship of the dissection flap to branch arteries and to determine the lumen from which each major branch arises. Pressures in the SMA, bilateral renal arteries, and bilateral external iliac arteries are measured simultaneously with pressures in the aortic root. Hand injections of contrast are performed in each branch vessel to establish that the location of each pressure measurement is peripheral to the distal extent of the false lumen, and to examine for arteriopathy or peripheral emboli. In the example of branch vessel malperfusion, true malperfusion is confirmed by a systolic gradient between the aortic root and the SMA or renal hilum of >15 mmHg, failure of a branch artery to fill during injection of contrast in the true and false lumen of the aorta, evidence of a "curtain-like" occlusion of the vessel origin or of the true lumen above the origin by IVUS, thrombosis, or peripheral emboli.

To perform endovascular aortic fenestration, an Amplatz wire is typically advanced through a Cobra catheter. The catheter is then withdrawn over the wire and exchanged for a Rosch-Uchida introducer set that is subsequently placed in the true lumen. The wire is removed and the trocar, in its encasing 5 Fr catheter, is advanced and thrust through the dissection flap using fluoroscopic and IVUS guidance. The trocar is exchanged for the Amplatz wire to allow balloon dilation of the flap and creation of a fenestration tear with a 14 mm diameter balloon. Other techniques to create or enlarge the fenestration have been described, including the use of a snare to have a stiff wire from the arm to the groin across the fenestration, similar to "flossing" in thoracic endografting, or using a double wire/one sheath "push" technique. Following creation of the tear, the configuration of the two lumens is observed using IVUS. If the true lumen remains collapsed or, in questionable cases, if a gradient between the root and the abdominal aorta persists, a large-diameter (16–22 mm) self-expanding stent is deployed entirely within the aortic true lumen taking care not to cover the renal or superior mesenteric artery origins. The stent should not be deployed through the fenestration tear, i.e. half in the true and half in the false lumen, which would greater complicate future transfemoral cardiopulmonary bypass or transfemoral access to the coronary arteries due to the shunting of blood into the false lumen through the stent. Note that compromise of the superior mesenteric artery should be treated before addressing compromise of the renal or iliac arteries.[5,10]

If there is evidence of static obstruction, branch vessel stenting should be attempted. (Figure 31-1A and B) A self-expanding bare stent is deployed under fluoroscopic and, in select cases, IVUS guidance. The stents are extended further into the aortic lumen (up to 5–10 mm) than is necessary when treating atherosclerotic stenoses.

Four studies in particular examining endovascular fenestration and stenting merit review. Patel et al. reported on 69 patients with complicated acute type B

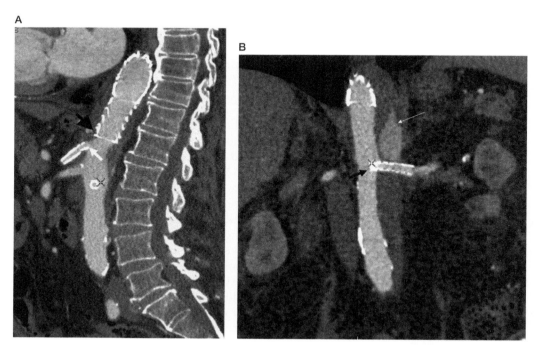

Figure 31-1. CT scan of a patient with a type B aortic dissection with **A**) a stent grafted celiac artery (white arrow) to seal a false lumen entry tear that had been covered proximally with a stent graft (black arrow). **B**) A stented left renal artery (black thick arrow) to treat a static dissection with malperfusion. The stent is placed in the aorta further than normal in an attempt to reach the true lumen. Note persistent flow in the false lumen of the dissection (thin white arrow).

dissection who underwent medical management along with fenestration and stenting at the University of Michigan.[13] The median time to intervention after onset of symptoms was one day. Multiple vascular beds were affected in 70% of patients by angiography for a total of 185 vascular beds at risk. Flow was successfully restored in 96% of these vascular beds. Stroke and paraplegia rates were 4.3% and 2.9% (2 patients), respectively. Both patients who suffered paraplegia had presented with paraparesis that was not improved following the procedure. Early mortality was 17% (12 patients) with 5 patients sustaining aortic rupture. All-cause mortality at mean follow up of 42 months was 36%.

Another study from the University of Michigan examined the outcomes of 165 patients presenting with aortic dissection, focusing on renal malperfusion.[14] This study included 56 patients with acute type A dissections, 59 with acute type B dissections, 19 with chronic type A dissections, and 31 with chronic type B dissections. Ninety patients were found to specifically have renal malperfusion. A total of 71 of these 90 patients underwent endovascular therapy to correct the renal malperfusion, including renal artery stenting, aortic fenestration and stenting. A total of 5 patients (7%) experienced procedure-related complications, all of which were minor. The 30-day mortality rate was 21% (15 patients), 3 of whom died of aortic rupture.

A study from Germany examined the role of endovascular fenestration and stenting to treat ischemia in 45 patients with aortic dissection.[15] Thirteen patients had type A dissections and 32 had type B. The study included both acute and chronic dissections. There were a total of 88 vascular beds compromised by the dissection: 33 involved the lower extremities, 25 the renal arteries, 22 the mesenteric vessels and 8 the spinal vessels. Three patients were able to be treated with stenting alone, while the other 42 underwent fenestration and stenting. The median duration of follow up was 37 months. Seven of the 25 patients with renal ischemia required dialysis, but all of the patients were able to be weaned off dialysis within three months following intervention. Two of the 8 patients (25%) with spinal cord ischemia did not have any improvement following intervention. The 30-day mortality rate was 6.7% (3 patients), with each of these three patients having acute dissections.

A study of long term outcomes following endovascular aortic fenestration of acute complicated aortic dissection reported on 20 patients with a mean follow up of 731 days.[16] Three patients had type A dissections who underwent surgical replacement of the ascending aorta prior to descending thoracic fenestration, while 17 had type B dissections. Branch vessel malperfusion improved in 18 of the patients (90%) following the procedure. Two patients showed partial thrombosis of the false lumen on follow up at 1 year. Two patients died within 30 days, for a mortality rate of 10%.

ENDOVASCULAR STENT-GRAFT THERAPY FOR ACUTE TYPE B DISSECTIONS

The first feasibility and safety trials of aortic stent-grafts for use the in the thoracic aorta began in 1992, with the primary goal of treating thoracic aortic aneurysms (TAAs). Since that time, several different companies have developed thoracic stent grafts for treatment of TAAs, with a number of stent grafts subsequently being FDA approved for this indication only. The concept of using an aortic stent graft to treat acute thoracic aortic dissection was first demonstrated by Dake and colleagues in 1999.[17] The rationale for using a stent-graft in this scenario is twofold. First, the stent-graft provides stability to the true lumen in the acute setting, preventing early rupture and in some cases relieving branch vessel obstruction (i.e. dynamic obstruction) without further intervention. (Figure 31–2) Second, covering the entry tear with a stent graft prevents blood flow into the false lumen, thereby allowing the true lumen to expand and promote thrombosis of the false lumen through stasis.[5] This theoretically helps to prevent late complications, such as dilation of the false lumen with possible aneurysm formation and rupture. Even if the false lumen does not completely thrombose, sheltering it from systemic systolic pressure may theoretically limit progression to aneurysmal dilatation.[17]

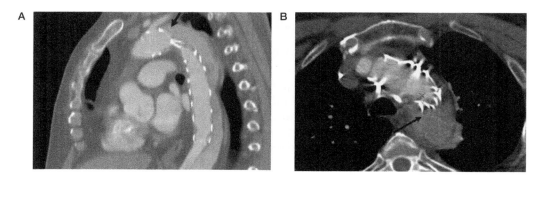

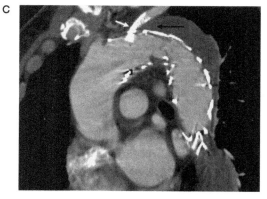

Figure 31-2. (**A**) CTA in a patient treated with a stent graft for an acute type B dissection who then developed a type 1A endoleak (dark arrow). (**B**) CTA 1 month latter showing diminished but persistent flow in the false lumen/aneurysm (dark arrow). (**C**) CTA following a laser fenestration and stent grafting (white arrow) of a proximal aortic cuff from the left subclavian artery. This approach sealed the type 1A endoleak (black arrow) and accelerated aneurysm shrinkage.

SINGLE CENTER STUDIES OF STENT-GRAFT THERAPY

In the initial report in 1999 by Dake and colleagues, aortic stent grafts were used to cover the entry tear in 15 patients with type B dissections, and in 4 patients with type A dissections with a primary entry tear in the descending thoracic aorta who suffered retrograde dissections (Table 31-1).[17] Stent-grafts were successfully placed in all 19 patients. There was complete thrombosis of the false lumen in 15 patients (79%) with partial thrombosis

TABLE 31-1. TRIALS OF STENT-GRAFT REPAIR OF COMPLICATED AND UNCOMPLICATED TYPE B AORTIC DISSECTIONS

Reference	No. of Patients	Type	Year	Technical Success (%)	Stroke (%)	Paraplegia (%)	30-day Mortality (%)
Dake[17]	19	4 type A	1999	100	0	0	16
		15 type B					
Leurs[21] (EUROSTAR/ UK)	131	7 type A	2004	89	1.5	0.8	8.4
		106 type B					
		18 N/A					
Bortone[36]	43	43 type B	2004	100	0	0	7
Dialetto[37]	28	28 type B	2005	100	0	0	10.7
Eggebrecht[38]	38	38 type B	2005	100	2.6	0	2.6
Eggebrecht[30] (meta-analysis)	609	24 type A	2006	98	1.9	0.8	5.3
		585 type B					
Song[2]	42	42 type B	2006	97	9.5	0	9.5
Xu[39]	63	63 type B	2006	95	1.6	0	3.2
Schoder[40]	28	28 type B	2007	86	0	3.6	10.7
Fattori[6]	66	66 type B	2008	N/A	3.4	1.5	10.6
Szeto[19]	35	35 type B	2008	97	2.8	2.8	2.8
Parker[31]	942	942 type B	2008	95	3.1	1.9	9
Kische[23]	180	9 type A	2009	98.3	3.9	2.8	5
		171 type B					
Cambria[22]	19	19 type B	2009	100	11	0	16
Nienaber[34] (INSTEAD Trial)	72	72 type B	2009	100	1.5	2.8	2.8
Feezor[18]	33	33 type B	2009	100	12	15	21
Zeeshan[20]	45	45 type B	2010	100	7	13	4
Zipfel[34]	91	76 type B	2011	95	2	4	8
VIRTUE[26]	100	100 type B	2011	98	8	2	8
White[2]	85	85 type B	2011	N/A	9.4	9.4	10.8
Ehrlich[24]	29	29 type B	2012	100	7	0	17
Lombardi[28]	40	40 type B	2012	100	7.5	2.5	5

in the other four. There were 3 deaths, all with complicated type B dissections, within the first 30 days following the procedure for an early mortality rate of 16%. However, there were no aneurysms, aortic ruptures, or deaths seen in the subsequent 13 months of follow up in the remaining patients. Additionally, there were no cases of paralysis. Thirty eight aortic branch vascular beds were ischemic due to the dissection in these 19 patients, with 28 of them being reperfused simply by covering the entry tear with a stent-graft. This study documented that the use of aortic stent-grafts to cover the entry tear in a dissection was feasible, suggesting further investigation of this concept was warranted.

A report from UCLA examined the use of the Medtronic AneuRx and Talent devices for the treatment of 42 patients with type B aortic dissections (Table 31-1).[2] There were 25 patients with acute dissections, and 17 with chronic dissections. All patients were ≥ASA class III. There were a total of 42 primary procedures and 18 secondary procedures. The risk of reintervention was four times higher in acute dissection compared to chronic, which was significantly different. Intravascular ultrasound (IVUS) was used in all cases to aid in placement of the endograft and to visualize the stagnation of blood flow in the false lumen following endograft placement. Technical success was achieved in 58 of the 60 procedures (97%). Thrombosis of the false lumen was seen in 61% of patients at 1 month and 88% at one year. Overall stroke rate was high at 9.5 % (4/42), with a procedural stroke rate of 6.7% (4/60). However, none of the patients developed paraplegia. A total of four patients developed a retrograde dissection following endograft placement, two after the primary procedure and two after a secondary procedure, requiring subsequent open repair with cardiopulmonary bypass. Three of these patients died and the fourth had an anoxic brain injury. The 30-day mortality for the entire group was 9.5% (n = 4), with an additional 5 late deaths, for an overall mortality rate of 21%.

A review of 33 patients with acute, complicated type B dissections treated with the Gore TAG device at the University of Florida from 2005–2007 revealed a 30-day mortality rate of 21% (Table 31.1).[18] The stroke rate was 12%, the spinal cord ischemia rate was 15% and there was a 76% major complication rate amongst all of the patients. Seventy-three percent of the patients who presented with malperfusion required branch vessel stenting in addition to aortic stent-graft placement. There was a 48% reintervention rate following endovascular repair and three patients required conversion to open repair due to persistent false lumen flow. Only 42% of the patients were discharged to home following an average of 17 days in the hospital, demonstrating the morbidity of the underlying pathology.

Szeto et al. from the University of Pennsylvania examined the use of stent-graft placement for the treatment of an acute, complicated type B dissection in 35 patients (Table 31.1). [19] Eighteen patients had evidence of rupture, while 17 had malperfusion. Technical success with coverage of the primary entry tear was achieved in 97% (34) of the patients. However, 12 patients (34%) required adjunct procedures, including bare metal stents in the infrarenal aorta, renal artery, celiac artery, or iliac artery. One patient suffered a stroke (2.8%), two patients (5.7%) had transient paraplegia, and one had permanent paraplegia (2.8%). The 30-day mortality rate was 2.8% (1 patient), while one-year survival was 93%.

In a subsequent study from the University of Pennsylvania, 77 patients with acute, complicated type B dissections between 2002 and 2010 were reviewed retrospectively. Forty-five patients underwent endovascular stent graft repair, 20 underwent open surgical repair, and 12 were treated with medical therapy alone.[20] The patients who had an endovascular repair had a 4% 30-day mortality compared to 40% for open surgical repair and 33% for medical therapy. This survival advantage for endovascular therapy persisted at 1, 3, and 5 years. There was a 7% stroke rate in the endovascular group, 17% in the medical therapy group, and none in the open surgical group. Paraplegia occurred in 13% of the TEVAR patients, 10% of the open patients, and 8% of the medical therapy only group. None of these differences reached statistical significance, particularly given the small numbers of patients in each group. Eighteen patients (40%) in the TEVAR group did require at least one adjunct procedure performed, most for visceral or ileofemoral stenting.

MULTI-CENTER STUDIES OF STENT-GRAFT THERAPY

The data from the European Collaborators on Stent Graft Techniques for the Thoracic Aortic Aneurysm and Dissection Repair (EUROSTAR) and the United Kingdom Thoracic Endograft registries was examined by Leurs et al. in 2004 (Table 31-1).[21] This review included 131 patients with acute aortic dissection over a 5 year period. There were 7 patients with a type A dissection, 106 with type B, and the classification was not available in 18. The descending thoracic aorta was involved in all patients. There was not a significant difference between the number of emergency and elective procedures performed, with 57% of patients having symptoms at the time of the procedure. Overall, there was an 89% primary technical success rate in stent grafting, with the others having incomplete coverage of the primary tear, persistent flow in the false lumen, no expansion of the true lumen, or endoleaks. One patient developed paraplegia (0.8%) and two had a stroke (1.5%). The 30-day mortality rate was 8.4%, without a significant difference between those undergoing elective versus emergency repair. The cumulative survival rate at 1 year was 90%.

A multicenter trial of the TAG device from Gore included 19 patients with acute complicated type B aortic dissections (Table 31-1).[22] Importantly, none of the patients suffered paraplegia. The 30 day mortality rate was 16% (3 patients), two of whom suffered a stroke, while one suffered aortic rupture. Seven patients had endoleaks following stent-grafting, with two requiring revisions. The one year mortality rate was 21%. False lumen thrombosis rate was not reported as a part of this study.

The Talent Thoracic Retrospective Registry, which includes data collected from 7 European referral centers, reported on 180 patients who received a Medtronic Talent stent graft for the treatment of aortic dissection (Table 31-1).[23] This group included 9 patients with type A dissection who had already undergone open ascending aortic repair and were being treated for a chronic "type B" dissection, and 171 patients with type B dissections, 29 of which were complicated. Overall, there was a 98% technical success rate in stent graft deployment. Stroke and paraplegia rates were 3.9% (7 patients) and 2.8% (5 patients), respectively. Paraplegia resolved in 2 of the 5 patients. Thirty-day mortality was 5% (9 patients), with an additional 11 late deaths. Overall survival was 95% at 30 days, 91% at 12 months, 91% at 24 months, and 82% at 36 months. The midterm results of the 29 patients who had complicated, acute type B dissections were recently published online (Table 31-1).[24] These patients had a hospital mortality of 17% with 6 late deaths. Two patients (7%) suffered a stroke and there were no cases of paraplegia. The survival at 1 year was 79% and was 61% at 5 years.

The RESTORE registry looked at the Bolton Relay stent-graft in patients with both type A and B dissections; however, most (84%) of the patients had type B dissections (Table 31-1).[25] Of the 76 patients with type B dissections, 30 were acute. There was a 93%

technical success rate in the patients with type B dissections. The 30-day mortality rate was 13% and the paraplegia rate 7% in the patients with acute type B dissections. There were 2 patients who suffered stroke, but the details of their aortic pathology are not given.

The VIRTUE registry enrolled 100 patients in Europe with both acute and chronic type B dissection who undergo repair with the Medtronic Valiant stent graft and the early results were recently reported (Table 31-1).[26] Fifty patients had an acute dissection, all of which were complicated. The technical success rate in the acute group was 98%. The 30-day mortality was 8%, the stroke rate 8%, and the paraplegia rate 2% in this group. There were no early deaths in the sub-acute and chronic dissection groups. There was only 1 case of paraplegia (3.8%) in the chronic dissection group, with no complications in the sub-acute group.

The Society for Vascular Surgery Outcomes Committee recently reported on the results of five investigator sponsored investigational device exemption clinical trials using endovascular stent grafts to treat acute, complicated, type B aortic dissection (Table 31-1).[27] Eighty-five patients were included. The stroke and paralysis rates were both 9.4%. The 30-day mortality was 10.8%, with a 1 year mortality of 29.4%.

Finally, the Study of Thoracic Aortic Type B Dissection Using Endoluminal Repair (STABLE) trial examined a unique device for the treatment of for the treatment of complicated type B dissection (Table 31-1).[28] This device consisted of a proximal TX2 endograft and a distal bare metal stent (Zenith Dissection Endovascular System) made by Cook. A total of 40 patients were enrolled across 10 centers. Twenty-four patients had acute dissection, 6 sub-acute, and 10 chronic dissections. The average time to treatment from the onset of symptoms was 20 days for the entire group. There was a 100% technical success rate with a 5% 30-day mortality rate. There was a 7.5% stroke rate and a 2.5% paraplegia rate. The one-year survival rate was 90%.

OPEN SURGERY VS. ENDOVASCULAR TREATMENT-COMPARISONS FROM IRAD

In 2006, IRAD investigators examined long-term survival in patients who presented with an acute type B dissection between 1996 and 2003.[29] A total of 242 patients were included with a mean follow-up time of 2.3 years. All patients had aggressive medical therapy. Twenty six (11%) also had open surgical intervention, while 27 (11%) received endovascular treatment. All of those who underwent further treatment had symptoms of ischemia or refractory pain. In-hospital mortality rate was 29% for surgical intervention, 11% for endovascular therapy, and 10% for medical management alone. The unadjusted survival rate at 1 and 3 years for those patients discharged alive from the hospital was 96% and 83% for surgery, 89% and 76% for endovascular treatment, and 90% and 78% for those patients treated with medical therapy alone. Thus, the mortality of an acute type B aortic dissection is relatively high, with almost 25% of patients dying within 3 years following discharge from the hospital, regardless of the initial therapy they received.

The IRAD investigators reported in 2008 on 66 patients who underwent endovascular treatment of acute type B dissections, including both fenestration and stenting along with stent-graft placement, in addition to aggressive medical management (Table 31–1).[6] These patients were compared to 59 patients who underwent open surgical treatment and 390 who were managed medically. A total of 43 patients had a stent-graft placed and 23 underwent endovascular fenestration. The patients who underwent endovascular therapy were significantly younger (58.8 years) than those undergoing open surgery (61.9 years) or who had medical management (65.5 years). The in-hospital complication rate was 21% in the endovascular group, compared to 40% in those undergoing open surgical treatment, which was also significantly different (p = 0.04). Stroke occurred in 2 patients (3.4%) in the endovascular group, compared to 4 (9.1%) in the surgical group. One patient suffered paraplegia in the endovascular group (1.5%) compared to 3 (5.1%) in the open repair group. The in-hospital mortality was also higher in the surgery group at 34%, compared to 11% in the endovascular group, which was significantly different (p = 0.002). The mortality rate for the group who received medical treatment alone was 8.7%.

META-ANALYSES OF ENDOVASCULAR STENT-GRAFT THERAPY

A meta-analysis published by Eggebrect et al. reflects the early cumulative experience with the use of stent grafts in the treatment of aortic dissection (Table 31-1).[30] This analysis included 39 studies published between January 1999 and May 2004, with a total of 609 patients. All studies included greater than 3 patients. All patients had an entry tear in the descending aorta, with 4% having a retrograde type A dissection and 96% with a type B dissection. There were 248 acute dissections from the data available. Technical success in endograft placement was achieved in 98% of patients, with 2.3% being converted to an open procedure at some point during their hospital stay. A total of 14% of patients had in-hospital complications, including 1.9% with retrograde extension of the dissection and 2.9% with neurologic complications. Of those who had neurologic complications, paraplegia occurred in 0.8% of patients and stroke in 1.9%. The in-hospital complication rate was higher in those undergoing stent-graft placement for acute dissection (22%) compared to chronic dissection (9%) (p = 0.005). Overall in-hospital mortality rate was 5.2%, with one death occurring after discharge, but within 30 days, giving a 30-day mortality rate of 5.3%. At a mean follow up of 19.5 months, 12% of patients required reintervention, with 2.5% undergoing open surgical intervention. The false lumen thrombosis rate was 76%. Overall survival was 93% at 30 days, 91% at 6 months, 90% at 1 year, and 89% at 2 years.[30]

A second meta-analysis encompassing the literature from 1997 to 2007 was recently conducted (Table 31-1).[31] This analysis included 29 studies, all of which reported on at least 10 patients, for a total of 942 patients. A technical success rate of 95% was achieved for all of the cases, and the conversion rate to open surgery was 0.6%. Stroke was the most common major complication, occurring in 3.1% of patients. Paraplegia occurred in 1.9%. Endovascular re-intervention was required in 7.6% of patients, and open surgical intervention was necessary in 2.8%. In-hospital mortality rate was 9%, while follow up at 20 months revealed a mortality rate of 12%.

A recent meta-analysis compared endovascular stent graft placement to open surgery for the treatment of acute type B aortic dissection.[32] The analysis only looked at controlled trials that compared endovascular to open repair. A total of 5 trials were ultimately analyzed which included 318 patients. The 30-day mortality was 11% for the TEVAR patients, and 35% for those undergoing open repair, a significant difference. The paraplegia rate was 8.6% in the endovascular group and 6.9% in the open group (p = not significant). Similarly, there was not a difference between the groups in the rates of stroke, renal failure, myocardial infarction, respiratory failure, bowel ischemia, or lower limb ischemia.

CHOICE OF ENDOVASCULAR FENESTRATION AND STENTING VS. ENDOGRAFT FOR ACUTE COMPLICATED DISSECTIONS

Efficacious treatment of acute complicated aortic dissection requires accurate anatomical knowledge of the aorta, branch arteries, limb and organ perfusion, and nature of the complication. In most cases this is provided by CTA, supplemented during the endovascular treatment procedure by fluoroscopy and intravascular ultrasound. In the setting of acute complicated dissection, fenestration and stenting ("fen-sten") is limited to treating malperfusion, but otherwise has broad anatomical application. It is appropriate for treating malperfusion accompanying type A, as well as type B dissections in certain settings. The fen-sten procedure is technically demanding and, if one is meticulous about documenting pressure gradients and examining peripheral arterial beds, time consuming.

Endografts have broader indications for use; they are indicated for impending rupture due to an unstable or leaking false lumen, as well as for malperfusion. However, currently available endografts have somewhat severe anatomical constraints, reflected by trial-protocol requirements of robust landing zones and uncertain knowledge about anatomical predispositions to device-complications, such as retrograde dissections.

In summary, fen-sten has narrow clinical indications, but broad anatomical applicability, whereas stent-grafts have broad clinical indications, but narrow anatomical applicability (Table 31-2). The choice of therapy for a given patient with complicated aortic dissection therefore depends on the nature of the complication and the individual patient's aortic and branch artery anatomy. Whatever the treatment choice, primary aortic treatment by fen-sten or stent-grafting, it should followed by evaluation of limb and distal organ perfusion.

STENT-GRAFTS FOR UNCOMPLICATED CHRONIC TYPE B DISSECTIONS

Given the relative success in the use of stent-grafts for acute dissection, further investigations have been conducted to examine the use of endografts in chronic dissections to prevent the late complication of aneurysm development and rupture. A single center report

TABLE 31-2. COMPARISON OF PERCUTANEOUS TREATMENTS OF AORTIC DISSECTION

	ENDOGRAFT VS FENESTRATION	
	ENDOGRAFT	FENESTRATION
INDICATION	COMPLICATED AD	MALPERFUSION
TECHNIQUE	SIMPLE	COMPLEX
TIME TO COMPLETION	SHORT	LONG
ANATOMICAL APPLICABILITY	<50%	NEARLY 100%
FATE OF FALSE LUMEN	VARIABLE	PERSISTS

AD = Aortic Dissection

Adapted from Table 16.4 in Williams, DM. "Aortic dissection: role of fenestration and stents in the endograft era" in Advanced Endovascular Therapy of Aortic Disease. Lumsden AB, Lin PH, Chen C, Parodi JC, eds. Malden, MA: Blackwell Futura, 2007.

This chapter was partially adopted from a review article: DiMusto PD, Williams DM, Patel HJ, Trimarchi S, Eliason JL, Upchurch GR Jr. Endovascular management of type B aortic dissections. J Vasc Surg. 2010 Oct;52(4 Suppl):26S-36S.

from the Cleveland Clinic with intermediate and long term outcomes after the use of the Cook Zenith TX1 and TX2 devices included 25 patients with chronic dissections with aneurysm formation.[33] The one year survival rate was 92% and the 5-year survival rate 88%. The secondary intervention rate was 12% at one year and 21% at 5 years. None of the devices migrated, which was a problem in patients treated with other aortic pathologies. The stroke and paraplegia rate was not reported separately for patients with aortic dissections.

The INSTEAD trial[34] randomized 140 patients with uncomplicated chronic (occurring 2 to 52 weeks before randomization) type B aortic dissections to endovascular stent-graft repair plus medical management versus medical management alone (Table 31.1). The analysis was done on an intention-to-treat basis. Seventy two patients were randomized to the endovascular group, with one death before intervention and one patient opting for medical management. Sixty eight patients were initially randomized to medical management alone, with two opting for endovascular stent-grafting. Technical success was achieved in all 70 patients who underwent endograft placement without a need for conversion to an open procedure. In the medical management group, 16% eventually required endovascular repair and 4.4% open repair of the aorta for aneurysmal dilatation greater than 6 cm. Two patients (2.8%) in the endovascular group developed paraplegia with one in the medical group (1.5%). One patient in the endovascular group also had a stroke for a stroke rate of 1.5%. Complete false lumen thrombosis was seen in 91% of the patients in the endovascular group. Two year survival was 89% in the endovascular group and 96% in the medical management group with no significant differences between the two groups. However, because the death rate was lower than expected, the study did not achieve statistical power. Further studies of this issue need to be conducted, but based on these results, the authors recommend reserving endovascular intervention for those patients who develop late complications after initial medical management.

FUTURE DIRECTIONS

Aortic stent-grafts for the thoracic aorta were initially developed to treat thoracic aortic aneurysms, which currently remains the only FDA approved indication. Their use to treat aortic dissections is relatively new. As manufacturers are developing dedicated devices tailored to this use, they will likely become less rigid and more flexible, reducing some of the problems with stent-graft migration and collapse.[33] Additionally, the development and use of branched thoracic endografts will allow their use in the aortic arch, particularly to treat left subclavian artery (LSA) involvement. The Society for Vascular Surgery guidelines currently recommend preoperative revascularization for patients whose anatomy requires covering the LSA with an endograft, unless the procedure is done emergently, in which case selective revascularization of the LSA is suggested.[35] Clearly, backflow from the LSA can cause an endoleak, and a branched endograft would eliminate the need for carotid-subclavian bypass.

SUMMARY

The optimal treatment of aortic dissections remains a challenging clinical dilemma. The treatment of type B aortic dissections, particularly those presenting with malperfusion, remains controversial despite recent unbridled enthusiasm in favor of stent-grafting. Open aortic fenestration and repair carries a high mortality rate, in addition to a high stroke and paraplegia rate. Endovascular fenestration and stenting represents a less invasive treatment option to restore perfusion to end organs compared to open surgical repair. However, the 30-day mortality rate remains high. This treatment also does not address the late complication of aneurysmal dilation requiring aortic repair to prevent rupture.

The concept of using aortic stent grafts to treat type B dissections is relatively new and continues to evolve as experience with this technique grows and technology improves. Device manufacturers continue to develop new endovascular devices specifically designed to treat aortic dissection and multi-center trials examining these devices are underway. In theory, treatment of a type B dissection with a stent graft not only treats the dynamic malperfusion created by the dissection, but also prevents late aneurysm degeneration. Based on these data, both endovascular fenestration and stenting, as well as stent-grafting, have a lower morbidity and mortality rate than open surgical repair, and appear to have complimentary roles in the treatment of this complex aortic pathology. The role of stent-grafting will likely expand given the familiarity with the procedure as more devices made specifically to treat aortic dissection are developed and enter clinical practice.

REFERENCES

1. Hiratzka L, Bakris G, Beckman J, et al. 2010 ACCF/AHA/AATS/ACR/ASA/SCA/SCAI/SIR/STS/SVM Guidelines for the Diagnosis and Management of Patients with Thoracic Aortic Disease. *Circulation.* 2010;121:e266–e369.
2. Song T, Donayre C, Walot I, et al. Endograft exclusion of acute and chronic descending thoracic aortic dissections. *J Vasc Surg.* 2006;43:247–258.
3. Nienaber C and Eagle K. Aortic dissection: new frontiers in diagnosis and management: part I: from etiology to diagnostic strategies. *Circulation.* 2003;108:628–635.
4. Tang D and Dake M. TEAR for acute uncomplicated aortic dissection: Immediate repair versus medical therapy. *Semin Vasc Surg.* 2009;22:145–151.
5. Swee W and Dake M. Endovascular Management of Thoracic Dissections. *Circulation.* 2008;117:1460–1473.
6. Fattori R, Tsai T, Myrmel T, et al. Complicated Acute Type B Dissection: Is surgery still the best option?: A report for the International Registry of Acute Aortic Dissection. *J Am Coll Cardiol Intv.* 2008;1:395–402.
7. Wheat Jr M. Acute Dissection of the Aorta. *Cardiovasc Clin.* 1987;17:241–262.
8. Doroghazi R, Slater E, DeSanctis R, et al. Long-terms survival of patients with treated aortic dissection. *J Am Coll Cardiol.* 1984;3:1026–1034.
9. Trimarchi S, Nienaber C, Rampoldi V, et al. Role and results of surgery in acute type B dissection: Insights from the International Registry of Acute Aortic Dissection (IRAD). *Circulation.* 2006;114:I357–I364.
10. Williams D, Lee D, Hamilton B, et al. The dissected aorta: percutaneous management of ischemic complications with endovascular stents and balloon fenestration. *J Vasc Interv Radiol.* 1997;8:605–625.
11. Erbel R, Oelert H, Meyer J, et al. Effect of medical and surgical therapy on aortic dissection evaluated by transesophageal echocardiography: implications for prognosis and therapy. *Circulation.* 1993;87:1604–1615.
12. Williams D, Lee D, Hamilton B, et al. The dissected aorta: part III. Anatomy and radiologic diagnosis of branch-vessel compromise. *Radiology.* 1997;203:37–44.
13. Patel H, Williams D, Meekov M, et al. Long-term results of percutaneous management of malperfusion in acute type B aortic dissection: implications for thoracic aortic endovascular repair. *J Thorac Cardiovasc Surg.* 2009;138:300–308.

14. Barnes D, Williams D, Daskia N, et al. A single-center experience treating renal malperfusion after aortic dissection with central aortic fenestration and stenting. *J Vasc Surg*. 2008;47:903–911.
15. Chavan A, Rosenthal H, Luthe L, et al. Percutaneous interventions for treating ischemic complications of aortic dissection. *Eur Radiol*. 2009;19:488–494.
16. Park K, Do Y, Kim S, et al. Endovascular treatment of acute complicated aortic dissection: Long-term follow-up of clinical outcomes and CT findings. *J Vasc Interv Radiol*. 2009;20:334–341.
17. Dake M, Kato N, Mitchell R, et al. Endovascular stent-graft placement for the treatment of acute aortic dissections. *N Engl J Med*. 1999;340:1546–1552.
18. Feezor R, Martin T, Hess P, et al. Early outcomes after endovasculat management of acute, complicated type B aortic dissection. *J Vasc Surg*. 2009;49:561–567.
19. Szeto W, McGarvey M, Pochettino A, et al. Results of a new surgical paradigm: Endovascular repair for acute complicated type B aortic dissection. *Ann Thorac Surg*. 2008;86:87–94.
20. Zeeshan A, Woo E, Bavaria J, et al. Thoracic endovascular aortic repair for acute complicated type B aortic dissection: Superiority relative to conventional open surgical and medical therapy. *J Thorac Cardiovasc Surg*. 2010;140:S109–115.
21. Leurs L, Bell R, Degrieck Y, et al. Endovascular treatment of thoracic aortic disease: Combined experience from the EUROSTAR and United Kingdom Thoracic Endograft registries. *J Vasc Surg*. 2004;40:670–680.
22. Cambria R, Crawford R, Cho J, et al. A multicenter clinical trial of endovascular stent graft repair of acute catastrophes of the descending thoracic aorta. *J Vasc Surg*. 2009;50:1255–1264.
23. Kische S, Ehrlick M, Nienaber C, et al. Endovascular treatment of acute and chronic aortic dissection: midterm results from the Talent Thoracic Retrospecitve Registry. *J Thorac Cardiovasc Surg*. 2009;138:115–124.
24. Ehrlich M, Rousseau H, Heijmen R, et al. Midterm results after endovascular treatment of acute, complicated type B aortic dissection: The Talent thoracic registry. *J Thorac Cardiovasc Surg*. 2012; In press.
25. Zipfel B, Czerney M, Funovics M, et al. Endovascular treatment of patients with types A and B thoracic aortic dissection using Relay thoracic stent grafts: Results from the RESTORE patient registry. *J Endovasc Ther*. 2011;18:131–143.
26. Investigators V. The VIRTUE registry of type B thoracic dissections—study design and early results. *Eur J Vasc Endovasc Surg*. 2011;41:159–166.
27. White R, Miller D, Criado F, et al. Report on the results of thoracic endovascular aortic repair for acute, complicated, type B aortic dissection at 30 days and 1 year from a multidisciplinary subcommittee of the Society for Vascular Surgery Outcomes Committee. *J Vasc Surg*. 2011;53:1082–1090.
28. Lombardi J, Cambria R, Nienaber C, et al. Prospective multicenter clinical trial (STABLE) on the endovascular treatment of complicated type B aortic dissection using a composite device design. *J Vasc Surg*. 2012;55:629–640.
29. Tsai T, Fattori R, Trimarchi S, et al. Long-term survival in patients presenting with type B acute aortic dissection: insights from the International Registry of Acute Aortic Dissection. *Circulation*. 2006;114:2226–2231.
30. Eggebrect H, Nienaber C, Neuhauser M, et al. Endovascular stent-graft placement in aortic dissection: a meta-analysis. *Eur Heart J*. 2006;27:489–498.
31. Parker J and Golledge J. Outcome of endovascular treatment of acute type B aortic dissection. *Ann Thorac Surg*. 2008;86:1707–1712.
32. Hao Z, Zhi-Wei W, Zhen Z, et al. Endovascular stent-graft placement or open surgery for the treatment of acute type B aortic dissection: A meta-analysis. *Ann Vasc Surg*. 2012;26:454–461.
33. Morales J, Greenberg R, Morales C, et al. Thoracic aortic lesions treated with the Zenith TX1 and TX2 thoracic devices: Intermediate and long-term outcomes. *J Vasc Surg*. 2008;48:54–63.

34. Nienaber C, Rousseau H, Eggebrect H, et al. Randomized comparision of strategies for type B aoric dissection; The INvestigation of STEnt Grafts in Aortic Dissection (INSTEAD) trial. *Circulation.* 2009;120:2519–2528.

35. Matsumura J, Lee W, Mitchell R, et al. The Society for Vascular Surgery pracice guidelines: Management of the left subclavian artery with thoracic endovascular aortic repair. *J Vasc Surg.* 2009;50:1155–1158.

36. Bortone A, De Cillis E, D'Agostino D, et al. Endovascular treatment of thoracic aortic disease—Four years of experience. *Circulation.* 2004;110:II-262–II-267.

37. Dialetto G, Covino F, Scognamiglio G, et al. Treatment of type B aortic dissection: endoluminal repair or conventional medical therapy? *Eur J Cardiothorac Surg.* 2005;27:826–830.

38. Eggebrect H, Herold U, Kuhnt O, et al. Endovascular stent-graft treatment of aortic dissection: determinants of post-interventional outcome. *Eur Heart J.* 2005;26:489–497.

39. Xu S, Huang F, Yang J, et al. Endovascular repair of acute type B aortic dissection: Early and mid-term results. *J Vasc Surg.* 2006;43:1090–1095.

40. Schoder M, Czerney M, Cejna M, et al. Endovascular repair of acute type B aortic dissection: Long-term follow-up of true and false lumen diameter changes. *Ann Thorac Surg.* 2007;83:1059–1066.

32

Simultaneous TEVAR and EVAR

Benjamin J. Herdrich, MD and Edward Y. Woo, MD

SCOPE OF THE PROBLEM: MULTILEVEL AORTIC ANEURYSMAL DISEASE

Disease of the aorta often occurs in multiple segments simultaneously. This was demonstrated by Crawford and Cohen in a review of 1,510 patients treated for aortic aneurysms between 1956 and 1982.[1] 9.1% of all patients had simultaneous multilevel disease, and considering that this study was done at a time when CT was not routinely available or widely used, that number may be an underestimate. Furthermore, they demonstrated that greater than 50% of patients with thoracic aortic aneurysms (TAA) have multilevel disease, and 12% of patients with abdominal aortic aneurysms (AAA) have TAA. Other studies have confirmed that there is a high incidence of concomitant multilevel aneurysmal disease, and this is likely a reflection of the fact that risk factors for aneurysm and other aortic disease, such as smoking, hypertension, hyperlipidemia, coronary artery disease, and genetic predisposition, can affect the aorta in its entirety.[2,3]

Different treatment strategies for patients with multilevel aortic disease exist, including a single-stage strategy where all areas of disease are addressed at one time and a multi-staged strategy where individual segments of diseased aorta are addressed separately with a recovery period between procedures. Traditionally, open surgical replacement of the affected aortic segment has been used in either a single-staged or multi-staged approach.[1,4] However, since the development of endovascular aortic repair (EVAR) and thoracic endovascular aortic repair (TEVAR), endografting has been used either alone or in combination with open surgery.[5-9] The optimal approach to patients with multilevel aortic disease is still controversial, but there are some important principles that can help to guide care.

The major risk associated with a multi-staged strategy is the potential for rupture of the untreated aneurysm prior to repair. This may occur during the normal interval between procedures or because patients become fearful and do not return for the subsequent staged procedure(s). Rupture of the untreated aneurysm may occur in the early or late post-operative periods and has been reported in as many as 24% of patients following an operation that leaves an untreated aneurysm.[1,4,9–11] Simultaneous repair of all aortic pathology has the benefit of decreasing the risk of rupture. Crawford and Cohen reported a significant survival benefit in patients treated with a single-staged procedure addressing all aortic pathology as opposed to a multi-staged approach, which prompted them to recommend that good risk patients be treated with simultaneous resection of all aortic aneurysmal disease.[1]

The major risk associated with the single-staged approach is the potential for added morbidity and mortality associated with a more complex procedure when all aortic disease is addressed simultaneously. Complications observed after these procedures may include respiratory failure, myocardial infarction, reoperation for bleeding, renal failure with or without the need for dialysis, spinal cord ischemia, stroke, sepsis, bowel obstruction, and venous thromboembolus. Gloviczki and colleagues demonstrated that 1/3 of patients died when they were treated with an open single-staged procedure to address multiple aortic aneurysms compared with a 4.4% mortality associated with a first stage procedure addressing only a single diseased segment.[4] Long-term mortality was not significantly different between the single and multi-staged approaches, and the authors generally favored a multi-staged strategy.

EVAR and TEVAR have become the preferred methods of treating aortic aneurysms in the abdominal and descending thoracic aorta. They have allowed for treatment of aortic aneurysms with decreased morbidity and peri-operative mortality. Although the experience using TEVAR and EVAR for patients with multiple aortic aneurysms is much less robust, they have the potential to decrease the morbidity and mortality associated with treating these patients. Moon et al. reported a hybrid approach to patients with abdominal and descending thoracic aortic aneurysms in which the AAA was treated with an open operation, and the TAA was treated with a TEVAR done at the same time.[5] 18 patients were treated in this fashion with an in hospital mortality of 6%, and no additional procedures were needed. Utilization of an endovascular approach appeared to decrease the mortality of a simultaneous procedure and eliminate the risk of rupture seen with a multi-staged approached.

A completely endovascular approach is now possible for these patients and has been described.[6–9] The experience with simultaneous TEVAR and EVAR is relatively limited but overall has been successful at treating both the abdominal and descending thoracic aorta at one time. A staged approach utilizing TEVAR and EVAR theoretically should also mitigate the risk of rupture of the untreated aneurysm between stages because with a quicker recovery time, the second stage should be completed sooner. There is no clear single best approach to patients with concomitant AAA and TAA, but simultaneous TEVAR and EVAR does currently offer a treatment advantage in a certain clinical situations. As the experience with simultaneous TEVAR and EVAR evolves, the indications will also likely evolve.

INDICATIONS FOR SIMULTANEOUS TEVAR AND EVAR

Assuming that a patient has concomitant AAA and TAA that are both anatomically amenable to endovascular repair, there are four major indications for simultaneous TEVAR and EVAR: (1) simultaneous symptomatic or ruptured aortic pathology in the thoracic and abdominal aortic segments, (2) poor iliac access, (3) the need for subsequent lifesaving procedures, and (4) the need to minimize the number of anesthetics.

In patients with concomitant AAA and TAA presenting with back pain, it can often be unclear which aneurysm is the symptomatic one (i.e. the etiology of the pain), and therefore, which one needs more urgent treatment. For these patients, a staged approach runs the risk of leaving a symptomatic aortic aneurysm untreated for a period of time at which it is at risk for rupture. Therefore, simultaneous treatment in these patients has a clear advantage and should be considered. This indication can also be extended to any patients with concomitant AAA and TAA who are high risk of rupture of both due to large size, uncontrollable hypertension, or radiographic findings suggesting impending rupture.

Poor iliac access is a major challenge in many patients with aneurysmal disease. Repeated instrumentation of the iliac arteries with large sheaths runs the risk of increased access complications. Some patients with poor access require adjunctive procedures for the delivery of the stent graft into the aorta which may include direct iliac artery access, a surgical conduit, iliac angioplasty, or iliac stenting. For these patients with poor iliac access, a simultaneous procedure minimizes the number of times diseased iliac arteries are instrumented and should decrease the risk of access complications, such as iliac rupture or lower extremity ischemia. In addition, one procedure may prevent another in terms of access. For example, the iliac limbs with EVAR may circumvent the ability to access the common iliac arteries for TEVAR.

It is not unusual for AAA or TAA to be discovered incidentally as part of a work-up for another disease. These patients may need treatment of their aortic aneurysms prior to definitive treatment for a malignancy or other life threatening condition. In this clinical situation, a staged approach would delay definitive treatment of a concurrent disease process. Simultaneous TEVAR and EVAR are indicated as they will minimize the recovery time and allow for treatment of concurrent pathologies in the most expeditious fashion.

Patients with aneurysmal disease often have a number of chronic comorbid conditions making them high risk for a general anesthetic. This may include patients with severe COPD at risk for ventilator dependence or patients with severe cardiac disease at risk for cardiac complications. Simultaneous TEVAR and EVAR have the benefit of minimizing the number of general anesthetics that the patient must undergo and should be considered in these situations.

TECHNICAL CONSIDERATIONS

There are a number of technical considerations that should be discussed in relation to simultaneous TEVAR and EVAR.

Preoperative preparations should focus on minimizing the risk of complications associated with the procedure. For elective indications, patients should undergo a full cardiovascular work-up as a high percentage of these patients have associated coronary artery disease. Our recommended preoperative work-up includes a stress test, echocardiogram, and carotid duplex. Any abnormalities may need to be addressed prior to treating the aortic aneurysms.

Patients undergoing TEVAR also have a risk of spinal cord ischemia that is on the order of 3–5% with risk factors that may elevate these risks.[12,13] To mitigate the risk of spinal cord ischemia, in elective cases, we recommend that a spinal drain should be placed preoperatively with initiation of a spinal drainage protocol should signs of spinal cord ischemia become evident either intraoperatively or post-operatively.[14] Intraoperative neurologic monitoring should be performed with somatosensory evoked potentials (SSEP) and/or motor evoked potentials (MEP). If patients show signs of spinal cord ischemia on intraoperative neuromonitoring, MAP augmentation and spinal drainage can be used to optimize spinal cord perfusion.[15] Furthermore, the response to treatment can be assessed by continued SSEP and MEP monitoring if clinical exam is unable to be performed. For emergent cases it is usually best to expedite the operation and reserve spinal drainage for patients who become symptomatic in the post-operative period as time may not allow for this to be done preoperatively.

In the conduct of the operation, we generally recommend that TEVAR be done first. This prevents the need to advance the thoracic stent graft delivery system through a freshly deployed abdominal stent graft and risk displacing the abdominal graft. Displacement of an abdominal stent graft in this fashion has the potential to create an endoleak or lead to coverage of a renal artery orifice. The second advantage of doing the TEVAR portion of the procedure first is that if the patient should develop signs of spinal cord ischemia after deployment of the thoracic stent graft, it can be treated before proceeding with the EVAR. In these instances, the collateral flow to the spinal cord from the lumbar arteries may be important. This may require ending the procedure after the TEVAR, if possible, and doing the EVAR in a staged fashion once the patient has recovered and there has been time for collateral flow to develop to the spinal cord. Access issues may also benefit from performing TEVAR first. The thoracic devices typically are larger and if retroperitoneal access to the iliac arteries is required, it is best done prior to placing the EVAR limbs. While it is our general approach to do the TEVAR first, there may be instances where it is advantageous to reverse the order and do the EVAR first. This needs to be individualized to the patient's clinical situation.

When both the thoracic and abdominal aorta are treated with stent grafts, the internal iliac arteries may be an important source of collateral flow to the spinal cord. Therefore, when performing a simultaneous TEVAR and EVAR, it is advantageous to preserve flow to the internal iliac arteries whenever possible. If the common iliac arteries are ectatic, techniques such as the bell-bottom technique, the sandwich/snorkeling technique, branched iliac stent grafting or external to internal iliac artery bypass are options that may be considered. Internal iliac embolization and coverage has been done in the setting of simultaneous TEVAR and EVAR in a single patient without complications, but this should only be done with the realization that it may increase the risk of spinal cord ischemia.[6]

Depending on the complexity of the anatomy, simultaneous TEVAR and EVAR has required contrast volumes ranging from 100–290 mL of non-ionic contrast.[7,9] While only 1/13 patients reported has suffered from post-operative renal failure, care should be taken to minimize the chances of contrast induced nephropathy. Patients should be adequately hydrated in the perioperative period. Infusion of sodium bicarbonate and the administration of n-acetylcysteine should be considered to minimize the risk to the kidneys. Intraoperatively, care should be taken to minimize the contrast usage especially if the patient has baseline renal insufficiency. Contrast can be diluted to half-strength, and the minimum volume needed should be used. Finally, utilization of intravascular ultrasound can be especially useful in minimizing contrast load.

OUTCOMES

There are only 15 reported cases of simultaneous TEVAR and EVAR in the literature, and full outcome data is reported for only 13 of these patients.[6–9] (Table 32-1) Even though the reported experience with simultaneous TEVAR and EVAR is relatively limited, the outcomes thus far have been encouraging. Follow-up for these 13 patients is an average of 19.0 months. The overall average procedure time is 157 minutes with a technical success rate of 100%. Average EBL is 255 mL. The average length of stay for all patients is 7.7 days. There is a 0% in hospital mortality and a 7.7% late mortality which was due to a type I endoleak and TAA rupture at 32 months in a single patient. Only 1/13 (7.7%) patients experienced symptoms of spinal cord ischemia, and they resolved with blood pressure augmentation.[6] No patient has been reported to have permanent neurological deficits. 1/13 (7.7%) patients developed post-operative renal failure, and no patient required dialysis. 2/13 (15.4%) patients developed endoleaks. One patient had a type II endoleak that was successfully coil embolized, and one patient developed a type I endoleak of the thoracic stent graft which led to TAA rupture.

TABLE 32-1. RESULTS FROM PUBLISHED CASE REPORTS OR SERIES OF SIMULTANEOUS TEVAR AND EVAR

	n	Procedure time (min)	EBL	Hospital LOS (days)	In hospital Mortality	Late Mortality	Spinal cord ischemia	Endoleaks	Follow-up (months)
Kirkwood et al.	8	173	325	8	0/8	0/8	1/8	1/8, Type II	20.3
Castelli et al.	4	94	105	8	0/4	1/4	0/4	1/4, Type I	16.5
Meguid et al.	1	285	300	4	0/1	0/1	0/1	0/1	18
Total	13	157	255	7.7	0% (0/13)	7.7% (1/13)	7.7% (1/13)	15.4% (2/13)	19.0

CONCLUSIONS

Patients with concomitant AAA and TAA would be best served with an approach that minimizes the risk of rupture of both aneurysms and minimizes the operative risk. Based on these criteria, the outcomes in a limited number of patients undergoing simultaneous TEVAR and EVAR have been very promising. The perioperative mortality of 0% for patients undergoing simultaneous TEVAR and EVAR compares very favorably to the perioperative mortality seen in simultaneous open repair which ranges from 14%–33% and that seen with simultaneous hybrid repair (6%).[1,4,5] The 7.7% risk of rupture following simultaneous TEVAR and EVAR also compares favorably against the risk of rupture reported for simultaneous open repair (5.2%) and staged open repairs (7.3–24%).[1,4] Furthermore, there is a low rate of spinal cord ischemia and renal failure and an average hospital LOS <8 days. Given the limited experience with simultaneous TEVAR and EVAR and the concern for increased complications with the increased complexity of a single-staged approach, the current indications are limited to simultaneous symptomatic abdominal and thoracic aortic pathology, patients with poor iliac access, the need for subsequent lifesaving procedures, and the need to minimize anesthetics. However, if more experience with simultaneous TEVAR and EVAR is gained, and the safety profile of the approach is maintained, the indications may be expanded to a greater number of patients with concomitant abdominal and thoracic aortic pathology requiring intervention.

REFERENCES

1. Crawford ES, Cohen ES. Aortic aneurysm: a multifocal disease. Presidential address. *Arch Surg.* 1982;117:1393–1400.
2. Bickerstaff LK, Pairolero PC, Hollier LH, et al. Thoracic aortic aneurysms: a population-based study. *Surgery.* 1982;92:1103–1108.
3. Pressler V, McNamara JJ. Aneurysm of the thoracic aorta. Review of 260cases. *J Thorac Cardiovasc Surg.* 1985;89:50–54.
4. Gloviczki P, Pairolero P, Welch T, et al. Multiple aortic aneurysms: the results of surgical management. *J Vasc Surg.* 1990;11:19–28.
5. Moon MR, Mitchell RS, Dake MD, et al. Simultaneous abdominal aortic replacement and thoracic stent-graft placement for multilevel aortic disease. *J Vasc Surg.* 1997;25:332–340.
6. Kirkwood ML, Pochettino A, Fairman RM, et al. Simultaneous thoracic endovascular aortic repair and endovascular aortic repair is feasible with minimal morbidity and mortality. *J Vasc Surg.* 2011;54:1588–1591.
7. Castelli P, Caronno R, Piffaretti G, et al. Endovascular repair for concomitant multilevel aortic disease. *Eur J Thorac Cardiovasc Surg.* 2005;28:478–482.
8. Aguiar Lucas L, Rodriguez-Lopez JA, Olsen DM, et al. Endovascular repair in the thoracic and abdominal aorta: no increased risk of spinal cord ischemia when both territories are treated. *J Endovasc Ther.* 2009;16:189–196.
9. Meguid AA, Bove PG, Long GW, et al. Simultaneous stent-graft repair of thoracic and infra-renal abdominal aortic aneurysms. *J Endovasc Ther.* 2002;9:165–169.
10. Plate G, Hollier LH, O'Brien P, et al. Recurrent aneurysms and late vascular complications following repair of abdominal aortic aneurysms. *Arch Surg.* 1985;120:590–594.
11. Crawford ES, Saleh SA, Babb JW, et al. Infrarenal abdominal aortic aneurysm. Factors influencing survival after operation performed over a 25-year period. *Ann Surg.* 1981;193:699–709.
12. Khoynezhad A, Donayre CE, Bui H, et al. Risk factors of neurologic deficit after thoracic aortic endografting. *Ann Thorac Surg.* 2007;83:S882–S889.
13. Buth J, Harris PL, Hobo R, et al. Neurologic complications associated with endovascular repair of thoracic aortic pathology: Incidence and risk factors. A study from the European Collaborators on Stent/Graft Techniques for Aortic Aneurysm Repair (EUROSTAR) registry. *J Vasc Surg.* 2007;46:1103–1110.
14. McGarvey ML, Mullen MT, Woo EY, et al. The treatment of spinal cord ischemia following thoracic endovascular aortic repair. *Neurocrit Care.* 2007;6:35–39.
15. Cheung AT, Pochettino A, McGarvey ML, et al. Strategies to manage paraplegia risk after endovascular stent repair of descending thoracic aortic aneurysms. *Ann Thorac Surg.* 2005;80:1280–1288.

33

Endovascular Repair of Mycotic Thoracic Aortic Aneurysms and Fistulas

Manuel Garcia-Toca, MD, Jill K. Johnstone, MD, and Jeffrey Slaiby, MD

INTRODUCTION

Dr. William Osler first described mycotic aortic aneurysms in 1885 after performing an autopsy on a patient who had malignant endocarditis and died of a ruptured mycotic aneurysm. The term mycotic is a misnomer. Dr. Osler used the term to describe the gross beaded appearance of the aneurysms since it resembled fungal growth, and not the actual cause of the aneurysm.[1] Infectious aneurysms develop due to inflammatory destruction of the arterial wall.[1,2] There are two factors that are necessary for the development of these aneurysms. The first is mural damage by embolism, atherosclerosis, obstruction of the vasa vasorum, congenital defects or external trauma. The second factor needed is sepsis from bacteremia, infected emboli or spread of a contiguous infection.[2] The majority of mycotic aortic aneurysms in the United States are caused by bacterial pathogens with *Staphylococcus aureus* being the most common, followed by *Streptococcus* and *Salmonella* species.[3]

Mycotic aortic aneurysms are a rare, yet life threatening disease, with their incidence ranging in the literature from 0.65% to 2% of all aortic aneurysms.[4–6] Mycotic thoracic aortic aneurysms (MTAAs) have an even smaller incidence. These aneurysms have a poor prognosis due to their tendency to expand rapidly and to rupture;[7] the patients who develop these aneurysms tend to have multiple co-morbidities, and to present with concomitant sepsis, making them a high surgical risk.

MTAAs tend to be symptomatic aneurysms, presentation can occur with constitutional symptoms (fevers, failure to thrive, weight loss), chest pain, or with symptoms attributable to adjacent organ development. The latter group often includes back pain from erosion into vertebrae, hemoptysis from aorto- bronchial fistulae, and hematemesis or odynophagia from aortoesophageal fistulae. The diagnosis is made based on clinical presentation, characteristic radio- graphic findings, and microbiologic data. The underlying aortic pathology in mycotic aneurysm is typically a saccular configuration. In contrast, fistulae between the thoracic aorta and adjacent organ systems can present with underlying fusiform, dissecting, or saccular aneurysms.

However their clinical presentation is insidious, making their diagnosis difficult and often delayed. This delay may lead to complications of their aneurysms such as aortic fistulae or rupture before the diagnosis is made, causing these patients to present with sepsis or hemodynamic compromise.[4,10]

Despite advancement in antibiotic regimens, purely medical management for mycotic aneurysms is inadequate due to persistent infection, subsequent aneurysm rupture and death.

TREATMENT OPEN VS. ENDOVASCULAR

Traditional treatment of MTAAs has consisted of intravenous antibiotic therapy with open surgical debridement of the aneurysm and surrounding infected tissue with revascularization using extra-anatomic or in situ bypass grafting.[8] Despite this treatment, morbidity and mortality for this disease remains high, with a mortality rate that ranges from 30 to 50%.[7] Such a high mortality rate can make this form of treatment prohibitive in patients with multiple co-morbidities.[4,9]

Endovascular repair of degenerative aortic aneurysms has been shown to be effective and safe,[10] however in the treatment of MTAA it leaves behind the infected aneurysm and surrounding tissue. This may cause continued inflammatory destruction of the arterial wall, reinfection or recurrent sepsis.[11] Even with these drawbacks, a less invasive alternative to open conventional surgery for repair of MTAA may reduce operative morbidity and mortality, especially in a high-risk surgical population.

There have been reports of endovascular repair of MTAA that demonstrate encouraging results,[6,11–15] however the questions of the durability of the repair and the rates of re-infection remain unanswered.

Semba et al. first described the use of enodovascular stent grafts for the treatment of mycotic aortic aneurysms in three case reports, all of which demonstrated successful aneurysm exclusion and no evidence of re-infection during his follow-up period of 17 months.[12] This disease process is rare and since the first report of endovascular repair of MAA the literature has consisted of case reports and small clinical series with limited follow-up. Several of the case series involve mycotic aneurysms of both the thoracic and abdominal aorta, which makes it difficult to compare outcomes for conventional open surgery with endovascular repair. Conventional open surgery for thoracic aortic aneurysms carries a higher mortality and morbidity than open surgery for abdominal aortic aneurysms, and by combining outcomes for both locations of aneurysms it may cause an underestimation of the benefit of thoracic endovascular aortic repair (TEVAR) for MTAA repair.[4]

The issue of the duration of antibiotic therapy is unclear. There is no consensus in the literature but in most series an antibiotic treatment of at least 6 months was performed some suggesting the need of lifelong therapy.

INSTITUTIONAL EXPERIENCE OF TEVAR FOR MTAA REPAIR

Between March 2001 and March 2011, seven consecutive patients with infected aneurysms of the thoracic aorta were treated with endovascular stent-graft repair at our institution.

The diagnosis of MTAA was based on the patients' clinical presentation, including the presence of fever (>101°F), leukocytosis (white blood cell count > 10,000/uL), pain or evidence of bronchoaortic fistula; positive blood cultures, and typical appearance of infected aneurysm on computed tomography (CT) imaging, including pseudoaneurysm or irregular aortic wall. Negative blood cultures, the presence of infected previous aortic graft or endograft and involvement of the aortic arch proximal to the left subclavian artery were considered exclusion criteria for this study.

The patients' demographic data, co-morbidities, symptoms, site of infected aortic aneurysm, and blood culture results were collected. All procedures were performed in an operating room angiosuite by board-certified vascular surgeons with advanced endovascular skills. The devices used to treat the MTAAs consisted of Gore thoracic aortic graft (TAG) (W. L. Gore & Associates) and commercially available endovascular abdominal aortic proximal extension cuffs (AneuRx, Medtronic/AVE, Santa Rosa, California). All of the patients received intravenous (IV) antibiotics pre-operatively, ranging from six weeks before surgery to the day of surgery and all patients received antibiotics post-operatively.

Patients were regularly assessed post-operatively with clinical examination, hematologic tests, including CBC and C-reactive protein and follow-up CT scans at one month and every six months thereafter. The details of the patients' treatment and the 30-day and mid-term morbidity and mortality are reported.

PATIENT DEMOGRAPHICS AND CLINICAL PRESENTATIONS

Seven patients were identified to have infected thoracic aortic aneurysms, three women and four men. Each patient was found to have a single myctoic aneurysm at the time of diagnosis. They had a mean age of 68 years with a range of 44 to 85 years. Five patients had significant co-morbidities that could increase their risk of infection, including leprosy with multi-drug induced neutropenia ($n = 1$), diabetes ($n = 3$), and ESRD requiring hemodialysis ($n = 2$). The patient demographics and co-morbidities are presented in Table 33-1.

All seven patients were symptomatic at presentation, with the most common symptom being pain ($n = 4$), including abdominal, back or chest pain. Three patients presented with fever (>101°F), two presented with hemoptysis from an aortobronchial fistula, and two presented with complaints of fatigue. Leukocytosis (white blood cell count > 10,000/uL) was found in four patients preoperatively. All seven patients had an elevated c-reactive protein (CRP) and six patients had an elevated erythrocyte sedimentation rate (ESR) at the time of diagnosis.

Positive blood cultures were present in all seven patients with results reported in Table 33-1. Three patients had culture isolates of *Staphylococcus aureus*, one of which was methicillin resistant. Of the remaining four patients, one of each had *Salmonella enteridis*, *Candida tropicalis*, *Burkholderia pseudomallei* and *Bacteroides fragilis*.

All seven patients had pre-operative CT scan imaging. Four patients had MTAAs of the proximal descending thoracic aorta described as pseudoaneurysms that ranged in size from 3 cm to 8 cm. Two of these patients were also described in their CT scan imaging to have mediastinal lymphadenopathy. Three patients had MTAAs of the distal descending thoracic aorta. Two of these were pseudoaneurysms and one was fusiform with marked irregularity of the aortic wall. Two patients were found to have contained aortic rupture on pre-operative thoracic CT scans. Patient 1 underwent

TABLE 33-1. PATIENT CHARACTERISTICS AND BACTERIOLOGY

Pt	Gender	Age	Comorbidities*	Presenting Symptoms	Blood Cx
1	M	81	CHF, DM, PVD< CVA, vertebral osteomyelitis	Chest pain	*Salmonella enteridis*
2	F	73	CAD, CHF, ESRD on hemodialysis	Lower back pain	*Candida albicans*
3	F	44	Scoliosis, s/p thoracolumbar laminectomy and fusion T10-L4	Lower back pain	*Staphylococcus aureus*
4	F	72	CAD, HTN, s/p total knee replacement	Hemoptysis	*Staphylococcus aureus*
5	M	58	DM, HTN	Malaise, fever, chest pain	*Burkholderia pseudomallei*
6	M	85	CAD, DM, ESRD on hemodialysis	Abdominal pain, fatigue	*Staphylococcus aureus*
7	M	65	Leprosy, neutropenic keratoidosis, uveitis	Hemoptysis	*Bacteroides fragilis*

*CAD, coronary artery disease; DM, diabetes mellitus; PVD, peripheral vascular disease; CVA, cerebral vascular accident; CHF, congestive heart failure; ESRD, end stage renal disease; HTN, hypertension

a tagged white blood cell scan in addition to a CT scan of his chest that showed an intense area of radiotracer activity at the area of the distal thoracic aortic pseudoaneurysm, further confirming the diagnosis of a MTAA.

TREATMENT AND PERI-OPERATIVE OUTCOMES

All seven patients were started empirically on broad-spectrum IV antibiotics pre-operatively and an infectious disease consultation was obtained. Two patients had antibiotics given the day of the endovascular repair; two patients had IV antibiotics started the day prior to their endovascular repair. The remaining three patients were determined to be stable and could undergo repair of their MTAAs electively, allowing more time for IV antibiotics to be given pre-operatively. One patient had IV antibiotics given for one week pre-operatively, one patient had IV antibiotics given for 2 weeks pre-operatively and one patient had IV antibiotics given for 6 weeks pre-operatively.

A Gore TAG stent graft was used in the treatment of six of the patients with MTAAs. One was combined with an AneuRx proximal extension cuff and one patient had two AneuRx proximal extension cuffs used alone. Exposure of the common femoral arteries was used as access routes in four patients. Three patients had iliac arteries that were not of adequate size to accept the sheath for the stent delivery system. They underwent either abdominal or flank incisions to expose the distal aorta or proximal iliac arteries for conduit anastomoses. All aneurysms were successfully excluded with an endograft at the initial intervention.

The 30-day survival rate was 85.7% (6 out of 7 patients). The patient who died within 30 days had co-morbidities consisting of coronary artery disease (CAD), diabetes, and end stage renal disease (ESRD) requiring hemodialysis. He presented with abdominal pain, leukocytosis, and fatigue and was found to have a distal descending MTAA with a contained rupture and blood cultures positive for *Staphylococcus aureus*. He was taken to the endovascular suite the same day as presentation and underwent a repair using Gore TAG stent grafts. He underwent exposure of his common iliac artery through an abdominal incision for anastomosis of a conduit graft. Post-operatively he was found to have paraplegia and multi-system organ failure and he died on post-operative day two. The remaining 6 patients had no in-hospital complications and their mean hospital stay was 9 days with a range of 7 to 10 days.

One patient on post-operative day 30 after endovascular repair of his proximal descending MTAA, was found to have a pseudoaneurysm proximal to his thoracic endograft on follow-up CT angiogram. The patient was afebrile, without complaints and had negative blood cultures at that time. He was taken back to the endovascular suite and had a Gore TAG graft proximal extension that excluded the pseudoaneurysm and its proximal landing zone was just distal to the take off of the left subclavian artery.

An infectious disease consult was obtained for all 7 patients to determine type of antibiotics and duration. There is currently no evidence in the literature for antibiotic regimens in the treatment of patients who have undergone endovascular repair of their MTAAs. Due to this lack of evidence, the post-operative antibiotic regimens in our patients were chosen based on doctor preference. The antibiotic type was tailored to the patients' blood culture results and sensitivities. The regimens varied and included 2 patients receiving life long antibiotics, one patient that received 2 weeks of IV and 6 months of oral antibiotics, and 4 patients that received 6 weeks of IV antibiotics.

In post-operative follow-up, 5 of the 7 patients had repeat CRP levels drawn. Four of the patients' CRP levels were decreased from the initial pre-operative levels and these were drawn at a range of 2 weeks to 2 months post-operation. There was one CRP level that was elevated above the pre-operative CRP level. This CRP level was drawn on the first post-operative day, and it was not followed further. All 5 patients who survived at one year post-operation had repeat CBC laboratory values that were within normal limits for their WBC counts.

The one-year survival rate for the study was 71.4%, with one death at 2 days post-operatively as previously described and one death occurring at 2 months after endovascular repair of a distal descending MTAA and blood cultures positive for *Salmonella enteridis*. He was admitted to the hospital at that time for shortness of breath and had a myocardial infarction that caused his death. All other surviving patients had no evidence of re-infection at one-year follow-up by both repeat blood work and imaging studies (Figure 33-1). Mean follow-up time was 25 months (range of zero to 72 months) with a survival rate at that time of 57.1% (4 of the 7 patients).

DISCUSSION

The largest case series of TEVAR for MTAA is from Patel et al with 27 patients that had infected thoracic aortic pathology (Table 33-2). Of those 27 patients, only 14 presented with MTAA. This study showed an in-hospital survival rate of 88.5%, and a 3-year survival of 57.8%.[15] This is comparable with our series that had 7 patients who presented with

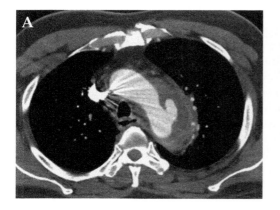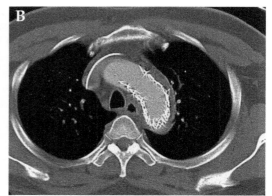

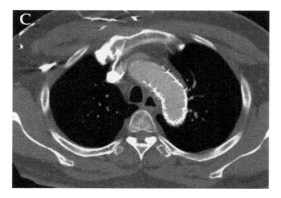

Figure 33-1. Pre-operative CT scan (**A**) showing a saccular aneurysm of the proximal descending aorta with transmural acute inflammation. The patient underwent endovascular repair of the saccular aneurysm. There was a follow-up CT scan at 3 months (**B**) that showed successful exclusion of the aneurysm. Follow up CT scan at 17 moths (**C**) that showed exclusion of the aneurysm with resolution of periaortic wall changes.

MTAAs. Our in-hospital survival rate was 85.7% with one patient dying of multi-system organ failure on post-operative day 2 from overwhelming sepsis. This patient was septic upon arrival to the hospital with multiple co-morbidities and was considered high risk for an open surgical repair. The one-year survival rate was 71.4% (2 patients in 7 died). The second patient died of a myocardial infarction while at home on post-operative day 53.

Late mortality in this high-risk group is often secondary to underlying pathology rather than to reinfection.

In our study, the mean follow-up time was 25 months and the survival rate at that time was 57.1% (3 patients in 7 died). The third patient died at 18 months

TABLE 33-2. CASE SERIES OF TEVAR FOR MTAA REPAIR

First Author	Pt number	30 day survival	1 year survival
Patel	21	85%	65.00%
Clough	16	87.50%	73%
Vallejo	5	80%	40%
Jones	7	87.50%	75%
Our series	7	85.70%	71.40%

of unknown causes. Of the two patients who died outside of the hospital, neither of them had signs of graft infection during their follow-up period. The remaining 4 patients have also been free of infection since their endovascular repair. These results are comparable to what has been presented by Patel et al and others in the literature for use of TEVAR in MTAA.

Long term biological monitoring is needed and usually involves measurement of the white blood cell count, erythrocyte sedimentation rate and C reactive protein level. Antibiotic therapy could be guided and discontinued when there is strictly normal biological monitoring, negative blood cultures and no signs of reinfection on follow up imaging after 6 months.

This studies and our experience show favorable short term and midterm outcomes in the use of TEVAR for treatment of MTAA with a broad range of infectious organisms. The major limitation of all this series are the small sample size, which is due to the rarity and lethality of this disease.

CONCLUSION

Endovascular repair of MTAAs is associated with favorable perioperative and mid-term mortality and morbidity. It should be considered a viable treatment option for patients who are a high surgical risk, however long-term follow-up is still needed to evaluate the effectiveness and durability of this treatment for MTAAs.

REFERENCES

1. Osler W. The Gulstonian lectures on malignant endocarditis. *Br Med J.* 1885;1:467–70.
2. Barker WF. Mycotic Aneurysms. *Ann Surg.* 1954;139:84–9.
3. Leon LR, Mills JL. Diagnosis and management of aortic mycotic aneurysms. *Vasc Endovasc Surg.* 2010;44:5–13.
4. Muller BT, Wegner OR, Grabitz K, et al. Mycotic aneurysms of the thoracic and abdominal aorta and iliac arteries: experience with anatomic and extra-anatomic repair in 33 cases. *J Vasc Surg.* 2001;33:106–13.
5. Vallejo N, Picardo NE, Bourke P, et al. The changing management of primary mycotic aortic aneurysms. *J Vasc Surg.* 2011;54:334–40.
6. Jones KG, Bell RE, Sabharwal T, et al. Treatment of mycotic aortic aneurysms with endoluminal grafts. *Eur J Vasc Endovasc Surg.* 2005;29:139–44.
7. Hsu RB, Lin FY. Infected aneurysm of the thoracic aorta. *J Vasc Surg.* 2008;47:270–6.
8. Gross C, Harringer W, Mair R, et al. Mycotic aneurysms of the thoracic aorta. *Eur J Cardiothorac Surg.* 1994;8:135–8.
9. Kyruakides C, Kan Y, Kerle M, et al. 11-year experience with anatomical and extra-anatomical repair of mycotic aortic aneurysms. *Eur J Vasc Endovasc Surg.* 2004;27:585–89.
10. Clough RE, Black SA, Lyons OT, et al. Is endovascular repair of mycotic aortic aneurysms a durable treatment option? *Eur J Vasc Endovasc Surg.* 2009;37:407–12.
11. Sorelius K, Mani K, Bjorck M, et al. Endovascular repair of mycotic aortic aneurysm. *J Vasc Surg.* 2009;50:269–74.
12. Semba CP, Sakai T, Slonim SM, et al. Mycotic aneurysms of the thoracic aorta: repair with use of endovascular stent-grafts. *J Vasc Interv Radiol.* 1998;9:33–40.

13. Kan CD, Lee HL, Yang YJ. Outcome after endovascular stent graft treatment for mycotic aortic aneurysm: a systematic review. *J Vasc Surg.* 2007;46:906–12.

14. Ting ACW, Cheng SWK, Ho P, et al. Endovascular stent graft repair for infected thoracic pseudoaneurysms—a durable option? *J Vasc Surg.* 2006;44:701–5.

15. Patel HJ, Williams DM, Upchurch GR, et al. Thoracic aortic endovascular repair for mycotic aneurysms and fistulas. *J Vasc Surg.* 2010;52:37S–40S.

34

Management of Late TEVAR Failures

Mark K. Eskandari, MD and Courtney M. Daly, MD

INTRODUCTION

The incidence of thoracic aortic aneurysms is 5.9/100,000. According to natural history studies, 74% of these progress to rupture with a median time to rupture of 2 years.[1]

The most common classification of thoracoabdominal aortic aneurysms is the Crawford system. This describes 5 different types of aneurysm. Type I is distal to the left subclavian artery extending to above the renal arteries. Type II is distal to the left subclavian artery to below the renal arteries. Type III is distal to the sixth intercostal space to below the renal arteries. Type IV is from the 13th intercostal space to the iliac bifurcation, and Type V is from below the 6th intercostal space to just above the renal arteries.

Traditional repair of thoracic aortic aneurysms is open surgical repair. This involves a thoracotomy and cross clamping the aorta. Depending on the extent of the aneurysm, it can require circulatory arrest and cardiopulmonary bypass.

Endovascular repair of thoracic aortic aneurysms was first described by Dake et al in 1994 as an alternative to open aortic repair.[2] The field of endovascular repair has grown rapidly since that time. The first commercially produced device, the Gore TAG endoprothesis, was approved by the FDA in 2005[3] followed by approval of two additional devices, the Zenith TX2 and the Medtronic Talent stent graft, in 2008.[4,5]

As thoracic endovascular aneurysm repair (TEVAR) is utilized more frequently in repair of thoracic aortic aneurysm and as more literature emerges regarding the long-term outcomes of these devices, we are seeing a new set of complications related to late failures of TEVAR. This chapter will provide an overview of these late failures and options for management.

MORTALITY

Most available long-term data on TEVAR show a similar long-term survival between open and endovascular repair. The Gore TAG trial demonstrates a 68% 5-year survival,[3] while the Zenith TX1 and TX2 trials demonstrate a 70% 5-year survival with >90% freedom from aneurysm mortality.[4] Although there are no randomized trials comparing open surgical repair and TEVAR, a meta-analysis was performed in 2010. This study reported a 5.8% 30-day mortality with TEVAR vs 13.9% 30-day mortality for open repair, which was significantly better, but the 1-year mortality of 16% following TEVAR and 21.9% following open repair failed to reach significance.[6]

NEUROLOGICAL COMPLICATIONS

Neurological complications are a devastating class of complications related to thoracic aortic repair. The most common neurological complications in TEVAR are stroke and spinal cord ischemia. Cheng et al reported overall combined neurologic complications of 8.9% in TEVAR vs 18.7% in open repair. When stratified by type, however, TEVAR had lower rates of paraplegia or paraparesis at 3.4% vs 8.2%, and permanent paraplegia of 1.4% vs 4.9%, whereas stroke rates were similar at 5.0% vs 6.2%.[6]

STROKE

Stroke is an important perioperative risk of TEVAR, although less significant in long-term follow-up. The manipulation of wires and catheters, especially in the area of the aortic arch, increases the risk of stroke. Another potential source of stroke is introduction of air through the sheaths and devices. This can be minimized by de-airing the grafts prior to insertion.

Most long-term data demonstrate the majority of the stroke risk lies within the perioperative period. In an analysis of neurological complications of TEVAR from the EUROSTAR database, the rate of stroke was 3.1% within the first month post procedure. Risk factors associated with stroke were increased duration of procedure and female sex.[7] In both the Gore TAG trial and the Zenith trial, there were no incidences of late stroke.[8]

SPINAL CORD ISCHEMIA

Spinal cord ischemia (SCI) is a devastating complication of aneurysm repair. It is most often seen in the perioperative period secondary to hypotension. The common risk factors for spinal cord ischemia are hypotension, length of aorta covered, and previous abdominal aortic repair. Perioperative SCI was shown to have occurred in 2.5% of patients in the EUROSTAR database. Risk factors included left subclavian artery coverage without revascularization, renal failure, concomitant AAA repair, and three or more stent grafts used.[7]

Though less of a focus in the literature, delayed SCI is a concern in TEVAR as well. Although adjunctive measures such as cerebrospinal fluid drainage and close management of blood pressure are protective in the perioperative period, patients can present with symptoms several months or even years postoperatively. Delayed SCI has been reported up to 1.5 years postoperatively following TEVAR.[8] The incidence of late spinal cord ischemia ranges from 2% to 12% in the literature. Risk factors have been found to be hypotension, amount of coverage of the aorta, previous AAA repair, use of an iliac conduit, and coverage of the hypogastric and left subclavian arteries. Another possible risk factor specific to TEVAR involves coverage of important inter-costal arteries. These may remain patent initially secondary to collateral flow through a type II endoleak, but when the endoleak seals, a neurological deficit can develop.[9] Delayed spinal cord ischemia is important to keep in mind, especially in patients who are anatomically at high risk, and patient education and medical alert bracelets may help providers manage acute problems.

ENDOGRAFT INFECTION

Endograft infection is a rare but challenging late complication. It is often associated with a high mortality rate (18–50%).[10,11] One retrospective study of both EVAR and TEVAR reported an endograft infection rate of 0.63%. When stratified by elective vs emergent cases, the rate was 0.56% for elective and 2.79% for emergent. Median time to infection was 115 days, with diagnosis within 30 days in 25% of cases, within 3 months in 42%, and within one year in 83% of patients.[10] Another single institution series describes an endo-graft infection rate of 0.26% with EVAR and 4.77% with TEVAR with a mean time to diag-nosis of 243.6 days.[11]

Signs and symptoms for endograft infection include abdominal pain, back pain, fever, chills, and early satiety. Laboratory studies suggestive of endograft infection include leukocytosis and elevated C-reactive protein. Cross-sectional imaging can be helpful in diagnosis including CT, which may show peri-aortic air or fluid collections or a rim-enhancing collection. PET scan and leukocyte scan are helpful as well.

The most common organism isolated from endograft infections is Staphylococcus, which may be attributed to the adherence to vascular prostheses of the Staphylococcus aureus species. Other organisms isolated include Staphylococcus epidermidis, streptococcus constellatus, pseudomonas, streptococcus viridans, Escherichia coli, Enterobacter, Wisteria, and propionibacterium.[10,11]

Endograft infection in EVAR is frequently treated with graft removal and extra-anatomic bypass or reconstruction with a cryopreserved arterial graft or an antibiotic soaked graft. Similar options are recommended for TEVAR. Although TEVAR is often not amenable to extra atomic bypass, one option includes ascending-to-distal-aortic bypass with explantation of the endograft. One series reports a two-stage procedure for a patient who was a poor operative candidate for aortic reconstruction in the setting of TEVAR infection. In the first stage, ascending-aorta-to-supraceliac-abdominal-aortic bypass was performed in addition to ascending-aorta- to-left-common-carotid-artery bypass with subsequent ligation of the aortic arch distal to the common carotid artery. During the second stage a few days later, the stent graft was explanted. This avoided a complete aortic reconstruction, but allowed removal of the infected graft material.[12] Alternatives include reconstruction with homograft or antibiotic soaked graft. Both of these options carry a high morbidity and leave the repair in the infected field, which may increase the chance of re-infection. Other options, if all infected graft cannot be removed or to protect graft insertion into an infected field, include the use of tissue flaps to protect the graft and close the dead space, the placement of catheters for infusion of perigraft antibiotics, or the use of life-long suppressive antibiotics. In the studies previously mentioned, not all patients were treated surgically. In one study, 6/11 patients were treated with surgery, with only 4/6 requiring surgical removal of the endograft. One used an aortic bi-iliac silver coated prosthesis, one required axillary-bifemoral bypass then graft explant and open reconstruction of the aorta with the deep femoral vein, and one used a combination of autologous vein and silver coated prosthesis.[10]

Another retrospective series describes infected EVAR repair with surgery, whereas, of the 5 TEVAR infections, only one was approached with surgical repair. Of the remaining 4, one was treated with IV antibiotics and transitioned to hospice. The remaining 3 resulted in early mortality, 2 due to mycotic aneurysm rupture and one due to multisystem organ failure.[11] In terms of antibiotic treatment, therapy is tailored to culture whenever possible. Patients are often treated with a long course of IV antibiotics and long-term suppressive therapy.

AORTOESOPHAGEAL FISTULA AND AORTOBRONCHIAL FISTULA

Closely related to endograft infection is fistulization to either the esophagus or bronchial tree. Suggested causes of fistulization include infection of the stent graft causing erosion into the nearby structures of either the esophagus or bronchial tree. Other suggested causes of aortoesophageal fistula include direct erosion of the stent graft struts into the esophagus, pressure necrosis of the esophageal wall, and ischemic necrosis of the esophagus secondary to coverage of aortic side branches.

One of the largest studies to date reports a 1.9% incidence of aortoesophageal fistula. Presenting symptoms include fever, chest pain, and often a sentinel episode of hematemesis followed by a massive gastrointestinal bleed. Survival is dismal with this series reporting 100% mortality.[13] Suggested conservative management involves IV antibiotics, either parenteral feeding or enteral feeding distal to the esophagus, and proton pump inhibitors. There are case studies that report success with this treatment,[14] but it often results in fatal mediastinitis or massive bleeding. Operative repair involves graft explanation with repair of the esophageal or bronchial erosion and aortic reconstruction in an infected field, which carries a high mortality and morbidity. See Figures 34-1 and 34-2.

Mechanistically, it seems that the chance of fistulization increases in the setting of contained rupture due to the presence of hematoma in the mediastinum. Dumfarth et al report that they perform a thoracotomy 2 days postoperatively in the setting of contained rupture to decompress the mediastinum and eliminate this factor in forming a postprocedure fistula.[15]

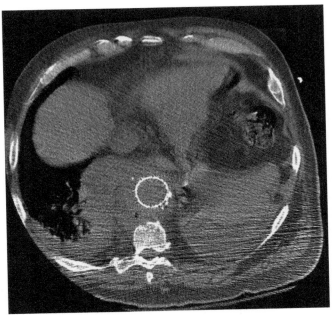

Figure 34-1. CT demonstrating peri-graft air suspicious for aortoesophageal fistula in a patient presenting with fevers and hematemesis.

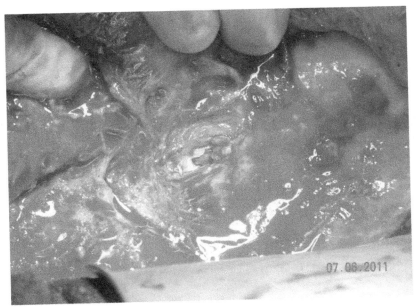

Figure 34-2. Intraoperative photos of infected endograft requiring explant; graft material can be seen at the fistula nidus.

RETROGRADE TYPE A AORTIC DISSECTION

Retrograde type A aortic dissection is a relatively rare complication of TEVAR, often thought to be relevant only in the perioperative period. It is most frequently seen in patients treated with TEVAR for aortic dissection. See Figures 34-3a and 34-3b.

Incidence of retrograde type A aortic dissection ranges from <1% to 3% with a majority occurring in a delayed fashion, outside of the acute perioperative period.[16,17,18,19] Several studies report cases occurring as far as 5 years out or greater.[16,17] Symptoms of retrograde type A aortic dissection include chest pain, dyspnea, syncope, stroke, cardiac tamponade, and sudden death, but up to 25% can be asymptomatic.[18,20] Diagnosis is most often made by CT, but transesophageal echocardiography (TEE), magnetic resonance imaging (MRI), and angiography are also optional imaging modalities.[18,20] Most retrograde type A aortic dissections are treated with open surgical repair, which involves total aortic arch replacement a majority of the time.[18,19] It is also often an emergency procedure, with a meta-analysis of TEVAR for chronic type B dissection reporting 64% of repairs for retrograde dissections emergent compared to 13% elective. Non-emergent cases were more likely to be managed conservatively.[18]

Causes of retrograde type A dissection in patients treated with TEVAR for type B dissection are classified into 5 different categories. These are procedure related, device related, unfavorable aortic dissection anatomy, patent false lumen, and natural progression of original aortic pathology. The first category is not exclusive to TEVAR and has been reported during cardiac catheterization as well. It involves injury from the manipulation of wires and catheters causing injury to the aortic wall. Device related causes have been related to the excessive radial force of oversizing, injury from semi-rigid devices in a tight arch causing injury to a fragile aortic wall, and bare metal proximal stents causing injury, especially in the setting of associated balloon dilation (specific to TEVAR). Some cases of retrograde aortic dissection are unable to be related to device or procedure related injury and may be attributed to progression of the original aortic disease.[20]

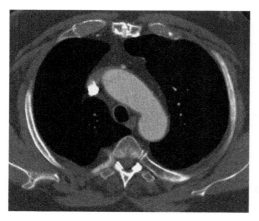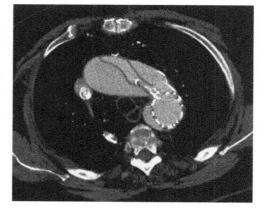

Figure 34-3. Preoperative (a) and one month postoperative (b) images depicting a retrograde type A dissection related to TEVAR.

The meta-analysis previously mentioned reports 60% of retrograde type A dissections as device induced whereas 15% were procedure related due to manipulation of wires and catheters and 15% were due to progression of the underlying disease. Patients with presumed stent graft injury were more likely to have emergency surgery at 81% compared to those with wire induced injury, which were managed conservatively 83% of the time. Patients with disease progression as a cause were most likely to undergo elective surgical repair at 57%.[18] Overall, retrograde type A aortic dissection is a rare but serious problem related to TEVAR. It carries a high mortality of up to 42%[18] and involves a morbid open repair when it occurs. The potential to present late and asymptomatically emphasizes the need for long-term surveillance in patients with TEVAR for type B aortic dissection. See Figures 34-4a and 34-4b.

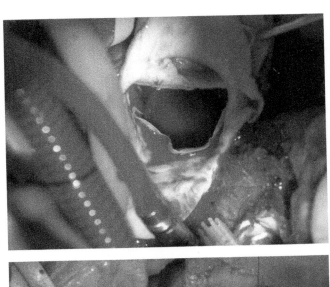

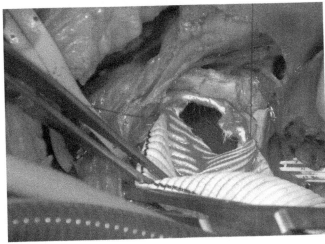

Figure 34-4. Intraoperative pictures depicting aortic arch repair for retrograde type A dissection **(a)** and subsequent repair **(b)**.

DEVICE FAILURE

TEVAR device failure can take several forms. The most common type of device failure is endoleak. Other types of device failures include device migration and device collapse. Although intervention for device failure is low, it can carry a high mortality. One series reports a 5% incidence of secondary surgical intervention for device failure with an in-hospital mortality of 19%, which was significantly higher in emergent operations (38%) than elective (7%). The majority of these failures could have been prevented by following strict indications for TEVAR, emphasizing the need for careful patient selection and attention to anatomy when planning thoracic aortic repair.[21]

DEVICE MIGRATION

According to the reporting standards for TEVAR, device migration is defined as migration of the stent graft either 10 mm proximal or 10 mm distal, while taking into account stent angulation.[21] Not all migrations have clinical consequences. The Gore TAG trial reported 4% of patients with stent graft migrations—3 were proximal migrations, 4 were component separations, and there were no associated endoleaks or interventions required.[3] The Valor trial reported 4 stent graft migrations—in 2 the proximal graft moved distally and in 2 the distal graft moved proximally; only 1 required intervention.[5] The one-year results of the Zenith TX2 trial reported a 2.8% migration rate with 2 caudal migrations of a proximal stent graft and one cranial migration of a distal graft. There were no associated endoleaks or secondary interventions. In both the Zenith TX2 trial and the Gore TAG trial, all migrations were associated with endografts that were oversized by less than 10% at the site of migration.[3,22]

ENDOLEAK

Endoleaks are classified by location of the leak. Type Ia endoleaks occur from the proximal landing zone of the stent graft. Type Ib endoleaks occur at the distal end of the graft. Type II endoleaks occur retrograde from excluded arteries into the aneurysm sac. Common sites of type II endoleaks are intercostal arteries, the left subclavian artery, and occasionally bronchial arteries. Type III endoleaks occur between device components or a fabric tear. Type IV endoleaks involve the porosity of the device fabric.[21]

Endoleaks are a common early complication following both EVAR and TEVAR. Rates of endoleak following TEVAR have been found to be similar to those after EVAR, ranging from 5% to 20%.[23,24] Most endoleaks are recognized either intraoperatively or at the first post-operative CT scan. One series reports 29% rate of endoleak, of which 90% were detected at the first post-operative CT scan at 30 days. There were only 2 endoleaks detected late. Overall, they reported 40% type I endoleak, 35% type II, 20% type III, and 5% with greater than one type of endoleak. Of the two detected late, the first one was a type II endoleak detected at 6 months and the second one was a type III endoleak detected at 2 years. No open repairs were required and 50% of the type 1 endoleaks required either distal or proximal extension. One of the type III endoleaks was repaired with a junctional stent with resolution. The remaining type III endoleaks demonstrated sac regression despite persistent endoleak, so no treatment was performed. Risk factors for endoleaks were found to include male sex, larger pre-operative aneurysm sac, length of aortic coverage, and number of stent grafts placed.[23]

Midterm results of the combined EUROSTAR and United Kingdom thoracic endo-graft databases demonstrated an endoleak rate of 4.2% in degenerative aneurysms, with one late rupture (1%) and 5.2% requiring a late intervention.

The degenerative process of aneurysmal disease may lead to degeneration of the landing zones. This may lead to late type I endoleaks and sac expansion. Sac enlarge-ment is seen more frequently in TEVAR compared with EVAR.[24] In the Gore TAG trial, there was a 7–14% rate of sac enlargement at one year, which increased to 20% at 5 years. 50% of patients demonstrated sac shrinkage, while the other patients had no change in the sac size. When this device was modified to ePTFE, which is less permeable, the rate of sac enlargement decreased to 2.9% at 2 years vs 12.9% in the original device.[8] Late presentation of endoleaks is often related to anatomy. Short proximal landing zone of <3 cm was found frequently in type Ia endoleaks, and placement of more than 3 stent grafts resulted in concomitant type III endoleaks. Steep arch angulation >90 degrees was also found to be associated with type Ia endoleaks, whereas steep thoracoabdominal transition was found to be associated with type Ib endoleaks. When more than one stent graft was placed, type III endoleaks were found in association with type Ib.[15]

Treatment of type Ia endoleak with proximal extension is often complicated by the fact that aortic arch vessels prevent further proximal extension. Options to address proximal extension into the region of the aortic arch vessels include extra-anatomic bypass with proximal extension, chimney grafts, branched grafts, and endograft explantation. Hybrid procedures with aortic arch vessel debranching either by bypass or transposition to more proximal landing zones are becoming a common alterna-tive to open aortic repair. Coverage of the left subclavian artery is the most common hurdle. There are well established guidelines for revascularization of the left subcla-vian, which include prior left internal mammary artery to coronary bypass, occluded or absent right vertebral artery, dominant left vertebral artery, or extensive coverage of the thoracic aorta.[25] Both carotid subclavian bypass and carotid subclavian transposi-tion are options for revascularization, but, in the presence of left internal mammary artery to coronary bypass, carotid subclavian bypass is required.[26] Chimney grafts were developed as a total endovascular approach to arch debranching. One series reports various indications for chimney, one of which was persistent type Ia endoleak after TEVAR. Chimney grafts are delivered through the brachial artery and the target supra-aortic vessel is cannulated with a long sheath. The chimney graft was deployed after placement of the TEVAR graft to 2–3 cm within the branch to 2 cm outside par-allel to the main endograft. This technique can lend itself to persistent endoleak due to perfusion of the gutter, thus the recommendation to leave at least 2 cm parallel to the aortic stent graft. A step beyond chimney grafts are fenestrated endografts and branched endografts, which allow a self expanding stent to be deployed through a fenestration or branch in the main body of the endograft into the branch vessel, thus expanding the proximal and distal landing zones by endovascular means.[27] Each of these techniques, although developed for hybrid placement of the original endograft, can be adapted for proximal extension to address type Ia endoleaks. Sometimes type Ia endoleaks cannot be repaired by endovascular means, which may result in graft explant. One series describes several indications for graft explants, one of which was a type Ia endoleak presenting 5 years post implant causing aneurysm expansion. This required endograft explantation and open thoracoabdominal aneurysm repair.[28]

Endoleaks are one of the most common early and late complications of TEVAR, and surveillance and management to prevent sac expansion is required. Although most type I endoleaks do require repair, it can often be accomplished by endovascular means. Type II and III endoleaks can often be observed but persistent sac expansion requires a low threshold to intervene. See Figures 34-5, 34-6a and 34-6b.

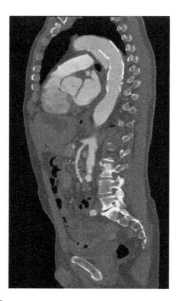

Figure 34-5. Type Ia endoleak on CT.

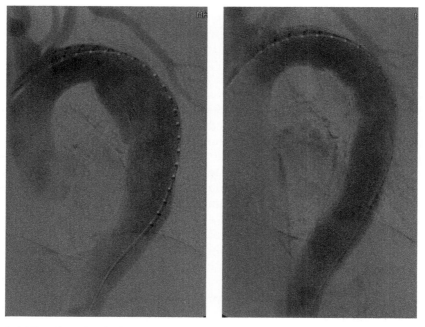

Figure 34-6. (a) Type Ia endoleak with placement of proximal stent graft component. **(b)** Completion aortogram demonstrates resolution.

DEVICE COLLAPSE

Endograft collapse is a serious complication following TEVAR placement as it can lead to acute aortic occlusion and multiorgan system failure. It is most commonly seen following repair for traumatic aortic injury, but can be seen following TEVAR for any aortic pathology. In a meta-analysis of endograft collapse the main causes of endograft collapse were oversizing by >20%, a small radius of curvature of the thoracic aorta, maldeployment, and progression of aortic disease. The median time to presentation of the collapse was 15 days, although this ranged from 1 day to 78 months, suggesting that device collapse can present as a late complication in addition to early. 65% of cases were diagnosed within the first month and 75% within the first three months. 59% of the patients with endograft collapse were asymptomatic, suggesting the need for surveillance imaging. Those that did present with symptoms presented with no or weak femoral pulses, thoracic pain, and acute renal failure. 87% of patients were offered an intervention, of which 68% were endovascular. The majority of endovascular repairs involved deployment of an additional endograft component to increase the radial force. 18% underwent surgical intervention, most often involving explanation of the endograft. Diagnosis of endograft collapse resulted in an 8.3% 30 day mortality, which was significantly higher in symptomatic patients. Among patients who received surgical or endovascular intervention, the 30-day mortality was 3.8% vs 38% in patients who did not receive an intervention. Beyond 30 days of diagnosis and repair, an additional 15% required a second reintervention, which included deployment of an additional endograft, bowel resection, embolization, and resection of aortoesophogeal fistula. Long-term results following endograft collapse report an estimated freedom from procedure related death of 77.5% at three years. The majority of the endografts resulting in collapse were the Gore TAG prosthesis; although it was the most commonly implanted device at the time of the publication.[29] Another review of the Gore TAG data addressed this topic directly. The authors reported a 0.4% incidence of endograft collapse, with 60.4% of the patients representing trauma patients. The average oversizing of the device was 33%, and diagnosis occurred at an average of 76 days following the procedure. Only 30% of the patients were symptomatic, presenting with chest or back pain, hypertension, oliguria, claudication, or paraplegia. There was a 7% mortality associated with device collapse, and 80% were successfully re-expanded endovascularly or removed surgically. The authors developed a classification of endograft collapse with suggested means of repair. Type Ia is proximal invagination and the suggested intervention is endovascular relining and balloon expansion. Type Ib is distal invagination, which can be relined or observed if there is no flow limitation. Type IIa involves proximal compression, which requires explanation or relining. Type IIb involves distal compression, which has not yet been reported as an isolated event. Type III is complete graft compression requiring complete device explanation.[30] One reason that may explain stent graft collapse in the early trials may relate to insufficient radial force. New generations of these devices such as the Gore c-TAG and the Medtronic Valiant have greater radial strength, more accurate delivery systems, and a wider range of sizes requiring less oversizing. A retrospective study of patients treated for blunt traumatic aortic disruption reported more appropriate oversizing (18% vs 24%), less morbidity (6.2% vs 18.7%), and decreased incidence of type Ia endoleak when comparing the newer generation devices to the original design.[31]

As a majority of patients with endograft collapse are young patients undergoing repair for traumatic injury who often present in the first month after implantation, it is important to have good surveillance and a high index of suspicion when following them postoperatively. Newer device technology with increased conformability and radial force, as well as smaller sizes, may be more appropriate for this population. See Figures 34-7, 34-8a and 34-8b.

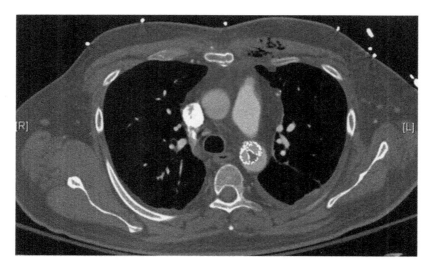

Figure 34-7. *CT* angiogram demonstrating device collapse.

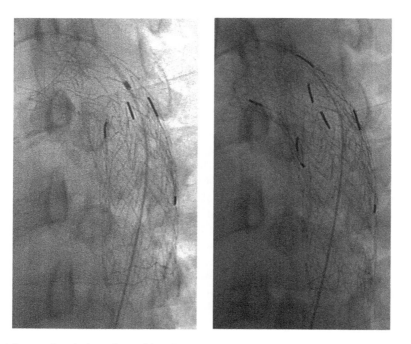

Figure 34-8. Intraoperative device collapse **(a)** and resolution with relining of the device with cuffs **(b)**.

CONCLUSIONS

Management of late TEVAR failures requires good postoperative surveillance and a high index of suspicion to recognize and address issues early. Device related failures such as migration, endoleak, or collapse can often be repaired by endovascular means. Proper patient and device selection is vital in preventing late failures.

REFERENCES

1. Bickerstaff LK, Pairolero PC, Hollier LH, et al. Thoracic aortic aneurysms: A population based study. *Surgery.* 1982;92:1103–1108.
2. Dake MD, Miller DC, Semba CP, et al. Transluminal placement of endovascular stent-grafts for the treatment of descending thoracic aortic aneurysms. *New Eng J Med.* 1994;331:1729–1734.
3. Makaroun MS, Dillavou ED, Kee ST, et al. Endovascular treatment of thoracic aortic aneurysms: Results of the phase II multicenter trial of the GORE TAG thoracic endoprosthesis. *J Vasc Surg.* 2005;41:1–9.
4. Matsumura JS, Cambria RP, Dake MD, et al. International controlled clinical trial of thoracic endovascular aneurysm repair with the Zenith TX2 endovascular graft: 1-year results. *J Vasc Surg.* 2008;47:247–257.
5. Fairman RM, Criado F, Farber M et al. Pivotal results of the Medtronic vascular Talent thoracic stent graft system: The VALOR trial. *J Vasc Surg.* 2008;48:546–554.
6. Cheng D, Martin J, Shennib H, et al. Endovascular aortic repair versus open surgical repair for descending thoracic aortic disease: A systematic review and meta-analysis of comparative studies. *J Am Coll Cardiol.* 2010;55:986–1001.
7. Buth J, Harris PL, Hobo R, et al. Neurologic complications associated with endovascular repair of thoracic aortic pathology: Incidence and risk factors. A study from the European Collaborators on Stent/Graft Techniques for Aortic Aneurysm Repair (EUROSTAR) registry. *J Vasc Surg.* 2007;46:1103–1111.
8. Chaer RA, Makaroun MS. Late failure after endovascular repair of descending thoracic aneurysms. *Semin Vasc Surg.* 2009;22:81–86.
9. Cho, JS, Rhee RY, Makaroun MS. Delayed paraplegia 10 months after endovascular repair of thoracic aortic aneurysm. *J Vasc Surg.* 2008;47:625–628.
10. Cernohorsky P, Reijnen MM, Tielliu IF, et al. The relevance of aortic endograft prosthetic infection. *J Vasc Surg.* 2011;54:327–333.
11. Heyer KS, Modi P, Morasch MD, et al. Secondary infections of thoracic and abdominal aortic endografts. *J Vasc Interv Radiol.* 2009;20:173–179.
12. Canaud L, Alric P, Gandet T, et al. Surgical conversion after thoracic endovascular aortic repair. *J Thorac Cardiovasc Surg.* 2011;142:1027–1031.
13. Eggebrecht H, Mehta RH, Dechene A, et al. Aortoesophagial fistula after thoracic aortic stent-graft placement: A rare but catastrophic complication of a novel emerging technique. *JACC Cardiol Interv.* 2009;2:570–576.
14. Kasai K, Ushio A, Tamura Y, et al. Conservative treatment of an aortoesophagial fistula after endovascular stent grafting for a thoracic aortic aneurysm. *Med Sci Monit.* 2011;17:CS39–42.
15. Dumfarth J, Michel M, Schmidli J, et al. Mechanisms of failure and outcome of secondary surgical interventions after thoracic endovascular aortic repair (TEVAR). *Ann Thorac Surg.* 2011;91:1141–1146.
16. Kang WC, Greenberg RK, Mastracci TM, et al. Endovascular repair of complicated chronic distal aortic dissections: Intermediate outcomes and complications. *J Thorac Cardiovasc Surg.* 2011;142:1074–1083.

17. Thrumurthy SG, Karthikesalingam A, Patterson BO, et al. A systematic review of mid-term outcomes of thoracic endovascular repair (TEVAR) of chronic type B aortic dissection. *Eur J Vasc Endovasc Surg*. 2011;42:632–647.

18. Eggebrecht H, Thompson M, Rousseau H, et al. Retrograde ascending aortic dissection during or after thoracic aortic stent graft placement: Insight from the European registry on endovascular aortic repair complications. *Circulation*. 2009;120[suppl 1]:S276–S281.

19. Lu S, Lai H, Wang C, et al. Surgical treatment for retrograde type A aortic dissection after endovascular stent graft placement for type B dissection. *Interact CardioVasc Thorac Surg*. 2012;14:538–542.

20. Bellos JK, Petrosyan A, Abdulamit T, et al. Retrograde type A aortic dissections after endovascular stent-graft placement for type B dissection. *J Cardiovasc Surg* (Torino). 2010;51:85–93.

21. Fillinger MF, Greenberg RK, McKinsey JF, et al. Reporting standards for thoracic endovascular aortic repair (TEVAR). *J Vasc Surg*. 2010;52:1022–1033.

22. Melissano G, Kahlberg A, Bertoglio L et al. Endovascular exclusion of thoracic aortic aneurysms with the 1- and 2-component Zenith TX2 TAA endovascular grafts: Analysis of 2-year data from the TX2 pivotal trial. *J Endovasc Ther*. 2011;19:338–349.

23. Parmer SS, Carpenter JP, Stavropoulos SW, et al. Endoleaks after endovascular repair of thoracic aortic aneurysms. *J Vasc Surg*. 2006;44:447–452.

24. Leurs LJ, Bell R, Degrieck Y, et al. Endovascular treatment of thoracic aortic diseases: Combined experience from the EUROSTAR and United Kingdom Thoracic Endograft registries. *J Vasc Surg*. 2004;40:670–680.

25. Criado FJ, McKendrick C, Criado FR. Technical solutions for common problems in TEVAR: Managing access and aortic branches. *J Endovasc Ther*. 2009;16(Suppl I):I63–I79.

26. Peterson BG, Eskandari MK, Gleason TG, et al. Utility of left subclavian artery resconstruction in association with endoluminal repair of acute and chronic thoracic aortic pathology. *J Vasc Surg*. 2006;43:433–439.

27. Brozzi NA, Roselli EE. Endovascular therapy for thoracic aortic aneurysms: State of the art in 2012. *Curr Treat Options Cardiovasc Med*. 2012;14:149–163.

28. Kirkwood ML, Pochettino A, Fairman RM, et al. Thoracic aortic endograft explant: A single center experience. *Vasc Endovasc Surg*. 2010;44:440–445.

29. Jonker FH, Schlosser FJ, Geirsson A, et al. Endograft collapse after thoracic endovascular aortic repair. *J Endovasc Ther* 2010;17:725–734.

30. Kasirajan K, Dake MD, Lumsden A, et al. Incidence and outcomes after infolding or collapse of thoracic stent grafts. *J Vasc Surg*. 2012;55:652–658.

31. Canaud L, Joyeux F, Berthet JP, et al. Impact of stent-graft development on outcome of endovascular repair of acute traumatic transection of the thoracic aorta. *J Endovasc Ther*. 2011;18:485–490.

SECTION **VIII**

Thoracoabdominal Disease

Disease Progression After Surgery for Takayasu Arteritis

Sung Wan Ham, MD and Fred A. Weaver, MD, MMM

HISTORY

At the 1908 Japan Ophthalmology Society Meeting held in Fukuoka, Japan; an ophthalmologist, Mikito Takayasu, reported a case of arteriovenous connections or "coronary anastomoses" of the retinal vasculature in a 21-year old Japanese woman with sudden vision loss.[1] At the same meeting, Katsutomo Onishi and Tsurukichi Kagoshima, presented two cases with similar ocular features, and the additional finding of absent radial artery pulses. Over the ensuing years additional cases were reported in Japan including a report by Shinmi in 1939 who named the condition "Takayasu Arteritis" (TA). The disease was introduced to Western medicine by reports from Shimizu and Sano who introduced "pulseless disease" into the English medical lexicon.

Ueda, in 1963, demonstrated TA to be an inflammatory process that involves segments of the aorta and main branches as well as the pulmonary and coronary arteries in selected patients. In 1975, the research committee of the Department of Health and Welfare in Japan officially named this condition "Takayasu Arteritis" (TA) as an acknowledgement of Mikito Takaysu's role in the recognition of the disease. Other commonly used synonyms include Onishi's disease, aortic arch syndrome, aortitis syndrome, young female arteritis, Martorell syndrome, and pulseless disease.

ETIOLOGY AND ANATOMIC DISTRIBUTION

TA is a nonspecific granulomatous inflammatory aortitis that affects the aorta, aortic branches; and pulmonary and coronary arteries to a varying extent and with characteristic patterns. Histopathology varies from an acute exudative inflammatory process of variable degree to intimal fibrosis and fibrous replacement of the elastic and muscles fibers in the media/adventitia of involved vessels. A definitive etiology for the inflammatory process

409

1994 Tokyo international conference classification of TA

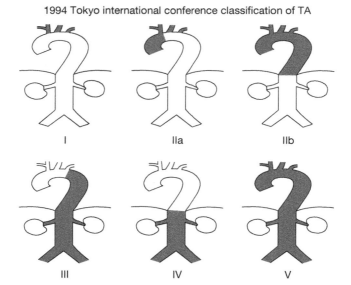

Figure 35-1. 1994 Tokyo International Conference Classfication of Takayasu's arteritis Disease classification is based on the initial aortogram.

has yet to be elucidated although a genetic predisposition has been suggested and is supported by Numano's report of twin sisters with TA.[2] Additional support for genetics as a causative factor is the higher prevalence in Japanese patients with TA of genetic antigens HLA-Bw52 and the haplotype of Bw52-Dw12 which confer a greater tendency for active inflammation.[3] However, the association between HLA antigens and disease severity has not been uniformly present and was absent in a group of North American patients diagnosed with TA.[4] Other proposed etiologies including infectious, familial, hormonal, and autoimmune have been suggested, yet a unifying causal relationship remains elusive.

The anatomic distribution of TA is currently classified using the 1994 Tokyo International Conference Classification which is based on the findings of the initial diagnostic aortogram.[5] (Figure 35-1). At our institution, the majority of patients have a Type V distribution with combined aortic arch, thoracic, and abdominal aortic disease. This is somewhat different from clinical series reported from Asia, where isolated brachiocephalic involvement is more common. Other classification systems have been developed by Ueno and Ueda.[6,7]

CLINICAL FEATURES

Relatively large series of patients with TA have been reported from Japan, Korea, Thailand, China, India, and Mexico.[8–10] Although TA can occur in males, it is rare with several series reporting an 80% or greater prevalence of females.[10,11] The clinical course of TA may include a prodromal four to six week "prepulseless phase," which is manifested by a variety of constitutional symptoms including pyrexia, weight loss, anorexia, night sweats, malaise, arthralgias, and myalgias. Because these symptoms are nonspecific, protean and not associated with peripheral pulse deficits, recognition of the acute arteritic process is often delayed or missed entirely.

For the vascular surgeon who is asked to see a patient with TA these constitutional symptoms are rarely present. Rather, the more commonly encountered clinical picture is one of a "burned-out" arteritis that is associated with peripheral pulse deficits, and specific end organ ischemia and dysfunction. In this clinical scenario, a minority of patients admit to a remote history of the typical, "prepulseless" prodromal symptom complex. When reported, it antedates the symptoms of end organ ischemia and dysfunction by 1 to 12 years.

TA arteriopathy leads to stenotic, occlusive and less commonly aneurysmal degeneration. Clinical manifestations include malignant hypertension, renal failure, stroke, ocular ischemia, extremity ischemia, aortic valve insufficiency, and aneurysm formation. Although the classic descriptions of TA focus on brachiocephalic involvement, the renal arteries are also commonly involved resulting in renovascular hypertension and ischemic nephropathy. TA induced renovascular hypertension is frequently associated with cardiac dysfunction and failure which can lead to premature death.[12-14]

Of the 40 patients treated at the University of Southern California Hospitals over the past 30 years, the most common symptom complex has been severe systemic hypertension associated with renal failure or varying degrees of cardiac failure (Table 35-1) Hypertension has been present in 34 patients and associated with overt cardiac failure in 2 and dialysis-dependent renal failure in 3. This preponderance of hypertension in the TA patient population is similar to more recent reports from many Asian countries.[8]

TABLE 35-1. DEMOGRAPHIC AND PATIENT CHARACTERISTICS

Characteristics	TA N = 40
Women, No. (%)	36 (90)
Age in years (mean ± SEM)	35±2.5
Race (%)	
Hispanic	25 (63)
Asian	10 (25)
White	5 (12)
Hypertension (%)	34 (85)
Renal Insufficiency[†] (%)	6 (15)
Dialysis dependent	3 (8)
CAD (%)	2 (5)
CHF (%)	2 (5)
Prior revascularization for TA	9 (23)
Follow-up (years)	
Mean ± SEM	6.41±1.2
Median	3.22
Range	0.03–30

TA, Takayasu's Arteritis; *SEM*, standard error of the mean; *meds*, medications; † Serum creatinine ≥1.5 mg/dL and does not include dialysis dependent patients, data not available for 3 patients; *CAD*, coronary artery disease; *CHF*, congestive heart failure; *mo*, months

SURGICAL MANAGEMENT

The value of surgical revascularization in correcting organ dysfunction and improving survival in patients with symptomatic TA has been demonstrated in numerous reports and is consistent with our own experience over the past 30 years.[15–22] Surgical revascularization is primarily accomplished by using autogenous or prosthetic bypass grafts, although early reports included the occasional endarterectomy. Endarterectomy has subsequently been abandoned due to the high rate of early re-occlusion, sometimes with catastrophic consequences. More recently, short term results of endovascular revascularization have been reported. These reports suggest a role for endovascular intervention as a temporizing measure or in situations where direct open surgical revascularization is not possible or advisable. But durability remains a concern in this predominantly young patient population and long term data concerning endovascular treatment is not readily available.

Surgical pre-operative planning requires angiography and the liberal use of CT imaging. The CT images provide information on vessel wall thickness and extent of involvement which complements the information provided by catheter based angiography. (Figures 35-2, 35-3, and 35-4) This permits the development of a successful operative strategy which is predicated on identifying inflow and outflow bypass target vessels minimally affected by the arteritic/inflammatory process. Placement of the

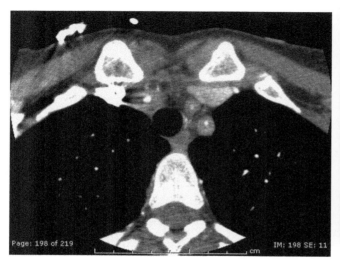

Figure 35-2. Axial CT image shows brachiocephalic arteritis.

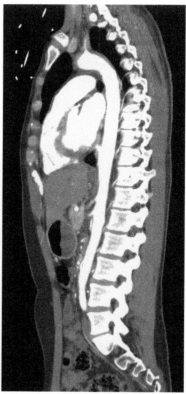

Figure 35-3. Sagittal CT image shows aortic arch and brachiocephalic arteritis.

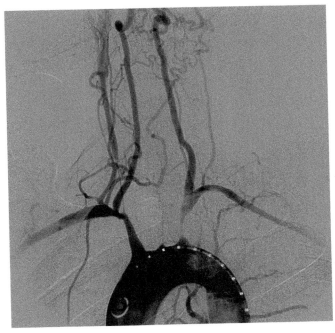

Figure 35-4. Arch aortogram of patient with the CT scan images found in Figure 35-1 and 35-2. Angiogram demonstrates the typical brachiocephalic disease pattern classically associated with Takayasu Arteritis. Note the hypertrophied verterbral arteries due to severe occlusive disease of the proximal common carotid arteries bilaterally.

bypass graft in a normal or minimally affected arterial segment may not be possible for the aortic inflow site, but is mandatory for the distal outflow vessel if long term bypass graft patency is to be maximized.

SURGICAL RESULTS AND DISEASE PROGRESSION

Since 1980, 40 patients with TA have undergone 64 primary vascular procedures for end organ ischemia at University of Southern California Hospitals. This experience includes 60 bypass procedures and 4 endovascular interventions with a mean follow-up of 77 months (Table 35-2). Longitudinal examination of this experience has permitted an assessment of the frequency of TA disease progression, the durability of the primary revascularization as well as the success of remedial procedures when required.

Four late deaths occurred following surgical revascularization providing a one and 5-year actuarial survival of 94% and 94%, respectively. In addition, during follow up, 16 patients have required 34 surgical procedures for either failure of the initial revascularization procedure or progression of disease. These procedures involved renal (12), extremity (8), cerebrovascular (8), aortic (5), and mesenteric (1) vascular beds (Table 35-2, 35-3). The mean time from revascularization to the remedial procedure was 5.8 years. The results of surgical intervention for either failure of the initial revascularization or progression of disease have been excellent overall with a primary graft patency of 85% at 5 years and a survival of 94% and 85% at 1 and 5 years respectively (Figure 35-5).

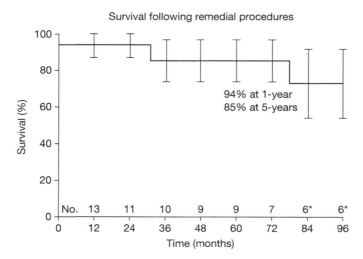

Figure 35-5. Kaplan meier estimates for survival for pateints with disease progression where time 0 begins from date of remedial procedure. *Standard error > 10%; No., number of patients remaining.

Recognition of the need for a remedial procedure was enhanced by routine patient follow up in combination with some form (usually duplex ultrasonography) of annual graft surveillance imaging. This allowed prompt correction of graft related problems by either direct repair or extension of the bypass to a more distal target. Pathologic material from these operative interventions demonstrated intimal hyperplasia as the cause of the anastomotic stenosis or graft occlusion. The value of imaging surveillance in detecting the failing graft before occlusion was evident since only two of the procedures were for an occluded graft whereas the remainder of the procedures were for either patent grafts with anastomotic stenoses or patent vessels with intrastent stenoses following endovascular intervention.

For patients with disease progression in a previously non-operated vascular bed, one procedure was required in five patients whereas 11 patients required two or more procedures. When progression occurs uncertainty exists as to whether it is due to a recurrence or flare of the arteritis or due to late vessel fibrosis as a consequence of the initial inflammatory insult. Our experience suggests the latter, since the Tokyo International Conference Classification of TA did not change for any patient with disease progression. In other words, disease progression occurred only in previously asymptomatic vascular beds with known lesions that were seen on the initial diagnostic angiogram or CT.

This observation is similar to that reported by Lagneau in a series of 33 patients treated surgically for TA. In his report, two patients had symptomatic and angiographic progression of disease that required surgical intervention during a mean 4 year follow up. One patient initially had a nephrectomy and then progression of existing lesions in both carotids and left subclavian artery 3 years later. The other patient who initially did not undergo an operation at diagnosis, presented 3 years later with symptomatic and angiographic progression of previously recognized aortic lesions that required an aortic-aortic bypass.[16] In another series of 25 patients

TABLE 35-2. INDEX AND REMEDIAL PROCEDURES FOR 40 PATIENTS

Index Procedure by Anatomic Location	N = 64	Remedial Procedure by Anatomic Location	N = 34
Renal	40	**Renal**	12
Aorto – Renal bypass	25	Aorto – Renal bypass	9
Visceral – Renal bypass	3	PTA ± stent	3
Ex Vivo	3		
Nephrectomy	5	**Extremity**	8
Percutaneous transluminal angioplasty	4	Lower extremity bypass	3
		Patch angioplasty/revisions	2
		PTA ± stent of lower extremity bypass graft	1
Aortic Reconstruction	12	LCC – LSA artery bypass	2
Aorto – Bi-iliac/femoral bypass	7		
Infrarenal Aortic replacement	3	**Cerebrovascular**	8
Thoracic aorto – Infrarenal aortic bypass	1	Aorto – Carotid bypass	5
		Carotid – Carotid bypass	1
Ascending aortic replacement/AVR	1	Carotid endarterectomy	1
		Femoral – Axillary bypass	1
Cerebrovascular	8		
Aorto – Carotid bypass	7	**Aortic Reconstruction**	6
Femoral – Axillary bypass	1	Ascending aortic replacement/AVR	2
		Para-anastomotic aneurysm repair	1
Extremity	4	Aorto – Bi-iliac/femoral bypass	2
LCC – LSA bypass/transposition	3	Aorto – mesenteric bypass	1
LCC – brachial artery bypass	1		

AVR, aortic valve replacement; *LCC*, left common carotid artery; *LSA*, left subclavian artery; *PTA*, percutaneous transluminal angioplasty;

reported by Robbs, one patient with type V who underwent thoracoabdominal aortic replacement with bilateral renal artery revascularization for aneurysm and refractory hypertension, had symptomatic progression at one year in an ectatic ascending aorta. Disease progression was manifested by new symptom onset only and occurred despite the patient taking chronic steroid therapy in the interim.[17]

A suggested strategy to prevent disease progression in TA has been the use of long term steroid/immunosuppressive therapy. The effect in our series of this management strategy was mixed. Of the 16 patients with disease progression, seven (44%) were on chronic medical therapy, versus nine (56%) receiving no medical therapy. Medical therapy consisted of corticosteroids alone or in combination with methotrexate, cyclophosphamide or azathioprine. Of the seven who were taking combination corticosteroid/immunosuppressive agents, disease progression in a previously asymptomatic vascular bed occurred in two, recurred in a previously operated bed in two, or recurred in a previously operated bed and progressed in

TABLE 35-3. DETAILS OF PATIENTS WITH RECURRENCE OR PROGRESSION OF DISEASE

Patient #	Gender	Age (Years)	Index Procedure	Medications [†]	Disease Extent [‡]	Procedures Required For Recurrence/ Progression Of Disease
1	F	45	Aorto-renal BYP	Cyclophospha-mide/pred	V	Femoral-femoral BYP, profunda-popliteal BYP, renal graft angioplasty + stent
2	F	19	Aorto-renal BYP	None	V	Aorto-iliac BYP, aorto-renal BYP, Spleno-renal BYP
3	F	33	Supraceliac aortoiliac, aorto-renal BYP	Pred	V	Contralateral aorto-renal BYP, aorto-renal graft revision
4	F	19	Supraceliac aorto-femoral BYP	None	V	Femoral graft revision, aorto-SMA BYP, femoral-renal BYP
5	F	50	Aorto-renal BYP	None	IV	Contralateral renal aorto-renal BYP
6	F	24	Femoral-axillary BYP	MTX/pred	V	Aorto-renal BYP, aorto-bicarotid BYP
7	F	31	Aorto-femoral, aorto-renal BYP	None	V	Carotid-subclavian BYP
8	F	13	Carotid-subclavian BYP	None	V	Asc aortic replace-ment, aorto-renal BYP, aorto-carotid
9	F	29	Aorto-renal BYP	Pred	V	Aorto-renal BYP
10	F	46	Renal/iliac angioplasty	Aziathioprine pred	III	Aorto-iliac BYP, aorto-renal BYP, carotid-carotid BYP, asc aortic replacement
11	F	23	Renal angioplasty	None	V	Carotid endarterectomy, aorto-renal BYP
12	F	59	Renal angioplasty	MTX/pred	IV	Contralateral renal angioplasty
13	F	15	Aorto-carotid BYP	None	I	Revision aorto-carotid BYP, femoral-axillary BYP, asc aortic replacement
14	F	15	Aorto-renal BYP	None	IV	Renal graft angioplasty, iliac angioplasty + stent
15	F	41	Aorto-bicarotid BYP	none	I	Redo aorto-bicarotid BYP
16	F	51	Supraceliac aorto-femoral BYP	Pred	III	Thoracotomy for para-anastomotic pseudoaneurysm at proximal anastomosis

BYP, bypass; pred, prednisone; *MTX*, methotrexate; *SMA*, superior mesenteric artery; *asc*, ascending; [†] type of immunosuppressive or steroid therapy taking at the time of index procedure; [‡] Extent of aortic involvement classified according to the 1994 Tokyo International Conference Classification of Takayasu Arteritis

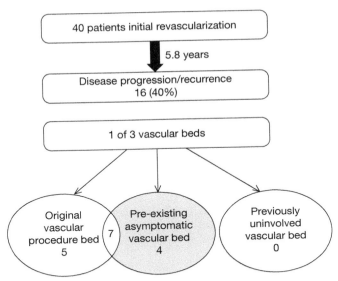

Figure 35-6. Disease progression or recurrence of all 40 patients over a mean 5.8 years. No disease progression in previously uninvolved vascular beds based on initial aortogram.

another vascular bed in three (Figure 35-6). The incidence of recurrence or disease progression was similar in those patients not receiving longitudinal medical therapy. This suggests chronic steroid/immunosuppressive therapy has minimal impact on the need for surgical reintervention or disease progression.

These results are consistent with another series of 42 patients with TA treated by surgical revascularization in which no difference in freedom from revision or disease progression was found when analyzed by the presence or absence of long-term steroid therapy. Moreover, there was no survival benefit over 10 years in the 22 patients (52%) who were on steroid therapy at the time of operation compared to the patients who were not.[23] As we found, disease progression or need for revision was as likely in patients on chronic steroid/immunosuppressive agents (44%) as those who were not.

The limited effect of medical therapy on disease progression and surgical outcomes suggests minimizing to eliminating medical therapy in the long term management of TA. However, this does not minimize the importance of corticosteroids in the acute phase of the disease where it has been shown to attenuate the systemic inflammatory insult thereby limiting the extent of vessel injury. How great a benefit this provides in the long term evolution of Takayasu Arteritis will require additional longitudinal studies.

CONCLUSION

The value of direct surgical revascularization for symptomatic manifestations of TA is well documented.[12,17,20,24–29] However, our experience indicates that remedial procedures are required in about a third of the patients who undergo surgical revascularization. Furthermore, the need for these procedures occurs on average about six years after the primary surgical procedure. The timing of failure of the initial revascularization or the development of disease progression underscores the importance of lifelong patient follow up coupled with surveillance imaging in patients with Takayasu Arteritis. When surgical re-intervention is required, it is effective and associated with acceptable late graft patency and survival. Finally, these beneficial late surgical results do not appear to be enhanced by long term steroid/immunosuppressive therapy.

REFERENCES

1. Takayasu M. A case with peculiar changes of the central retinal vessels. *Acta Soc Ophthalmol Jpn*. 1908;12:554.
2. Numano F, Isohisa I, Kishi U, et al. Takayasu's disease in twin sisters. Possible genetic factors. *Circulation*. 1978;58(1):173–7.
3. Isohisa I, Numano F, Maezawa H, et al. HLA-Bw52 in Takayasu disease. *Tissue Antigens*. 1978;12(4):246–8.
4. Khraishi MM, Gladman DD, Dagenais P, et al. HLA antigens in North American patients with Takayasu arteritis. *Arthritis & Rheumatism*. 1992;35(5):573–5.
5. Hata A, Noda M, Moriwaki R, et al. Angiographic findings of Takayasu arteritis: New classification. *Int J Cardiol*. 1996;54(Suppl):S155–63.
6. Ueno A, Awane Y, Wakabayashi A, et al. Successfully operated obliterative brachiocephalic arteritis (Takayasu) associated with the elongated coarctation. *Jpn Heart J*. 1967;8(5):538.
7. Ueda H, Morooka S, Ito I, et al. Clinical observation of 52 cases of aortitis syndrome. *Jpn Heart J*. 1969;10(4):277–88.
8. Numano F, KT, Chang YH. Takayasu arteritis. *Heart Vessels* 1992;7(suppl):1–178.
9. Herrera EL, TG, Marcushamer J, et al. Takayasu's arteritis: Clinical study of 107 cases. *Am Heart J*. 1977;93:94–103.
10. Cong XL, Dai SM, Feng X, et al. Takayasu's arteritis: Clinical features and outcomes of 125 patients in China. *Clin Rheumatol*. 2010;29(9):973–81.
11. Chung JW, Kim HC, Choi YH, et al. Patterns of aortic involvement in Takayasu arteritis and its clinical implications: Evaluation with spiral computed tomography angiography. *J Vasc Surg*. 2007;45(5):906–14.
12. Numano F, Kobayashi Y. Takayasu arteritis—beyond pulselessness. *Intern Med*. 1999;38(3):226–32.
13. Sharma BK, Jain S, Radotra BD. An autopsy study of Takayasu arteritis in India. *Int J Cardiol*. 1998;66 Suppl 1:S85–90; discussion S1.
14. Koide K. Takayasu arteritis in Japan. *Heart Vessels Suppl*. 1992;7:48–54.
15. Giordano JM. Surgical treatment of Takayasu's arteritis. *Int J Cardiol*. 2000;75(suppl 1):S123–8.
16. Lagneau P, Michel JB, Vuong PN. Surgical treatment of Takayasu's disease. *Ann Surg*. 1987;205(2):157–66.
17. Robbs JV, Abdool-Carrim AT, Kadwa AM. Arterial reconstruction for non-specific arteritis (Takayasu's disease): Medium to long term results. *Eur J Vasc Surg*. 1994;8(4):401–7.
18. Miyata T, Sato O, Koyama H, et al. Long-term survival after surgical treatment of patients with Takayasu's arteritis. *Circulation*. 2003;108(12):1474–80.
19. Ogino H, Matsuda H, Minatoya K, et al. Overview of late outcome of medical and surgical treatment for Takayasu arteritis. *Circulation*. 2008;118(25):2738–47.
20. Taketani T, Miyata T, Morota T, et al. Surgical treatment of atypical aortic coarctation complicating Takayasu's arteritis—experience with 33 cases over 44 years. *J Vasc Surg*. 2005;41(4):597–601.
21. Weaver FA, Yellin AE, Campen DH, et al. Surgical procedures in the management of Takayasu's arteritis. *J Vasc Surg*. 1990;12(4):429–37; discussion 38–9.

22. Weaver FA, Yellin AE. Surgical treatment of Takayasu arteritis. *Heart Vessels Suppl.* 1992;7:154–8.
23. Fields CE, Bower TC, Cooper LT, et al. Takayasu's arteritis: Operative results and influence of disease activity. *J Vasc Surg.* 2006;43(1):64–71.
24. Tada Y, Kamiya K, Shindo S, et al. Carotid artery reconstruction for Takayasu's arteritis the necessity of all-autogenous-vein graft policy and development of a new operation. *Int Angiol.* 2000;19(3):242–9.
25. Kieffer E, Chiche L, Bertal A, et al. Descending thoracic and thoracoabdominal aortic aneurysm in patients with Takayasu's disease. *Ann Vasc Surg.* 2004;18(5):505–13.
26. Weaver FA, Kumar SR, Yellin AE, et al. Renal revascularization in Takayasu arteritis-induced renal artery stenosis. *J Vasc Surg.* 2004;39(4):749–57.
27. Kieffer E, Piquois A, Bertal A, et al. Reconstructive surgery of the renal arteries in Takayasu's disease. *Ann Vasc Surg.* 1990;4(2):156–65.
28. Ando M, Kosakai Y, Okita Y, et al. Surgical treatment for aortic regurgitation caused by Takayasu's arteritis. *J Card Surg.* 1998;13(3):202–7.
29. Matsuura K, Ogino H, Kobayashi J, et al. Surgical treatment of aortic regurgitation due to Takayasu arteritis: Long-term morbidity and mortality. *Circulation.* 2005;112(24):3707–12.

36

Hybrid Endovascular Repair of Thoracic and Thoracoabdominal Aortic Aneurysms

Gustavo S. Oderich, MD and Bernardo C. Mendes, MD

INTRODUCTION

Endovascular aortic aneurysm repair (EVAR) has gained widespread acceptance and is currently considered the first treatment option for most patients with abdominal and thoracic aneurysms. Prospective trials have demonstrated several short-term advantages over open repair, including less blood loss, operative time, hospital stay, mortality and morbidity.[1,2] The presence of short neck or involvement of the visceral arteries continues to limit the application of endovascular approaches. In these patients, open conventional repair remains the standard treatment, but technical complexity increases with more extensive dissection, higher clamp site, prolonged visceral ischemia and more extensive reconstruction. It is logical to speculate that the advantages achieved with endovascular repair of infra-renal aneurysms will pale in comparison to the potential for reduction in morbidity and mortality for treatment of more complex aneurysms that involve the visceral segment.

Contemporary series have shown that open repair of thoracoabdominal aortic aneurysms (TAAAs) can be performed with acceptable results in centers of excellence.[3,4] Mortality and spinal cord injury are the most frequently analyzed outcome measures, but other important end points are renal insufficiency, morbidity rates, quality of life and functional status after the operation. Coselli and associates reported 2,286 patients treated by open TAAA repair, with an operative mortality of 6.6% and spinal cord injury in 4%.[4] Other reports from large volume aortic centers have shown mortality rates in the range of 4.6% to 14.6%.[3,5] However, 'real world' data using national and regional datasets have demonstrated more ominous results. The Mayo Clinic group has reported elective TAAA repair in 300 patients, with spinal cord injury of 9% with and 12% without epidural cooling. Mortality at 30 days was 7% and 15%, respectively.[6] In the study by Rigberg and associates on 797 Medicare beneficiaries who underwent elective open TAAA repair in the State of California the mortality was 19% at 30-day and 31% in 1 year.[7]

ENDOVASCULAR STRATEGIES

Endovascular approaches to TAAAs have evolved during the last decade. The initial experiences with fenestrated and branched endografts have shown that total endovascular repair is effective and may reduce morbidity rates in patients with arch, thoracoabdominal and pararenal aneurysms.[8–11] The Cleveland Clinic group has recently reported on their updated clinical experience with the first 633 patients treated by fenestrated and branched endografts. Operative mortality was 1.8% for pararenal, 5.2% for types I–III and 2.3% for type IV TAAAs.[8] Nonetheless, these devices are not yet widely available and still require a period of customization of six to eight weeks. While "off-the-shelf" devices are likely to allow treatment of >60–80% of patients with complex aneurysms, standardized designs have not yet been tested clinically in large number of patients with longer follow up. In the absence of widely available endograft designs, a number of centers have reported creative techniques to incorporate the visceral arteries, including 'chimney', 'sandwich', 'octopus', 'periscope' and physician-modified endografts.[5,12] However, these approaches are limited by off label indication, lack of quality control, violation of basic engineering concepts, and questionable durability.

HYBRID ENDOVASCULAR REPAIR

Hybrid procedures have been introduced as a less invasive alternative to open conventional repair, avoiding the need for a thoracotomy and in many patients aortic cross clamping. The first report was by Quinones-Baldrich and associates from UCLA in 1999.[13] The operation aimed to reduce the anatomic and physiologic stress to the patient by avoiding several shortcomings of open surgery: thoracotomy, single lung ventilation, aortic cross clamping, and prolonged end-organ ischemia.

Since its introduction, hybrid procedures have been widely adopted as an alternative to open surgery. Its current role in the treatment of patients with complex aortic aneurysms has evolved, and most centers with easy access to fenestrated and branched endografts have relegated hybrid procedures to high-risk patients who are neither candidates for total endovascular repair or open surgery. It is likely that hybrid repair will be replaced by total endovascular techniques in most centers; its future applications may be in patients who fail total endovascular repair or in centers with no access or experience with fenestrated and branched endografts. Patient selection, case planning and technical aspects of the procedure are key for successful outcomes.

CLINICAL RISK ASSESSMENT

A comprehensive evaluation of cardiac, pulmonary and renal performance is crucial to optimize patient selection. These operations are often indicated in the sickest patient, but clinical data suggests that prohibitively high-risk patients and those with limited life expectancy are not ideal candidates for hybrid procedures. The evaluation should include non-invasive cardiac stress test (DSE or Sestamibi study), pulmonary function tests and carotid ultrasound. The Society for Vascular Surgery (SVS) clinical comorbidity score system can be used to stratify operative risk, but the criteria has not been validated prospectively in patients undergoing complex aortic surgery.[14] Nonetheless, most agree that factors associated with increased risk include unstable angina, symptomatic or poorly controlled ectopy, recurrent CHF, ejection fraction <25%, myocardial infarction <6 months, vital capacity <1.8 liters, FEV1 <800 ml, DLCO <30%, resting pO2 <60 mmHg and pCO2 >50 mmHg, and serum creatinine >2.5 mg/dL.

AORTIC IMAGING AND PLANNING

A basic tenet of endovascular repair is the presence of adequate seal zone. A hybrid procedure should only be considered if the extra-anatomic bypass would provide adequate proximal and/or distal sealing zones. In most centers, computed tomography angiography (CTA) is the preferred imaging modality to plan the operation (Figure 36-1); less frequently, magnetic resonance angiography (MRA) can also be used. The presence of a conic calcified and angulated neck compromises seal. A minimum length of 2-cm of parallel aortic wall without excessive calcification or thrombus is required in the thoracic aorta, and longer seal zones may be needed in the aortic arch. Distal attachment is equally important and most often can be achieved in the common iliac arteries, infrarenal aorta or prior aortic graft. If the common iliac arteries are aneurysmal, preservation of pelvic flow is critical to minimize risk of spinal cord injury.[15] Similarly, proximal debranching of the subclavian artery may reduce rates of paraplegia in patients who need extensive coverage of the thoracic aorta.

Aortic side branches requiring incorporation should also be analyzed for presence of occlusive disease, excessive calcification or thrombus, unusual or aberrant anatomy. Small sized, calcified or multiple renal arteries pose a challenge and may require complex reconstruction. The quality of the inflow site, which is typically located in the distal common and proximal external iliac artery, should be reviewed for presence of occlusive disease. It is critical to assure optimal inflow to the visceral grafts and enough length within the common iliac artery for attachment of the endografts. The presence of any abnormal venous anatomy (e.g. left sided vena cava, retro-aortic renal vein, etc) should be noted to avoid inadvertent injury. Finally, it is critical to assure adequate iliac access, which ideally should be planned in the opposite side. Nonetheless, ipsilateral access remains an alternative and can be done with a conduit, which is tied at the end and buried within the retroperitoneum for second stage procedure.

TECHNICAL TIPS

The debranching procedure can be done using midline trans-peritoneal or retroperitoneal incision, either in one or two stages followed by aortic stent graft coverage. The two-stage approach may minimize morbidity and mortality rates, particularly in the higher risk patient or in those who require difficult open surgical reconstructions. However, single

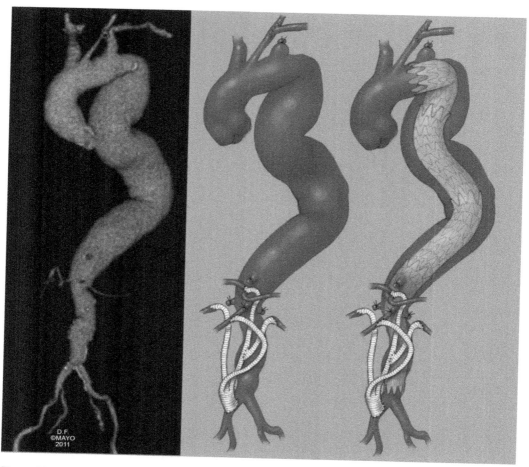

Figure 36-1. Computed tomography angiography with 3-dimensional reconstructions on a patient treated for a type II thoracoabdominal aortic aneurysm. The illustration demonstrates a four-vessel debranching based on the right common iliac artery, followed by aortic stent graft coverage as a staged procedure.

stage procedures eliminate the risk of rupture in between stages, and should be considered in those patients who have uneventful debranching, excessively large aneurysms and require more limited extent of aortic coverage. The source of inflow for extra-anatomic reconstruction is usually the distal common iliac artery extending into the proximal external iliac artery. Other alternative sites are the infrarenal aorta, previous aortic grafts, or the hepatic and splenic arteries. A variety of graft configurations have been described (Figure 36-2). Our preference is to use a trifurcated graft from one of the common iliac arteries, with an added limb depending on the patient anatomy. Alternatively, a bifurcated graft can be anastomosed with a short main body and graft limbs to the right renal and superior mesenteric arteries (Figure 36-3).[16] Separate graft limbs can be added for the celiac axis and left renal artery as needed, allowing selection of the ideal position for the graft limb and avoiding kinks, which can occur with pre-fashioned trifurcated grafts. A modification of the technique, VORTEC, was described by Lachat and associates and allows a sutureless anastomosis using Viabahn stent grafts (WL Gore, Flagstaff, AZ).[17]

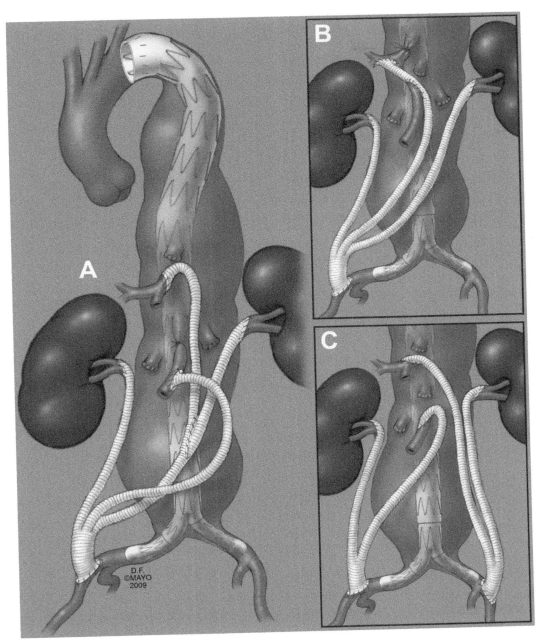

Figure 36-2. Configurations of 4-vessel visceral debranching. These included use of a pre-fashioned trifurcated graft with a separate side limb (**A**), trifurcated graft with side-to-side anastomosis into the superior mesenteric artery (**B**), and bilateral bifurcated grafts (**C**), as well as a variety of other creative configurations.

Perigraft fluid collections have been described in 54% of patients treated by hybrid repair. These can represent perigraft seromas with benign course or frank graft infection. Predictors of perigraft fluid include impaired renal function or advanced age, and PTFE grafts as opposed to polyester graft. Therefore, our preference has been to

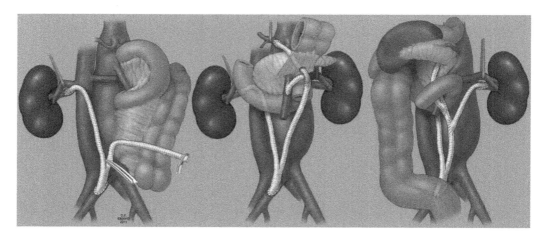

Figure 36-3. Four-vessel debranching based on a bifurcated right common iliac graft to avoid kinks and allow position of separate side limbs anastomosed in one of the limbs of the bifurcated graft.

use polyester grafts and to cover the grafts by retroperitoneal tissue and/or omentum to prevent graft enteric erosion.[18]

RESULTS

Single-Center Experiences

Despite logical advantages over open repair and early successes, results of hybrid procedures have been tempered by high morbidity and mortality rates in several centers (Table 36-1).[5,19] The UCLA and University of Michigan groups have reported two of the largest experiences with remarkably low mortality rates of 0% and 3.4%, respectively.[20,21] Others (Cleveland Clinic, Mayo Clinic, Mass General Hospital, Methodist Hospital Houston) have shown higher mortality rates in the range of 10% to 25%. Lin and associates reported high mortality rates for hybrid repair of TAAAs using single or two-stage approaches in a center with large referral of open TAAAs.[22] Spinal cord injury occurs in 2 to 25% and correlates with extent of aortic coverage, preservation of flow into the subclavian and hypogastric arteries and periprocedural hypotension.[5] Rates of type I and II endoleak have been reported in the range of 3% to 15% and 5% to 25%, respectively.

Systematic Reviews

Two systematic reviews of the available literature have been published on hybrid repair of TAAAs.[23,24] Bakoyiannis and associates reviewed the outcomes of 108 patients from 15 reports between 1999 and 2008. Technical success was 92% and 30-day mortality 10%.[23] In this report, 19 patients (17%) had primary endoleaks and other three (3%) developed secondary endoleaks. Spinal cord injury occurred in three patients (3%) and renal insufficiency in 12 (11%). After a mean follow up of 10 months, 97% of the visceral grafts remained patent and 24% of patients died of unrelated causes.

A more recent review by Moulakakis and associates included 507 patients and 19 reports published since 1999. There were 319 male (64%) and 188 female patients with mean age of 70 years old. Aneurysm extent was classified as type I in 14%, type

TABLE 36-1. RESULTS OF REPORTED CLINICAL SERIES OF HYBRID REPAIR OF THORACOABDOMINAL AORTIC ANEURYSMS.

Author	Year	n	Mortality[a]	Morbidity	Spinal Cord Injury[b]	Dialysis	Endoleak	Reintervention	Mean Follow-Up
					Percent				Months
Fulton et al.	2005	10	0	50	0	0	10	10	8.7
Resch et al.	2006	13	38	23	31	15	23	38	23
Black et al.	2006	29	21	69	0	7	38	10	8
Donas et al.	2007	8	12	37	0	12	0	25	21
Lee et al.	2007	17	23	23	0	12	12	12	8
Gawenda et al.	2007	6	0	0	0	0	17	0	12
Ballard et al.	2008	4	25	50	25	25	0	0	12
Van de Mortel et al.	2008	16	31	19	0	12	12	0	13
Quinones–Baldrich et al.	2009	17	0	53	6	0	23	29	16.6
Biasi et al.	2009	18	22	22	5	0	33	5	23
Da Rocha et al.	2009	9	44	33	11	11	0	0	79.2
Donas-Lachtat et al.	2009	58	26	c	3	0	12	7	22.1
Drinkwater et al.	2009	107	15	3	12	26	31	c	c
Kabbani et al.	2010	36	17	30	3	11	44	19	6
Patel et al.	2010	29	3	3	3	17	34	7	30.5
Kuratani et al.	2010	86	4	7	1	0	10	7	88.5
Chiesa et al.	2010	41	17	15	7	0	10	2	23.3
Smith et al.	2011	24	12	62	8	17c	8	37	11.7
Lin et al.	2012	58	24	52	c	10	3	3	27.3
Hughes et al.	2012	47	8	36	4	13	0	0	19.3
NACAAD Registry	2012	208	14	73	10	7	13	39	23
Total		841	15	33	6	12	16	15	

NACAAD – **N**orth **A**merican **C**omplex **A**bdominal **A**ortic **D**ebranching

a. Overall mortality
b. transient or permanent.
c. non-specified

II in 27%, type III in 34%, type IV in 14% and type V in 11%. A single stage procedure was used in 55% and two-stage in 45%, with mean period of 28 days between the two stages. Thirty-day or in-hospital mortality was 13% and the most common causes of death were multisystem organ failure, ischemic colitis, respiratory failure and aneurysm rupture prior to a second stage procedure. Pooled rates of spinal cord injury were 7.5%, with irreversible paraplegia in 4.5%. After a mean follow up of 35 months, a total of 111 patients (22%) had endoleaks and visceral graft patency was 96%.[24]

North American Complex Abdominal Aortic Debranching (NACAAD) Registry

The preliminary results of the NACAAD registry were presented at the 2011 Vascular Annual meeting. This study included 208 patients treated for complex abdominal aortic aneurysms in 14 academic centers of North America. There were 118 male (57%) and 90 female patients with mean age of 71 years old. Cardiovascular risk factors included hypertension in 86%, cigarette smoking in 78%, hyperlipidemia in 60%, coronary artery disease in 58%, chronic pulmonary disease in 43%, prior aortic repair in 42%, and chronic kidney disease stage >3 (eGFR <60 ml/hr/ 1.73m^2) in 28%. Aneurysm diameter averaged 6.6 ± 1.3 cm and aneurysm extent included 163 TAAA (type I in 6%, type II in 25%, type III in 31% and type IV) and 45 pararenal aneurysms. A total of 659 visceral arteries were reconstructed using single stage debranching in 92 patients (44%) or two stage approach in 116 (56%). Arch debranching was needed in 22 patients (11%) to provide adequate proximal landing zone. The inflow for visceral reconstruction was based on the iliac arteries in 63%, aorta or aortic graft in 29% or a hepatic/ splenic artery in 8%. Extent of visceral reconstruction includes one- or two vessels in 58 patients (28%) and three or four vessels in 150 (72%).

Thirty-day or in-hospital mortality was 14% for all patients, 16% for TAAAs and 9% for pararenal aneurysms. Mortality rates ranged from 0% to 21% in centers with >10 cases. In this study, mortality was associated with severity of comorbidities as determined by SVS clinical scores: 3% for low risk patients (SVS score <9) and 17% for high-risk patients (score >9). Independent predictors of early mortality included >3vessel reconstruction, coronary artery disease, CHF, high SVS scores and chronic kidney disease stage >3. Any morbidity occurred in 73% of the patients, most commonly pulmonary (22%), renal (19%), and gastrointestinal complications (14%). Spinal cord injury occurred in 21 patients (10%) and ischemic colitis in 13 (6%). The mean length of hospital stay was 21 days. Patient survival at 1- and 5-years were 77 ± 3% and 61 ± 5% and predictors of late mortality included chronic kidney disease (stage >3), high SVS scores and >3 vessel reconstruction. After a median follow up of 21 months, 70% of the patients had repeat aortic imaging. Endoleaks occurred in 23 patients (13%) and were classified as type I in 3%, type II in 8% and type III in 1%. Primary visceral graft patency and freedom from re-interventions were 90 ± 2% and 85 ± 3% at 1-year, respectively.[25]

CONCLUSION

Hybrid procedures have several advantages over conventional open repair including avoiding thoracotomy, single-lung ventilation, aortic cross clamping and minimizing end-organ ischemia. Shortcomings are the need for extensive dissection in multiple abdominal areas and prolonged operative time. Patient selection is key for optimal results. A few centers have adopted hybrid procedures as their primary treatment option in intermediate and high-risk patients with good results. However, several centers with large complex aortic volume, systematic reviews and a national registry have shown that hybrid procedures carry high mortality rates. It is likely, that once fenestrated and branched endografts will receive FDA approval for clinical use, indications for hybrid repair of complex aortic aneurysms will further diminish.

REFERENCES

1. EVAR Trial Participants. Endovascular aneurysm repair versus open repair in patients with abdominal aortic aneurysm (EVAR trial 1): Randomised controlled trial. *Lancet*. 2005;365:2179–86.
2. Prinssen M, Verhoeven EL, Buth J, et al. A randomized trial comparing conventional and endovascular repair of abdominal aortic aneurysms. *N Engl J Med*. 2004;351(16):1607–18.
3. Conrad MF, Crawford RS, Davison JK, et al. Thoracoabdominal aneurysm repair: A 20-year perspective. *Ann Thorac Surg*. 2007;83(2):S856–61; discussion S90–2.
4. Coselli JS, Bozinovski J, LeMaire SA. Open surgical repair of 2286 thoracoabdominal aortic aneurysms. *Ann Thorac Surg*. 2007;83(2):S862–4; discussion S90–2.
5. Oderich GS, Mendes BC, Gloviczki P, et al. Current role and future directions of hybrid repair of thoracoabdominal aortic aneurysms. *Perspect Vasc Surg Endovasc Ther*. 2012;24(1):14–22.
6. Gloviczki P. Surgical repair of thoracoabdominal aneurysms: Patient selection, techniques and results. *Cardiovasc Surg*. 2002;10(4):434–41.
7. Rigberg DA, McGory ML, Zingmond DS, et al. Thirty-day mortality statistics underestimate the risk of repair of thoracoabdominal aortic aneurysms: A statewide experience. *J Vasc Surg*. 2006;43(2):217–22; discussion 23.
8. Greenberg R, Eagleton M, Mastracci T. Branched endografts for thoracoabdominal aneurysms. *J Thorac Cardiovasc Surg*. 2010;140(6 Suppl):S171–8.
9. Greenberg RK, Lu Q, Roselli EE, et al. Contemporary analysis of descending thoracic and thoracoabdominal aneurysm repair: A comparison of endovascular and open techniques. *Circulation*. 2008;118(8):808–17.
10. Nordon IM, Hinchliffe RJ, Holt PJ, et al. Modern treatment of juxtarenal abdominal aortic aneurysms with fenestrated endografting and open repair–A systematic review. *Eur J Vasc Endovasc Surg*. 2009;38(1):35–41.
11. Verhoeven EL, Vourliotakis G, Bos WT, et al. Fenestrated stent grafting for short-necked and juxtarenal abdominal aortic aneurysm: An 8-year single-centre experience. *Eur J Vasc Endovasc Surg*. 2010;39(5):529–36.
12. Oderich GS, Ricotta JJ, Hofer J, et al. Surgeon-modified fenestrated and branched stent graft for high risk patients with juxtarenal, paravisceral and thoracoabdominal aortic aneurysms: Comparison with open abdominal debranching in a single center. *J Vasc Surg*. 2009;49 (supplement): S48–9.
13. Quinones-Baldrich WJ, Panetta TF, Vescera CL, et al. Repair of type IV thoracoabdominal aneurysm with a combined endovascular and surgical approach. *J Vasc Surg*. 1999;30(3):555–60.
14. Chaikof EL, Fillinger MF, Matsumura JS, et al. Identifying and grading factors that modify the outcome of endovascular aortic aneurysm repair. *J Vasc Surg*. 2002;35(5):1061–6.
15. Drinkwater SL, Goebells A, Haydar A, et al. The incidence of spinal cord ischaemia following thoracic and thoracoabdominal aortic endovascular intervention. *Eur J Vasc Endovasc Surg*. 2010;40(6):729–35.
16. Lall P, Kalra M, McKusick MA. Hybrid endovascular and open surgical repair of a Crawford type III thoracoabdominal aneurysm in a high-risk patient. *Perspect Vasc Surg Endovasc Ther*. 2006;18(3):255–8.
17. Lachat M, Mayer D, Criado FJ, et al. New technique to facilitate renal revascularization with use of telescoping self-expanding stent grafts: VORTEC. *Vascular*. 2008;16(2):69–72.

18. Hurie J, Patel HJ, Criado E, et al. Postoperative fluid collection after hybrid debranching and endovascular repair of thoracoabdominal aortic aneurysms. *J Vasc Surg.* 2011;54(6):1623–8.

19. Hughes GC, Barfield ME, Shah AA, et al. Staged total abdominal debranching and thoracic endovascular aortic repair for thoracoabdominal aneurysm. *J Vasc Surg.* 2012. Epub ahead of print May 9.

20. Patel HJ, Upchurch GR, Jr., Eliason JL, et al. Hybrid debranching with endovascular repair for thoracoabdominal aneurysms: A comparison with open repair. *Ann Thorac Surg.* 2010;89(5):1475-81.

21. Quinones-Baldrich W, Jimenez JC, DeRubertis B, et al. Combined endovascular and surgical approach (CESA) to thoracoabdominal aortic pathology: A 10-year experience. *J Vasc Surg.* 2009;49(5):1125–34.

22. Lin PH, Kougias P, Bechara CF, et al. Clinical outcome of staged versus combined treatment approach of hybrid repair of thoracoabdominal aortic aneurysm with visceral vessel debranching and aortic endograft exclusion. *Perspect Vasc Surg Endovasc Ther.* 2012;24(1):5–13

23. Bakoyiannis C, Kalles V, Economopoulos K, et al. Hybrid procedures in the treatment of thoracoabdominal aortic aneurysms: A systematic review. *J Endovasc Ther.* 2009;16(4):443–50.

24. Moulakakis KG, Mylonas SN, Avgerinos ED, et al. Hybrid open endovascular technique for aortic thoracoabdominal pathologies. *Circulation.* 2011;124(24):2670–80.

25. Oderich GS, Farber M, Quinones-Baldrich W, et al. Abdominal debranching with aortic stent grafts for complex aortic aneurysms: Preliminary results of the North American Complex Abdominal Aortic Debranching (NACAAD) registry. Presented at the 2011 Vascular Annual Meeting, Chicago IL, June 18 2011.

37

Chimney, Snorkel, Periscope Combined with EVAR/TEVAR

Chandu Vemuri, MD and Luis A. Sanchez, MD

INTRODUCTION

The endovascular treatment of abdominal and thoracic aortic pathology has significantly evolved since Parodi and colleagues published their data on endovascular repair of aortic aneurysms (EVAR) in 1991.[1] This technology has been embraced in the treatment of AAAs and randomized trials have demonstrated lower morbidity and mortality in the short-term, although longer term data suggest higher cost and no further reduction in mortality.[2,3]

Since Dake et al. published their revolutionary series for the endovascular management of thoracic aneurysms in their 1994 article discussing TEVAR, the success of TEVAR has been documented in multiple industry sponsored trials, single-center experiences and registries.[4] Walsh et al published a meta-analysis in 2008 which revealed that TEVAR had a lower mortality and rate of neurologic complications compared to open surgical repair.[5]

To date EVAR accounts for >60% of the treatment of infra-renal AAAs and for 50% of thoracic aneurysms. The data on EVAR and TEVAR lag behind the rapid development of devices, improvements in the technical aspects of the procedure and the introduction of adjunctive procedures. Additionally, knowledge and understanding of the anatomical limitations of EVAR/TEVAR has increased and new techniques have evolved to attempt to overcome them. Aortic neck length, for EVAR >10 mm and for TEVAR >15 mm, remains the most significant limitation for the successful use of endovascular devices. Many are used outside the devices' IFU in patients with short and angulated necks. Retrospective studies have shown that this results in a higher rate of both early and late Type I endoleaks which require additional interventions to maintain exclusion of the aneurysm.[6]

In an attempt to better treat patients unfit for open surgery for juxtarenal/suprarenal abdominal aortic aneurysms or complex thoracic aneurysms near the major branches, there has been an increase in the creative use of endovascular technology.[7] Aggressive proximal deployment techniques in patients with challenging landing

431

zones can be complicated by covering of major branches of the thoracic and abdominal aorta and endovascular rescue techniques were developed to re-establish flow such as the placement of chimney grafts, snorkeling and periscope grafts. As the experience with these techniques grew they began to be used prophylactically at the time of initial operation to increase graft attachment and decrease endoleak rates. Fenestrated and branched endografts have been developed to address this problem. However, they have limited availability and devices currently require weeks to construct and tailor for each patient whereas the chimney/snorkel/periscope technique can be readily used with off-the-shelf components.[8,9]

We will review the current concepts and data behind the use of chimney grafts, the snorkel technique and periscope grafts as adjunctive procedures in EVAR/TEVAR for the treatment of abdominal and thoracic aortic pathologies.

CHIMNEY GRAFTS AND THE SNORKEL TECHNIQUE

Concept

The "snorkel" and "chimney graft" techniques are named after the physical appearance of the deployed stents. The purpose is to maintain flow to a visceral or aortic branch vessel with a stent that begins in the target vessel, runs parallel to the main body of the graft and then extends into the aortic lumen.

ABDOMINAL AORTIC ANEURYSMS

In patients with a short proximal neck seal zone, there are ultimately two options for treatment: open abdominal thoracic/aortic aneurysm repair or, in those unfit for surgery, complex endovascular repair. Treatment in some of these patients may require placement of the device at or above the level of the renals or require coverage of multiple visceral branches. To preserve blood flow to the renal arteries Greenberg et al. described a procedure in which stents can be placed into the renal arteries alongside the main body of the graft to allow flow to the renals while permitting more proximal placement of the endograft to potentially improve the seal zone. Specifically, they described deploying the proximal portion of the graft a few millimeters over the ostium of the lowest renal artery. Prior to the main body deployment they had attained access to the renal artery retrograde through a brachial approach. If renal flow was compromised by the main body they would deploy a self expanding stent. If they had not gained access to the renal artery first, they would gain access via the contralateral limb and would deploy a balloon expandable stent. Regardless of the technique, this essentially raises the orifice of the renal arteries. If there was a persistent type IA endoleak they would deploy an aortic Palmaz stent to obtain a proximal seal. (7) This technique has come to be called snorkeling or placement of a chimney graft. In general, snorkels are short covered/uncovered balloon expandable stents used to maintain patency of an aortic branch allowing more proximal placement of the endograft by a short distance (<2 cm). Chimney grafts are longer, parallel, self-expanding covered stents used to maintain patency of aortic branches that are covered by the endograft for a long distance (>2 cm). Although they are technically different, these terms are often used interchangeably.

Since that initial report, many groups have published individual/institutional case series. In 2008 Ohrlander et al. described chimney graft placement in the renal and superior mesenteric (SMA) arteries. For thoracic aortic branches they described placement of chimney grafts in the left subclavian artery (LSA), left common carotid artery (CCA) and the innominate artery. Planned cannulation of the aortic arch branches was achieved in a retrograde fashion while the abdominal aortic branches were accessed antegrade from above. The main body of the endograft was deployed followed by chimney grafts. In the event of inadvertent coverage of aortic branches an antegrade or retrograde approach was used to gain access to the vessels and in one instance laparotomy for retrograde cannulation of the SMA was described.[10] Since then they have reported completing a total of 25 cases in the abdominal aorta and multiple in the thoracic aorta. For the abdominal cases 8 were elective and the remaining were ruptured or symptomatic. 2/25 patients had an SMA stent in addition to renal stenting. Almost all patients had a balloon-expandable stent placed. They had three deaths in the ruptured patients with 2 from multi-organ failure and 1 from a persistent type IA endoleak. With a mean follow-up of 10 months, they had only one chimney graft occlusion and three type I endoleaks, of which one required intervention.[11]

Another large case series was published by Hiramoto et al. in 2009 and discussed their management of 29 patients who underwent EVAR with Zenith endografts and renal artery stenting. In this study a chimney graft or snorkel was utilized when there was a preoperative plan to nearly cover or "encroach" upon the renal arteries. Access to the renal artery was attained via a brachial approach. Their stent choice covered the full range of balloon-expandable, self-expanding, bare-metal and covered stents. They suggest that balloon-expandable stents are better as they track more easily, can be deployed precisely and have better radial force than self-expanding stents. Furthermore, they commented that covered stents are more difficult in these circumstances as their increased bulkiness leads to stiffness and renders them more difficult to deploy. If a renal ostium is partially covered they gained access either antegrade or retrograde depending on patient specific anatomy. Three additional technical points regarding the encroachment technique from this study warrant discussion. The first is understanding that access to the renal arteries was gained through the interstices of the uncovered proximal stent. However, the interstices may be narrow or wide and they verified that they had entered through a workable route by checking for passage of a 5 French sheath. If they were unable to place a sheath, they would withdraw and began renal access again. The second point is that the proximal stent does not need to be fully deployed for the encroachment technique. Renal access can be obtained even in a partially opened state. Lastly, in the encroachment technique they always used balloon-expanding stents as the radial force in self-expanding stents was felt to be insufficient and they ensured that 5 mm of the stent was protruding into the aorta. They reported an intraoperative type I endoleak rate of 17.2% (5 patients) and they were able to successfully treat four of these with a Palmaz stent. Of technical note, the balloons should be inflated in the renal stents at the same time as Palmaz stent deployment so they are not crushed. 10.3% of patients had a new type I endoleak on a postoperative CT scan all of which resolved without intervention. They reported no restenosis during their followup and 100% primary assisted patency at a median follow-up of 12.5 months.[12]

Troisi et al. published their experience using the Endurant graft in 2010. They treated 156 patients in total and 14 patients (9%) needed utilization of the chimney graft technique. While the technical details are not fully elaborated upon, they discuss that chimney grafts were used in patients with a <5 mm proximal aortic neck. They reported successful completion of the technique and a type I endoleak rate of 1.3%. Furthermore, they had one renal artery thrombosis and a type III endoleak. Therefore, they concluded that the technique provides immediately acceptable results, but the long term efficacy was unclear.[13]

A more recent series was published by Lee et al. in April 2012. They reviewed patients treated with the chimney graft technique from 2009–2011. Over that time period they placed 56 chimney grafts in 28 patients. Of significance only 5 were unilateral renal grafts, 17 were bilateral renal grafts and 6 were multi-visceral grafts. Their technical success rate was 98.2% with the only failure due to loss of wire access to a renal vessel. Over a mean follow-up of 10.7 months they reported a thirty-day mortality of 7.1%, permanent hemodialysis in 3.6%, 98.2% graft patency, and 25% early endoleaks with one requiring endovascular re-intervention.[14]

Two review articles summarize the majority of the published literature to date. The first was in 2012 from Moulakakis et al which analyzed the data from 15 studies with a mean followup of 9 months +/− 1 month. A total of 93 patients were treated and 77.4% had a chimney graft for abdominal aneurysmal disease, 5.4% for TAAAs, one for a Marfan's patient with dissection, 8.6% for para-anastomotic aneurysm in patients who had a prior open repair, 6.4% for correction of endoleak and in 2.1% for occlusive disease. While the Zenith (Cook Inc) and Excluder (W.L. Gore and Associates) grafts were the most commonly used endografts, other FDA approved grafts were also used. In the aggregate group of patients, 134 chimney grafts were placed. The majority, 108, were placed in a renal artery and 26 in the mesenteric vasculature. All the chimney grafts were successfully placed however there were immediate and mid-term complications. Specifically, an overall type I endoleak rate of 14%, 10 postoperatively detected endoleaks (4 require re-intervention) and 3 graft thromboses. They analyzed endoleak rate by the number of chimney grafts placed and found 7% were in those with one, 15.6% in those with two, 0% in those with three and 100% (1/1) for four. A statistically insignificant correlation between the use of covered stents and endoleak was reported. In regards to major morbidity and mortality 11.8% had renal impairment, 2.1% myocardial infarction, 3.2% ischemic stroke and 30 day in-hospital mortality was 4.3%.[15] Tolenaar et al. also published an insightful review in 2012 in which they reviewed eight studies on the chimney procedure. They summarized the aggregate data on 75 patients (52 AAA, 23 TAAA) who had 96 chimney grafts placed (7 innominate arteries, 13 left common carotid, three left subclavian, 11 superior mesenteric arteries, 62 renal arteries). The full range of FDA approved aortic endografts was used with a combination of chimney grafts and the follow-up ranged from 2 days to 54 months. The analysis revealed 6.7% (5) type I endoleaks and in regards to late complications they found one SMA stent occlusion, three deaths (1 from MI, 1 from stroke, 1 from overstenting of the SMA resulting in mesenteric ischemia) and two chimney graft occlusions requiring open thrombectomy.[16]

The review articles discussed are representative of the existing data on the use of chimney grafts. While there have been no randomized control trials to date, Bruen et al. published a study comparing open repair (21 patients) versus endovascular repair (21 patients) of juxta and suprarenal aneurysms in anatomically matched patients. Those patients suitable for open repair were treated as such and those not suitable for open repair were evaluated for endovascular repair with planned chimney grafts. They limited the endovascular repairs to patient who would require no more than two chimney grafts based on preoperative planning. Technical points from this study include the use of 7 French sheaths advanced over Rosen wires (Cook, Inc, Bloomington, Indiana) into the target visceral vessel, followed by deployment of the main body endograft, deployment of iCast chimney grafts (Atrium, Hudson, NH) with 20 mm in the visceral vessel and 5–10 mm into the renal arteries above the covered portion of the main body endograft. They then performed triple "kissing-balloon" deployment as others have done by inflating the proximal balloon in the aortic endograft simultaneously with balloons in the visceral stents. The thirty-day in hospital mortality was 4.8% for both groups and late survival was also similar at 87–89%. As expected, operative blood loss, ICU and hospital LOS and transfusions were significantly less in the endovascular group. The endovascular group had two strokes whereas the open repair group trended towards higher pulmonary complications. In regards, to renal function 29% (6) patients in the endovascular group had acute kidney injury whereas five patients in the open group had either acute kidney injury or acute renal failure with two patients requiring chronic hemodialysis. Acute kidney injury in the endovascular group was not related to the volume of contrast but renal preservation was correlated with maintenance of renal vessel patency. Primary chimney graft patency was 84% at 12 months and there was only one type Ia endoleak which resolved spontaneously. Ultimately, this study revealed that in the short-term endovascular repair with chimney grafts was not inferior to open repair and demonstrated decreased morbidity. Furthermore, it provided a feasible therapeutic alternative to those patients deemed unfit for surgery.[17]

AUTHORS' TECHNICAL POINTS

Successful endovascular repair of juxtarenal and suprarenal aneurysms requiring major branch coverage requires careful patient selection with meticulous preoperative planning. As highlighted by the data, the risks of renal failure and mesenteric ischemia must be discussed with the patients. Once the decision has been made to proceed, there are a few technical tips that enhance success. Reviewing and understanding the specific visceral/renal arterial morphology is essential to deciding whether to approach the vessel antegrade or retrograde. Once access is obtained, a Rosen or other stiff wire provides reliable access to the vessel with minimal trauma. One must advance a sheath into the target vessel prior to deployment of the main body of the endograft. Furthermore, the size of sheath the vessel allows may limit stent choices. Covered, balloon-expandable stents are preferable for snorkels for reasons discussed above which include easy tracking, precise deployment and strong radial force. I would recommend that at least 15–20 mm of the stent be in the target vessel with 5 mm above the covered portion of the main endograft. Following deployment of the snorkel graft the sheath should be re-advanced into the target vessel as the balloon is deflated to allow continued access to the vessel. The triple kissing balloon concept is essential to accomplish the duel goals of proximal seal and chimney graft patency. Chimney grafts using self-expanding covered stents are best for longer segments (>2 cm) and run parallel to the aortic endovascular reconstruction. If compression of the covered stent or poor transition into the target vessel is noted, an additional self-expanding stent should be added to the chimney graft.

THORACIC AORTIC ANEURYSMS

Treatment of thoracic aortic pathology is traditionally associated with significant morbidity and mortality although significant advances have been made in the past two decades. As discussed previously, TEVAR may allow patients unfit for surgery to undergo treatment and may evolve to become the primary treatment modality as data matures. However, a significant portion of patients cannot undergo traditional TEVAR due to lack of an adequate proximal or distal landing zone of 15–20 mm. Specifically, in order to obtain a seal and treat the aortic pathology the main body of the stent graft may need to extend across one or multiple aortic arch and/or mesenteric branches. To provide endovascular repair for these patients a variety of techniques have evolved: 1. Planned endovascular coverage of aortic branch vessels with surgical bypass, 2. Branched endovascular devices, 3. Unmodified endovascular devices with placement of chimney grafts.

In 1999, Inoue et al. described the use of branched endovascular thoracic stent grafts in fifteen patients. Fourteen had an endograft with one branch, and one patient had an endograft with three branches. They were able to achieve complete thrombosis of the aneurysm in 73% of treated patients with 4 leaks, one intra-operative external iliac rupture, one incidence of peripheral microembolization and one patient with a cerebral infarction. This early series demonstrated the feasibility of this technique.[18] Criado et al. published a description of the multiple re-vascularization options available via extra-anatomic bypasses when coverage of aortic branches is planned at the time of TEVAR.[19] In 2003, Chuter et al. published a description of hybrid technique that involved a modular graft with a limb into the innominate and extra-anatomic bypasses for reconstruction of the left carotid and left subclavian vessels.[20]

The chimney graft technique has also been employed at the time of TEVAR to treat thoracic aortic pathology. Much like the data on chimney grafts in the endovascular treatment of abdominal aortic pathology, case reports comprise the available literature.

Larzon et al. published a case series of two patients with thoracic aortic aneurysms where exclusion required covering the left subclavian artery and encroaching on the ostium of the left carotid. In these patients, they first performed a left carotid to subclavian bypass with an 8 mm graft and then placed a 7Fr sheath through the left carotid artery to maintain access. Once the main body thoracic aortic stent graft, Gore TAG® (W.L. Gore and Associates Inc, Flagstaff, AZ, USA) was deployed, the chimney graft into the left common carotid was deployed. Of note, they also coiled embolized the subclavian arteries. Both patients did well with no significant, persistent endoleaks or cerebrovascular events.[21]

In 2007, Criado et al. published a series of 8 patients to discuss a technique centered on the percutaneous deployed of chimney grafts for aortic arch branches. The main body thoracic aortic endografts were all Talent grafts and they performed the procedure only if coverage or encroachment of the aortic branches would result in obtainment of a 20 mm proximal seal zone. They used a micropuncture technique to gain percutaneous access to the left common carotid artery and placed a wire through the ostium into the arch. They then deployed the main body of the thoracic aortic endograft and if encroachment/coverage was found on subsequent imaging they proceeded to chimney graft placement. To do this they exchanged the wire over the micropuncture sheath for a 0.035 stiff guidewire (Storq or Wholey) and introduced a

6 french sheath. They then used a 6 or 7 x 40 mm balloon to expand the ostium and also to help in determining the size of the stent needed. They then would place an 8.0 or 9.0 by 29 or 39 mm balloon-expandable, uncovered stent with minimal protrusion of the stent into the aortic lumen. Left subclavian chimney grafts were placed using a similar technique with percutaneous access obtained via access to the brachial artery in the ante-cubital fossa. They reported excellent results with 100% technical success, 100% primary patency, 0% stroke, 0% mortality at follow-up ranging from 10–32 months in 6 patients.[22]

Another important series is from Sugiura et al. in 2009. They discuss their experience in the management of 11 patients who required a TEVAR with a chimney graft. The thoracic aortic pathologies being treated were: acute complicated type b dissection (2), ruptured arch aneurysm (1), ruptured descending aortic aneurysm (2), traumatic aortic transection (1), aortoesophageal fistula (1), rescue of overstented aortic branch vessel (4). The distribution of chimney grafts into the branch vessels was: innominate (3), left common carotid (7), left subclavian (1). They used covered stents when the purpose was to extend the proximal seal zone and uncovered stents when the purpose was to re-establish flow to an inadvertently overstented vessel. Access to the innominate and left carotid was via open exposure and the left subclavian via percutaneous access. Two technical points are the use of a carotid-carotid bypass with all innominate chimney grafts and the use of balloon-expandable stents inside self-expanding stents to increase the radial force. With a mean follow-up of 20.1 months they reported 100% technical success, 100% chimney graft patency with no compression or kinking, two deaths, two type Ia endoleaks, one case of transient paraplegia, one iliac artery rupture and no cases of postoperative aneurysm sac enlargement. Of the two deaths one was from lung cancer and the other a fatal, intraoperative stroke in a patient who had a TEVAR and left common carotid chimney graft who had unknown total right internal carotid occlusion. Of the two type Ia endoleaks, both were in patients with chimney grafts in the innominate artery, one was treated successfully with coil embolization and the second patient was awaiting treatment at the time of publication.[23]

AUTHORS' TECHNICAL POINTS

TEVAR for thoracic aortic pathologies has many crucial technical points. In regards to chimney grafts, as with EVAR patient selection and preoperative planning are essential. In elective cases, with planned use of the chimney graft technique, establishing access to the target vessel and placing a sheath through the ostium into the aortic lumen is a key protective maneuver. In cases where it is not for certain that a chimney graft would be needed, establishing this access will protect against a situation with inadvertent coverage of an aortic branch vessel where flow cannot be re-established. In regards to stent selection, balloon-expandable stents are preferred for the same reasons of trackability, precise deployment and strong radial force. Covered stents are applicable in situations where a proximal seal is the goal and uncovered stents in situations where re-establishing flow is the goal. Self-expanding stents are most useful if a significant parallel course (>2 cm) is necessary to obtain a seal in the aortic neck similar to the situation with suprarenal aneurysms.

PERISCOPE GRAFTS

Concept

The principle of these grafts is similar to the overall concept to snorkeling or placing chimney grafts in that a stent is placed in a vessel to maintain patency and allow for sealing of an endograft. The key differences are that this is used to help extend the distal landing zone and that the flow in these grafts is retrograde. Self-expanding, covered stents are the usually the stent of choice.

Literature

The data on the periscope technique is less mature than that on the chimney graft technique. Although there are several case reports of complex endovascular repair of thoracic and abdominal aortic pathology, we will limit this discussion to case series in which the periscope graft technique was used.

Rancic et al. published their initial experience on the periscoping technique in 2010. They attained percutaneous, retrograde access to the target vessel. An 8 french sheath was left in place and a balloon-expandable stent was placed over a Rosen guidewire. The main body thoracic or abdominal aortic graft was then placed and deployed. The periscope grafts were then deployed and extended if needed. As with the chimney grafts the triple-kissing-balloon technique was employed to obtain a distal seal of the endograft while maintaining patency of the periscope grafts. They described two patients they treated in this fashion. The first was a 58 year-old male with an acute, ruptured Crawford type III TAAA who already had occlusion of the celiac trunk, SMA and left renal artery. They deployed the thoracic main body and maintained perfusion of the mesenteric vasculature via a Viabahn (W.L. Gore and Associates Inc, Flagstaff, Ariz) into the IMA and right renal flow with a Palmaz Blue stent (Cordis Endovascular, Warren, NJ) and a Viabahn stent graft. The patient's family ultimately withdrew care due to ongoing issues with infection, but they reported patency of the periscope grafts TAAA on autopsy. The second patient was a 40 year-old male with a Crawford type I and after deployment of the main body they maintained celiac and SMA perfusion via the periscope technique. Immediate post-operative imaging revealed a type Ib leak that spontaneously sealed and remained so at six months. Of note both patients were hemodynamically unstable and determined to not be candidates for open surgery. The authors discuss that their preference is for covered stents as bare metal stents could produce type Ib endoleaks. The also discussed their preference of Viabahn stents for their flexibility. Thirdly, they discuss an issue specific to the periscope technique in that the aortic endograft may impinge on the periscope grafts and cause reduced flow and similarly the periscope grafts may reduce the distal aortic lumen. For this reason they recommend routinely performing pressure measurements and augmenting periscope graft flow with additional stenting or augmenting distal aortic flow with axillofemoral bypass as indicated by the pressure measurement.[24]

Pecoraro et al. published their series of nine patients treated with this technique. Specifically they treated six ruptured TAAAs, two para-renal AAAs and one infrarenal AAA with a combination of chimney grafts ($n = 7$) and at least one periscope graft ($n = 17$). The chimney graft and periscope graft techniques were similar to those in the above mentioned studies. They reported one technical complication of a dislodged renal graft and flow was not able to be re-established, one postoperative death from multi-organ system failure, six patients had early endoleaks of which two required endovascular re-intervention. At 10 months of mean follow-up 5/8 were living (mortality of 11%), no patients had aneurysm growth, all the chimney and periscope grafts were patent, one type III endoleak which was untreated as there was no aneurysm growth and one persistent type Ib endoleak which also was managed conservatively as there was no aneurysm growth. Of technical note, they mention only considering this technique if the target vessel for chimney/periscope grafts is at least 4 mm in diameter and there is a landing zone of at least 10 mm.[25]

Dias et al. published their experience in 2011. They treated four patients with TEVAR and periscope grafts into the SMA. Three patients had TAAAs and one had a type B dissection. They had 100% technical success, one perioperative death in a patient with a ruptured TAAA, and at followup of 7, 12, 14 months, the patients had patent SMA grafts with no abdominal symptoms. Of note the TAAAs were excluded in 2/3 patients and the third dissection patient had flow in the false lumen but was rendered asymptomatic. The authors point out the necessity of ensuring a patent pancreaticoduodenal arcade to ensure that with a covered celiac trunk, a periscope graft in the SMA will provide adequate flow to the SMA and celiac trunk distributions and long term exclusion of the aneurysm being treated.[26]

CONCLUSION

The treatment of abdominal and thoracic aortic pathologies is in rapid evolution. The diffusion of existing technology along with the development of new technology has made the field challenging and exciting. Currently, there are no randomized trials evaluating the chimney graft or periscope technique. However, case series have shown that the techniques are safe, feasible and efficacious. Importantly they can be done emergently or urgently using readily available off-the-shelf-components. While the learning curve is significant, adhering to some of the key principles outlined above can improve immediate technical success. There are significant concerns regarding the long-term patency of these grafts, specifically long chimney grafts, as well as the long-term exclusion of the aneurysm being treated. Thus, the future of these techniques depends on what long term data reveals. As fenestrated and branched endografts become available as custom devices and subsequently "off-the-shelf", these techniques may becomes less common in the elective setting. However, these techniques can still be very useful in the emergency setting.

REFERENCES

1. Parodi JC, Palmaz JC, Barone HD: Transfemoral intraluminal graft implantation for abdominal aortic aneurysm. *Ann Vasc Surg.* 1991;5:491–499.
2. Greenhalgh RM, Brown LC, Kwong GP, et al. Comparison of endovascular aneurysm repair with open repair in patients with abdominal aortic aneurysm (EVAR trial 1), 30-day operative mortality results: randomized controlled trial. *Lancet.* 2004;364:843–848. for the EVAR trial participants.

3. Blankensteijn JD, de Jong S, Prinssen M, van der Ham A. Two year outcomes after conventional or endovascular repair of abdominal aortic aneurysms. *N Engl J Med.* 2005;352:2398–2405.

4. Dake MD, Miller DC, Semba CP, et al. Transluminal placement of endovascular stent-grafts for the treatment of descending thoracic aortic aneurysms. *N Engl J Med.* 1994;331:1729–1734.

5. Walsh SR, Tang TY, Sadat U, et al. Endovascular stenting versus open surgery for thoracic aortic disease: systematic review and meta-analysis of perioperative results. *J Vasc Surg.* 2008;47:1094–1098.

6. AbuRahma AF, Campbell J, Stone PA, et al. The correlation of aortic neck length to early and late outcomes in endovascular aneurysm. *J Vasc Surg.* 2009;50:738–748.

7. Greenberg RK, Clair D, Srivastava S, Bhandari G, Turc A, Hampton J, et al. Should patients with challenging anatomy be offered endovascular aneurysm repair? *J Vasc Surg.* 2003;38:990–6.

8. Greenberg R, Eagleton M, Mastracci T. Branched endografts for thoracoabdominal aneurysms. *J Thorac Cardiovasc Surg.* 2010;140(6 Suppl):S171–8.

9. Anderson JL, Adam DJ, Berce M, et al. Repair of thoracoabdominal aortic aneurysms with fenestrated and branched endovascular stent grafts. *J Vasc Surg.* 2005;42:600e7.

10. Ohrlander T, Sonesson B, Ivancev K, et al. The chimney graft: a technique for preserving or rescuing aortic branch vessels in stent-graft sealing zones. *J Endovasc Ther.* 2008;15:427e32.

11. Resch TA, Sonesson B, Dias N, et al. Chimney Grafts: Is there a Need and Will They Work? *Perspect Vasc Surg and EndovascTher.* 2001;23(3):149–153.

12. Hiramoto JS, Chang CK, Reilly LM, et al. Outcome of renal stenting for renal artery coverage during endovascular aortic aneurysm repair. *J Vasc Surg.* 2009;49:1100e6.

13. Troisi N, Torsello G, Donas KP, et al. Endurant stent-graft: a 2-year, single-center experience with a new commercially available device for the treatment of abdominal aortic aneurysms. *J Endovasc Ther.* 2010;17:439–448.

14. Lee JT, Greenberg JI, Dalman RL. Early experience with the snorkel technique for juxtarenal aneurysms. *J Vasc Surg.* 2012;55:935–46.

15. Moulakakis KG, Mylonas SN, Avgerinos E, et al. The chimney graft technique for preserving visceral vessels during endovascular treatment of aortic pathologies. *J Vasc Surg.* 2012;55:1497–1503.

16. Tolenaar JL, van Keulen JW, Timarchi S, et al. The chimney graft, a systematic review. *Ann Vasc Surg.* 2012 April 20 (Epub).

17. Bruen KJ, Feezor RJ, Daniels MJ, et al. Endovascular chimney techniques versus open repair of juxtarenal and suprarenal aneursysms. *J Vasc Surg.* 2011;53:895–905.

18. Inoue K, Hosokawa H, Iwase T, et al. Aortic arch reconstruction by transluminally placed endovascular branched stent graft. *Circulation.* 1999;100(Suppl 2):316–321.

19. Criado FJ, Barnatan MF, Rizk Y, et al. Technical strategies to expand stent-graft applicability in the aortic arch and proximal ascending aortic dissection. *J Endovasc Ther.* 2002;9(Pt II):32–38.

20. Chuter TA, Schneider DB, Reilly LM, et al. Modular branched stent graft for endovascular repair of aortic arch aneurysm and dissection. *J Vasc Surg.* 2003;38:859–863.

21. Larzon T, Gruber G, Friberg O, et al. Experiences of intentional carotid stenting in endovascular repair of aortic arch aneurysms-- two case reports. *Eur J Vasc Endovasc Surg.* 2005;30:147–51.

22. Criado FJ. A percutaneous technique for preservation of arch branch patency during thoracic endovascular aortic repair (TEVAR): retrograde catheterization and stenting. *J Endovasc Ther.* 2007;14:54–8.

23. Sugiura K, Sonesson B, Akesson M, et al. The applicability of chimney grafts in the aortic arch. *J Cardiovasc Surg. (Torino)* 2009;50:475–81.

24. Rancic Z, Pfammatter T, Lachat M, et al. Periscope graft to extend distal landing zone in ruptured thoracoabdominal aneurysms with short distal necks. *J Vasc Surg.* 2010;1:1293–6.

25. Pecoraro F, Pfammater T, Mayer D, et al. Multiple periscope and chimney grafts to treat ruptured thoracoabdominal and pararenal aortic aneurysms. *J Endovasc The.r* 2011;18:642–649.
26. Dias NV, Resch T, Sonesson B, et al. Single superior mesenteric artery periscope grafts to facilitate urgent endovascular repair of acute thoracoabdominal aortic pathology. *J Endovasc Ther.* 2011;18:656–660.

38

Branched and Fenestrated TEVAR for Thoracoabdominal Disease

Mark A. Farber, MD and Raghuveer Vallabhaneni, MD

INTRODUCTION

Thoraco-abdominal, juxtarenal and pararenal aortic aneurysms pose complex problems for vascular surgeons involved in their management. Development of endovascular repair of aortic aneurysms has been associated with low perioperative morbidity and mortality even with high-risk patients. Recent publications reveal that as many as 45% of patients have aneurysms that are not amenable to endovascular techniques based on the instructions for use for infrarenal aortic devices.[1] Until recently EVAR has not been available for these types of patients in the United States outside of IDE studies. Exclusion may be because of short, non-existent, or angulated necks precluding adequate proximal seal. Good surgical candidates may tolerate the complex open procedures necessary to exclude these aneurysms, but many patients with serious cardiac, pulmonary or renal comorbidities are unlikely to fully recover from the extensive open procedure. These patients may be best served by a minimally invasive approach to aneurysm exclusion, with the most appropriate treatment determined by an experienced surgeon after consideration of each patient's risk profile.

HISTORY

Since the initial reports of endovascular stent grafting for AAA exclusion by Juan Parodi and associates in 1991,[2] there has been significant adoption of endovascular techniques to treat aortic pathology in nearly every subset of patients. However, despite advances in almost all aspects of endovascular technology including preoperative imaging, wires, catheters, balloons, and delivery systems, all available devices in the United States are limited by the proximal neck characteristics (length, diameter, angulation, shape, thrombus lining) required to achieve and maintain an effective proximal seal.[3] Of the devices approved by the US Food and Drug Administration (FDA) for treatment of abdominal aortic aneurysms (Cook Zenith [Cook Inc, Indianapolis, IA], Gore Excluder [WL Gore, Flagstaff, AZ], AneurRx [Medtronic Inc, Santa Rosa, CA], Endurant and Talent [Medtronic Inc], and Endologix Powerlink [Endologix, Irvine, CA], all must have a minimal proximal neck length of 1.5 cm for adequate sealing, except the Endurant and Talent device, which is approved for 1 cm neck lengths. In juxtarenal aneurysms where the neck length is shorter than these approved lengths, the visceral vessels may be accommodated by making fenestrations in the proximal sealing zone, thus lengthening this area. Since the first report of AAA repair with fenestrated devices in 1996 by Park and associates,[4] there have been considerable innovations and improvements in this technology as well. With the recent approval of the Cook Fenestrated device in the United States, advanced devices are now becoming more readily available and several "off-the-shelf" designs are being examined with respect to their applicability and real world use. In this chapter we will give an overview of the current status and data available regarding fenestrated and branched repair of TAAA.

INDICATIONS

Fenestrated stent-grafts were originally developed as a minimally invasive alternative to open repair to treat complex aneurysm morphology in patients considered to be unfit or at high risk for open surgery. The criteria for treatment with a fenestrated device are in evolution as the safety and efficacy of available devices and techniques are determined. Generally accepted high-risk characteristics include old age, severe medical comorbidities, prior aortic reconstruction, and the need for suprarenal aortic crossclamping.[5] Until recently, there were no FDA approved fenestrated devices approved for general use in the US. The device approved for use is the Cook Zenith Fenestrated device. This device is indicated for use in aneurysms with a 4–12 mm neck and less than 45 degree of angulation at the neck. Two additional devices are undergoing, or about to begin, clinical trial investigation and involve "off-the-shelf" designs. These are the Ventana from Endologix and the P-branch device from Cook.

The currently approved custom fenestrated device requires a 3 to 4-weeks manufacturing period, which has led to advances in seeking "off-the-shelf" fenestrated stent-grafts. In addition outside the US or through physician sponsored investigations, thoracoabdominal branched devices are available for implantation. As the results of seminal work done by the Chuter and his colleagues[6] a standard four branched design has been proposed that will accommodate greater than 85% of patients with TAAA and incorporated standardized locations for all visceral vessels.

OUTCOME MEASURES IN FENESTRATED AORTIC ENDOGRAFTING

There are several important outcome measures to evaluate when assessing the utility of fenestrated stent-grafts for repair of juxtarenal and thoraco-abdominal aneurysms.

Definitions

Aortic aneurysms in the region of the renal arteries are grouped collectively as pararenal aneurysms and further classified into juxtarenal and suprarenal subtypes. There is no universally agreed upon definition of the term "juxtarenal aneurysm," however it is commonly used to describe a complex AAA with either a short infrarenal neck or one which encroaches upon the renal segment of the aorta. Suprarenal aneurysms involve the renal arteries and extend up to the splanchnic arteries. Type IV thoraco-abdominal aortic aneurysms extend to a variable abdominal length, but always involve the visceral aortic segment. Heterogeneity of definitions throughout the literature lends some ambiguity to the terms and makes comparison of clinical studies difficult. Type I-III thoracoabdominal aortic aneurysms have been more clearly defined in the literature and do not need redefining.

The terms fenestrated and branched endovascular repair describe two similar uses of the same technique. The term fenestrated endovascular repair is used when the visceral branch target vessels arise from the sealing region of the stent-graft in the normal aorta. In the case of juxtarenal aneurysms there is typically no gap between the device and the target vessel. This is contrasted with a branched endovascular repair, in which the target arteries arise from aneurysmal aorta, and there is a gap between the device and the aortic wall at the vessel origin. In branched devices these can either be separated into fenestrated branch-stent graft in which a reinforced fenestrated device uses a stent-graft to traverse the aneurysmal sac to the visceral branch or more typically, a directional cuff attached to the device, which facilitates the placement of the branch artery stent-graft.[7]

Branch Patency

Branch vessel patency is a critically important endpoint for fenestrated and branched stent-graft repair. The original designs for fenestrations had either no stent placed in the visceral vessel or a bare metal stent placed but more recently covered stent grafts have been used because of a potentially decreased risk of in stent restenosis.[8] More recently there has been an increase in covered-stent usage in this location to reduce the branch vessel complication rate.

Renal Function

Renal function following FEVAR is an important determinant of success. Many things are performed during a FEVAR that may cause deterioration of renal function (nephrotoxic contrast, wire manipulation, micro embolization, etc.). Up to one third of patients may have deterioration in renal function perioperatively, but the majority of these patients may return to near their baseline renal function at 6 months.[9]

Endoleak and Component Separation

The integrity of the seal between components is also very important. As the number of components required for repair increases, a corresponding increased risk of endoleak from component separation ensues.

REVIEW OF THE LITERATURE

The first fenestrated aortic endograft was placed and reported by Park and associates in 1996.[4] Since that time many case series and some randomized controlled trials have been reported about outcomes of fenestrated endografts. The first series of patients treated with fenestrated endografts utilized modified Cook Zenith platforms. Anderson et al. in 2001 reported on the implantation of 13 fenestrated endografts in patients who were unable to receive an infrarenal EVAR for pararenal aneurysms. They used Palmaz bare metal stents for fixation in the visceral arteries and had a 100% technical success rate in 33 visceral arteries targeted being perfused at follow up of 3–24 months.[10] Since that study there have been several other studies reporting outcomes of fenestrated devices. A summary of the largest studies is included in Table 38-1.[11–18] Many studies include both juxtarenal and TAAA of different varieties and both branched and fenestrated devices. This makes it difficult to include these studies to compare outcomes. The final results of the US Cook fenestrated trial have not been published as of the writing, but should be forthcoming.

30 DAY PERIOPERATIVE MORTALITY

The ranges of overall perioperative mortality was 0–3.4% with a cumulative perioperative mortality of 1.8%.

Branch Patency

The overall branch patency ranges from 90.5% to 96.6% in short and midterm follow-up. The group from the Cleveland Clinic has analyzed its data in renal stenting in both fenestrated and branched devices and their outcomes.[8] During a 5-year period they treated 518 renal arteries with covered or uncovered renal stents in 287 patients. The estimated freedom from stenosis at 12, 24, and 36 months were 95% (95% confidence interval [CI] 93–98), 92% (89–96), and 89% (85–93) for uncovered stents, and 98% (96–100), 97% (95–100), and 95% (91–100) for covered stents (log rank $P < .04$).8 They concluded that covered stent grafts have a decreased risk of restenosis. Therefore it is recommended that covered stent grafts be used in FEVAR for visceral artery perfusion even if no gap exists between the graft and the aortic wall.

TABLE 38-1. SUMMARY OF OUTCOMES OF FENESTRATED ENDOGRAFTS IN JUXTARENAL ANEURYSMS

	30 day mortality n (%)	Branch vessel patency (%)	Late Mortality n (%)	Follow up months (range)
Semmens et al (2006)	2/58 (3.4)	90.5	6/58 (10.3)	16.8 (3–30)
Muhs et al (2006)	1/30 (3.3)	92	NA	25.8 (13–39)
O'Neill et al (2006)	1/119 (0.8)	90.7	15/119 (12.6)	19 (0–42)
Halak et al (2006)	0/15 (0)	NA	1/15 (6.7)	20.5 (4–40)
Ziegler et al (2007)	1/63 (1.6)	92.2	14/63 (22.2)	22 (5–41)
Scurr et al (2008)	1/45 (2.2)	96.6	4/35 (8.8)	24 (1–48)
Haulon et al (2010)	2/80 (2.5)	95	4/80 (5)	10 (1–38)
Verhoeven et al (2010)	1/100 (1)	93.3	22/100 (22)	24 (1–87)

Renal Function

As mentioned previously, up to a third of patients after FEVAR may have deterioration of renal function. In a recent review by Nordon et al. 14.9% of FEVAR patients had an increase in serum creatinine of >30%.[19] This risk is higher in patients with preoperative renal insufficiency. In a review of patients undergoing FEVAR at the Cleveland Clinic, the risk of perioperative renal insufficiency was 16% in patients that had normal preoperative eGFR (>60 ml/min/1.73 m^2) and 39% in those patients with preexisting renal insufficiency. Baseline renal insufficiency was also a strong predictor of mortality (p < 0.2) with an increased relative risk of 8.52.[9] In this study 59% of patients who had perioperative worsening in renal function, had this occur within the first month postoperatively with the majority of them returning to their mean eGFR within 6 months.

Although early on in FEVAR, fenestrations to the renals were not always stented if there was good apposition of the graft to the aortic wall, there has been some evidence that this may lead to a higher incidence of occlusion of the renal arteries. It is recommended that all renal arteries be stented, even in scalloped grafts.[11] As mentioned previously, covered stent grafts appear to have lower rates of in stent restenosis when compared to uncovered stents.

Open Surgical Repair versus Endovascular Fenestrated Repair of Juxtarenal Aneurysms

No randomized controlled trial has compared fenestrated/branched endovascular aneurysm repair with conventional open repair. However, multiple case series and cohort studies have documented the safety and efficacy of the technique. In a recent review, Nordon and associates analyzed 8 studies with a total of 368 cases of FEVAR and compared them with 12 studies representing 1164 open repairs of juxtarenal aneurysms. Cumulative mortality was similar in the two groups. There was statistically significant increase in transient renal failure in the open group compared with the FEVAR group, however there was no difference in the rate of dialysis requirement in the two groups (1.4% in both).[19] The open surgical group did have a significantly lower reintervention rate of only 2.6% vs. 15% for FEVAR.

Endoleak and Component Separation

With more components in fenestrated/branched modular devices there is an increased risk of type III endoleaks in between the components. This potential problem was evaluated at the Cleveland Clinic.[20] Out of 106 patients who were treated with fenestrated or branched modular devices that were followed for more than one year, 13% of patients had greater than 10 mm component movement. There were 8 patients that had component separation (defined as less than 2 stent overlap). All of the patients with component separation also had >10 mm component movement. There were 29 endoleaks: 6 Type I; 17 Type II and 6 Type III. The endoleaks occurred in 50% of the patients that had component movement.[20] Following component movement and component separation may help identify patients at risk for endoleaks.

TECHNIQUES

The technique of fenestrated repair has undergone considerable evolution since its inception. This description represents the current standards, but it subject to change as dictated by a rapidly improving technique.

The most important component of successful fenestrated aneurysm repair is careful and accurate advance planning of the procedure and of the graft construction. Computed tomography (CT) angiography allows measurements of distances using centerline of flow analysis and of the clock position of the target vessel using axial measurements. The criteria for device implantation are essentially unchanged from standard endovascular repairs. The proximal landing zone must consist of at least 2 cm of normal parallel aortic wall, <32-mm in diameter for juxtarenal aneurysms and <38-mm for thoraco-abdominal aneurysms. The centerline measurement from the top of the landing zone to the center of the target vessel origin is recorded, as are the clock position, orientation, and diameter of each target vessel origin. The device configuration can consist of single or multiple fenestrations, depending of patient characteristics. Fenestration can be construction of varying sizes. Small fenestrations (6 mm × 6 mm or 6 mm × 8 mm) are preferentially designed for the renal vessels. Large fenestrations (8 mm, 10 mm, or 12 mm) are used preferentially for the celiac or superior mesenteric arteries. Scallops are typically provided in varying widths depending upon the device manufacturer and design.

Regardless of the presence of a gap between the graft and the aortic wall, all fenestrations are bridged with a balloon-expandable stent or stent graft to reduce any misalignment between the fenestration and the vessel origin. The device design for internationally available Cook Zenith or TX2 platform fenestrated devices is based on these measurements, and customized devices based on individual patient specifications are available from the manufacturer in 3–4 weeks.

Branched endovascular aortic repairs are accomplished by implanting the main aortic component from the femoral region. After insertion, the target branched vessel are connected thru a high axillary approach instead of the femoral approach used for fenestrated repairs. Branched designs are slightly more forgiving than fenestrated devices and cuffs attached to the main aortic device are planned 1–2 cm above the target vessel and preferably oriented toward the target vessel. Covered self-expanding stents are preferably used to connect the main aortic device with the branched target vessel.

Prior to commencing any complex endovascular aneurysm repair, it is imperative that the surgeon have access to excellent imaging equipment and a complete endovascular inventory. A wide range of catheters, wires, sheaths, stents, and stent grafts may be required to safely and effectively complete this procedure. Preoperatively, the patient is medically optimized. Consideration for preoperative hydration with or without bicarbonate infusion and oral acetylcysteine is appropriate in the patient with baseline renal insufficiency. Intraoperatively, contrast is routinely diluted to 50% strength with normal saline. Attempts are made to minimize contrast administration by using hand injections for selective arteriographies. A spinal drain should be considered in patients in whom extensive aortic coverage will be required or in those patients with other risk factors for paraplegia including those with prior aortic grafting or hypogastric artery occlusion.

Graft implantation generally requires bilateral femoral and occasionally left brachial or axillary arterial access. The larger femoral artery is generally used for main body device implantation and the contralateral femoral artery is used for the target vessels. A large sheath is introduced via the contralateral femoral artery, and the sheath valve is accessed with multiple 5-French sheaths. These sheaths are used for selective catheterization of the renal and superior mesenteric arteries. The target vessels are then catheterized using selective contrast injections. Once all target branches are accessed, the main stent graft is oriented and introduced via the femoral artery.

Via a sheath, a balloon-expandable stent graft is introduced into each target vessel after it has been selectively catheterized through the stent-graft fenestration. Once all bridging stent grafts are in place, the main body stent graft is fully deployed. The balloon-expandable stent grafts are then deployed to profile and flared proximally with a balloon.

A high level of endovascular surgical expertise is required to safely perform these complex aortic procedures. It is imperative that the surgeon be facile with salvage or "bail out" maneuvers that may be required for device design or deployment errors. Access to the target vessel cannot always be regained when significant misalignment occurs. Some authors describe the use of a flush catheter left between the main aortic stent graft and the aortic wall during the entire procedure. In the case of device misalignment, this catheter may be exchanged for a balloon, allowing enough space for wire and catheter manipulation to make catheterization of the target vessel possible.[10] Use of microcatheters, microwires, and a variety of catheter shapes may be necessary.

FUTURE DIRECTIONS

Endovascular repair of aneurysms involving the visceral aorta has become a reality. More than 5000 cases have been performed worldwide with midterm results that demonstrate safety and success. Continued success with fenestrated and branched endografting will require continued appropriate patient selection, high-resolution imaging, proper device design, and technical expertise on the part of the endovascular surgeon. However, as technology and techniques evolve, the endovascular treatment of TAAA and juxtarenal aneurysms is certain to become more commonplace. The continued efforts to provide safe, prefabricated devices available to more patients will certainly allow greater ease of treating patients.

REFERENCES

1. Arko FR, Filis KA, Seidel SA, et al. How many patients with infrarenal aneurysms are candidates for endovascular repair? The Northern California experience. *J Endovasc Ther*. 2004 Feb.;11(1):33–40.
2. Parodi JC, Palmaz JC, Barone HD. Transfemoral intraluminal graft implantation for abdominal aortic aneurysms. *Ann Vasc Surg*. 1991 Nov.;5(6):491–499.
3. Carpenter JP, Baum RA, Barker CF, et al. Impact of exclusion criteria on patient selection for endovascular abdominal aortic aneurysm repair. *J Vasc Surg*. 2001 Dec.;34(6):1050–1054.
4. Park JH, Chung JW, Choo IW, et al. Fenestrated stent-grafts for preserving visceral arterial branches in the treatment of abdominal aortic aneurysms: preliminary experience. *J Vasc Interv Radiol*. 1996 Oct.;7(6):819–823.
5. Dias NV, Ivancev K, Malina M, et al. Does the wide application of endovascular AAA repair affect the results of open surgery? *Eur J Vasc Endovasc Surg*. 2003 Aug.;26(2):188–194.
6. Sweet MP, Hiramoto JS, Park K-H, et al. A standardized multi-branched thoracoabdominal stent-graft for endovascular aneurysm repair. *J Endovasc Ther*. 2009 Jun.;16(3):359–64.
7. Oderich GS. Reporting on fenestrated endografts: surrogates for outcomes and implications of aneurysm classification, type of repair, and the evolving technique. *J Endovasc Ther*. 2011 Apr.;18(2):154–156.

8. Mohabbat W, Greenberg RK, Mastracci TM, et al. Revised duplex criteria and outcomes for renal stents and stent grafts following endovascular repair of juxtarenal and thoracoabdominal aneurysms. *J Vasc Surg.* 2009 Apr.;49(4):827–37; discussion 837.

9. Haddad F, Greenberg RK, Walker E, et al. Fenestrated endovascular grafting: The renal side of the story. *J Vasc Surg.* 2005 Feb.;41(2):181–190.

10. Anderson JL, Berce M, Hartley DE. Endoluminal aortic grafting with renal and superior mesenteric artery incorporation by graft fenestration. *J Endovasc Ther.* 2001 Feb.;8(1):3–15.

11. Semmens JB, Lawrence-Brown MMD, Hartley DE, et al. Outcomes of fenestrated endografts in the treatment of abdominal aortic aneurysm in Western Australia (1997–2004). *J Endovasc Ther.* 2006 Jun.;13(3):320–329.

12. Muhs BE, Verhoeven ELG, Zeebregts CJ, et al. Mid-term results of endovascular aneurysm repair with branched and fenestrated endografts. *J Vasc Surg.* 2006 Jul.;44(1):9–15.

13. Halak M, Goodman MA, Baker SR. The fate of target visceral vessels after fenestrated endovascular aortic repair--general considerations and mid-term results. *Eur J Vasc Endovasc Surg.* 2006 Aug.;32(2):124–128.

14. O'Neill S, Greenberg RK, Haddad F, et al. A prospective analysis of fenestrated endovascular grafting: intermediate-term outcomes. *Eur J Vasc Endovasc Surg.* 2006 Aug.;32(2):115–123.

15. Ziegler P, Avgerinos ED, Umscheid T, et al. Fenestrated endografting for aortic aneurysm repair: a 7-year experience. *J Endovasc Ther.* 2007 Oct.;14(5):609–618.

16. Scurr JRH, Brennan JA, Gilling-Smith GL, et al. Fenestrated endovascular repair for juxtarenal aortic aneurysm. *Br J Surg.* 2008 Mar.;95(3):326–332.

17. Haulon S, Amiot S, Magnan P-E, et al. An analysis of the French multicentre experience of fenestrated aortic endografts: medium-term outcomes. *Ann Surg.* 2010 Feb.;251(2):357–362.

18. Verhoeven ELG, Vourliotakis G, Bos WTGJ, et al. Fenestrated stent grafting for short-necked and juxtarenal abdominal aortic aneurysm: an 8-year single-centre experience. *Eur J Vasc Endovasc Surg.* 2010 May;39(5):529–536.

19. Nordon IM, Hinchliffe RJ, Holt PJ, et al. Modern treatment of juxtarenal abdominal aortic aneurysms with fenestrated endografting and open repair—a systematic review. *Eur J Vasc Endovasc Surg.* 2009 Jul.;38(1):35–41.

20. Dowdall JF, Greenberg RK, West K, et al. Separation of components in fenestrated and branched endovascular grafting--branch protection or a potentially new mode of failure? *Eur J Vasc Endovasc Surg.* 2008 Jul.;36(1):2–9.

39

Spinal Cord Protection After Open Thoracoabdominal Aortic Aneurysm Repair

Ali Azizzadeh, MD, Maria Codreanu, MD, Anthony L. Estrera, MD, Kristofer Charlton-Ouw, MD, and Hazim J. Safi, MD

INTRODUCTION

The surgical repair of thoracoabdominal aortic aneurysms (TAAA) remains a challenging procedure performed in major aortic centers with acceptable morbidity and mortality. One of the most dreaded complications that can follow even a technically successful operation is neurological deficit related to spinal cord ischemia. A conventional repair of the diseased thoracic or thoracoabdominal aorta can be complicated by paraplegia or paraparesis in up to 22% of cases[1], especially in type II TAAA repair. The quality of life is severely affected by spinal cord ischemia and the life expectancy at 5 years decreases from 62% to 44%.[2]

HISTORY

In the late 19th century, the standard treatment for an aortic aneurysm was simple ligation, which led to distal body gangrene and death. Dr. Samuel Etheredge performed the first successful thoracoabdominal aortic aneurysm repair using a homograft in 1954.[3] Dr. Michael DeBakey and colleagues subsequently devised an ingenious method of using an end to side Dacron tube graft from the descending thoracic to the infrarenal aorta and sequentially bypassed the celiac axis, superior mesenteric artery, and both renal arteries. This technique both decreased the load on the heart as well as the ischemic time to the bowels and kidneys.[4] Dr. E. Stanley Crawford's repair of thoracoabdominal aortic aneurysm incorporated three principles of vascular surgery: the Matas inclusion technique, whereby the aneurysm sac is opened but not resected;[5] the reattachment of the intercostal arteries to the graft (as described in an animal model by Dr. Frank Spencer and colleagues in 1950);[6] and the reattachment of the small arteries into a large artery, attributed to Alexis Carrell in 1906. Crawford accrued 28 cases by 1973 and published his results of a large group of aneurysm cases treated for the first time with the clamp-and-sew technique.[7] This technique depended on expeditious repair with short aortic clamp times since the spine and visceral vessels suffered ischemia during repair. Several adjunctive methods for spinal cord and visceral protection later emerged, including distal aortic perfusion, cerebrospinal fluid (CSF).[8–10]

cerebrospinal fluid (CSF) drainage,[11] and systemic or regional profound hypothermia.[12]

By the end of the 1980s, the preferred method of treatment was still the clamp-and-sew technique, but it continued to be associated with high complication rates, predominantly due to spinal neurological deficits and renal failure. Since 1992, supported by animal models and clinical experience, we abandoned the clamp-and-sew technique, except in emergency situations, in favor of left atrio-femoral bypass with the addition of perioperative CSF drainage and moderate passive hypothermia. The aim of this chapter is to review the techniques involved in reducing the risk of spinal cord ischemia during TAAA repair.

CLASSIFICATIONS

Thoracoabdominal aortic aneurysms are classified in five categories. (Figure 39-1) Extent I is from the left subclavian to above the most proximal renal artery. Extent II is from the left subclavian artery to below the renal arteries. Extent III is from the 6th intercostal space to below the renal arteries. Extent IV is from T12 to below the renal arteries. Extent V, which was introduced by our group in the last two decades, is from T6 to just above the renal arteries. The importance of the classification scheme is that it correlated with the incidence of neurological deficits and mortality, especially when using the clamp-and-sew technique.

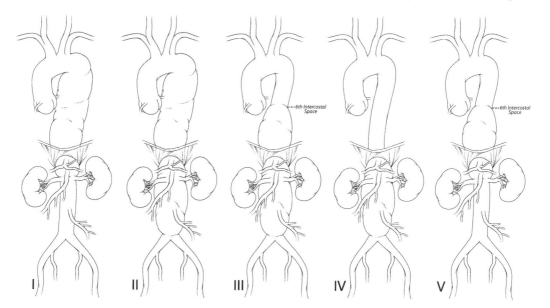

Figure 39-1. Classifications of Thoracoabdominal aortic aneurysms (TAAA).

The definition of the neurological deficit associated with repair of TAAA is not uniform among studies, and any new neurological deficit should be considered spinal cord ischemia until proven otherwise. The primary clinical scale used to quantify the degree of spinal cord ischemia after repair of thoracic aorta is the Modified Tarlov scoring system.[13] A score of 0-2 represents paraplegia and a score of 3-4 paraparesis.

0-no lower extremity motions
1-lower extremity motions without gravity
2-lower extremity motions against gravity
3-able to stand with assistance
4-able to walk with assistance
5-able to walk without assistance

ETIOLOGY

Spinal cord ischemia during thoracic aortic aneurysm repair occurs due to cessation of blood flow to intercostal arteries, inadequate collateral circulation, reperfusion injury, and decreased cerebrospinal perfusion pressure. The incidence of spinal cord ischemia after TAAA repair varies between 5-11% in recent studies.[14–17] However, it is particularly high after extent II TAAA repair, with a reported incidence of 22% in a 2008 study.[18] Although several risk factors are currently recognized as increasing the incidence of neurologic injury, spinal cord ischemia remains unpredictable. An understanding of the potential risk factors, however, provides the basis for applying a uniform protocol for the prevention of spinal cord injury.

Vascular Anatomy of the spinal cord

The supply to the spinal cord originates in the aorta at the level of the cervical, thoracic and lumbar branches. These in turn give off the segmental radicular arteries from which the anterior and two posterior spinal arteries originate. The largest radicular artery is known as the artery of Adamkiewicz, which originates from the intercostal arteries T8-L1 level but varies in position from T7 to L4.[19] It originates in the left thoracic or lumbar branch in 68-73% of cases and from the 9th-12th intercostals in 62-84%.[20] It supplies the lower part of the spine and has a poor connection with the superior portion of the spinal cord. Other collaterals supplying the spine are coming from the subclavian arteries, the iliac arteries and the vertebral arteries.

Duration of Aortic Cross Clamping

Previously, the duration of aortic cross-clamping was recognized as the most important predictor of spinal cord ischemia. In Crawford's studies that used the clamp-and-sew technique, an aortic cross-clamp time of more than 30 minutes was associated with an incidence of spinal cord ischemia of 27%.[21] Reduction of aortic cross-clamp time to < 30 min reduced the incidence to 8%. That prompted an expedient surgery with emphasis on surgical skills. However, recent work with adjuncts of distal aortic perfusion and CSF drainage has reduced the effect of aortic cross-clamp time on risk of spinal cord injury.[22] Although we still support the approach of expeditious repair during the aortic cross-clamp time period, the application of the adjuncts has reduced the effect of "clamp time" on spinal cord injury, providing more time for repair.

Extent of the Aortic Replacement

Neurological outcomes correlate with aneurysm extent based on the modified Crawford classifications of TAAA. Specifically, extent IV and V are associated with a low risk (0% to 4.8%) for developing spinal cord ischemia [22–25] while extent III in itself is considered a risk factor for neurologic deficit.[26] Prior to reclassification of some extent III cases as extent V, extent III cases was not considered high risk for spinal cord ischemia. With the modification of the Crawford classification, extent III has now become a significant risk factor for development of spinal cord ischemia after open repair.

Aortic Dissection

Aortic dissection was previously considered high risk for paraplegia in the era of the cross-clamp and go.[27] Aortic dissection is sub-classified as either acute (less than 2 weeks from onset) or chronic (greater than 2 weeks from onset). It was previously thought that in acute dissection, the incidence of spinal cord ischemia is greater than in cases of chronic dissection. The primary reason for this was related to the inability to reattach pertinent intercostal arteries in an acutely dissected aorta. With further analysis, however, chronic dissection was determined not be a risk factor for spinal cord injury with use of adjuncts of distal aortic perfusion and CSF fluid drainage.[28]

SPINAL CORD PROTECTION

Our spinal protective adjuncts are CSF drainage, mild-to moderate-passive hypothermia, and distal aortic perfusion (left atriofemoral bypass). We reduce the spinal cord ischemic time by sequential clamping, increase spinal cord tolerance to ischemia by passive hypothermia, augment spinal cord perfusion by deliberate hypertension, and detect and reverse spinal cord ischemia as early as possible.

Increase spinal cord tolerance to ischemia: hypothermia

At a normal temperature, the central and peripheral nervous system have a poor tolerance for ischemia. Hypothermia is an external intervention that can reduce the ischemic insult on the brain and the spinal cord by decreasing metabolic demand. Newer studies have also shown a membrane stabilization effect as well as an anti-inflammatory response. Hypothermia for spinal cord protection can be divided in 3 groups: mild hypothermia (32-34°C, passive, achieved by the simple exposure of the body, the most commonly used method, including by us), deep or profound systemic hypothermia (10-18° when cardiopulmonary bypass is used for more proximal repair of the arch or ascending aorta) and regional spinal cord hypothermia (26°C, through an epidural catheter placed in the T11,T12 vertebral interspace). Regional spinal cord hypothermia precludes the use of intra-operative neuromonitoring.

Augmentation of spinal cord perfusion

The spinal cord perfusion pressure is equal to the difference between the mean arterial pressure (MAP) and the intracranial pressure (ICP), (SCPP= MAP - ICP). Our protocol for deliberate hypertension involves keeping the MAP higher than 80 mmHg to maintain a SCPP of at least 70 mmHg. The factors taken into account to accomplish this task are an optimal volume status, adequate cardiac, and a normal to high hemoglobin (>12 g) to optimize oxygen delivery. In addition, we drain the CSF to a pressure <10 mm Hg (see discussion on spinal drain). In addition, we do re-implantation of intercostals arteries when necessary. Revascularization of arteries around the T8 to T12 level may well be most important in reducing the risk of spinal cord ischemia. Large segmental arteries with little or no back bleeding are particularly important for spinal cord perfusion. Alternatively, occlusion or oversewing of segmental arteries that back-bleed have been advocated to improve spinal cord perfusion by preventing arterial steal. We have used a selective approach to revascularization by reimplantation only when signs of frank spinal cord ischemia are seen intraoperatively manifested by changes in somatosensory evoked potentials (SSEPs) or motor evoked potentials (MEPs).[29]

Early detection of spinal cord ischemia

Our protocol involves intraoperative monitoring of SSEPs as well as MEPs. Monitoring allows for early detection of spinal cord ischemia as well as identification of spinal cord vessels that need to be reimplanted. It also establishes a baseline optimal MAP necessary to ensure good spinal perfusion. They are used as a rough estimate, however, as they do not correlate in an exponential manner with the rate of postoperative paraplegia. This is because monitoring may be influenced by a number of other factors that are independent of the local spinal cord ischemia, such lower extremity malperfusion, stroke, and other anesthesia protocols. Among the two monitoring modalities, the MEPs are more sensitive and specific than SSEPs. However, more susceptible to anesthesia protocols.[29-31] In addition, we perform serial postoperative neurologic examination and take necessary corrective measures.

CSF DRAINAGE

The proposed effect of CSF drainage is to lower the CSF pressure, thereby increase blood perfusion pressure. Our institutional protocol involves preoperative placement of a lumbar drain by the anesthesia team. We believe that placement of the drain a day before the operation unnecessarily increases the indwelling time and its complication rate. The drain consists of an 80 cm (1.6 mm OD) silicone elastomeric multi-orifice catheter introduced between L2 and L5 in the subarachnoid space via a 14-gauge thin-walled Tuohy needle. The tip of the catheter is placed 5-10 cm into the subarachnoid space and attached to a pressure gauge. The fluid is drained intra- and postoperatively in a sterile reservoir with the goal to maintain the measured pressure below 10 mmHg.

We awaken the patient as soon as possible postoperatively to ascertain neurologic status. The goal for mean arterial pressure is greater than 80 mm Hg and the CSF pressure goal is less than 10 mm Hg. A maximum of 15 mL of CSF is drained each hour to prevent intracranial hypotension and hemorrhage when the patient is neurologically intact. If blood is noted in the effluent, the drain is capped and any coagulopathy corrected. In addition, we obtain a CT scan of the head as well as a neurological consultation to rule out intracranial hemorrhage. We routinely remove the drain on the third postoperative day if neurologically intact. Neurologic function is frequently assessed to detect delayed deficit.

TABLE 39-1. COMPLICATIONS OF CEREBROSPINAL FLUID (CSF) DRAINAGE

Complication	Frequency (%)
CSF leak without spinal headache	0.1%
CSF leak with spinal headache	0.54%
Intracranial hemorrhage	0.45%
Meningitis	0.2%
Spinal headache without CSF leak	0.2%
Fractured catheter	0.1%

Complications of CSF drainage are low but include CSF leak, headache, and intracranial hemorrhage. (Table 1) [32] The overall complication rate was 1.5% in over 1100 patients. Serious complications occurred in less than 1%. The most common complication was CSF leak with spinal headache. Most CSF leaks required hydration and blood patch but resolved without additional invasive management. Meningitis occurred in two patients (0.2%) who developed delayed neurologic deficit with prolonged catheter insertion. We have not noted intracranial hemorrhage in our recent cases since limiting the CSF drainage to 15 mL per hour in neurologically intact patients.

A meta-analysis found that use of CSF drainage in thoracic aortic aneurysm repair led to an absolute risk reduction in neurologic deficit of 9%.[33] We believe the risk reduction is even greater since the meta-analysis included older studies that limited CSF drainage to 50 mL intraoperatively.[34]

DISTAL AORTIC PERFUSION

The aim of distal aortic perfusion (left atriofemoral bypass) is to maintain spinal cord, mesenteric and renal perfusion during aortic clamping. The decreased risk of spinal cord ischemia during clamping with the use of distal perfusion is secondary to maintaining blood flow to the iliac arteries which serve as a source of collateral blood flow to the spinal cord. It can be accomplished via a passive shunt (which relies on a pressure gradient), a bypass with interposed roller or centrifugal pumps or a total cardiopulmonary bypass. The most widely used technique is the left atrial-femoral bypass; the left atrium is used as a source of oxygenated blood while the femoral artery is the perfused artery distal to the aorta. If this artery is not usable, then the distal abdominal aorta or distal thoracic aorta is used. The body temperature is allowed to drift passively to the range of 33°-34°C.

OPERATIVE TECHNIQUE

The patient is placed in the thoracoabdominal position with the shoulder blades at right angles to the edge of the table and the hip tilted 60° for access to both groins. (Figure 39-2) The incision is made and is tailored to the extent of the aneurysm. With regard to extent II, III, or IV, the skin incision begins just above the symphysis pubis and extends from the umbilicus to the costal cartilage as shown in the graphic. It is extended 2 cm below the angle of the scapula parallel to the vertebral border of the scapula. The latissimus dorsi and the serratus anterior muscles are cut. The 6th rib is usually removed. Once the

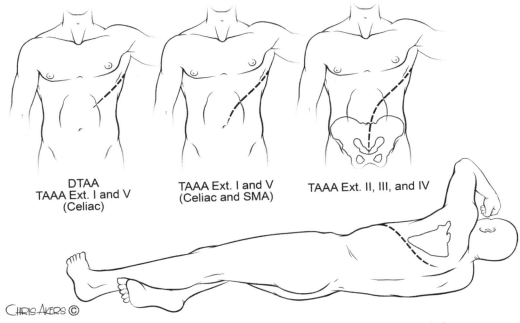

DTAA
TAAA Ext. I and V
(Celiac)

TAAA Ext. I and V
(Celiac and SMA)

TAAA Ext. II, III, and IV

CHRIS AKERS ©

Figure 39-2. Right lateral decubitus position for modified thoracoabdominal incision (dashed line).

pleural cavity is entered, the costal cartilage is excised in wedge fashion and the muscular portion of the diaphragm is cut. Medial rotation of the viscera—the spleen, kidneys, and intestines–exposes the crus of the diaphragm as well as the abdominal aorta, including the orifices of the celiac axis, superior mesenteric artery, and both renal arteries. With the patient exposed, and with a self-retaining retractor in place, the crus of the diaphragm is cut around the aorta allowing the passage of the graft. The lower pulmonary vein is exposed using 3–0 Prolene suture. A cannula is inserted directly into the left atrium or left lower pulmonary vein. This is connected to a centrifugal pump and in-line heat exchanger. The femoral artery is cannulated after exposing it through a longitudinal groin incision. Schematics of left atriofemoral bypass is shown in Figure 39-3. Then, in cephalad fashion, we dissect from the hilum at the wall of the aorta and parallel to vagus, and that leads into the atretic ligamentous. Care is taken to protect the recurrent laryngeal nerve. If the neck is distal to the left subclavian artery, this is the area that will be clamped. If it is proximal to the left subclavian artery, then we prepare the distal arch for clamping.

The patient is anti-coagulated using 1 mg of heparin per kg of body weight. The clamp is applied either proximal or distal to the left subclavian artery and the mid-descending thoracic aorta. The area in between is opened and the walls are retracted with #2 self-retracting sutures. The proximal descending thoracic aorta distal to the left subclavian artery is excised and lifted away from the esophagus to prevent esophageal aortic fistula. (Figure 39-4) A graft that is appropriate to the size of the aorta is selected and sutured with 3-0 polypropylene sutures. When this is done, the mid-descending thoracic aortic clamp is repositioned on the abdominal aorta at the level of the celiac axis and the remainder of the aorta is opened. The aortic hiatus is retracted using a skinny retractor. The lower intercostal arteries from T8 to T12 will be preserved if they are patent as guided by neuromonitoring. In the past, we cut a side-hole into the graft and the

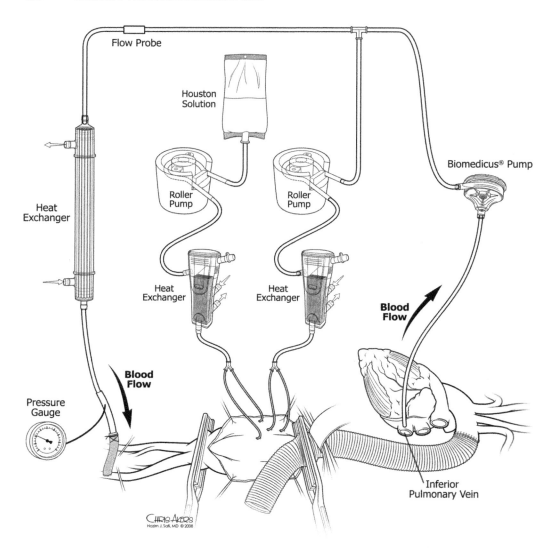

Figure 39-3. Schematics of left atriofemoral bypass. Inflow is usually from the left inferior pulmonary vein and roller pumps can provide perfusion via visceral cannulas. Outflow is usually via a graft placed end-to-side on the left common femoral artery. Visceral perfusate is cold blood. Renal perfusate is cold crystalloid solution via a separate roller pump.

graft is sutured around the lower intercostal artery with 3-0 polypropylene sutures. However we currently apply the reattachment as a loop graft in a side-to-side fashion. (Figure 39-5) Following completion of the intercostal anastomosis, we move the clamp from the proximal to the distal left subclavian artery on the graft and the flow is restored to the intercostal arteries.

Next, we apply the clamp onto the infrarenal abdominal aorta, if possible. If this is not possible, we instead clamp the iliac artery and open the remainder of the abdominal aorta. We identify the celiac axis, superior mesenteric artery, and both renal arteries. A balloon-tip catheter is used to perfuse the celiac axis, superior mesenteric artery, and both renal arteries. Two separate pumps are used. We also monitor

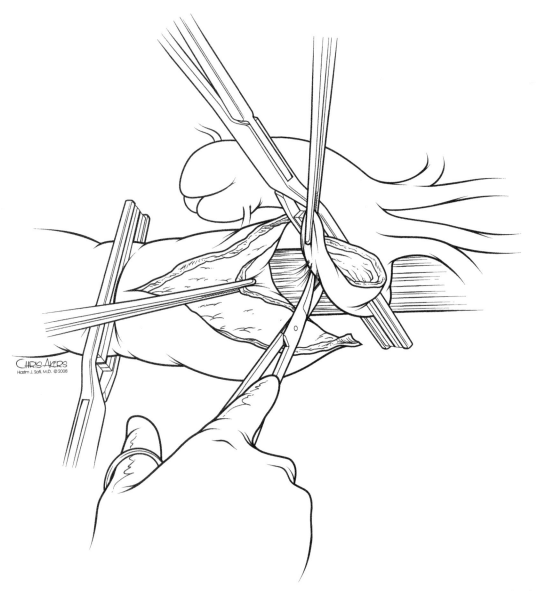

Figure 39-4. Illustration of separation of the aorta from the underlying esophagus in preparation for the proximal anastomosis.

the left renal artery blood pressure, distal femoral artery pressures, and the amount of blood excreted during the clamp. We then retrieve the other end of the graft in the abdominal portion of the aorta by cutting an elliptical hole opposite the visceral vessels. (Figure 39-6) We anastomose the side-hole into the vessels with 3-0 polypropylene sutures. At this point, we clamp the visceral flow, remove the cannula, and finish the anastomosis. The patient is placed in the head-down position and the graft is flushed to remove all air and debris. We then restore pulsatile flow to the viscera and clamp distal to the visceral patch and anastomosis. Following that, the graft will be

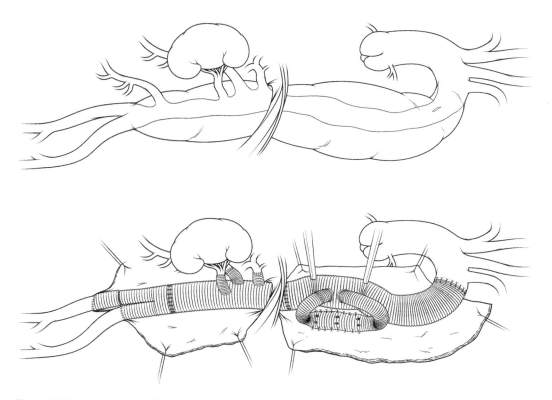

Figure 39-5. Reattachment of intercostal arteries using a loop graft.

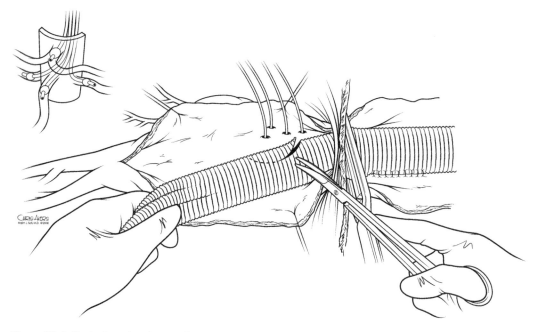

Figure 39-6. Illustration of graftotomy for the visceral patch.

cut to an appropriate length and sutured to the infrarenal abdominal aorta above the aortic bifurcation with running 3-0 polypropylene sutures. When that is finished, the clamp is released and pulsatile flow is restored to the viscera and lower extremities. Rewarming is begun until the patient's nasopharyngeal temperature is 36°C. Once that is achieved and all of the bleeding sites are secured and the patient is hemodynamically stable, the pump is stopped. The cannulae are removed from the superior pulmonary vein and femoral artery. The suture on the pulmonary vein is secured and the femoral artery is repaired using a 5-0 polypropylene suture. The hole in the superior pulmonary vein is secured and removed from the femoral artery and the femoral artery is repaired using 3-0 or 4-0 polypropylene sutures.

The closing is achieved in the usual fashion. We like to insert 3 #36 Argyll chest tubes. The pericostal space will be approximated with 2-0 Ticron. The muscular layers are approximated with #1 PDS. The diaphragm and the linea alba are closed with #1 Prolene. The skin will be approximated with interrupted skin staples. Once this is done and the patient is hemodynamically stable, the patient is placed in the supine position and the double-lumen tube is exchanged for a single-lumen tube. The patient is then transferred to intensive care for postoperative care.

DELAYED NEUROLOGICAL DEFICIT

Our current rate of delayed neurologic deficit is 3% in cases of descending thoracic and thoracoabdominal aortic aneurysm repair.[29] If delayed neurologic deficit occurs, several maneuvers—identified by the COPS acronym (CSF drain status/oxygen delivery/patient status)—are performed with the goal of increasing the spinal oxygenation and perfusion

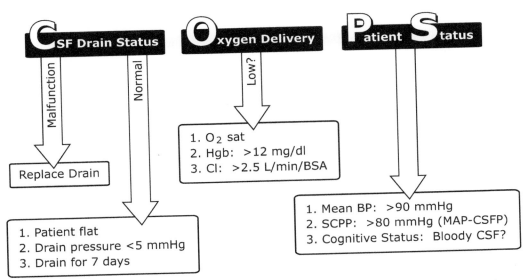

Figure 39-7. The COPS protocol for treatment of patients with delayed neurological deficit: CSF drainage, supplemental oxygen, maximixing patient status (increasing blood pressure and spinal cord perfusion pressure).

pressure (Figure 39-7).[32] Supplemental oxygen is given and the patient is kept supine. The mean arterial pressure goal is raised to greater than 90 mm Hg and the cardiac index is kept greater than 2.5 L/min/BSA. Blood transfusions are given to keep the hemogloblin level above 12 mg/dL. The CSF drain is opened to keep CSF pressure less than 5 mm Hg. The drain is kept in place for 7 days in cases of delayed deficit.

RESULTS

Using the adjuncts CSF drainage, mild to moderate passive hypothermia, and distal aortic perfusion, we have successfully reduced the incidence of spinal cord ischemia. In the clamp-and-sew era, the incidence of neurological deficits in TAAA was 15% in extent I, 31% in extent II, 7% in extent III, and 4% in extent IV.[35] In addition to aneurysm extent, other predictors of neurologic deficit in the clamp-and-sew era included aortic clamp time and preoperative renal insufficiency. The use of adjuncts has mitigated aortic clamp time as a risk factor for immediate neurologic deficits. In more than 1000 TAAA repairs by the authors, aortic clamp times increased by an average of 34 seconds per year while the risk of neurologic deficit significantly decreased in extent II cases from 1 in 5 to 1 in 30.[36] The strongest risks for postoperative spinal paralysis or paraparesis – collectively termed neurologic deficits – were extent II, preoperative renal insufficiency, current smoking, and clamp-and-sew technique.[36] Thus, for the purpose of neurologic risk stratification in the modern era, we can separate the groups into extent II and non-extent II. In our most recent series, we reported postoperative neurologic deficit rates of 4% in extent II and 1.1% in non-extent II cases.[37]

CONCLUSION

Open thoracoabdominal aortic aneurysm repair remains a surgical challenge. Neurological deficit secondary to spinal cord injury remains a dreaded complication. Current adjunctive techniques including CSF drainage, mild to moderate passive hypothermia, and distal aortic perfusion have successfully reduced the risk of spinal ischemia to acceptable levels even in high-risk patients. Aneurysm extent remains an important risk predictor.

REFERENCES

1. Greenberg RK, Lu Q, Roselli EE, et al. Contemporary analysis of descending thoracic and thoracoabdominal aneurysm repair: a comparison of endovascular and open techniques. *Circulation.* 2008; 118(8):808–17.
2. Svensson LG, Patel V, Robinson MF, et al. Influence of preservation or perfusion of intra-operatively identified spinal cord blood supply on spinal motor evoked potentials and paraplegia after aortic surgery. *J Vasc Surg.* 1991; 13(3):355–65.
3. Etheredge SN, Yee J, Smith J, et al. Successful resection of a large aneurysm of the upper abdominal aorta and replacement with homograft. *Surgery.* 1955; 38:1071–1081.

4. DeBakey ME, Cooley DA, Crawford ES, et al. Clinical application of a new flexible knitted Dacron arterial substitute. *Arch Surg*. 1957; 74:713–724.
5. Matas R. I. An Operation for the Radical Cure of Aneurism based upon Arteriorrhaphy. *Ann Surg*. 1903;37:161–96.
6. Spencer FC. The influence of ligation of intercostal arteries on paraplegia in dogs. *Surg Forum*. 1950;9:340.
7. Crawford ES, Snyder DM, Cho GC, et al. Progress in treatment of thoracoabdominal and abdominal aortic aneurysms involving celiac, superior mesenteric, and renal arteries. *Ann Surg* .1978;188:404–22.
8. Harris EJ, Connolly JE, Bruns DL. Surgical management of dissecting aneurysm; the use of a simplified bypass. *Calif Med* .1959;91:127–30.
9. Wakabayashi A, Connolly JE. Prevention of paraplegia associated with resection of extensive thoracic aneurysms. *Arch Surg*. 1976;111:1186–9.
10. Carlson DE, Karp RB, Kouchoukos NT. Surgical treatment of aneurysms of the descending thoracic aorta: an analysis of 85 patients. *Ann Thorac Surg*. 1983;35:58–69.
11. McCullough JL, Hollier LH, Nugent M. Paraplegia after thoracic aortic occlusion: Influence of cerebrospinal fluid drainage. Experimental and early clinical results. *J Vasc Surg*. 1988;7:153–60.
12. Cambria RP, Davison JK, Zannetti S, et al. Clinical experience with epidural cooling for spinal cord protection during thoracic and thoracoabdominal aneurysm repair. *J Vasc Surg*. 1997;25:234–41; discussion 41–3.
13. Estrera AL, Miller CC, Huynh TT, et al. Preoperative and Operative Predictors of Delayed Neurologic Deficit following repair of Thoracoabdominal aortic aneurysms. *J Thorac Cardiovasc Surg*. 2003 Nov; 126(5):1288–94.
14. Hollier LH, Money SR, Naslund TC, et al. Risk of spinal cord dysfunction in patients undergoing thoracoabdominal aortic replacement. *Am J Surg*. 1992; 164(3):210–3; discussion 213–4.
15. Coselli JS, LeMaire SA, Miller CC 3rd, et al. Mortality and paraplegia after thoracoabdominal aortic aneurysm repair: A risk factor analysis. *Ann Thorac Surg*. 2000 Feb;69(2):409–14.
16. Estrera AL, Miller CC 3rd, Huynh TT, et al. Neurologic outcome after thoracic and thoracoabdominal aortic aneurysm repair. *Ann Thorac Surg*. 2001 Oct;72(4):1225–30; discussion 1230–1.
17. Cambria RP, Clouse WD, Davison JK, et al. *Ann Thorac Surg*. Thoracoabdominal aneurysm repair: results with 337 operations performed over a 15-year interval. *Ann Surg*. 2002;236(4):471–9; discussion 479.
18. Greenberg RK, Lu Q, Roselli EE, et al. Contemporary analysis of descending thoracic and thoracoabdominal aneurysm repair: a comparison of endovascular and open techniques. *Circulation*. 2008; 118(8):808–17.
19. Yoshika K. MR angiography and CT angiography of the artery of Adamkiewicz: state of the art. *Radiogr*. 2006 Oct; 26 Suppl 1:S63–73.
20. Uotani K, Yamada N, Kono AK, et al. Preoperative visualization of the artery of Adamkiewicz by intra-arterial CT angiography. AJNR Am J Neuroradiol. 2008 Feb; 29(2):314–8. Epub 2007 Nov 1.
21. Svensson LG, Crawford ES, Hess KR, et al. Deep hypo- thermia with circulatory arrest. Determinants of stroke and early mortality in 656 patients. *J Thorac Cardiovasc Surg*. 1993;106:19–25.
22. Safi HJ, Estrera AL, Miller CC, et al. Evolution of Risk for Neurologic Deficit After Descending and Thoracoabdominal Aortic Repair. *Ann Thorac Surg*. 2005 Dec; 80(6): 2173–2179.
23. Bicknell CD, Riga CV, Wolfe JH. Prevention of paraplegia during thoracoabdominal aortic aneurysm repair. *Eur J Vasc and Endovasc Surg*. 2009; 37(6):654–60.
24. Patel VI, Ergul E, Conrad MF, et al. Continued favorable results with open surgical repair of type IV thoracoabdominal aortic aneurysms. *J Vasc Surg*. 2011; 53(6):1492–8.

25. Weigang E, Hartert M, von Samson P, et al. Thoracoabdominal aortic aneurysm repair: interplay of spinal cord protecting modalities. *Eur J Vasc and Endovasc Surg.* 2005; 30(6):624–31.

26. Estrera AL, Miller CC 3rd, Huynh TT, et al. Neurologic outcome after thoracic and thoracoabdominal aortic aneurysm repair. *Ann Thorac Surg.* 2001; 72(4):1225–30; discussion 1230–1.

27. Svensson LG, Crawford ES, Hess KR, et al. Experience with 1509 patients undergoing thoracoabdominal aortic operations. *J Vasc Surg.* 1993; 17:357–68; discussion 68–70.

28. Huynh TT, Porat EE, Miller CC 3rd, et al. The effect of aortic dissection on outcome in descending thoracic and thoracoabdominal aortic aneurysm repair. *Semin Vasc Surg.* 2002 Jun; 15(2): 108–15.

29. Estrera AL, Sheinbaum R, Miller CC 3rd, et al. Neuromonitor-guided repair of thoracoabdominal aortic aneurysms. *J Thorac Cardiovasc Surg.* 2010 Dec;140(6 Suppl):S131–5; discussion S142–S146.

30. Achouh PE, Estrera AL, Miller CC, 3rd, et al. Role of somatosensory evoked potentials in predicting outcome during thoracoabdominal aortic repair. *Ann Thorac Surg* .2007;84:782–7; discussion 7–8.

31. Keyhani K, Miller CC 3rd, Estrera AL, et al. Analysis of motor and somatosensory evoked potentials during thoracic and thoracoabdominal aortic aneurysm repair. *J Vasc Surg.* 2009 Jan; 49(1):36–41. Epub 2008 Oct 1.

32. Estrera AL, Sheinbaum R, Miller CC, et al. Cerebrospinal fluid drainage during thoracic aortic repair: safety and current management. *Ann Thorac Surg.* 2009; 88:9–15; discussion

33. Cina CS, Abouzahr L, Arena GO, et al. Cerebrospinal fluid drainage to prevent paraplegia during thoracic and thoracoabdominal aortic aneurysm surgery: a systematic review and meta-analysis. *J Vasc Surg.* 2004; 40:36–44.

34. Crawford ES, Svensson LG, Hess KR, et al. A prospective randomized study of cerebrospinal fluid drainage to prevent paraplegia after high-risk surgery on the thoracoabdominal aorta. *J Vasc Surg.* 1991; 13:36–45; discussion -6.

35. Svensson LG, Crawford ES, Hess KR, et al. Variables predictive of outcome in 832 patients undergoing repairs of the descending thoracic aorta. *Chest.* 1993;104:1248–53.

36. Safi HJ, Estrera AL, Miller CC, et al. Evolution of risk for neurologic deficit after descending and thoracoabdominal aortic repair. *Ann Thorac Surg.* 2005; 80:2173–9; discussion 9.

37. Safi HJ, Estrera AL, Azizzadeh A, et al. Progress and future challenges in thoracoabdominal aortic aneurysm management. *World J Surg.* 2008; 32:355–60.

Complex Venous Problems

40

Technical Tips for Renal Cell Cancer Caval Tumor Thrombus Removal

Chin Chin Yeh, MD and R. Clement Darling III, MD

INTRODUCTION

Renal cell carcinoma (RCC) constitutes 2% of all adult neoplasms and its incidence has been increasing in the Western population over the last 30 years.[1] Unfortunately, RCC has a unique feature of intraluminal growth into renal venous circulation. In four to 10% of patients, this feature of venous invasion extends beyond the renal vein into the inferior vena cava (IVC). Direct venous wall involvement is rare and unfortunately carries a much poorer prognosis.[2] The treatment of choice for patients presenting with renal cell carcinoma invading the vena cava is usually radical nephrectomy with enbloc thrombectomy. Surgery can be curative, cytoreductive or palliative. In cases where the tumor can be removed in total, there is over 60% five-year survival.[3]

From a clinical standpoint, venous extension may be suspected if the patient develops lower extremity edema; a varicocele that does not collapse when the patient is supine; dilated superficial abdominal veins; development of a pulmonary embolism or a right atrial mass; loss of kidney function; or proteinuria.

STAGING

Staging of RCC has been shown to be a significant predictor of overall survival in patients. In the absence of metastases or lymph node involvement, complete surgical excision offers a 69% 5-year survival. When metastases are present, 5-year survival is reduced to 0–20%. (2) Therefore, accurate staging to fully identify tumor and assess its extent is essential. (Figure 40-1)

In addition to TNM classification, extension or invasion of the IVC is also classified. Level I thrombus is found in the renal vein and extends <2 cm within the IVC.

TABLE 1 2010 AJCC TNM clinical staging system for renal cell carcinoma

Tumor status.
- **TX:** The primary tumor cannot be evaluated.
- **T0:** There is no evidence of a primary tumor in the kidney(s).
- **T1:** The tumor is found only in the kidney and is 7 centimeters (cm) or smaller in size at its largest area. There has been much discussion among doctors whether this classification should only include a tumor 5 cm and under.
  - **T1a:** The tumor is found only in the kidney and is 4 cm or smaller in size at its largest area.
  - **T1b:** The tumor is found only in the kidney and is between 4 cm and 7 cm at its largest area.
- **T2:** The tumor is found only in the kidney and is larger than 7 cm in size at its largest area.
  - **T2a:** The tumor is only in the kidney and is more than 7 cm but 10 cm or less at its largest area.
  - **T2b:** The tumor is only in the kidney and is more than 10 cm at its largest area.
- **T3:** The tumor has grown into major veins or perinephric tissue (connective, fatty tissue around the kidneys). It has not grown into the adrenal gland (gland on top of each kidney that produces hormones and adrenaline to help control heart rate, blood pressure, and other body functions) on the same side of the body as the tumor, and it has not spread beyond Gerota's fascia (an envelope of tissue that surrounds the kidney).
  - **T3a:** The tumor has spread to the large vein leading out of the kidney, called the renal vein, or the muscles of the vein, or it has spread to the fat surrounding the kidney and/or the fat inside the kidney. The tumor has not grown beyond Gerota's fascia.
  - **T3b:** The tumor has grown into the large vein leading out of the heart, called the vena cava, below the muscle known as the diaphragm under the lungs that helps breathing.
  - **T3c:** The tumor has spread to the vena cava above the diaphragm or the walls of the vena cava.
- **T4:** The tumor has spread to areas beyond Gerota's fascia and extends into the adrenal gland on the same side of the body as the tumor.

Nodal status. The 'N' in the TNM staging system stands for lymph nodes. Lymph nodes near the kidneys are called regional lymph nodes. Lymph nodes in other parts of the body are called distant lymph nodes.
- **NX:** The regional lymph nodes cannot be evaluated.
- **N0:** The cancer has not spread to the regional lymph nodes.
- **N1:** The cancer has spread to regional lymph nodes.

Distant metastasis. The 'M' in the TNM system indicates whether the cancer has spread to other parts of the body. Common areas where kidney cancer may spread include the bones, liver, lungs, brain, and distant lymph nodes.
- **M0:** The disease has not metastasized.
- **M1:** The cancer has spread to other parts of the body beyond the kidney area.

Used with the permission of the American Joint Committee on Cancer (AJCC), Chicago, Illinois. The original source for this material is the AJCC Cancer Staging Manual, Seventh Edition (2010) published by Springer Science and Business Media LLC, http://www.springer.com.

Figure 40-1. Staging Table (reproduced with permission by John Wiley & Sons. Source material from BJU International online journal "Important surgical considerations in the management of renal cell carcinoma (RCC) with inferior vena cava (IVC) tumour thrombus"). Original source material from the AJCC Cancer Staging Manual, Seventh Edition (2010) published by Springer Science and Business Media LLC, http://www.springer.com used with permission by BJU from the American Joint Committee on Cancer (AJCC), Chicago, IL.

Level II is infrahepatic thrombus, while level III is infrahepatic. Finally, level 4 represents thrombus extension above the level of the diaphragm. (Figure 40-2)

DIAGNOSIS

Preoperative planning is of course crucial to the surgical management of RCC patients who are undergoing a resection. In fact, it has been shown that a larger IVC diameter is associated with wall invasion. Knowing the level of the thrombus also allows for careful planning of the operation itself and can indicate whether a multidisciplinary group of different surgeons are necessary.

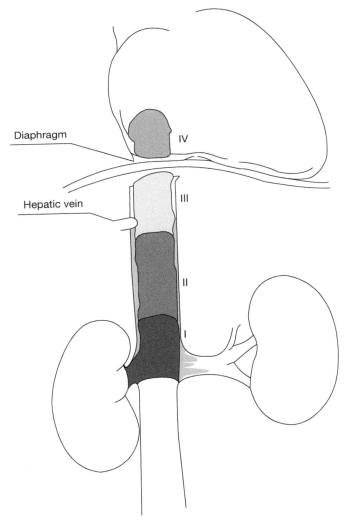

Figure 40-2. Classification of IVC tumor thrombus levels according to the Novick staging system (reproduced with permission by John Wiley & Sons. Source material from BJU International online journal "Important surgical considerations in the management of renal cell carcinoma (RCC) with inferior vena cava (IVC) tumour thrombus").

Ultrasonography is commonly used to evaluate patients. Ultrasound, unfortunately, is largely dependent on the technician, and it has been shown a sensitivity of 68%.[3] Another disadvantage is that ultrasound is not very sensitive in detecting tumor thrombosis.

Currently, MRI represents the "gold standard" in terms of accurate assessment of IVC involvement. It has replaced traditional venacavography. MRI has a sensitivity level of 100%. MRI also has the advantage of avoiding radiation to the patient. It also offers multiplanar views which allows us to see the relationship of the thrombus and assess the relationship of the thrombus with other parts of the body.

Computed tomography has not been shown to be accurate; its accuracy is around 65% in determining the extent of the tumor or thrombus. However, multidetector CT (MDCT) may replace MRI as a precise diagnostic modality. MDCT has a sensitivity of 93% and a specificity of 80%. However, recent studies suggest that the timing of the study preoperatively may be more important; for example, Woodruff et al. demonstrated that obtaining imaging less than 14 days before surgery is ideal. The longest interval from imaging to resection should be no longer than 30 days.[2]

In 30 to 40% of cases, a distinct arterial supply exists that supplies the tumor thrombus. This arterial supply is best identified by a renal arteriogram. In the past, there is also the practice of pre-operative embolization that may shrink the tumor and facilitate excision; however, recent studies have not supported this practice except in specific cases.[4] Otherwise, it does not appear to facilitate tumor excision and may cause perioperative complications.

SURGICAL CONSIDERATIONS

Surgical planning for resection of RCC that has extended into the IVC requires a multidisciplinary approach, often determined by the level of the IVC thrombus. Ayyathurai et al. examined how the presence of bland tumor combined with tumor thrombus affected outcomes for patients who undergo surgical resection for RCC. They found their perioperative mortality to be 2.3% and that only the level of the tumor thrombus predicted the presence of associated bland thrombus.[5]

Because embolization of bland or tumor thrombus can be a fatal complication of surgical resection, there has been debate over the usefulness of IVC filter placement. While there have been some case reports that suggest placement of an IVC filter can prevent embolization, the most important concern for a surgeon is the incorporation of the filter into the thrombus, which would increase the level of complexity of surgical resection. For these reasons, an IVC filter may be considered in only level I or II tumors when anticoagulation is not feasible.[6]

There is mixed literature on the use of preoperative renal artery embolization in order to decrease blood loss during the resection. If one is to contemplate preoperative embolization, resection has to occur within 24 to 48 hours after embolization in order to have some positive effect. If one waits longer, collateral formation can occur and it may be more difficult to control rather than a singular renal artery.[7]

As mentioned before, the extent of the tumor in the IVC also affects the type of surgical resection. For level I and II tumors, the resection is usually easily performed below the liver; however, in those tumors that extend up to the hepatic veins, full control of the suprahepatic cava as well as the hepatic veins may be necessary in order to minimize blood loss. Obviously, those tumors that extend to the right atrium need to be evaluated preoperatively with a cardiac surgeon to see if the patient needs to have a median sternotomy and/or cardiopulmonary bypass. In our experience, in the majority of patients who have had tumors ascend to the right atrium, the tumor can be removed without putting the patient on cardiopulmonary bypass; however, a median sternotomy does make access to the tumor much easier. Usually in these cases, either the use of a Fogarty balloon or just gentle finger compression under transesophageal echocardiography (TEE) can milk the tumor down below the atrium and a clamp can then be placed on the cavoatrial junction.

Unfortunately, it is extremely difficult to assess whether the vein wall is involved, so at the time of surgery one must be prepared to not only do a local resection with primary reconstruction but also have different options for patching, replacing, or ligating the vena cava while preserving flow to the contralateral renal vein. Typically in our experience, PTFE has worked well whether we were patching or reconstructing the vena cava.

TECHNICAL CONSIDERATIONS

Once one has drawn up a perioperative surgical plan, the management is relatively straightforward. The three major concerns are: 1) how to minimize embolization from the tumor, 2) how to minimize engorgement of the organs and control hypotension during vena cava clamping, and 3) how to minimize blood loss. Our approach to optimize vena cava resection and minimize trauma to the patient has been to obtain control above the tumor. The incision for level I and level II are subcostal or chevron incisions and a thoracoabdominal incision is used for level II and III. In the vast majority of cases we have gone to the suprahepatic cava as well as dissected at the hepatic veins in order to minimize embolization. This requires mobilization of the left lobe of the liver, incising the triangular ligament, and opening up the bare area of the right lobe of the liver. This allows complete access of the retrohepatic cava, suprahepatic cava, as well as the short hepatic veins, and decreases the risk of embolization as well as blood loss. It does require somewhat more dissection, but we feel in those tumors that extend up to the hepatic veins, it is much safer and more controlled.

Once we do obtain proximal control, we move the clamp down to the infrahepatic IVC as soon as technically possible to minimize hemodynamic instability, a situation similar to moving the clamp down from supraceliac aorta to infrarenal aorta during a ruptured aortic aneurysm. One technology that we have used extensively in many of the level III and IV tumors that I feel strongly should be used in all tumors is the transesophageal echocardiogram (TEE). This allows visualization of the extent of the tumor in real time, as well as evaluate if any embolization or air has been extruded into the circulation. Most recently, this has helped us clamp lower in the vena cava than we had previously done as we can see the entire extent of the tumor. This visualization then allows us to "milk" the tumor down and then place a clamp just above the area with almost complete assurance that we have not embolized or compromised our resection.

One also has to be cognizant of the short hepatic veins which can be ripped or torn during dissection and/or removal of the tumor and equally as important, is the large lumbar veins which can cause a significant amount of blood loss once one opens up

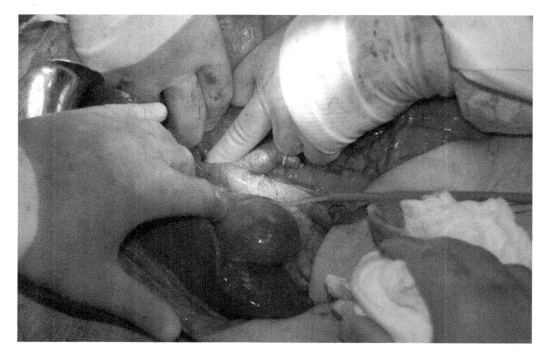

Figure 40-3. Exposure of the infrahepatic and infrarenal vena cava and contralateral renal vein.

the vena cava. We most commonly do not use a side bending clamp unless we have a good sense that the tumor has been pulled back and we can partially occlude the cava. More frequently we use umbilical tape and Rummel clamps above and below the tumor in order to minimize the amount of trauma on the veins (Figure 40-3) and also allows us to inspect the entire inside of the vena cava in order to make sure there is no further tumor. (Figure 40-4).

In a small amount of cases there has been tumor into the lumbar veins which had to be resected in the posterior portion of the cava closed separately from the venotomy that was made in order to remove the intraluminal tumor. If one used a partial occluding clamp, one may not be able to evaluate it effectively and thus in order to maximize the patient's lifespan and make it a complete tumor resection, we feel we should have the ability to inspect the interior of the vena cava.

When dissecting out the hepatic veins, one has to be careful as they can be easily damaged. One also needs to know the anatomy well. The first maneuver we perform is ligating the renal artery. Next, we control the porta hepatis and place an umbilical tape and Rummel clamp in order to occlude the arterial inflow. In cases of extreme blood loss or difficult dissection, one can get supraceliac control of the aorta but we usually find this unnecessary except for patients who are significantly hemodynamically unstable. The middle hepatic vein emerges variably either directly off the vena cava or off the right or left hepatic veins. If the branching of the hepatic veins is intra hepatic, then obviously we may choose not to dissect them out individually.

Once the liver has been dissected off the cava or off its lateral and medial attachments, one can get around the suprahepatic cava by dividing portions of the retroperitoneum and crus. This again allows a right angle to be placed around it and

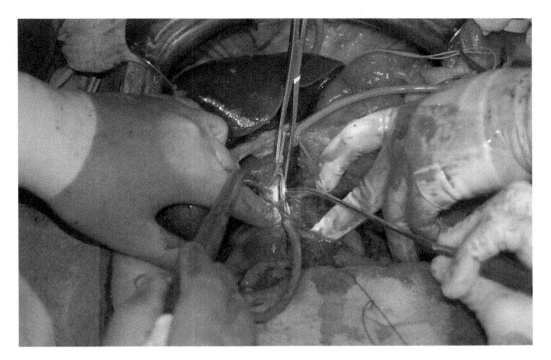

Figure 40-4. Inspection of Vena cava after tumor resection.

an umbilical taper and Rummel clamp to be utilized to obtain suprahepatic control. Similarly, we obtain control of the intrahepatic vena cava, contralateral renal vein, and infra renal vena cava below the tumor. If the patient has an extensive DVT, one has to consider one of two things: either thrombectomy of the proximal iliacs and vena cava or ligation as a secondary therapy. The latter we use very infrequently, and only in cases of patients who have a significant amount of vena cava tumor that has a backup of red thrombus that cannot be removed in total.

After we have control of the vena cava above the level of the tumor and the contralateral renal vein, we evaluate the vena cava for gonadal veins and lumbar veins. When these structures have been identified, we place either a Cooley clamp or a Rummel clamp around it. The lumbar veins tend to be somewhat friable, especially if they are dilated from tumor engorgement; therefore, one has to be very careful about venous injury.

The clamping sequence can be somewhat variable. First, we clamp the arterial inflow as this will decrease hepatic engorgement. Secondly, under TEE, we compress cephalad above the tumor and then place a clamp on the contralateral renal vein, the infrarenal cava, and then either the suprahepatic or infrahepatic cava depending on location of the tumor. We then clamp all the lumbars or accessory veins. Once the vessels are clamped, we make sure the patient is hemodynamically stable, and when this appears to be the case, a 15 blade is used to incise an oval around the renal vein orifice. This opening can be extended cephalad. If the tumor is adherent, we take a rim of tissue to make sure there are no tumor cells on the closure of the vena cava. If the tumor extends cephalad, one can also use a Fogarty catheter in order to bring it down, but in the vast majority of cases it comes out in one piece and does not need much assistance.

In those extreme circumstances, one has to do an endovenectomy to remove the tumor as a thin layer of reactive tissue is between the tumor and the vena cava wall. This can be done much like one would do a carotid endarterectomy.

Once the tumor is removed and the inside of the vena cava is inspected, a 5–0 prolene suture can be used to close the vena cava in a one or two-layer closure. The one-layer closure is simple linear baseball stitch tied on either end. More frequently we use a first layer of horizontal mattresses and then run the suture back and tie it to itself. Once this is performed we "de-air" the cava by releasing the contralateral renal vein and lumbar veins, and then unclamping the infrarenal vena cava in order to make sure there is no air within the reconstruction. This can also be evaluated through the TEE and once we are comfortable, we release the infra or suprahepatic cava clamps. Inspection of the suture line is imperative and we usually tolerate up to 30% decrease in diameter. Many vena cava are distended secondary to chronic tumor obstruction so a complete tumor resection can usually be performed without significant luminal reduction. As was mentioned earlier, we use PTFE for patch or reconstruction when necessary (in about 10–20% of resections).

Throughout the clamping and un-clamping routine, the vascular surgeon must communicate with the anesthesia team in order to make sure the patient is kept hemodynamically stable. Intraoperative fluid management and judicious use of cardiotonic medications will maximize patient outcomes.

In our experience of close to 100 resections, patients have tolerated the procedure well and we have had no in-hospital or 30-day mortality. A multidisciplinary approach with urologists, vascular surgeons, anesthesia, radiology, oncology, occasionally cardiac surgery, and especially the patient and their family will result in a smooth perioperative course and optimal outcomes.

REFERENCES

1. Lopez CM, Esteban E, Astudillo A, et al. Predictive factors for response to treatment in patients with advanced renal cell carcinoma. Springer Science + Business Media, LLC, Published online May 27, 2012.
2. Lawindy SM, Kurian T, Kim T, et al. Important surgical considerations in the management of renal cell carcinoma (RCC) with inferior vena cava (IVC) tumour thrombus. *BJU International.* February 2012:1–14.
3. Ciancio G, Manoharan M, Katkoori D, et al. Long-term survival in patients undergoing radical nephrectomy and inferior vena cava thrombectomy: Single-center experience. *Eur Urol.* 2010;57:667–672.
4. Guo HF, Song Y, Na YQ. Value of abdominal ultrasound scan, CT and MRI for diagnosing inferior vena cava tumour thrombus in renal cell carcinoma. *Chin Med J.* (Engl) 2009; 122:2299–302.
5. Subramanian VS, Stephenson AJ, Goldfarb DA, et al. Utility of preoperative renal artery embolization for management of renal tumors with inferior vena caval thrombi. *Urology.* 2009;74:154–159.
6. Ayyathurai R, Garcia-Roig M, Gorin MA, et al. Bland thrombus association with tumour thrombus in renal cell carcinoma: analysis of surgical significance and role of inferior vena caval interruption. *BJU International.* January 2012:1–7.
7. Woodruff DY, Van Veldhuizen P, Muehlebach G, et al. The perioperative management of an inferior vena caval tumor thrombus in patients with renal cell carcinoma. *Urol Oncol.* 2009;122:2299–2302.

41

Inferior Vena Cava Filters: The Challenges of Potentially Retrievable Devices

Robert K. Ryu, MD and Anthony M. Esparaz, BA

Inferior vena cava filters (IVCF) are indicated for the prevention of recurrent or primary pulmonary embolism (PE) in patients with a contraindication to anticoagulation.[1,2] Expanded indications for caval filtration include prophylactic clinical situations including trauma patients, major orthopaedic or neurosurgical procedures, and bariatric patients. Potentially retrievable IVC filters (prIVCFs) provide mechanical protection from PE in patients who need caval filtration for a defined period of time. They are designed to be retrieved when the patient can restart anticoagulation safely or when the risk of PE is diminished. Their potential removal offers the notional benefit of avoiding the long-term complications associated with permanent IVC filters. There has been a recent expansion of prIVCF use in the United States: over the past three years, several reports describe an annual prIVCF placement rate exceeding that of permanent filters.[3,4] In 2012, it is estimated that 259,000 IVC filters will be placed in the United States with over 75% being potentially retrievable.[5]

As response to an alarming increase in the incidence of prIVCF-related complications, the United States Food & Drug Administration (FDA) issued an "Alert and Notice" on August 9, 2010 entitled "Removing Inferior Vena Cava Filters: Initial Communication."[6] The FDA specifically recommended "that implanting physicians and clinicians. . . consider removing the filter as soon as protection from [pulmonary embolism] is no longer needed."

For many practitioners, the FDA recommendation came as no surprise; this was an institutional acknowledgement that currently available prIVCF and permanent IVCF (pIVCF) are not equivalent in terms of device-related complications and durability, despite the fact that the FDA approval process had been for the most part identical for the two types of devices. Fundamentally, retrievable filters are engineered differently from permanent devices. The design of prIVCF is inherently paradoxical: although

FDA approved for use as permanently implanted devices, prIVCF are specifically designed to be retrievable and, therefore, "impermanent" implantations. Alternatively, if designed to be more stable during the implantation period, retrievable devices become more difficult to remove and are, therefore, more likely to be permanently implanted.

Unfortunately, the marketing of these devices suggests a "one size fits all" strategy. Given their permanent implantation indication, they offer the advantage of less device inventory (although, generally speaking, prIVCF are more costly than their permanent counterparts) and more purported clinical decision-making flexibility. Additionally, by using a prIVCF, the labeling of these devices effectively absolves the implanting physician of responsibility for actually retrieving the device since it is technically labeled as a permanent device. Permanent devices are now widely perceived as outdated technology. Proponents of retrievable devices are quick to refer to the conclusions of Decousus et al, making a "stronger" case for the widespread adoption of retrievable devices.[1]

In response to the FDA recommendation, several publications subsequently focused on improving historically poor retrieval rates (as low as 5%) by establishing specific IVCF clinics. By focusing on better patient follow up, the study's authors were able to achieve significantly improved IVCF retrieval rates.[7,8]

Interestingly, what also became clear in these studies was the fact that a significant proportion of patients who received potentially retrievable devices were patients with a clear indication for a permanent device. In our own institutional experience, we have published a study of 100 retrievable filters; of the 40 potentially retrievable devices that were not retrieved (deemed as permanent), a clear majority were declared permanent (82.5%), rather than failed retrieval (12.5%) or lost to follow up (2.5%).[7]

An important conclusion to be drawn from this experience is that "retrospectively-oriented interventions," like improved patient tracking after placement, can improve retrieval rates, however their impact is inherently limited by the following scenario: a retrievable filter is placed in a patient who really should receive a permanent device. Therefore, to further incrementally improve retrieval rates, additional attention must be paid to the "prospective" or decision-making process of whether a patient has a defined time-limited need for caval filtration and should have a prIVCF placed, versus a patient who should receive a permanent device.

In a prospective study at our institution, we carefully analyzed the prIVCF vs pIVCF choice decision by prospectively comparing the IR consultant choice versus the referring physician's choice.[9] Decisions were classified as concordant (device choice agreement between IR and referring physician) or discordant (disagreement over device choice). In addition, the consulting IR prospectively estimated the likelihood of retrieval (0–100%) for all prIVCFs at the time of placement.

Of the 66 devices placed during the study period, 16 (24%) were discordant. Of the 16 discordant devices, seven were retrievable. Six of the seven (86%) retrievable devices were later declared permanent (no attempt was ever made to retrieve). The prospective estimate of the likelihood of retrieval for these seven patients was 6.4% (range 0–15%). In the concordant group, 36 patients had prIVCF implanted. 31 of the 36 (86%) were retrieved. The prospective estimate of the likelihood of retrieval for these 36 patients was 88.3% (range 80–100%). Of the five concordant devices that were not retrieved, two of the patient died while three were declared permanent (no attempt was ever made to retrieve).

The study concluded that prospective consultation yields higher retrieval rates. With improved retrieval rates after consultation, it is evident that device utilization is improved, which leads to cost savings: prIVCF devices are marginally more costly than permanent devices. It is important to note that increased scrutiny of device-related expenditures is to be expected in today's increasingly precarious healthcare finances.

To further optimize our device choice decision-making, we undertook a single institution study of 265 prIVCF patients over a 31 month period in an attempt to identify key patient parameters that could be used to quantitatively predict the need for a permanent or retrievable device.[10] Four parameters were statistically more likely to be present at the time of prIVCF placement whose devices were later deemed permanent: advanced age, male gender, underlying malignancy, and failure of anticoagulation therapy. A nine-predictor logistic model was fitted to the data to test the relationship between the likelihood that an optional filter would remain permanent and the selected patient parameters. This logistic regression prediction equation produces the probability that a prIVCF will become a permanent device. As anticipated, according to the model, the natural log of the odds of a pfIVCF being deemed permanent was positively related to: patient age, male gender, presence of underlying malignancy, and failure of anticoagulation therapy.

TECHNICAL CONSIDERATIONS FOR IVCF RETRIEVAL

Even with optimized prospective and post-procedural monitoring, successful filter retrievals may ultimately be limited by technical challenges. It is impossible to predict which patient and which filter may become firmly embedded and, therefore, resistant to conventional methods of retrieval. Anecdotally, the duration of the implantation period seems to loosely correlate with difficulty of retrieval. However, even filters that have only been implanted for 3–4 weeks can be extremely difficult to retrieve.

It is important to master adjunctive techniques for successful retrieval of a "challenging" prIVCF. "Challenging" features should prompt appropriate preparation for adjunctive retrieval methods. Specific features that may predict a technically difficult retrieval include: duration of implantation, significant tilting, malposition, migration, fracture, and strut penetration.[11] Iliescu et al have authored an exhaustive review of adjunctive techniques (including angioplasty balloon-assisted retrieval, looped guidewires through the apex, use of endobronchial forceps, and other methods). Readers are encouraged to familiarize themselves with their described techniques.[12]

A unique principle for choosing the appropriate approach to the challenging prIVCF retrieval is the concept of the fibrin cap that entraps or embeds the retrieval hook at the apex of the filter device. The mechanism behind fibrin cap formation lies in endothelial injury induced by the filter, which leads to focal desquamation of vessel wall lining.[13] The underlying endothelial connective tissue becomes exposed, causing adherence and aggregation of platelets and activation of thrombin from prothrombin.[14] Thrombin acts to convert the glycoprotein dimer fibrinogen to fibrin monomers that aggregate into a fibrin mesh. We hypothesize that it is this fibrin mesh or cap that forms over the filter apex which, in turn, prevents filter hook engagement.

Filter retrieval histology itself has been relatively underreported. Nevertheless, there are studies that describe the adherence of fibrin to retrieved filters. Kuo et al. described surgical pathological evaluation of tissue adherent to an Optease filter device (Cordis Endovascular, Miami Lakes, FL) retrieved after 52 days of implantation.[15] Analysis of the specimen revealed evolving stages of an organizing thrombus with a fibrin band overlaid with granulation tissue. However, in their larger series of 26 complex retrievals, nine of the filters had histologic evidence of "scant caval tissue."[16]

IVCF tilting >15% is a common phenomenon, seen in over 13% in our review of 476 implanted devices.[17] An even greater proportion of filters tilt to a lesser degree. Device tilting is theorized to results in turbulent blood flow near the apex of the filter which may promote further tilting and subsequent formation of a fibrin cap (figure 41-1). The presence of a fibrin cap, which may or may not be radioopaque (figure 41-2), can prevent successful engagement of the retrieval hook with a conventional endovascular snare device. Some of the methods in Iliescu et al indirectly address fibrin caps.[12] We have described a more direct method of disrupting the fibrin cap to facilitate filter retrieval.[18] By engaging the radiolucent fibrin cap with a reverse curve catheter (figure 41-3), a hydrophilic guidewire can be looped around the fibrin cap (figure 41-4). The fibrin cap can then be disrupted by either advancing a sheath over the looped guidewire, or applying manual traction to the looped guidewire. The filter can then be removed using conventional means.

We have successful employed this strategy in 16 patients who have failed conventional retrieval methods. The challenging aspect of this approach is probing for the fibrin cap with the reverse curve catheter to find an effectively invisible structure. However, in our experience, this can be successfully performed repeatedly, quickly, and with minimal use of fluoroscopy.

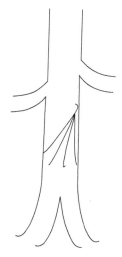

Figure 41-1. Filter tilt will promote fibrin cap formation and adherence of the retrieval hook to the caval wall.

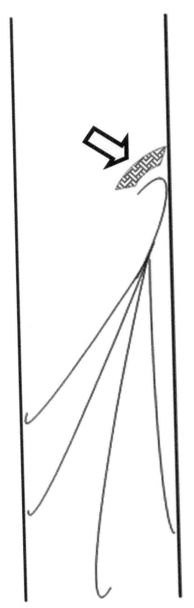

Figure 41-2. The fibrin cap (arrow) prevents engagement of the retrieval hook with an endovascular snare device.

EXCIMER LASER-ASSISTED FILTER RETRIEVAL

Rarely, conventional and adjunctive methods of filter retrieval fail. The causative factor is often excessive scarring at the points of contact between the filter device and the caval wall. To date, there are no known patient parameters that can predict excessive scarring which results in a firmly embedded filter. A novel method of fibrinolysis has been described, utilizing sheath-mediated application of focused photothermal laser energy. Kuo et al

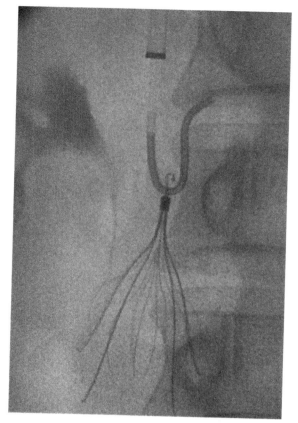

Figure 41-3. Subtle resistance to fluoroscopically guided probing of the caval wall around the retrieval hook with a reverse curve catheter can result in looping of a hydrophilic guidewire around the radiolucent fibrin cap.

subsequently published a series of 25 patients with IVCF with a mean implantation period of well over 500 days, with a range of 71 days to over 18 years.[19] They reported a 96% successful extraction rate with one major complication (in situ thrombosis requiring thrombolysis), three minor complications (focal self-limited extravasation, not requiring treatment) and one adverse event (coagulopathic retroperitoneal hemorrhage).

The Spectranetics SLS II laser sheath (Spectranetics Inc, Colorado Springs, CO) is FDA approved for cardiac pacer lead extraction and comes in 12F, 14F, and 16F diameters. The application of the device for removal of embedded IVCF is off label. The laser fibers run the length of the sheath and are arrayed at the tip of the sheath in a circular configuration. When activated, the 308 nm ultraviolet laser generates low temperature energy that ablates adjacent soft tissue to an estimated depth of 50 microns.

Our own preliminary experience with the Spectranetics SLS II laser sheath has mirrored Kuo et al. We have attempted four excimer laser-assisted retrievals with a mean implantation time of 638 days (range 135–1664 days) with a 100% success rate. There have been no major complications. Pathologic analysis of the devices reveals organized thrombus, fibrinoconnective tissue and scar, but no endothelial elements (figure 41-5).

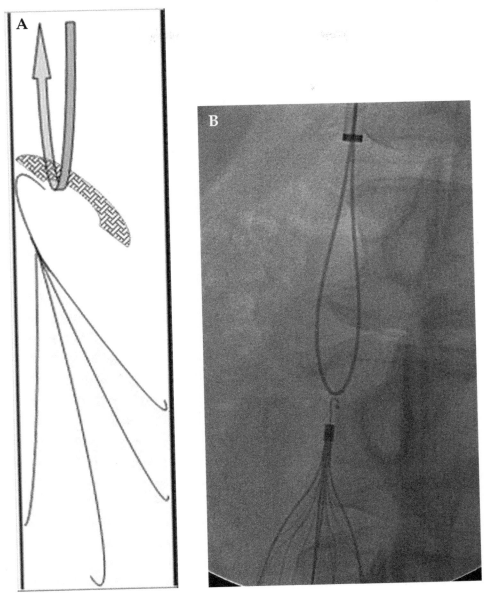

Figure 41-4a. Hydrophilic guidewire (curved arrow) is looped around the fibrin cap. **b.** Radiographic image showing a looped hydrophilic guidewire around a radiolucent fibrin cap. Note that the guidewire is clearly not engaged on the retrieval hook.

SUMMARY

Potentially retrievable IVCF are an evolving technology. Although engineered differently from permanently implanted devices, they are comparably effective in preventing pulmonary embolism. However, their intrinsic design feature is to be relatively easy to retrieve from the IVC. This dichotomy led to a recent recommendation from the FDA to remove

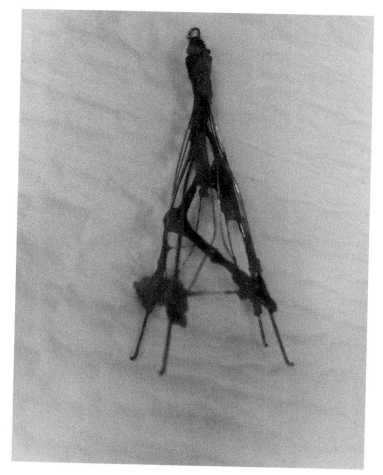

Figure 41-5. Tulip filter that was removed with excimer laser assistance two years after implantation. Note the excessive scar around the filter apex and at the points of contact between the filter struts and caval wall.

prIVCF as soon as possible. There is still a role for permanent devices in current practice, especially in those patients with an open-ended need for caval prophylaxis and specific clinical parameters. The critical parts of any IVCF clinical practice are careful prospective device decision-making and meticulous patient tracking.

Various adjunctive techniques have been described for removal of embedded IVCF. The concept of the fibrin cap is an important cornerstone to the understanding of the etiology of an embedded IVCF and can positively impact outcomes. More aggressive methods like excimer laser-assisted retrieval show promise in small, preliminary studies; however, further controlled investigation is warranted.

REFERENCES

1. Decousus H, Leizorovicz A, Parent F, et al. A clinical trial of vena caval filters in the prevention of pulmonary embolism in patients with proximal deep-vein thrombosis. *N Engl J Med.* 1998;338:409–415.

2. Greenfield LJ. The PREPIC study group. Eight-year follow-up of patients with permanent vena cava filters in the prevention of pulmonary embolism: The PREPIC randomized study. *Perspect Vasc Surg Endovasc Ther.* 2006;18:187–188.

3. Van Ha TG, Chien AS, Funaki BS, et al. Use of retrievable compared to permanent inferior vena cava filters: a single-institution experience. *Cardiovasc Intervent Radiol.* 2008;31:308–315.

4. Yunus TE, Tariq N, Callahan RE, et al. Changes in inferior vena cava filter placement over the past decade at a large community-based Academic Health Center. *J Vasc Surg.* 2008;47:157–165.

5. Smouse B, Johar A. Is market growth of vena cava filters justified? A review of indications, use, and market analysis. *Endovasc Today.* 2010;9(2):74–77.

6. Food and Drug Administration (2010) Removing retrievable inferior vena cava filters: Initial communication. http://www.fda.gov/MedicalDevices/Safety/AlertsandNotices/ucm221676.htm

7. Minocha J, Idakoji I, Riaz A, et al. Improving inferior vena cava filter retrieval rates: Impact of a dedicated inferior vena cava filter clinic. *J Vasc Interv Radiol.* 2010;21:1847–1851.

8. Lynch FC. A method for following patients with retrievable inferior vena cava filters: results and lessons learned from the first 1,100 patients *J Vasc Interv Radiol.* 2011;22:1507–1512.

9. Ryu RK, Parikh P, Gupta R, et al. Optimizing IVC filter utilization: A prospective study of the impact of IR consultation. *J Am Coll Radiol.* 2012 in press.

10. Eifler AC, Lewandowski RJ, Gupta R, et al. Optional or permanent?: Clinical factors that optimize IVC filter utilization 2012. *J Vasc Interv Radiol.* 2012 in press.

11. Geisbüsch P, Benenati JF, Peña CS, et al. Retrievable inferior vena cava filters: Factors that affect retrieval success. *Cardiovasc Intervent Radiol.* 2011 Nov 1 [ePub ahead of print].

12. Iliescu B, Haskal ZJ. Advanced techniques for removal of retrievable inferior vena cava filters. *Cardiovasc Intervent Radiol.* 2011 June 15 [ePub ahead of print].

13. Harker LA, Ross R, Slichter SJ, et al. Homocystine-induced arteriosclerosis. The role of endothelial cell injury and platelet response in its genesis. *J Clin Invest.* 1976;58:731–741.

14. Roberts HR, Monroe DM, Oliver JA, et al. Newer concepts of blood coagulation. *Haemophilia* 1998;4:331–334.

15. Kuo WT, Tong RT, Hwang GL, et al. High-risk retrieval of adherent and chronically implanted ivc filters: Techniques for removal and management of thrombotic complications. *J Vasc Interv Radiol.* 2009;20:1548–1556.

16. Kuo WT, Robertson SW, Odegaard JI, et al. Complex retrieval of fractured, embedded, and penetrating IVC filters: A prospective study with histologic and electron microscopic analysis *J Vasc Interv Radiol.* 2012;23(3S):S27.

17. Lewandowski RJ, Ryu RK, Riaz A, et al. A prospective study of 467 IVC filter placements: Is there a difference between optional and permanent filters? *J Vasc Interv Radiol.* 2012;23(3S):S25.

18. Esparaz A, Ryu RK, Gupta R, et al. Fibrin cap disruption: An adjunctive technique for inferior vena cava filter retrieval *J Vasc Interv Radiol.* 2012 in press.

19. Kuo WT, Odegaard JI, Louie JD, et al. Photothermal ablation with the excimer laser sheath technique for embedded inferior vena cava filter removal: Intitial results from a prospective study *J Vasc Interv Radiol.* 2011;22(6):813–823.

42

Venous Reconstructions after Malignant Resections

Thomas C. Bower, MD

INTRODUCTION

Venous reconstructions for malignancies involving the central and peripheral veins now play an important role in treatment. However, early detection and better adjuvant therapy remain keys to improve survival, because most patients with tumors of the vena cava and iliac veins have advanced local, regional, or metastatic disease by the time diagnosis is made.[1] Malignancies involving the superior vena cava (SVC) rarely are operable, and treatment of venous obstruction often is relegated to stenting.[2] Renal cell carcinoma, retroperitoneal sarcoma, and abdominal cancers of the inferior vena cava (IVC) are most common. The accrued data from several centers have now firmly established the technical feasibility of tumor resection and IVC graft replacement for patients with isolated disease and a good performance status.[3–13] Tumors of the peripheral veins usually arise from the adjacent bone or soft tissues, which mandates resection of these structures, either with or without replacement of the axial veins.[14–16]

TUMOR TYPES

Primary and secondary vena cava malignancies are shown in Table 42-1. Venous leiomyosarcoma is the most common primary tumor, and was first described in the IVC by Perl in 1871.[17] Venous leiomyosarcoma occurs more often than sarcomas of the arteries, but represent 2% or less of all leiomyosarcomas.[1] Primary venous leiomyosarcoma (PVL) involves the suprarenal IVC in over 40% of cases, but may arise from any caval segment or in other abdominal veins.[1,18]

These tumors are polypoid, nodular, and typically attach to the vein wall. Growth pattern is intraluminal for most, but with advanced disease, the tumor may invade through the vein wall and into adjacent structures. This characteristic makes it difficult to differentiate them from other retroperitoneal sarcomas. Distant metastases to the

TABLE 42-1. TUMORS OF THE INFERIOR VENA CAVA (IVC)

Primary

- IVC leiomyosarcoma

Secondary

- Retroperitoneal soft tissue tumors
  - Liposarcoma
  - Leiomyosarcoma
  - Malignant fibrous histiocytoma
- Hepatic tumors
  - Cholangiocarcinoma
  - Hepatocellular carcinoma
  - Metastatic (e.g., colorectal)
- Pancreaticoduodenal cancers
- Osteosarcoma, osteochondroma, or chordomas involving the lumbar spine or sacrum

Secondary Tumors that may have Tumor Thrombus

- Renal cell carcinoma
- Pheochromocytoma
- Adrenocortical carcinoma
- Sarcomas of uterine origin
  - Leiomyomatosis
  - Endometrial stromal cell
- Germ cell tumors
  - Embryonal
  - Teratocarcinoma

lung, liver, kidney, or bone are evident in one half of patients when diagnosis is made. For this reason, median survival is measured in months.[18,19]

Lung cancer with mediastinal adenopathy is the most common cause of secondary SVC obstruction, although other mediastinal malignancies such as lymphoma, follicular or medullary thyroid cancer, teratoma, thymoma, angiosarcoma and synovial cell sarcoma may also cause venous obstruction. Together, these tumors account for 60–85% of cases of malignant SVC obstruction.[2]

Extra-luminal cancers or sarcomas which obstruct or invade the IVC are more common than PVL, and affect the caval segment in proximity to the site of origin of the malignancy.[1] Some tumors grow intraluminally as tumor thrombus into the IVC toward the heart. Renal cell cancer (RCC) is the most common malignancy to exhibit this behavior, and this problem occurs in 4–15% of patients. The right kidney develops tumor thrombus more often than the left one, but in most cases, it is large cancers that have this characteristic. The extent of IVC thrombus is classified by its proximity to the diaphragm and hepatic veins. Only 10% of patients have renal cell cancer tumor thrombus in the right heart.[1]

The great saphenous vein is the most common site of peripheral PVL.[19] Lower extremity tumors also are nodular and mobile. If the tumor originates in the deep veins, there is often invasion of adjacent soft tissues. Sarcomas of the bone, cartilage, or muscle are the most common secondary malignancies, but venous invasion is seen in some individuals with malignant melanoma or fibrous histiocytoma.[14–16]

CLINICAL PRESENTATION

The symptoms and signs of patients with tumors of the vena cava are shown in Table 42-2. Primary venous leiomyosarcoma of the IVC occurs at a mean patient age of 50 to 60 years, and is more common in women. Early detection of IVC leiomyosarcoma is rare, with only 4 of 144 patients reported by Mingoli et al, having the tumor discovered before metastases were present.[18] Abdominal pain occurs in 66–96% of these patients, whereas an abdominal mass, lower extremity edema, Budd-Chiari or nephrotic syndrome, and constitutional symptoms occur in less than 50% of patients. Deep vein thrombosis is rare with caval malignancies, but is a common finding with tumor involvement of the iliac or lower extremity veins.[1,18] Secondary caval tumors occur in patients between the ages of 40 and 70 years. A variety of symptoms and signs are possible in these patients, depending on tumor location and whether there is venous outflow obstruction from a major organ.

EVALUATION

We favor a multidisciplinary team composed of medical and surgical oncologists, and vascular, urologic, orthopedic, neurologic or cardiothoracic surgeons as clinically indicated.[1,3,7,9] Medical and radiation oncologists determine if neo-adjuvant therapy is needed prior to operation, or after it. The goals of evaluation are to define the type and extent of the tumor, search for metastases, and assess the degree of venous obstruction and the extent of venous collaterals. All of these assessments are important to determine prognosis and plan operation.

TABLE 42-2. CLINICAL PRESENTATIONS RELATED TO VENA CAVA OBSTRUCTION

Level of Vena Cava	Symptoms and Signs
Superior Vena Cava	Headache, upper extremity swelling, facial swelling or cyanosis, syncope, shortness of breath when leaning forward
Inferior Vena Cava	
Suprahepatic	Cardiac arrhythmias, syncope, pulmonary embolism
Suprarenal	
Retrohepatic with hepatic vein involvement	Budd Chiari syndrome, ascites
Retrohepatic between hepatic and renal veins	Abdominal pain, biliary symptoms, nausea (nonspecific)
At renal vein confluence	Renal insufficiency, nephrotic syndrome
Infrarenal	Pain, dilated veins on abdominal wall, palpable mass, lower extremity edema, motor or sensory neuropathy

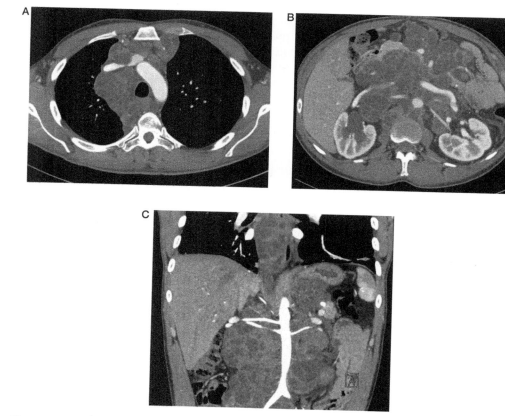

Figure 42-1. Axial and coronal images of a patient with extensive teratoma in the mediastinum and abdomen. While seemingly unresectable, the patient has undergone staged resections of the tumor, without the need for venous or arterial replacement.

Computed tomographic (CT) or magnetic resonance (MR) angiography with venous phase imaging are the primary diagnostic modalities. These studies have supplanted the use of venacavagraphy, which only is used if a biopsy is needed. CT and MR scans provide axial, coronal, and sagittal images which define the three dimensional anatomy of the tumor (Figure 42-1).[1] Ultrasonography may be used to assess obstruction or patency of the peripheral veins, but is less ideal for assessment of the iliac veins and the vena cava in our opinion. Magnetic resonance imaging is almost 100% sensitive for detecting intracaval tumor thrombus associated with renal cell or other cancers, with false positives due to flow artifact. Multidetector or helical electron beam CT also has excellent sensitivity and accuracy. Transesophageal echocardiography is used to corroborate proximal extent of the tumor thrombus prior to operation, and to intraoperatively assess patency of the IVC.[1,20,21]

TREATMENT

Patients with localized disease, satisfactory cardiopulmonary function, and a good performance status are offered operation. Operative treatment and approach depends on the

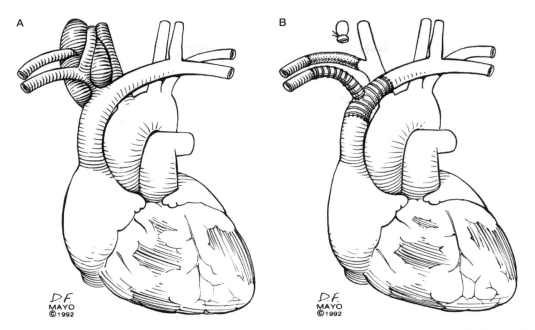

Figure 42-2. (A) Recurrent medullary thyroid carcinoma involving the right subclavian artery and vein, innominate vein, and upper superior vena cava **(B)** Reconstruction was done with an ePTFE graft from the left innominate vein to the superior vena cava and interposition grafts for the right subclavian vein and artery. (With permission from Mayo Foundation.)

location, type, and extent of the tumor and the vena cava involvement; the degree of caval obstruction and the status of collateral veins; and body habitus. Malignancies involving the SVC, if resectable, are approached through a median sternotomy with the incision extended toward either side of the neck as needed to complete the resection and perform a venous reconstruction. The suprahepatic or retrohepatic IVC can be approached through a right thoracoabdominal incision over the top of the 8th or 9th rib; a bilateral subcostal incision if the costal flare is wide; and on occasion, a midline abdominal incision. Individuals with intracaval tumor thrombus can be approached through a midline or bilateral subcostal incision, extended into a median sternotomy if there is cardiac involvement. The infrarenal IVC and the iliac veins are best approached through a midline incision.[1]

Malignant obstruction of the SVC is most often treated by stenting because of advanced stage of disease at diagnosis.[2] If a disease free resection is possible and the SVC requires reconstruction, it can be either done with a patch or an interposition graft, with the latter comprised either of femoral vein, spiral saphenous vein, or prosthetic (Figure 42-2). We prefer externally-supported expanded polytetrafluoroethylene (ePTFE) grafts for SVC or IVC reconstructions.[1,3,7,9] Prosthetic is a simpler choice for SVC reconstruction except for the occasional patient in whom concomitant tracheal or esophageal resection is needed. In that circumstance, femoral vein is a good alternative.

The need to resect and segmentally replace the IVC depends on the segment of vein involved by the tumor, and whether venous collaterals will be sacrificed during operation. Patients with chronic infrarenal IVC occlusion, well-developed venous collaterals, and no lower extremity edema do not require IVC replacement. Our preference is to replace the IVC at or above the renal veins in all patients, even if concomitant renal vein re-implantation or graft interposition is needed.[1,3,7,9] While some authors report

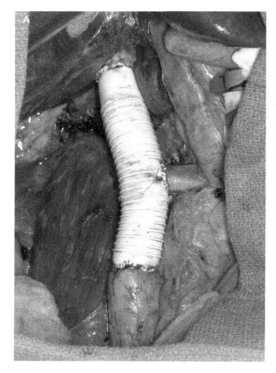
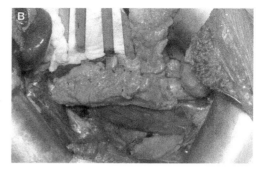
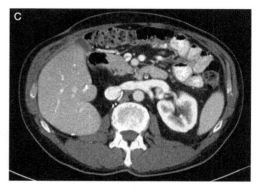

Figure 42-3. Intraoperative photographs **(A, B)** and postoperative axial CT image **(C)** in a patient who underwent resection of a large right retroperitoneal sarcoma involving the right kidney. A portion of the suprarenal and infrarenal vena cava required replacement. The left renal vein was reimplanted onto the graft. The graft is covered with omentum, taking care that it does not compress the renal vein. The CT scan shows a widely patent left renal vein.

cases in which the pararenal IVC is resected and neither renal vein is reconstructed, the surgeon must be confident that there is adequate collateral outflow through left renal vein tributaries.[1] If in doubt, it is safest to reimplant or reconstruct the renal vein with a short interposition ePTFE graft of 10 to14 mm in diameter (Figure 42-3). Moreover, if the patient becomes anuric or has poor urine output following IVC resection, renal vein reconstruction is needed.

There is a growing literature on the role for retrohepatic IVC replacement, even combined with major liver resection.[3–6, 9–13] This operation is the most challenging of all the caval reconstructions. While both in situ and ex situ liver perfusion techniques have been used during resection of malignancies with perihepatic IVC involvement, it is our opinion that in situ resection and IVC graft replacement has broader applicability, versatility, and similar efficacy as those done with ex situ techniques.[9] The latter is useful if a patient requires a combination of complex hepatic vein, portal vein, and/or IVC reconstruction. There is a risk of salvage orthotopic liver transplantation in a few patients treated with this technique.[12,13]

We have standardized our approach and operative technique to patients who need combined liver resection and retrohepatic IVC replacement (Figure 42-4).[3,9] The key steps in operation include total vascularization of the liver; selective use of veno-venous bypass to maintain hemodynamics if patients do not respond to volume loading only; a secure position for the upper caval crossclamp, whether that be

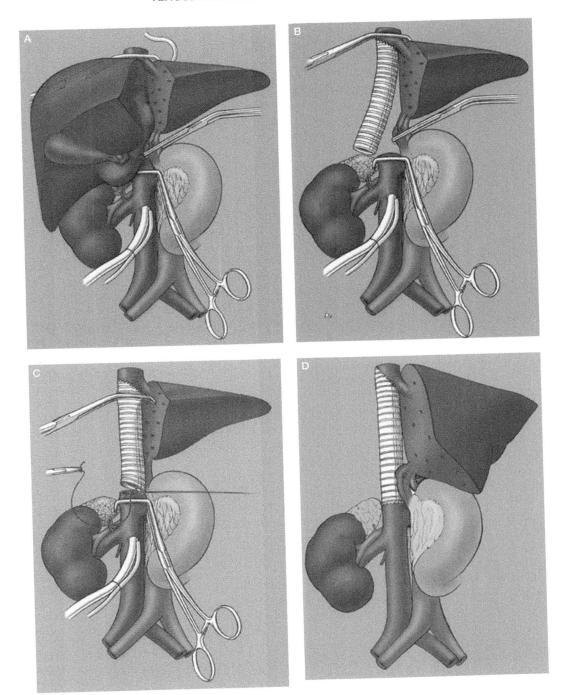

Figure 42-4. (A) Vascular isolation of the liver just prior to completion of tumor and IVC resection **(B)** Upper caval anastomosis performed with vascular isolation of the liver. Some patients require venovenous bypass to maintain stable hemodynamics **(C)** Blood flow is reestablished through the liver and the lower caval anastomosis is completed **(D)** Completed graft reconstruction with reattachment of the ligaments of the liver to avoid torsion of the hepatic venous outflow. (With permission from Mayo Foundation.)

subdiaphragmatic or in a supradiaphragmatic extrapericardial position; early ligation of the afferent and efferent lobar vasculature prior to parenchymal division, and appropriate repositioning of the liver remnant to avoid torsion and hepatic vein outflow obstruction. The operation begins with thorough abdominal exploration and intraoperative ultrasonography to exclude occult multicentric intraparenchymal liver disease. Hepatic resection using the Cusa device (Valley Lab, Boulder, Colorado) helps to minimize the blood loss and is initiated after a 5-minute period of inflow vascular occlusion of the liver which serves as ischemic preconditioning. Patients with significant parenchymal bleeding, prior hepatectomy, or polycystic liver disease may require additional periods of vascular inflow occlusion. We prefer to test clamp the suprahepatic IVC before completing the tumor resection. It is rare to need veno-venous bypass, though this technique may be necessary in patients over the age 60 years who have cardiopulmonary dysfunction. If the systolic blood pressure cannot be maintained at or over 100 mm Hg, we institute veno-venous bypass from the infrarenal IVC via a cannula inserted at the gonadal vein confluence through a large-bore jugular venous catheter. Total vascular isolation is instituted when the surgeon is ready to transect the vena cava to complete the en bloc tumor resection. Our order of crossclamping is infrarenal or suprarenal IVC depending on the caudal extent of resection, followed by inflow occlusion of the hepatic artery and portal vein in the gastrohepatic ligament, and then the suprahepatic IVC. This provides a bloodless field, except for the rare patients with a replaced left hepatic artery. The upper caval anastomosis is performed first, and may include incorporation of the hepatic vein remnant. Rarely, we have sewn the remnant hepatic vein(s) to a button hole in the IVC graft, and then placed the graft in normal anatomic position for an end-to-end anastomosis to the IVC at the diaphragmatic hiatus. Once the proximal anastomosis is completed, the patient is placed in a head-down position, the lungs are inflated to 30 mm Hg to avoid air embolism, and the hepatic inflow occlusion clamp is released to allow efflux of acid metabolites. Clamps are transferred onto the graft; the graft is cut to length and sewn to the lower IVC. Two technical mishaps are possible at this point. First, there is a tendency to cut the graft too long. This problem is eliminated by checking graft length during maximum inspiration and expiration before it is cut to fit. The second is torsion of the graft which may obstruct outflow from the hepatic vein(s). This problem is avoided by allowing the liver remnant to return to its normal anatomic position and then marking the graft to avoid a twist. To date, we have not had to perform a separate autologous vein interposition graft to reconstruct the remnant hepatic vein. The primary limitation of in situ liver resection and caval replacement is warm hepatic ischemia time. In most cases, this liver ischemia can be kept below 20 minutes. We have utilized allopurinol and other agents to enhance ischemic tolerance in select cases, but do not have enough experience with those medications to know if they are valuable.[9]

The most common operation on the IVC involves removal of tumor thrombus secondary to renal cell carcinoma. For most patients, this thrombus is removed en bloc with the cancer by open thrombectomy. The cavotomy is closed primarily or with a bovine pericardial patch if primary closure will narrow the IVC. Figure 42-5 shows the calculations necessary to size the patch to the caval defect, as the tendency is to make the patch too narrow. In general, the patch assumes a broad oval shape, but can be tailored if the IVC has been distended by the tumor thrombus, to allow better size match between the lower uninvolved IVC and the suprarenal IVC. IVC wall invasion should be anticipated if the caval diameter exceeds 40 mm, thrombus extends to the

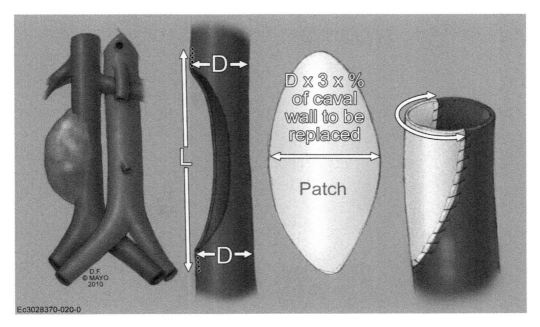

Figure 42-5. Schematic diagram showing a bovine pericardial patch of the vena cava, and the calculations needed to make the patch the right size. The width of the patch is calculated by estimating the circumference of the vena cava (diameter x 3) multiplied by the percent of wall of the vena cava that is resected (or to be replaced). For example, if one-half of a 20 mm diameter vena cava was resected, the circumference of the vena cava would be 60 mm, and the width of the patch would have to be 30 mm. (With permission from Mayo Foundation.)

suprahepatic level or into the heart (level III and IV), or the renal vein ostium is more than 14 mm in diameter.[22] Patients with intra-cardiac extension of tumor thrombus are treated by cardiopulmonary bypass, with or without hypothermic circulatory arrest. The suprahepatic and retrohepatic IVC can be inspected under direct vision. Intraoperative transesophageal echocardiography is used after removal of tumor thrombus in anyone in whom there has been retrohepatic or intra-cardiac extension of thrombus. The technique allows for interrogation of both the IVC and the hepatic veins.

The IVC is replaced with an interposition ePTFE graft if more than 60% of the caval circumference requires resection. Others have used polyester or cryopreserved large-diameter vein instead of using ePTFE. In most cases, a 20 mm ePTFE graft accommodates the vena cava diameter nicely. Some authors suggest smaller diameter grafts because the theoretic increase in blood flow velocity is felt to enhance patency.[8] We do not support that concept. The rings of the graft are kept close to the anastomosis, even if a bevel is cut in the graft. This prevents collapse of any unsupported part of the graft (Figure 42-6). All of our patients receive low dose intravenous heparin prior to caval replacement at any level, but that dose depends on body weight and the amount of blood loss to that point in the operation. Postoperatively, subcutaneous heparin is administered for the first 48 hours as long as platelet counts are in normal range. We anticoagulate patients with warfarin for a goal International Normalized Ratio of between 2 and 3, and do so for at least 6 months. Some patients with IVC grafts in a suprarenal position can stop anticoagulation at that point if CT imaging shows a widely patent caval reconstruction. Those who undergo concomitant major liver

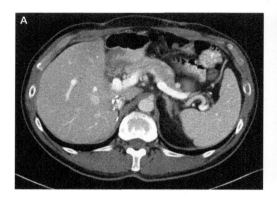
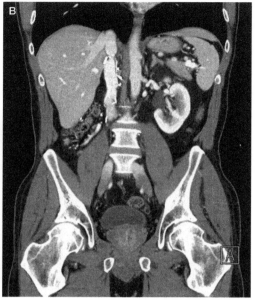

Figure 42-6. Postoperative axial **(A)** and coronal **(B)** CT images of a patient who had replacement of the para-renal vena cava. Note the stenosis at the upper caval-graft anastomosis where the graft was not supported by rings. We have changed our practice and keep the rings as close to the anastomosis as possible, even if the graft has to be beveled. This patient will be treated with a venous stent.

resection have elevation of liver function tests for the first few days after operation. If liver enzymes remain elevated beyond 4 to 5 days, ultrasound or CT imaging should be performed to ensure patency of the IVC graft and the hepatic and portal veins.[1,3,9]

Some patients present with both intracaval tumor thrombus and bland thrombus below. Unless the bland thrombus in the infrarenal IVC or iliac veins can be completely removed, we favor caval interruption to avoid pulmonary embolism. Blute et al, followed 40 patients who had IVC interruption by ligation or Greenfield filter, among 160 cases of renal cell cancer with level II-IV thrombus.[23] They found long-term venous disability to be satisfactory when scored by the American Venous Forum International Consensus Committee Standards. Twenty-eight patients had no or class I disability, 12 had class II and no one had class III disabilities.

OUTCOMES

Many factors affect patient outcome. Tumor type, completeness of resection, perioperative complications such as multisystem organ failure or cardiopulmonary dysfunction, and the location and length of vena cava replacement all influence recovery and survival. Since most reports of IVC resection and/or replacement have small numbers of patients, and tumor types vary between the studies, comparison of outcomes is difficult. Moreover, patients with circumferential IVC resection and graft replacement are often lumped with those who had primary patch closure of the vena cava. These are important distinctions because the hemodynamic and physiologic consequences of partial resection or segmental replacement of the infrarenal IVC vary considerably to individuals who need retrohepatic

TABLE 42-3. CONTEMPORARY SERIES OF PRIMARY AND SECONDARY INFERIOR VENA CAVA MALIGNANCIES

	N	Type		Location			Liver Resection	Tumor size (cm)	Graft	Mortality n (%)
				IR	SR/RH	SH				
Illuminati (2008)	11	PVL		8	3	0	-	15	11	0
Kieffer (2006)	22	PVL		3	13	4	4	21	13	4 (20)
Ito (2007)	20	PVL		6	13	1	1	10.7	5	0
Bower (2000)	29	PVL	2	10	19	0	13	-	29	2 (6.9)
		Secondary	27							
Sarmiento (2003)	19	Cholangiocarcinoma	9	0	19	0	19	-	18	1 (5)
		Metastatic	5							
		Sarcoma	3							
		HCC	2							
Kuehnl (2007)	35	Secondary	20	5 (4)	7 (3)	14 (2)	-	-	-	2 (6)
		PVL	6							
Delis (2007)	12	Colorectal	6	0	12	0	12	-	12	0
		HCC	4							
		Cholangiocarcinoma	2							

*9 SVC and 26 IVC tumors. The location of the 9 pts with grafts shown in parentheses

PVC = Primary venous leiomyosarcoma

IR = Infrarenal segment

SR/RH = Suprarenal-retrohepatic segment

SH = Suprahepataic segment

HCC = Hepatocellular carcinoma

IVC replacement in conjunction with major liver resection, and those who require cardiopulmonary bypass and circulatory arrest for tumor removal.[1,9] Some of the larger and more contemporary surgical series are listed in Table 42-3. The Kieffer series reports a 20% mortality rate, but these tumors were large. Thirteen of the 20 patients treated had suprarenal or retrohepatic IVC involvement, and 4 the suprahepatic segment.[4] In contrast, the report from Brigham and Women's Hospitals report no mortality among 20 patients treated for primary venous leiomyosarcoma. Only 1 patient had involvement of the IVC above the hepatic vein or needed a partial liver resection, and 5 required prosthetic graft replacement.[5] The University of Rome group also has excellent results, with no mortality among 11 patients with IVC graft replacement, but 8 of those involved the infrarenal segment.[6] These differences account for the disparity in mortality rates. Major adverse events are common and occur in 17-33% of patients. Cardiopulmonary problems, medically managed liver dysfunction, bile leak, chylous or pleural effusions, pulmonary emboli and graft thrombosis or infection have all been reported.[1-3,23,24] Among the series listed in Table 42-3, only one graft infection is reported. Prosthetic graft patency is excellent and ranges from

85–100% over follow-up ranging from 1.5 to 4 years.[1,3–13] The last detailed Mayo Clinic report showed overall survival to be 89% at 1 year, 80.3% at 2 years, and 75% at 3 years.[3] Segment of IVC replacement affected survival, with the longest survivors in those who had infrarenal IVC replacement. Although our updated analysis is ongoing, there is one survivor with a patent IVC graft 16 years after implantation. To date, we are aware of 3 graft occlusions and 2 graft infections among 90 patients who have had IVC replacement.

The large database compiled by Mingoli and colleagues for patients with primary leiomyosarcoma of the IVC has been used to analyze variables affecting survival.[25] Mean survival is 3 months without operation to approximately 3 years with radical resection. The IVC segment involved, extraluminal or intraluminal growth, size and histologic grade, and the use of adjuvant therapy all influenced outcome. Limited versus extensive resection had no impact on 5 and 10 year survival rates. Resection with negative microscopic margins stands as the most important predictor of recurrence and survival.

Operative morbidity and mortality rates for patients treated for renal cell carcinoma and IVC tumor thrombus have improved over time, and are the lowest at high volume centers. For example, the report by Blute et al, from Mayo Clinic, showed the mortality rate among 435 patients with RCC to be 8.1% for the period 1970–1989, and only 3.8% for 105 patients treated between 1990–2000.[24] Five-year cancer-free survival is lower if there is regional nodal spread, perinephric fat invasion, tumor necrosis, and sarcomatoid features. Survival in those with tumor thrombus ranges from 30–72% at 5 years if there is no metastatic disease, but drops considerably if there is distant spread.[1,24]

There are few data on patient performance status or quality of life after these operations. Several studies from Mayo Clinic suggest that at least 80% of patients operated for primary and secondary malignancies involving the IVC are able to function with minimal restriction in daily activities.[3] Patients seem able to maintain this performance status even if they later develop distant metastases or local recurrence.

SURGICAL TREATMENT OF SECONDARY TUMORS OF THE ILIAC AND PERIPHERAL VEINS

Resection of malignancies involving the iliac and peripheral veins also depends on the extent of tumor, and whether adjacent arteries and nerves are encased.[14–16] Long segment, chronic occlusions of the iliac veins rarely require venous replacement, unless a large number of collateral veins are sacrificed. In the extremity, axial venous reconstruction often is done using contralateral saphenous vein, especially if preoperative imaging shows few collaterals draining the ipsilateral deep and saphenous systems.[1] Venous reconstruction should follow arterial reconstruction if both vessels are resected. Patency rates with autogenous reconstructions approach 80% as long as 2 to 5 years after operation, but prosthetic carries a lower patency rate.[15,16] While the femoral vein can be resected and not replaced in select patients, venous reconstruction is needed at the common femoral and popliteal vein level.

Management of the iliac veins during sacral resections or hemipelvectomies can be challenging. For patients undergoing sacral resection, the anterior stage of the operation often is done first. If the resection will extend to the L5 vertebral body, the lower aorta and IVC require mobilization. Patients may have between one and three small

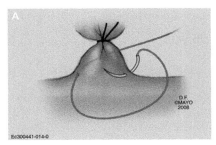
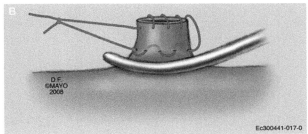

Figure 42-7. Short, broad branches of the iliac veins or inferior vena cava require suture ligature techniques for control, as illustrated in **(A)** and **(B)**. The distal vein can be ligated while the proximal portion of the branch is controlled with a prolene suture passed behind the branch at its confluence with the major vein, and then brought forward to secure the contralateral edge of the vein. The branch can be divided and the suture ligature tied. The combination of a running horizontal mattress and a whip stitch is another technique for control. (With permission from Mayo Foundation).

vein branches at the iliac vein-caval confluence, which can be thin-walled or broad-based. Simple ligation of these branches is ineffective, and suture ligation is needed. Mobilization of the common and external iliac arteries affords exposure of the adjacent iliac veins. Control of the common and external iliac veins is done before attempting dissection of the internal iliac artery and vein branches. Individual ligation of as many internal iliac artery and vein branches as possible reduces blood loss during the bone resection. The internal iliac artery branches are first ligated, followed by those of the internal iliac veins. In some patients with high sacral resection, an effort is made to preserve the posterior division branches of the internal iliac artery. I prefer to control, but not ligate, the main internal iliac vein trunk(s), while the more caudal and posterior branches are isolated and ligated. This prevents distention of the distal branches, many of which are thin-walled, and can cause troublesome bleeding if inadvertently injured. Several techniques can be used to control and ligate or oversew short, broad-based internal iliac vein branches as shown in Figure 42-7. Patch angioplasty of the external or common iliac vein is preferred over graft replacement whenever possible. We use ePTFE 12 or 14 mm diameter grafts if segmental resection is done. However, replacement of both common iliac veins is rarely done if they are both encased by tumors. If prosthetic is used, omentum, adjacent soft tissue or bovine pericardium is used to cover the graft.

In summary, primary and secondary malignancies of the vena cava, iliac, or peripheral veins can be safely treated in select patients. A team comprised of oncologists and surgeon specialists, meticulous preoperative planning and choice of incision, and precise execution of the tumor resection with venous reconstruction are the keys to good outcomes.

REFERENCES

1. Bower TC. Venous tumors. In: Cronenwett JL, Johnston KW (ed). Rutherford's Vascular Surgery, 7th edition. Philadelphia, PA: Elsevier Saunders; 2010:983–995.
2. Gloviczki P, Kalra M. Superior vena cava obstruction: Surgical treatment. In: Cronenwett JL, Johnston KW (ed). Rutherford's Vascular Surgery, 7th edition. Philadelphia, PA: Elsevier Saunders; 2010:963–973.

3. Bower TC, Nagorney, DM, Cherry KJ Jr., et al. Replacement of the inferior vena cava for malignancy: An update. *J Vasc Surg*. 2000:31:270–281.

4. Kieffer E, Alaoui M, Piette JC, Cacoub P, Chiche L. Leiomyosarcoma of the inferior vena cava: Experience in 22 cases. *Ann Surg*. 2006:244:289–295.

5. Ito H, Hornick JL, Bertagnolli MM, George S, et al. Leiomyosarcoma of the inferior vena cava: Survival after aggressive management. *Ann Surg Oncol*. 2007;14:3534–3542.

6. Illuminati G, Calio FG, D'Urso A, et al. Prosthetic replacement of the infrahepatic inferior vena cava for leiomyosarcoma. *Arch Surg*. 2008;141:919–924.

7. Bower TC, Nagorney DM, Toomey BJ, et al. Vena cava replacement for malignant disease: Is there a role. *Ann Vasc Surg*. 1993;7:51–62.

8. Sarkar R, Ellber FR, Gelabert HA, et al. Prosthetic replacement of the inferior vena cava for malignancy. *J Vasc Surg*. 1998;28:75–83.

9. Sarmiento JM, Bower TC, Cherry KJ, et al. Is combined partial hepatectomy with segmental resection of the inferior vena cava justified for malignancy? *Arch Surg*. 2003;138:624–630.

10. Kuehnl A, Schmidt M, Hornung HM, et al. Resection of malignant tumors invading the vena cava: Perioperative complications and long-term follow-up. *J Vasc Surg*. 2007;46:533–540.

11. Delis S, Madariaga J, Ciancio G. Combined liver and inferior vena cava resection for hepatic malignancy. *J Surg Oncol*. 2007;96:258–264.

12. Oldehafer KJ, Lang H, Schlitt HJ, et al. Long-term experience after ex situ liver surgery. *J Surg*. 2000;127:520–527.

13. Lodge JPA, Ammori BJ, Prasad KR, et al. Ex vivo and in situ resection of inferior vena cava with hepatectomy for colorectal metastases. *Ann Surg*. 2000;127:520–527.

14. Bonardelli S, Nodari F, Maffeis R, et al. Limb salvage in lower-extremity sarcomas and technical details about vascular reconstruction. *J Orthop Sci* .2000;5:555–560.

15. Schwarzbach MHM, Hormann Y, Hinz U, et al. Results of limb-sparing surgery with vascular replacement for soft tissue sarcoma in the lower extremity. *J Vasc Surg*. 2005;42:88–97.

16. Nishinari K, Wolosker N, Yazbek G, et al. Venous reconstructions in lower limbs associated with resection of malignancies. *J Vasc Surg*. 2006;44:1046–1050.

17. Perl L. Ein fall von sarkom der vena cava inferior. *Virchow's Arch (A)* 1971;53:378–83.

18. Mingoli A, Feldhaus RJ, Cavallaro A, et al. Leiomyosarcoma of the inferior vena cava: Analysis and search of world literature on 141 patients and report of three new cases. *J Vasc Surg*. 1991;14:688–99.

19. Dzsinich C, Gloviczki P, van Heerden JA, et al. Primary venous leiomyosarcoma: A rare but lethal disease. *J Vasc Surg*. 1992;15:595–603.

20. Welch TJ, LeRoy AJ. Helical and electron beam CT scanning in the evaluation of renal vein involvement in patients with renal cell carcinoma. *J Comput Assis Tomogr*. 1997;21:467–471.

21. Laissey JP, Menegazzo D, Debray MP, et al. Renal carcinoma: Diagnosis of venous invasion with GD-enhanced MR venography. *Eur Radiol*. 2000;10:1138.

22. Zini L, Destrieux-Garnier L, Leroy X, et al. Renal vein ostium wall invasion of renal cell carcinoma with inferior vena cava tumor thrombus: Prediction by renal and vena caval vein diameters and prognostic significance. *J Urol*. 2008;179:450–454.

23. Blute ML, Boorjian SA, Leibovich BC, et al. Results of inferior vena caval interruption by Greenfield filter, ligation or resection during radical nephrectomy and tumor thrombectomy. *J Urol*. 2007;178:440–445.

24. Blute ML, Leibovich BC, Lohse CM. The Mayo Clinic experience with surgical management, complications and outcome for patients with renal cell carcinoma and venous tumor thrombus. *BJU International*. 2004;94:33–41.

25. Mingoli A, Sapienza P, Cavallaro A, et al. The effect of extent of caval resection in the treatment of inferior vena cava leiomyosarcoma. *Anticancer Res*. 1997;17:3877–3882.

43

Technical Tips for Treatment of Nutcracker Syndrome

Efthymios D. Avgerinos, MD, Geetha Jeyabalan, MD, and Rabih A. Chaer, MD

INTRODUCTION

The nutcracker syndrome (NCS) occurs in the setting of symptomatic compression of the left renal vein (LRV), most commonly between the superior mesenteric artery (SMA) anteriorly and the abdominal aorta posteriorly. Compression of the LRV between the SMA and the aorta was first described by Grant in 1937 who found the anatomy analogous to a nut in a nutcracker.[1] The first patient with NCS was described in 1950,[2] although the compression was documented by venography only two decades later when this entity was first venographically described in the 70's, confirming LRV compression.[3,4]

The diagnosis of NCS is a challenging one for several reasons, and is often time made by exclusion. In addition to being a rare condition, specific diagnostic clinical features or criteria are absent and a high degree of suspicion must be exercised by the clinician in the appropriate setting. Moreover, noninvasive imaging must be followed by other invasive diagnostic modalities to rule out urologic etiologies and confirm hemodynamically significant LRV compression using renocaval pullback pressure gradient measurements.

The management of NCS has ranged from surgical correction of the anatomy to endovascular treatment of the extrinsic compression on the LRV. The purpose of this chapter is to review the clinical presentation and diagnostic algorithm, and the outcomes of surgical and endovascular therapies.

ETIOLOGY & PATHOPHYSIOLOGY

The terms nutcracker *syndrome* and nutcracker *phenomenon* are frequently used interchangeably in the literature. However the nutcracker anatomy is not always associated with clinical manifestations and may actually represent a normal anatomic variant. In these cases it is refered to as nutcracker phenomenon.

The etiology of the NCS can be better appreciated by understanding the anatomy of the region. The LRV arises from the left kidney and drains into the inferior vena cava after 5 to 9 cm. Typically, in its distal part, the LRV courses between the anterior aspect of the juxtarenal aorta and the posterior aspect of the proximal segment of the SMA. The main tributaries of the LRV are the left gonadal vein, the left ureteral vein, capsular veins, lumbar veins, and the ascending lumbar vein, while the left middle suprarenal vein and the inferior phrenic vein communicate from above. There are also connections with the left hemiazygos vein and with the internal and external vertebral plexuses.[5] The LRV can rarely (<3%) have a retroaortic course, or be doubled in a pre- and a retro- aortic course in a circumaortic configuration (0.3–5.7%).[5-7] Typically, the SMA runs ventrally for 4–5 mm in an almost rectangular configuration and then caudally. Its origin is separated by a distance of 2–4 mm from the LRV and the distance between SMA and abdominal aorta is in the range of 0.6–2.6 cm.[5-7] This anatomical arrangement normally prevents compression of the LRV by the SMA.

Several theories have been proposed to explain the nutcracker syndrome, implicating either LRV or SMA anomalies. A steep caudal SMA descent may cause compression of the LRV on the aorta, representing the most typical nutcracker morphologic feature, known as anterior nutcracker. Rarely, anterior nutcracker may co-occur when the third portion of the duodenum courses in front of the LRV between the aorta and the SMA (Wilkie syndrome). The posterior nutcracker may occur when the LRV has a retro-aortic course between the abdominal aorta and the vertebral body. Nutcracker syndrome can also occur in the setting of a circumaortic LRV, with entrapment of both the anterior and posterior LRV.[8,9] Contributory or exclusive factors include an asthenic body habitus with paucity of retroperitoneal fat is postulated to result in LRV compression by narrowing the aortomesenteric angle and/or stretching the LRV secondary to posterior ptosis of the kidney, excessive fibrous tissue at the origin of the SMA, pancreatic and retroperitoneal tumors, para-aortic lymphadenopathy and overarching testicular artery.[10]

The compression, which is aggravated by the standing position due to bowel weight, induces venous obstruction of the LRV. This phenomenon leads to increase in proximal venous pressure, which induces the development of varicose veins and collateral pathways. The pressure gradient between the left renal vein and vena cava may rise up to 3 mmHg (normal 1 mmHg) leading to rupture of thin walled septum between the small veins and the collecting system in the renal fornix manifesting ashematuria. It has also been proposed that hematuria may be the result of communication between dilated venous sinuses and adjacent renal calices.

The NCS shares similarities with the Cockett or May-Thurner syndromes (compression of the left iliac vein by the right iliac artery). Findings of spurs, thickening, and membranes at the site of compression and associated varices have been described in both clinical entities.[6,7,10,11]

It should be also noted that some elements of the pathophysiology of NCS are likely unknown, since surgical ligation of the LRV during aortic aneurysm repair is well described and almost always well tolerated. It is unclear why patients who undergo ligation of their LRV do not develop the NCS, suggesting that other elements are at play that lead to this clinical presentation.

CLINICAL PRESENTATION

The typical patient with NCS, though highly unpredictable, is a female in the second or third decade of life, with an above average height and an asthenic built.[6,7,10,11] The severity of symptoms and extent of various findings that are enough to warrant the designation of a clinical syndrome are not defined, but they all probably reflect an evolutionary process, starting from asymptomatic microhematuria up to severe pelvic congestion.

The usual clinical symptoms are primarily flank pain and hematuria. It should be noted though that hematuria is not always present, and can be microscopic or macroscopic. The pain is exacerbated by sitting, standing, walking, or riding a "shaking" vehicle or can even manifest as left ureteral colic, from the passing of blood clots down the ureter.[10] Additional symptoms include left-sided varicocele in males, pelvic congestion syndrome in females, orthostatic proteinuria, fatigue, lower limb varices and vague gastrointestinal symptoms.[12–15] Symptoms may also be triggered or aggravated by pregnancy and multiparity, and symptoms of pelvic congestion are often aggravated by a bladder distention, and can be partially relieved through relieving the compression of the pelvic varices by voiding. Finally, systemic manifestations have also been reported in adolescents including headache and tachycardia mimicking an orthostatic disturbance.

Symptoms are often chronic as the diagnosis is elusive. A common pattern of presentation involves a patient on chronic opioid therapy for pain control, who has underwent multiple diagnostic tests including endoscopy, laparoscopy, endometrial resection, ovarian cyst resection, cystoscopy and uretroscopy, among others, before the diagnosis is made.

Pelvic Congestion Syndrome

A distinct mode of presentation of the NCS is a symptom complex called pelvic congestion syndrome (PCS) characterized by chronic pelvic pain associated with dyspareunia, dysuria, dysmenorrhea, increased frequency of polycystic changes of the ovaries and demonstrable varicoceles.[11,12] In a study by Scultetus et al,[11] 9 of 51 patients with PCS were diagnosed as having NCS.

DIAGNOSIS

The diagnosis of Nutcracker syndrome is often delayed as the entity is quite rare. Alongside, although primarily a vascular disorder its manifestations are predominantly urological or gynaecological. Most cases present either to urologists or to gynecologists and infrequently to vascular surgeons if patients manifest lower limb varices as their main presenting complaint. A high index of suspicion is therefore necessary and the primary diagnostic test should be careful clinical examination and elicitation of history.

Diagnosis is frequently reached by an exclusion process. The more common renal conditions of hematuria are ruled out by blood tests, urinalysis, cytology, cystoscopy, urography, imaging of kidneys with ultrasound (US), computed tomography (CT) or magnetic resonance (MR) and even renal biopsy. When NCS is suspected, the initial non-invasive workup includes a Doppler US followed by CT or MR venography.

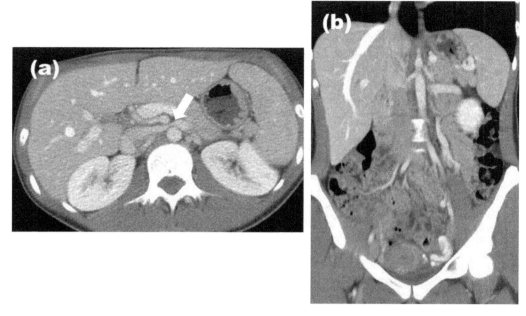

Figure 43-1. CT venography. (**a**) Tight stenosis of the left renal vein compressed by the overlying SMA, (**b**) Multiple enlarged pelvic venous collaterals are visualized.

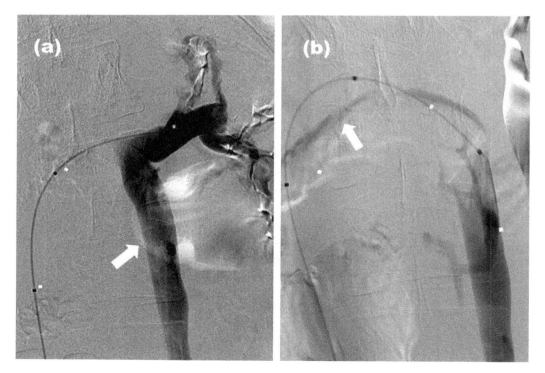

Figure 43-2. Invasive retrograde venography. (**a**) The guidewire has crossed the left renal vein and venogram reveals a dilated gonadal vein. (**b**) Poor refluxing of dye into the vena cava indicates a severe LRV stenosis.

Duplex ultrasound provides hemodynamic data, which may assist in the diagnosis. In particular, elevated peak velocity ratio of the renal vein ($\geq$4) at the aortomesenteric junction and the hilum do appear to be indicative of the syndrome. Axial imaging MR or CT can demonstrate compression of the left renal vein, (Figure 43-1) evaluate venous congestion and collateralization and rule out other sources of flank pain and hematuria.

Once NCS is strongly considered, invasive retrograde venography and cine video-angiography with reno-caval pressure gradient measurement is accepted as the gold standard for final diagnosis, (Figure 43-2), particularly when the gradient is significant (>3 mm Hg).

TREATMENT

Treatment of Nutcracker syndrome is indicated when patients are suffering from severe hematuria or intractable flank pain and should generally be guided by the expected reversibility of symptoms, the stage of the syndrome and the patient's age. Management options range from observation to nephrectomy, with several open surgical and endovascular options in between these two extremes. There are no clear selection criteria and given the limited reports and outcomes following intervention for NCS, the standard of care remains ill-defined. Nevertheless, the aim of any intervention is to reduce LRV hypertension, while others aim to reduce pelvic venous reflux and congestion.

Conservative Treatment

A conservative approach with surveillance should be maintained in pubertal patients because of higher likelihood of spontaneous remissionpossibly due to physical development. This approach may also be sufficient in older patients with tolerable or atypical symptoms. Low doses of aspirin have been suggested as a possible treatment option, as well as angiotensin inhibitors in improving orthostatic proteinuria. Their routine use, however, remains questionable.

Surgical Treatment

The main established surgical options include left renal vein transposition, renal venous bypass, autotransplantation of the kidney, and mesoaortic transposition.[12–18] Less popular but documented techniques targeting to alleviate LRV hypertension include medial nephropexy with excision of renal varicosities, gonadocaval bypass, resection of fibrous tissue and placement of a synthetic wedge at the aortomesenteric angle, external stenting with ringed polytetrafluoroethylene graft interposition around the LRV (open or laparoscopically) and laparoscopic splenorenal venous bypass.[7,10–14] In cases of persistent hematuria nephrectomy has been suggested. Venous reflux alone (varicoceles, leg varicosities, pelvic congestion) can be managed by gonadal vein interruption by laparoscopic ligation.

LRV Transposition

LRV transposition seems to be the most commonly performed surgical intervention for the NCS.[6,10] The procedure is performed through a midline transperitoneal approach (mini laparotomy). The small and large bowels are packed away, and the retroperitoneum is opened in the midline, inferior to the transverse mesocolon. The LRV is completely mobilized, and the left adrenal vein is routinely ligated and divided to facilitate this. Under systemic heparinization, a side-biting clamp is applied on the IVC across the LRV confluence, and the LRV is transected with a small cuff of IVC. Before LRV clamping some authors suggest renal artery clamping and external kidney cooling, following administration of 20 mg furosemide and 125 mg mannitol, although this practice is not commonly used given the associated renal ischemia time The LRV is then re-anastomosed to the left lateral aspect of the IVC in a more distal situation in a tension-free end-to-side manner with continuous or interrupted sutures of 4.0 or 5.0 polypropylene (Figure 43-3). Care should be taken to avoid twisting of the LRV and perform a tension free anastomosis to minimize compression by the aortic pulsation. Ongoing compression by the SMA can be also minimized by transposing the LRV as distally as possible from its most inferior initial location.

Renal Venous Bypass

In contrast to renal vein transposition, limited exposure of the regional lateral wall of the LRV and IVC is enough for left renocaval venous bypass. This markedly decreases the surgical technical difficulty and venous bleeding risks. The inferior adrenal vein, left ovarian/

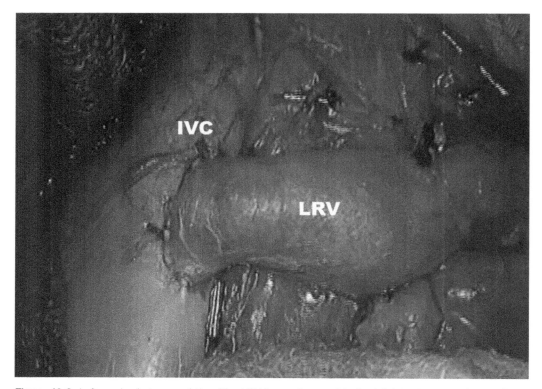

Figure 43-3. Left renal vein transposistion. The LRV is anastomosed to the left lateral aspect of the IVC in a tension-free end-to-side manner with continuous polypropylene suture.

testicular vein, and lumbar veins do not need to be ligated if they are not varicose and do not affect the anastomosis. A side-biting clamp is applied approximately 10 cm away from LRV confluence and the proximal end of the saphenous vein is primarily anastomosed. By again placing a side-biting clamp on the LRV the distal end of the saphenous vein is anastomosed. Another advantage of the renal venous bypass is that there is no need for renal circulation compromise, as the LRV is partially clamped and the left renal artery does not require clamping.[8]

Autotransplantation

Renal auto-transplantation involves nephrectomy as in live donors and transplantation of the kidney into either ipsilateral or contralateral iliac fossa. It is potentially a more complete procedure and would correct concomitant posterior ptosis. However, it involves a much more extensive dissection, longer period of renal ischemia, and two additional anastomoses (renal artery and ureter) with potential for more complications.

Mesoaortic Transposition

Transposition of the superior mesenteric artery entails transection of the SMA at its junction with the abdominal aorta and re-anastomosis to the abdominal aorta at a lower position away from the left renal vein. It has been argued that the advantages of such a procedure are the limitation of the surgical exposure to the retroperitoneum and avoidance of left renal vein thrombosis due to extensive dissection and mobilization. However, consequences of possible SMA thrombosis are devastating and the higher post-operative complication rate have minimized the popularity of the technique.[16]

Outcomes of Surgical Treatment

Surgical outcomes are generally satisfying but may be less impressive in patients with lower pressure gradients. Left renal vein transposition appears to be safe and efficacious, although it has been reported that select patients may have persistent symptoms despite relief of the venous obstruction.[13,16] Long-term results with this procedure demonstrate a reasonably high rate of resolution of symptoms of flank pain and hematuria.[13,19] In a series described by Glovicski and colleagues, out of 11 patients who underwent LRV transposition 3 required reintervention 2 of which had been found intraoperatively to have LRV thrombosis.[13] Within a mean follow up of 70 months (range 11–19) results were good or excellent in 10/11 patients. Hematuria was relieved immediately/or early in all patients, while relief from flank pain was immediate in eight patients and gradual in two. Two of three patients with preoperative varicocele had recurrent, symptomatic varicoceles following LRV transposition, so the authors concluded that patients presenting with varicocele in the setting of NCS may need independent repair. In agreement with these outcomes, Hartung et al reviewed open surgical procedures for NCS and reported excellent results in 35 of 42 patients, while 17 of 18 patients undergoing LRV transposition were asymptomatic with recurrent hematuria in one patient.[19] Finally, Ahmed et al described 57 patients with NCS and concluded that LRV transposition and autotransplantation were associated with the best results.[6]

ENDOVASCULAR TREATMENT

Stenting

Endovascular approaches using angioplasty and stenting for the initial treatment of NCS are increasingly described.[9,10,19–21] The first stent attempted for this condition was the Wallstent (Schneider, Minneapolis, MN) in 1996. Since then, several others, such as the spiral Z-stent (Cook Medical, Bloomington, IN), Niki stent, Palmaz stent (Johnson & Johnson, Providence, RI), and Smart Control stent (Cordis, Johnson & Johnson, Miami, FL) have been tried with good technical success.[19–21] Self-expanding stents may be preferable given their increased flexibility and less likelihood of occlusion fromthe dynamic compression by the underlying aorta.

Under local anesthesia, percutaneous access of the right or left common femoral vein is obtained and eventually elective catheterization of the left renal vein is performed. Confirmation of the diagnosis can be made on venography (using valsalva) by visualization of contrast wash and well-developed collaterals as well as by renocaval pressure gradient measurements. In equivocal cases, IVUS can be invaluable not only to establish the diagnosis through pull back imaging but also to obtain accurate measurements of the renal vein diameter for proper stent sizing.

Once NCS is confirmed and before proceeding to the definite management some authors suggest administration of general anesthesia, since stent deployment and angioplasty can be very painful in the setting of NCS.[19] An appropriately sized sheath is inserted into the common femoral vein and the wire is changed for a stiff guidewire, which should be placed downwards into the left gonadal vein for increased purchase and to allow the stent to cross the stenosis. The guidewire should then be retrieved and pushed cautiously into the renal vein before stent deployment. Long stents that lean on both sides of the stenosis should be used, preferably 60 mm and their usual diameter is suggested at 16 mm. Partial protrusion of the stent in the inferior vena cava does not seem to cause any complication and is generally advocated. Diameter sizing is critical since undersizing can result in stent migration, usually into the IVC. This can be avoided by sizing the LRV under valsalva to fully distend it, or by using IVUS.

The role of balloon pre- or post- dilation controversial, but the more reasonable approach would be to use it post- stent deployment and only to treat a residual stenosis.

Endovascular treatment can be an even more rational approach in symptomatic patients with restenosis following LRV transposition, since it avoids a redo surgical exposure.[22] (Figure 43-4)

Coil Embolization

The left gonadal vein or other intra-extra pelvic tributaries can be embolized to improve symptoms (varicocele or PCS) in patients without renal manifestations.[7,23]

The endovascular technique follows the general principles described in the previous section. Stainless steel, platinum microcoils, (Figure 43-5) and/or sclerosants are the most frequently used embolic agents. The first few coils should be oversized to avoid untoward distal embolization. The procedure is typically done via femoral venous access; altought jugular access can also be utilized. Imaging of the LRV should be performed after the coiling is completed, to ensure ongoing drainage of the left

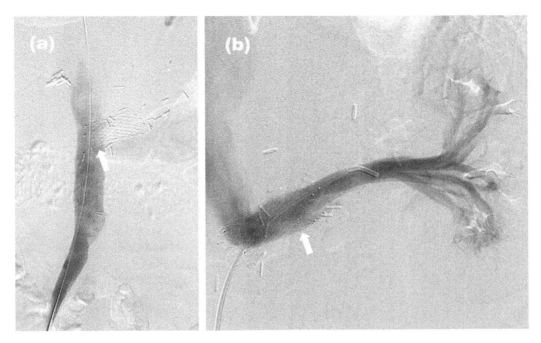

Figure 43-4. Left renal vein stenting following LRV transposition and symptomatic anastomotic restenosis. (**a**) A self-expanding 12 mm diameter stent partially protrudes in the IVC, (**b**) a widely patent left renal vein with complete coverage of the stenotic area.

kidney since patients with severe LRV compression may be very dependent on the pelvic outflow.

Outcomes of Endovascular Treatment

Although endovascular stenting is a simple and attractive option its role in the management of NCS remains to be established. Stents in the venous system can cause fibromuscular hyperplasia, in-stent restenosis and occlusion. The effect of the ongoing arterial compression on the stent structural integrity is also unclear. Another possible complication is proximal migration or embolization.[9,19,20,24]

Interestingly though, a recent large retrospective series of 61 patients treated with stenting showed symptom relief in 59 patients within 6 months and no significant restenosis within an average 66-month follow up. The authors advocate adequate stent sizing, avoidance of balloon dilatation and operator experience as driving factors of short and long term success.[20] This series currently remains the largest one with long-term data available. However, such recommendations and outcomes have not been widely reported yet, and remain confined to single institutions.

Coil embolization of gonadal veins in patients with pelvic congestion syndrome and demonstrable pelvic varicoceles may provide symptomatic improvement in 56% to 98% of patients.[10] However, it seems that addressing venous reflux alone by gonadal interruption, has usually temporary alleviating effects, so combined treatments including LRV decompression are more durable.[12] In fact, gonadal veins may be outflow conduits, and their interruption may worsen NCS symptoms.[25]

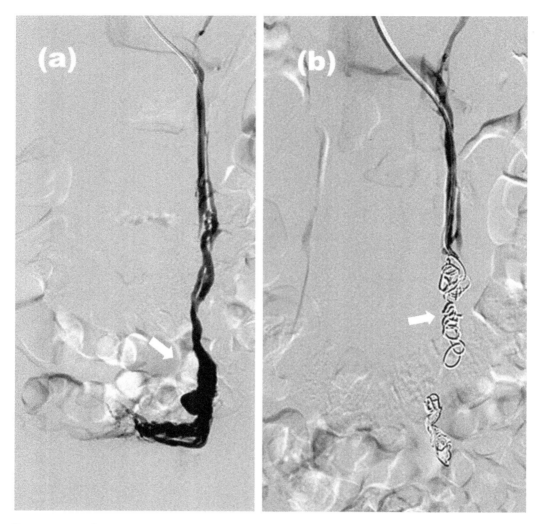

Figure 43-5. (a) Gonadal vein reflux in a patient with LRV compression and PCS. (b) Coil embolization from a right jugular approach is performed, resulting in occlusion of the left gonadal vein and pelvic symptom resolution.

CONCLUSIONS

The nutcracker syndrome is a rare condition demanding a high index of suspicion upon careful history delineation. The gold standard for definite diagnosis remains venography with measurement of reno-caval pullback pressure gradient. Treatment is mainly guided by the severity of symptoms. It appears that for the majority of centers, surgery remains the first-line therapy, although few reports have recently described favorable long term outcomes with endovascular treatments. However, longer-term follow-up and multicenter experience are needed to determine the durability of endovascular therapy. Close duplex surveillance for recurrent stenosis is warranted in this typically young patient population.

REFERENCES

1. Grant JCB. *A Method of Anatomy, Descriptive and Deductive* 3rd ed. Baltimore (MD): The Williams and Wilkins Company; 1944.
2. El-Sadr AR, Mina E. Anatomical and surgical aspects in the operative management of varicocele. *Urol Cutaneous Rev.* May 1950;54:257–62.
3. Chait A MK, Fabian CE, Mellins HZ. Vascular impressions on the ureters. *Am J Roentgen Rad Ther.* 1971;3:729–49.
4. de Schepper A. "Nutcracker" phenomenon of the renal vein and venous pathology of the left kidney. *J Belge Radiol.* 1972;55:507–11.
5. Satyapal KS. The renal veins: a review. *Eur J Anat.* 2003;7S1:43–52.
6. Ahmed K, Sampath R, Khan MS. Current trends in the diagnosis and management of renal nutcracker syndrome: a review. *Eur J Vasc Endovasc Surg.* 2006;31:410–6.
7. Alimi YS, Hartung O. Iliocaval venous obstruction; In: Cronenwett JL, Johnston W, eds. *Rutherford's,Vascular Surgery,* Philadelphia, Elsevier 2010.
8. Shaper KR, Jackson JE, Williams G. The nutcracker syndrome: an uncommon cause of haematuria. *Br J Urol.* 1994;74:144–6.
9. Cohen F, Amabile P, Varoquaux A, et al. Endovascular treatment of circumaortic nutcracker syndrome. *J Vasc Interv Radiol.* 2009;20:1255–7.
10. Kurklinsky AK, Rooke TW. Nutcracker phenomenon and nutcracker syndrome. *Mayo Clin Proc.* 2010;85:552–9.
11. Scultetus AH, Villavicencio JL, Gillespie DL. The nutcracker syndrome: its role in the pelvic venous disorders. *J Vasc Surg.* 2001;34:812–9.
12. Rudloff U, Holmes RJ, Prem JT, et al. Mesoaortic compression of the left renal vein (nutcracker syndrome): case reports and review of the literature. *Ann Vasc Surg.* 2006;20:120–9.
13. Reed NR, Kalra M, Bower TC, et al. Left renal vein transposition for nutcracker syndrome. *J Vasc Surg.* 2009;49:386–93.
14. Menard MT. Nutcracker syndrome: when should it be treated and how? *Perspect Vasc Surg Endovasc Ther.* 2009;21:117–24.
15. Wang L, Yi L, Yang L, et al. Diagnosis and surgical treatment of nutcracker syndrome: a single-center experience. *Urology.* 2009;73:871–6.
16. Zhang H, Li M, Jin W, et al. The left renal entrapment syndrome: diagnosis and treatment. *Ann Vasc Surg.* 2007;21:198–203.
17. Chuang CK, Chu SH, Lai PC. The nutcracker syndrome managed by autotransplantation. *J Urol.* 1997;157:1833–4.
18. Thompson PN, Darling RC 3rd, Chang BB, et al. A case of nutcracker syndrome: treatment by mesoaortic transposition. *J Vasc Surg.* 1992;16:663–5.
19. Hartung O, Grisoli D, Boufi M, et al. Endovascular stenting in the treatment of pelvic vein congestion caused by nutcracker syndrome: Lessons learned from the first five cases. *J Vasc Surg.* 2005;42:275–80.
20. Chen S, Zhang H, Shi H, et al. Endovascular Stenting for Treatment of Nutcracker Syndrome: Report of 61 Cases With Long-Term Followup. *J Urol.* 2011;186:570–5.
21. Venkatachalam S, Bumpus K, Kapadia SR, et al. The Nutcracker Syndrome. *Ann Vasc Surg.* 2011; 25:1154–64.
22. Baril DT, Polanco P, Makaroun MS, Chaer RA. Endovascular management of recurrent stenosis following left renal vein transposition for the treatment of Nutcracker syndrome. *J Vasc Surg.* 2011;53:1100–3.
23. Bittles MA, Hoffer EK. Gonadal vein embolization: treatment of varicocele and pelvic congestion syndrome. *Semin Intervent Radiol.* 2008;25:261–70.
24. Kim SJ, Kim CW, Kim S, et al. Long-term follow-up after endovascular stent placement for treatment of nutcracker syndrome. *J Vasc Interv Radiol.* 2005;16:428–31.
25. Rogers A, Beech A, Braithwaite B. Transperitoneal laparoscopic left gonadal vein ligation can be the right treatment option for pelvic congestion symptoms secondary to nutcracker syndrome. *Vascular.* 2007;15:238–40.

44

Open Surgical Options for Infrainguinal and Iliocaval Venous Occlusions

Nitin Garg, MBBS, MPH and Peter Gloviczki, MD

Chronic venous insufficiency (CVI) is secondary to infrainguinal, femoral or iliocaval obstruction in a select subgroup of patients. Venous reconstruction may be required in patients with post-thrombotic venous occlusion, who fail conservative management. Reconstruction of large veins may also be needed in patients with acute traumatic or iatrogenic venous injuries or in those who undergo excision of primary or metastatic malignant tumors invading the ilio-caval segments.

Endovascular treatment for iliocaval obstruction has progressed rapidly, and venous stenting is the primary choice for treatment of benign iliac, iliofemoral or iliocaval venous occlusions in patients, although infrainguinal endovascular interventions have limited applicability. In the last two decades results of open surgical reconstructions have improved, and symptomatic patients who are not candidates or who failed endovascular reconstructions can be treated with venous bypasses to relieve venous outflow obstruction.[1]

ETIOLOGY

Venous obstruction can be the result of primary venous disease, like May-Thurner syndrome,[2] or it can be the result of a previous acute deep venous thrombosis (DVT). Uncommon causes include retroperitoneal fibrosis; iatrogenic, blunt, or penetrating trauma; placement of IVC filter, congenital venous anomalies like deep vein agenesis or hypoplasia and benign or malignant tumors. May and Thurner observed secondary changes, such as an intraluminal web or "spur," in the proximal left common iliac vein in 20% of 430 autopsies. The most frequent primary malignant tumor originating from large veins is leiomyosarcoma; secondary tumors invading the vena cava include adenocarcinoma or liposarcoma. Renal carcinoma may extend into the IVC, although invasion of the

IVC wall is rare. Congenital suprarenal caval occlusion can occur due to webs or caval coarctation that may also present with associated hepatic vein occlusion (Budd-Chiari syndrome).[3,4]

PATHOPHYSIOLOGY

During the acute phase of DVT, the thrombus in the vein activates the inflammatory cascade, which in turn promotes partial lysis of the thrombus and leads to recanalization. However, recanalization is incomplete in most situations and these processes are also responsible for damage to the vein wall and to the venous valves, leading to chronic obstruction and valvular incompetence. If collateral venous circulation in occlusion is inadequate, ambulatory venous hypertension develops due to a functional venous outflow obstruction. In postthrombotic syndrome (PTS), deep reflux and obstruction of multiple venous segments often coexists.

PRESENTATION

Limb swelling and pain during and after exercise that is relieved with rest and leg elevation (venous claudication) is the typical presentation of patients with chronic venous obstruction.[5] Patients with obstruction may also have similar symptoms as those with primary valvular incompetence, such as varicosities, edema, skin changes or venous ulcers, although claudication and edema are usually more severe with venous obstruction and relief with limb elevation is not as pronounced.

Depending on the extent of the collateral circulation, patients with outflow obstruction will have pain, swelling and heaviness of the limb, and the most severe forms of venous obstruction may even interfere with the viability of the limb. Obstruction alone may also result in skin changes and venous ulcerations. Most patients have long lasting symptoms before surgical treatment is offered, and the mean duration of symptoms was six years in a recent series.[1]

CLINICAL EVALUATION

Detailed medical history may help establish the diagnosis of primary, secondary, or congenital venous problems. Previous history of DVT or thrombophlebitis, abdominal or pelvic interventions, trauma, tumor or symptoms of malignancy, personal or family history of thrombophilia, medication history (particularly oral contraceptive pills), smoking, obstetric history, and a family history of venous disorders (most patients with varicose veins would be able to relate to their parents or grandparents disease) should be addressed in all patients.

Perineal, vulvar, or groin varicosities can be seen in iliac vein obstruction or internal iliac vein or gonadal vein incompetence causing pelvic congestion syndrome. Scrotal varicosity may be a sign of gonadal vein incompetence, left renal vein compression between the superior mesenteric artery and the aorta (Nutcracker syndrome) or, occasionally, even IVC lesions or renal carcinoma. An abdominal mass or lymphadenopathy can provide a clue to venous compression and outflow obstruction.

INVESTIGATIONS

Duplex Scanning

This is a safe, noninvasive, cost-effective, and reliable test and is recommended as the first diagnostic test for all patients with suspected CVD.[6–8] Duplex scanning is excellent for evaluation of both infrainguinal venous obstruction and valvular incompetence.[9] Venous duplex scanning should be performed in all patients with symptoms of CVI to help define the location, cause, and severity of the underlying problem.

The four essential components of a complete venous duplex scanning are visibility, compressibility, venous flow, and augmentation. Typical appearance of a post-thrombotic vein at duplex scanning is that of a thickened, poorly compressible vessel with damaged, incompetent valves and variable degrees of venous flow due to partial recanalization. Asymmetry in flow velocity, lack of respiratory variations in venous flow, and waveform patterns at rest and during flow augmentation in the common femoral veins may indicate proximal obstruction. Obesity and bowel gas may prevent good visualization of the common hepatic veins and the IVC with ultrasound.

Plethysmography

Venous plethysmography is rarely used in current practice but it is a useful tool that provides information on venous function in patients with CVI and is complementary to duplex scanning. Air or strain gauge plethysmography is designed to evaluate the global leg hemodynamics by measuring reflux, obstruction, and calf pump function. This quantifies venous reflux and obstruction and has been used to monitor functional changes and assess physiologic outcome of venous patients after surgical treatments.[10,11] These studies are especially helpful in patients with suspected outflow obstruction but normal duplex findings or those suspected of having venous disease due to calf muscle pump dysfunction, but no reflux or obstruction is noted on duplex scanning.

CT and MR Venography

Advanced imaging studies after duplex ultrasonography are rarely indicated in early venous disease (CEAP C1-2) unless clinical evaluation is suggestive of secondary venous disease. CT and MR imaging have progressed tremendously in the last decade, and provide excellent three-dimensional imaging of the venous system. Both modalities are suitable for identifying pelvic or iliac vein obstruction in patients with lower limb varicosity, when proximal obstruction or iliac vein compression (May-Thurner syndrome) is suspected.[12] Venous phase examination helps to identify any obstructing mass or tumor, and provides sufficient information in most patients about venous anatomy, obstruction or stenosis.

Contrast Venography and Hemodynamic Studies

Ascending or descending (or both) contrast venography for CVI is performed only selectively in patients with suspected or known deep venous obstruction, post-thrombotic syndrome, pelvic congestion syndrome, nutcracker syndrome, vascular malformations, venous trauma, tumors and if invasive treatment is planned. Descending venography to study associated venous valve incompetence with Valsalva maneuver is classified to grade the severity of reflux (Grade 1–4, 1 = to upper thigh, 2 = to distal thigh, 3 = popliteal reflux, 4 = reflux to tibials and perforators) but rarely performed nowadays.[13,14] Ascending venography is performed in a standing position to evaluate patency of the superficial and/or deep venous system. Ascending venography is useful as a "road map" of the deep veins of the limb; it defines the sites of obstruction, and images the collateral venous circulation and the patterns of preferential flow.

Contrast venography is routinely used in CVD to perform endovenous procedures, such as angioplasty or venous stenting or open venous reconstructions. Pressure gradient across iliofemoral obstruction at rest in the supine patient (3 mmHg) or 10 mmHg after exercise is indicative of functional venous obstruction. Exercise consists of 10 dorsiflexions of the ankles or 20 isometric contractions of the calf muscle. Arm/foot venous pressure test, and ambulatory venous pressure (AVP) measurement in a dorsal foot vein are additional tests that can be performed. Detailed descriptions and techniques for these tests are beyond of the scope of this chapter and the reader is referred to the consensus statement for details.[15]

Intravascular Ultrasound (IVUS)

IVUS can be used in veins with obstruction without occlusion to assess the venous wall morphology and mural thickness, identify trabeculations and recanalization, frozen valves, and external compression. Some of these lesions, as emphasized by Raju and Neglen, are not seen with conventional contrast venography; IVUS provides dynamic measurements in assessing the degree of stenosis.[12] In addition, IVUS confirms the position of the stent in the venous segment and the resolution of the stenosis.[12]

Laboratory Evaluation

Selective patients, based on their history, with recurrent DVT, thrombosis at a young age, or thrombosis in an unusual site, or those with family history of thrombotic disorders should undergo screening for thrombophilia.[8]

TREATMENT

Conservative Management

Compression therapy and local wound care of venous ulcerations, if present, are the first line of treatment for symptomatic chronic deep venous obstruction. Compression is recommended in addition to lifestyle modifications that include weight loss, exercise, and elevation of the legs whenever possible. The rationale of compression treatment is to compensate for the increased ambulatory venous hypertension. Pressures to compress the superficial veins in supine patients range from 20 to 25 mmHg, while in the upright position, pressures around 35 to 40 mmHg have been shown to narrow the superficial veins, and pressures higher than 60 mmHg are needed to occlude them.[16] Ambulatory compression techniques and devices include elastic compression stockings, paste gauze boots (Unna boot), multilayer elastic wraps, dressings, and elastic and non-elastic bandages and non-elastic garments. Pneumatic compression devices (e.g. IPC), applied primarily at night, are also used in patients with refractory edema and venous ulcers.[17] Compression techniques result in variable degrees of success and mandate strict patient compliance, which in a hot climate can be both distressing and difficult. Patients with persistent disabling symptoms, such as venous claudication, severe swelling, and non-healing or recurrent ulcers not responding to conservative treatment, should be considered for endovascular or open surgical reconstruction.

Endovascular Treatment

Iliac or iliocaval stenting has become the primary treatment for chronic nonmalignant venous occlusions. Early and midterm results of endovascular techniques, such as angioplasty and stenting, using most frequently self-expandable stents, have been good. Outcomes are better for stenosis versus occlusions.

Hybrid Reconstruction

In patients with common femoral vein obstruction and proximal disease, conventional venous stenting is frequently not possible. Endovenous recanalization and stent placement, however, can be combined in selected cases with femoral vein endophlebectomy and patch angioplasty, using bovine pericardial patch. Balloon angioplasty and stenting is performed prior to or at completion of the patch angioplasty. Jugular vein access is obtained for retrograde recanalization as an alternative to or in combination with femoral access. The stent is extended proximally to the healthy vein and across the inguinal ligament distally. With recent experience, we extend the distal end of the stent into the venous patch.[1] Others have reported good patient outcomes with the hybrid technique, using saphenous vein patch for closure.[18]

We do not recommend hybrid reconstructions poor inflow even to the profunda femoris vein or if there are other contraindications for stenting.[19]

Open Surgical Treatment

Patients who are not candidates (e.g. congenital hypoplasia or aplasia of veins) or those who failed endovascular reconstructions can be treated with venous bypasses to relieve symptomatic venous outflow obstruction. Venous reconstruction is also performed in those patients who undergo excision of malignant tumors invading the vena cava or iliac veins or in patients with traumatic or iatrogenic injury with subsequent ligation.

We do not recommend open surgical reconstructions in cases where a prosthetic graft has to be anastomosed to an infrainguinal inflow and an arterio-venous fistula (AVF) is contraindicated due to arterial disease, or in acute presence of acute DVT or poor surgical candidates.[19]

Sapheno-popliteal bypass

First described independently by May and Husni, this procedure is indicated for femoral or proximal popliteal vein obstruction. The GSV, which most commonly is the major outflow from the leg via collaterals in these patients, is exposed above the knee joint and a direct anastomosis is performed between the GSV and popliteal vein (end to side). Alternatively, a free vein conduit can be used in case the ipsilateral GSV is not suitable.

Crossover Saphenous Vein Transposition (Palma Procedure)

Patients with symptomatic unilateral iliac vein obstruction are candidates for Palma procedure (Figure 44-1). With this technique, the contralateral saphenous vein is used for a crossover bypass to decompress venous congestion in the affected limb. The common femoral vein on the affected side is exposed first through a 6- to 8-cm long longitudinal groin incision. The collateral veins should be preserved if possible. The great saphenous vein of the contralateral leg is dissected through a 3- to 5-cm incision made in the groin crease, starting just medial to the femoral artery pulse. Tributaries of the saphenous vein are ligated and divided and the saphenous vein is mobilized in a length of about 20–25 cm using a skip incision in the upper thigh. The vein is ligated and divided and flushed after delivering it in the groin incision. Alternatively, endoscopic harvesting of the saphenous vein can also be performed, although this likely results in increased vein wall damage and that may affect patency.

It is essential to free up the saphenofemoral junction completely and dissect at least the anterior wall of the common femoral vein around the saphenous vein so there is no kink or buckle when the saphenous vein is pulled into the suprapubic tunnel. In

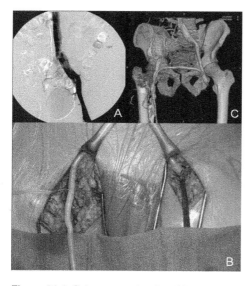
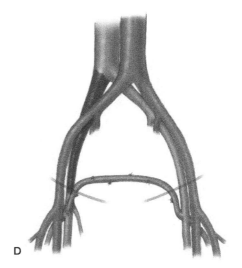

Figure 44-1. Palma procedure in a 38 year old male with post thrombotic syndrome. **A)** Chronic right iliofemoral obstruction after multiple failed attempts at endovenous recanalization. **B)** A right to left femoral vein bypass with left GSV (Palma procedure). **C)** Follow up CT venogram at 2 months. **D)** Schematic representation of the procedure (Reproduced with permission from Mayo Clinic Foundation) (Adapted from Garg N, Gloviczki P, Karimi KM, et al. Factors affecting outcome of open and hybrid reconstructions for nonmalignant obstruction of iliofemoral veins and inferior vena cava. *J Vasc Surg* 2011; 53(2):383–93)

some patients with a low saphenofemoral junction a kink is unavoidable. Excision of the saphenous vein with a 2-mm cuff from the common femoral vein and reanastomosis to the femoral vein with running 6/0 polypropylene suture, after turning the junction upwards 180 degrees can be performed in this situation. Before tunneling, a small Satinsky clamp is placed on the common femoral vein to allow distention of the saphenous vein and the saphenofemoral junction under gentle pressure using heparinized papaverine-saline solution. The vein is then tunneled subcutaneously in the suprapubic space over to the contralateral side using an aortic clamp to ensure a large tunnel without any constriction of the graft whatsoever. Saphenous vein graft in morbidly obese patients is not recommended because of the high chance of external compression of the vein. The common femoral vein is cross clamped with small vascular clamps or bulldogs and the vein is opened longitudinally in a length of about 2 cm. End to side anastomosis is performed between the saphenous vein and ipsilateral common femoral vein. This anastomosis can be spatulated onto the ipsilateral GSV if the femoral or deep femoral veins are diseased and the GSV is the predominant outflow in the affected leg. The anastomosis between the saphenous vein and the femoral vein is performed with running 6/0 polypropylene suture. A vein, at least 5 mm in diameter is required to achieve a satisfactory result and provide high venous flow to treat the basic problem of poor venous emptying in these patients.

Although few large series have been reported, overall patency of Palma grafts in nine series ranged between 70% and 83% at 3 to 5 years.[3] Results were better in patients who had no or minimal infrainguinal venous disease in those with May-Thurner syndrome without previous deep vein thrombosis. We observed a 70% primary and a 78% secondary patency rate at 5 years in 25 Palma vein grafts.[1] Endoscopic vein harvest was associated with decreased primary but not secondary patency rates.

Crossover Femoral Venous Prosthetic Bypass

An externally supported 10–12 mm diameter PTFE graft is used if the GSV is inadequate, <5 mm in diameter or of poor quality (Figure 44-2). Similarly to the autologous femoral suprapubic bypass, the femoral veins are exposed bilaterally, the ePTFE graft is positioned in the subcutaneous suprapubic tunnel, and an end-to-side anastomosis is performed to the common femoral veins at each side. A distal arteriovenous fistula (AVF) on the affected side is routinely added to the procedure using a 4- to 5-mm PTFE graft for the fistula between the PTFE graft and the superficial femoral artery. Sottiurai recommended cutting out a small window rather than just making a longitudinal cut in cross-femoral graft at the hood of the femoral anastomosis to optimize inflow and decrease intimal hyperplasia of the AVF.[20]

Variable patency rates of ePTFE grafts in this location have been reported and range between 0% and 100%.[21] In the authors' experience, the secondary patency of these bypasses is only 50% and preference still should be given to saphenous crossover grafts.

Femorocaval or Complex Bypass

Long bypasses from the femoral vein to the inferior vena cava (IVC) have poor results due to the hemodynamics of flow across the femoral vein. Most of these patients also have extensive post-phlebitic changes in the femoral and distal veins, making these procedures

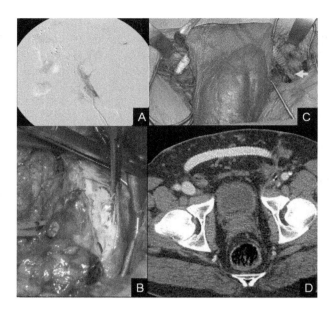

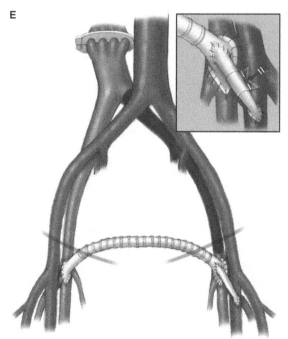

Figure 44-2. Femoro-femoral crossover ("Palma" prosthetic) bypass in a young patient with history of post traumatic left iliofemoral DVT and chronic venous ulceration. **A)** Venogram demonstrating occluded venous stent, that could not be recanalized. **B)** Chronic scarring and post thrombotic changes in the left CFV. **C)** Left to right femoral vein bypass with 12 mm externally supported PTFE (prosthetic "Palma" procedure), with a left SFA to graft AV fistula (arrow). **D)** CT venogram preformed at one year demonstrated a patent bypass. **E)** Schematic image demonstrating the bypass (Reproduced with permission from Mayo Clinic Foundation) (Adapted from Garg N, Gloviczki P, Karimi KM, et al. Factors affecting outcome of open and hybrid reconstructions for nonmalignant obstruction of iliofemoral veins and inferior vena cava. *J Vasc Surg* 2011; 53(2):383–93)

technically challenging and prone to failure due to poor inflow. Patients with bilateral disease or those with obstruction of supra-renal or supra-hepatic IVC, who have failed endovascular intervention, are evaluated for a complex reconstruction using either a bifurcated graft or tube graft with contralateral jump graft.

For in-line reconstruction of iliocaval or caval occlusions, an ePTFE graft with external support is the preferred conduit. Short, large-diameter (12-mm) grafts are used most frequently; a diameter of 12 to 14 mm is used for iliocaval bypasses and at least 10 mm for femorocaval bypass. The upper portion of the infrarenal IVC at and immediately distal to the renal veins is best approached transperitoneally through a midline incision, reflecting the ascending colon medially and mobilizing the duodenum using the Kocher maneuver. The low IVC just above the iliac bifurcation is well approachable through a right flank incision retroperitoneally (Figure 44-3). If the occlusion is limited to the right common iliac vein, the same incision is used to expose the external iliac vein for the distal anastomosis. Inflow is obtained from the iliac vein, exposed via a flank incision or femoral vein, through a standard groin incision. The graft is tunneled under the ureter. If a femorocaval graft is placed, the graft is tunneled under the inguinal ligament. To all grafts originating from the femoral vein and to most long iliocaval grafts, an arteriovenous fistula is added at the groin (Figure 44-3).

The use of autologous vein for femoroiliac or femorocaval reconstruction is also an option. Because of a relatively small size, saphenous vein in this location can only rarely be used. If short segment of the common femoral or iliac vein has to be reconstructed, a better size match is a spiral saphenous vein graft, prepared using the contralateral saphenous vein (Figure 44-4). The excised vein is opened longitudinally, the valves are excised, and the graft is wrapped around a 28- or 32-mm argyle chest tube. The edges are approximated with running 6/0 polypropylene sutures or with stainless steel non-penetrating vascular clips. The internal or external jugular veins are other conduits that can be considered for venous reconstruction. The femoral vein is also an alternative for reconstruction of abdominal veins, although morbidity of removing this vein in many of these patients with underlying thrombophilia or postthrombotic syndrome is high and other options are recommended. Cryopreserved saphenous or femoral vein has also been reported for venous reconstruction, but long-term patency of these grafts for venous replacement has been poor.

Experience with femorocaval or iliocaval PTFE bypass grafts for benign disease has been limited. In one series, published by Sotturai, long-term patency of 77% was reported.[20] We observed five year primary and secondary patency of 31% and 57%, respectively for femoro-infrahepatic IVC bypasses.[1]

Femoro- iliac or Ilio-caval Bypass

The iliac vein is exposed via a flank incision and femoral vein through a standard groin incision as detailed above. In cases with common iliac vein (CIV) occlusion, infra-hepatic cava is used as outflow, exposed through a midline incision or the right flank incision. These "short "bypasses have a hemodynamic advantage due to the length and high flow. We prefer an externally supported 10-14 mm PTFE graft for these bypasses. Among 17 patients who underwent a short bypass, we observed five year primary and secondary patency of 63% and 86% respectively.[1]

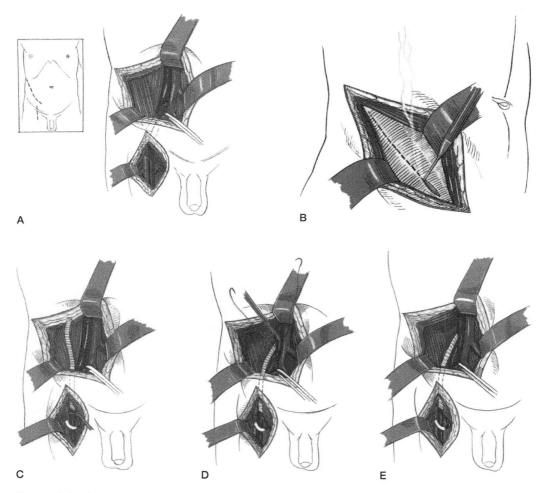

Figure 44-3. A) Location of the incisions of a right femorocaval bypass. The common femoral vein and the proximal saphenous vein is exposed through a 6- to 8-cm vertical incision at the groin. **B)** The distal inferior vena cava is exposed retroperitoneally through a right oblique anterolateral flank incision, transecting the abdominal muscles and the transversalis fascia. The ureter is retracted medially. **C)** The femoral arteriovenous fistula is performed first in this case with a large tributary of the saphenous vein and the femoral artery. The distal anastomosis is performed then in an end-to-end fashion between the common femoral vein and the 10-mm externally supported polytetrafluoroethylene graft. The graft is tunneled under the inguinal ligament **D)** The anastomosis between the graft and the inferior vena cava is performed in an end-to-end fashion using 5/0 polypropylene suture. Air is carefully flushed from the graft before removing the clamp from the inferior vena. **E:** Completed femorocaval bypass with a saphenofemoral arteriovenous fistula. (By permission of Mayo Foundation for Medical Education and Research. All rights reserved)

Inferior Cavoatrial Bypass

Patients with symptomatic short membranous occlusion of the IVC or longer congenital or acquired narrowing (caval coarctation) without or with hepatic venous outflow obstruction (Budd-Chiari syndrome) can be treated by cavoatrial bypass when attempts at percutaneous angioplasty or stenting have failed. The largest experience for the treatment of Budd Chiari syndrome comes from the Asian countries and multiple modalities have been described to treat associated caval occlusion. Some of the preferred techniques include

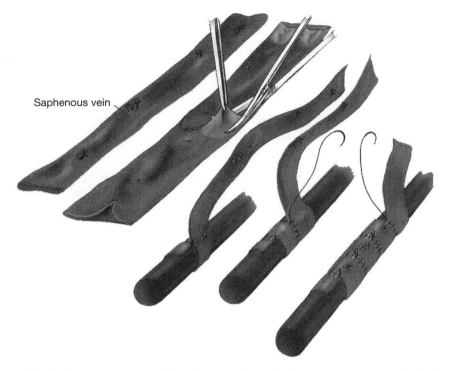

Figure 44-4. Technique to prepare a spiral saphenous vein graft. The vein is opened longitudinally, venous valves are excised, and the vein is wrapped around a 28F or 32F argyle chest tube. Vein edges are approximated using running 6/0 polypropylene sutures, with interrupted stitches after each circle to minimize purse stringing. Alternatively, non-penetrating vascular clips can be used for this purpose. (By permission of Mayo Foundation for Medical Education and Research. All rights reserved)

membranotomy, endovenectomy with patch angioplasty, cavo-caval bypass or meso-atrial bypass with or without caval limb.[4,22] Results of these techniques are encouraging with greater than 85% long term success in appropriately selected patients. Recent data suggests significantly better outcomes with meso-atrial caval bypass compared to mesocaval bypass,[23] and originating one limb from the superior mesenteric vein has higher patency rate as compared to splenic vein.[24]

The suprahepatic inferior vena cava or right atrium is approached through an anterolateral right thoracotomy (Figure 44-5a–d). The pericardium is opened anterior to the phrenic nerve. If the membranous occlusion is short and is located to this area, a short PTFE interposition graft can be performed from this exposure. If the occlusion extends distal to the hepatic veins, the abdomen is entered through the same thoracotomy, transecting the diaphragm circumferentially and mobilizing the liver forward and medially. Division of the triangular and the right coronary ligament will help mobilization of the liver. The adrenal gland and the kidney are left in their bed and dissection is moved more medially. Excellent exposure of the suprarenal IVC can be achieved through this approach. If the distal anastomosis has to be made more distally, a separate right subcostal or midline incision can be performed as previously described.

For a cavoatrial bypass an end-to-side anastomosis to the IVC is performed and the graft is routed under the liver parallel to the IVC. The graft is then anastomosed

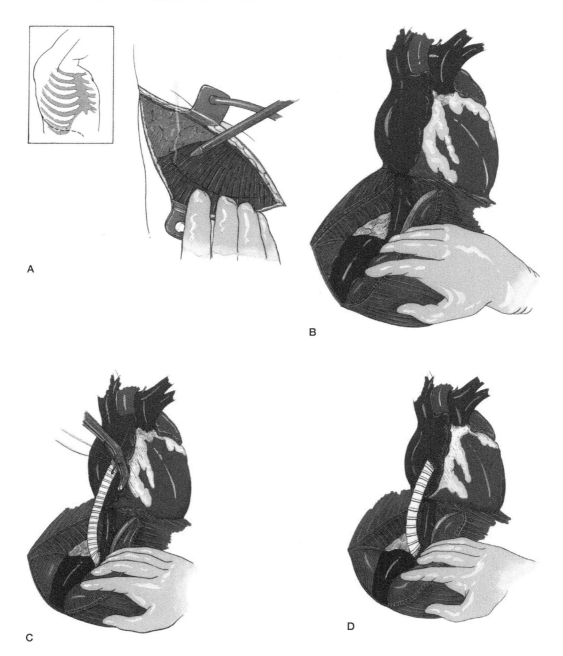

Figure 44-5. Cavoatrial bypass for suprarenal caval occlusion. **A)** The thorax is entered through the eighth intercostal space performing an anterolateral thoracotomy. The costal arch is sharply divided through the eight and ninth ribs but the abdomen is not entered. The inferior pulmonary ligament is divided and the diaphragm is circumferentially incised and the abdomen is entered. **B)** The triangular and right coronary ligament is divided and the right lobe of the liver is mobilized medially and anteriorly. **C)** The suprarenal inferior vena cava is dissected and partially cross clamped. A 14- or 16-mm externally supported polytetrafluoroethylene (PTFE) graft is anastomosed first to the cava, then to the right atrium. Air is carefully flushed before opening up flow in the graft. **D)** Completed cavoatrial PTFE bypass. (By permission of Mayo Foundation for Medical Education and Research. All rights reserved)

end to side to the suprarenal IVC or the lower portion of the right atrium. Partially occluding clamps are used to perform the anastomosis, and cardiopulmonary bypass is not needed. Traumatic or iatrogenic occlusions can also be managed by this technique. The use of a 16- to 20-mm externally supported PTFE graft is recommended.

The reported clinical success rate with cavoatrial grafts is about 77%, with a perioperative mortality of 3% and 2-, 5-, and 10-year patency rates of 86%, 78%, and 57%, respectively.[21,25]

SPECIAL CONSIDERATIONS

Endophlebectomy

Postthrombotic femoral veins frequently have multiple lumens due to partial recanalization of the thrombus. Excision of the organized and fibrotic thrombus will enlarge the lumen, although the exposed collagen in the media of the vein wall is more thrombogenic than the intact venous wall. Still, careful endophlebectomy will improve inflow to a great extent; attention, however, must be paid to avoid injury to the thin residual venous wall. In patients who have localized high-grade stenosis of the common femoral vein, this operation alone is sufficient to improve venous outflow. This procedure has also been performed combined with deep venous valve transplantation in patients with PTS. The defect is closed with a patch using a segment of the saphenous vein or bovine pericardium. The endophlebectomized segment can also be used to improve inflow for iliocaval stenting (see hybrid procedures) or for a cross-femoral or femoro-caval bypass. In a series of patients who underwent endophlebectomy, early results showed 77% primary patency of the operated segments at 8 months and 93% secondary patency rate.[26]

Valve Repair

CVI resulting from post-thrombotic reflux in the infrainguinal deep veins has been managed with limited endovenectomy and valve repair or transposition with variable success. Readers are referred to a recent review on outcomes.{Bond, 2012 #13883}

Arterio-venous Fistula

Caval reconstructions or short iliocaval grafts, including prosthetic bypasses do not need an adjunctive temporary AVF to maintain patency, except in case of poor inflow and distal anastomosis at the level of common femoral vein. Even in these distal cases, additional benefit provided by AVF to prevent early thrombosis is questionable.[1]

Prevention of Complications

In general, large vein reconstructions for benign disease are performed in good surgical candidates only, with a low risk of systemic complications. Of the local, nonvascular complications, wound infection, hematoma and lymphatic leaks (fistula, lymphocele) are the most frequent, and atraumatic surgical technique, antibiotic prophylaxis, and standard surgical principles are helpful in prevention. Intraoperative air embolism, especially during caval reconstruction, is a potentially fatal complication and may be prevented by meticulous flushing of the grafts before re-establishment of the circulation and passive Valsalva maneuver (30 mmHg) as well as Trendelenburg position before release of the proximal clamp.

Deep venous thrombosis and pulmonary embolism are serious systemic vascular complications. During 64 procedures that we performed for non-malignant disease there was no mortality and no pulmonary embolism.[1] Although early graft thrombosis rate was high (20%), and re-interventions were needed, 96% of the patients left the hospital with a patent graft after open surgical bypass. Perioperative anticoagulation with heparin and warfarin, the use of elastic stockings, intermittent pneumatic compression pumps, and early ambulation help prevent thromboembolic complications, which are fortunately rare. Local vascular complications are specific to venous reconstructions and include graft stenosis or thrombosis, perioperative bleeding, graft infection, and injury to the surrounding vascular and nonvascular structures.

Anticoagulation

Grafts placed in the venous system have a higher rate of thrombosis than arterial grafts due to a low venous flow. Presence of thrombophilic disorders and thrombogenic surface of any prosthetic graft increases the risk of graft failure. Infrainguinal venous obstruction and valvular incompetence further decrease inflow to the graft, and it is a major contributing factor to failure. For these reasons, perioperative anticoagulation is indicated in patients undergoing reconstructive venous surgery for deep venous obstruction.

The patient is fully heparinized during reconstruction and protamine is avoided at the completion of the procedure. Unfractionated heparin infusion is started immediately in the post-operative period. Complete postoperative systemic heparinization is achieved by 48 hours, and full-dose low-molecular-weight heparin is continued subcutaneously for another 3 to 5 days, given simultaneously with warfarin. The incidence of postoperative bleeding has been between 5% and 10%, mainly as a result of anticoagulation. Warfarin is continued indefinitely in most patients with prosthetic grafts and in all with a known underlying coagulation abnormality.

FOLLOW-UP AND RE-INTERVENTIONS

Duplex scan on the first postoperative day or contrast venography is performed to confirm graft patency. Stenosis or thrombosis is corrected immediately after recognition. If thrombosis occurred in a graft without fistula, thrombectomy is done with addition of a fistula. Graft stenosis discovered during surveillance in the late postoperative period is treated first with angioplasty or venous stenting. Late graft thrombosis is treated with thrombolysis, angioplasty, and stenting. Surgical revision is usually limited to patch angioplasty of the stenotic portion of the graft, although occasionally aneurysmal dilation of the saphenous crossover graft may also need surgical correction. On long term follow up, about half of the patients require some kind of re-intervention. More than 60% of the patients had no venous claudication and no or minimal swelling on long term follow-up.

REFERENCES

1. Garg N, Gloviczki P, Karimi KM, et al. Factors affecting outcome of open and hybrid reconstructions for nonmalignant obstruction of iliofemoral veins and inferior vena cava. *J Vasc Surg.* Feb 2011;53(2):383–393.
2. May R, Thurner J. [A vascular spur in the vena iliaca communis sinistra as a cause of predominantly left-sided thrombosis of the pelvic veins]. *Z Kreislaufforsch.* Dec 1956;45(23–24):912–922.
3. Jost CJ, Gloviczki P, Cherry KJ, Jr., et al. Surgical reconstruction of iliofemoral veins and the inferior vena cava for nonmalignant occlusive disease. *J Vasc Surg.* Feb 2001;33(2):320–327; discussion 327–328.
4. Inafuku H, Morishima Y, Nagano T, Arakaki K, Yamashiro S, Kuniyoshi Y. A three-decade experience of radical open endvenectomy with pericardial patch graft for correction of Budd-Chiari syndrome. *J Vasc Surg.* Sep 2009;50(3):590–593.
5. Langer RD, Ho E, Denenberg JO, Fronek A, Allison M, Criqui MH. Relationships between symptoms and venous disease: the San Diego population study. *Arch Intern Med.* Jun 27 2005;165(12):1420–1424.
6. Cavezzi A, Labropoulos N, Partsch H, et al. Duplex ultrasound investigation of the veins in chronic venous disease of the lower limbs—UIP consensus document. Part II. Anatomy. *Eur J Vasc Endovasc Surg.* Mar 2006;31(3):288–299.
7. Coleridge-Smith P, Labropoulos N, Partsch H, Myers K, Nicolaides A, Cavezzi A. Duplex ultrasound investigation of the veins in chronic venous disease of the lower limbs—UIP consensus document. Part I. Basic principles. *Eur J Vasc Endovasc Surg.* Jan 2006;31(1):83–92.
8. Gloviczki P, Comerota AJ, Dalsing MC, et al. The care of patients with varicose veins and associated chronic venous diseases: clinical practice guidelines of the Society for Vascular Surgery and the American Venous Forum. *Journal of vascular surgery: official publication, the Society for Vascular Surgery [and] International Society for Cardiovascular Surgery, North American Chapter.* May 2011;53(5 Suppl):2S–48S.
9. Labropoulos N, Tiongson J, Pryor L, et al. Definition of venous reflux in lower-extremity veins. *J Vasc Surg.* Oct 2003;38(4):793–798.
10. Rhodes JM, Gloviczki P, Canton L, Heaser TV, Rooke TW. Endoscopic perforator vein division with ablation of superficial reflux improves venous hemodynamics. *J Vasc Surg.* Nov 1998;28(5):839–847.
11. Park UJ, Yun WS, Lee KB, et al. Analysis of the postoperative hemodynamic changes in varicose vein surgery using air plethysmography. *J Vasc Surg.* Mar 2010;51(3):634–638.
12. Neglen P, Raju S. Intravascular ultrasound scan evaluation of the obstructed vein. *J Vasc Surg.* Apr 2002;35(4):694–700.
13. Masuda EM, Kistner RL. Long-term results of venous valve reconstruction: a four- to twenty-one-year follow-up. *J Vasc Surg.* Mar 1994;19(3):391–403.
14. Kistner RL, Ferris EB, Randhawa G, Kamida C. A method of performing descending venography. *J Vasc Surg.* Nov 1986;4(5):464–468.
15. Nicolaides AN. Investigation of chronic venous insufficiency: A consensus statement (France, March 5–9, 1997). *Circulation.* Nov 14 2000;102(20):E126–163.
16. Partsch B, Partsch H. Calf compression pressure required to achieve venous closure from supine to standing positions. *J Vasc Surg.* Oct 2005;42(4):734–738.
17. Moneta G, Partsch B. Compression therapy for venous ulceration. In: Gloviczki P, ed. *Handbook of venous disorders.* Vol 1. Third ed. London: Hodder Arnold; 2009:348–358.
18. Vogel D, Comerota AJ, Al-Jabouri M, Assi ZI. Common femoral endovenectomy with iliocaval endoluminal recanalization improves symptoms and quality of life in patients with postthrombotic iliofemoral obstruction. *J Vasc Surg.* Jan 2012;55(1):129–135.
19. Gloviczki P, Kalra M, Duncan AA, Oderich GS, Vrtiska TJ, Bower TC. Open and hybrid deep vein reconstructions: to do or not to do? *Phlebology.* Mar 2012;27 Suppl 1:103–106.
20. Sottiurai V. Results of Deep-Vein Reconstruction. *Vasc Surg.* 1997;31:236–238.

21. Ricotta JJ, 2nd, Gloviczki P. Surgical treatment of chronic venous insufficiency. In: Hallett JW, Jr., Mills JL, Earnshaw J, Reekers JA, eds. *Comprehensive Vascular and Endovascular Surgery*. 2nd ed. Philadelphia: Elsevier; 2009:783–806.

22. Xu PQ, Ma XX, Ye XX, et al. Surgical treatment of 1360 cases of Budd-Chiari syndrome: 20-year experience. *Hepatobiliary Pancreat Dis Int*. Aug 2004;3(3):391–394.

23. Chen H, Zhang F, Ye Y, Cheng Y, Chen Y. Long-term follow-up study and comparison of meso-atrial shunts and meso-cavo-atrial shunts for treatment of combined budd-Chiari syndrome. *J Surg Res*. Jun 1 2011;168(1):162–166.

24. Zhang Y, Zhao H, Yan D, Xue H, Lau WY. Superior mesenteric vein-caval-right atrium y shunt for treatment of budd-Chiari syndrome with obstruction to the inferior vena cava and the hepatic veins — a study of 62 patients. *J Surg Res*. Jul 2011;169(1):e93–99.

25. Gloviczki P, Pairolero PC, Toomey BJ, et al. Reconstruction of large veins for nonmalignant venous occlusive disease. *J Vasc Surg*. Nov 1992;16(5):750–761.

26. Puggioni A, Kistner RL, Eklof B, Lurie F. Surgical disobliteration of postthrombotic deep veins—endophlebectomy—is feasible. *J Vasc Surg*. May 2004;39(5):1048–1052; discussion 1052.

SECTION **X**

Upper Extremity Disease

45

Pectoralis Minor Muscle Syndrome

William H. Pearce, MD, Marlon Lee, MD, and Suman Annambhotla, MD

The pectoralis minor muscle syndrome (PMS) is a component of a broader diagnosis of thoracic outlet syndrome (TOS). Sixty years ago, physicians were more accurate in the description of the neurovascular compression that occurs in the thoracic outlet. Shoulder girdle symptoms or TOS included cervical ribs,[1] scalenus anticus syndrome,[2] costoclavicular syndrome[3] and the syndrome of prolonged hyperabduction described by Wright.[4] The prolonged hyperabduction syndrome was specific to PMS, but could overlap with other syndromes. In recent years, all of these different neurovascular compressions that occur in the upper extremity have been lumped together as TOS. Because of the generalization of the topic, physicians and surgeons rapidly forgot the importance of the pectoralis minor muscle and focused their attention on more proximal anatomic structures such as the scalene triangle or costoclavicular space. There has been a great deal of literature that is focused on operations that relieve this proximal compression, either by removing the first rib, performing a scalenectomy or by doing both. It has been only recently that attention has been drawn to the pectoralis minor muscle and its importance in patient symptomatology.[5-9]

In 1956, Lord and Stone described pectoralis minor tenotomy and scalenectomy for hyperabduction syndrome and after subclavian vein thrombosis.[10] In this article he refers to Wright's original description of, "postural hyperabduction that occurs when the arms are brought together above the head with the elbows flexed". In this paper, they describe five patients who have had improvement to their symptoms with resection of the pectoralis minor muscle tendon. This report lay dormant for almost fifty years, until it was rediscovered by Sanders and Rao who describe six patients with similar symptoms in 2007.[9] However, Sanders gives credit to Dr. George Thomas of Seattle who rekindled his interest in the pectoralis minor muscle as a cause of both venous and neurogenic thoracic outlet syndromes.[8]

PATHOPHYSIOLOGY

The shoulder girdle is a remarkable structure that allows for a wide range of motion. The range of motion is guided by numerous muscles that connect the scapula to the chest wall and to the upper extremity. As a result of this dynamic structure, there is opening and closing of many spaces through which the neurovascular bundle of the upper extremity passes. The most recognized and understandable space is the costoclavicular space (junction of the first rib and clavicle). The costoclavicular space includes not only the first rib and clavicle, but also the subclavius muscle. The pectoralis minor muscle plays an important role in closing this space, in that it is a depressor of the coracoid at the tip of the scapula and clavicle. Similarly, the subclavius muscle depresses the clavicle and hypertrophies with certain exercises. In addition, the pectoralis minor muscle forms a tight band that passes directly over the second portion of the axillary artery, vein and nerves. Resection of the muscle has been possible in some high performance athletes with good results.[11]

The scapula has eighteen muscle insertions or origins. Malfunction of any one of these muscles may result in abnormal shoulder girdle function and the occurrence of symptoms. Careful physical examination and understanding of the dysfunction of the shoulder girdle may lead to accurate diagnosis. The pectoralis minor muscle originates from the third, fourth and fifth ribs and converges to form a flat tendon, which is inserted on the coracoid process of the scapula (Figure 45-1). The pectoralis minor

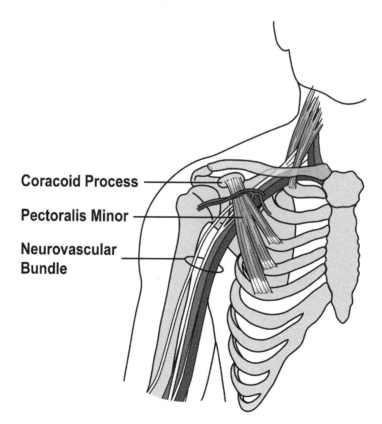

Coracoid Process

Pectoralis Minor

Neurovascular Bundle

Figure 45-1A. The pectoralis minor muscle arises from the 3–5 ribs to form a narrow tendon then attaches to the coracoid process of the scapulae.

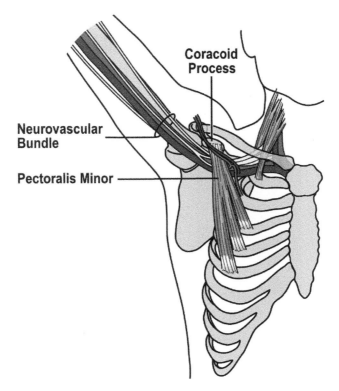

Figure 45-1B. With abduction and external rotation (hyperabduction) the pectoralis minor muscle stretches across the chest wall impinging the neurovascular bundle.

muscle depresses the shoulder, pulling the scapula anteriorly and inferiorly. Pectoral nerve branches pass through the muscle belly of the pectoralis minor muscle.

DIAGNOSIS

In patients with TOS the goal is to identify the muscles in spasm and that are tender, as well as the neurogenic symptoms with dynamic positioning. Patients with neurogenic TOS tend to have tenderness over the scalene muscle, the trapezius and the levator scapula. The physical examination is generally unremarkable except for a positive Roos or EAST test. The patients have rapid onset of their symptoms with their arms abducted and externally rotated. In general, these patients do not have tenderness over their anterior chest wall particularly in the location of the coracoid and the pectoralis minor muscle.

Contrary to patients with TOS caused by the first rib and anterior scalene muscles, the patients with PMS tend to have a depressed shoulder and tenderness of the pectoralis minor muscle. The pectoralis minor muscle is reached by pushing into the axilla and pushing forward. These patients also have more symptoms when their chest wall is hyperabducted.

However, the most important diagnostic test for determining the location of the impingement is the use of scalene muscle blocks and/or pectoralis minor muscle blocks. In our practice the muscle blocks are performed under ultrasound guidance by the anesthesia service. In other practices these are performed by the surgeon. A good response to the block is a significant predictor of improvement with surgery. More recently, Sucher described ultrasound findings predictive of PMS with "bowing" of the muscle. In addition, he showed impingement of the neurovascular bundle by the pectoralis minor muscle with abduction.[12] Dynamic CTA imaging is useful as seen in Figure 45-2A and 45-2B.

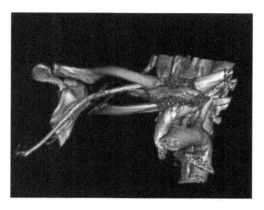

Figure 45-2A. CTA demonstrating a normal axillary artery with the arm in neutral position.

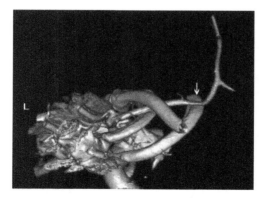

Figure 45-2B. CTA demonstrating a compressed axillary artery (arrow) with the arm hyperabducted.

Here a patient with neurogenic PMS demonstrates arterial flattening in the region of the pectoralis minor muscle with the arm abducted and externally rotated.

OPERATIVE APPROACHES AND RESULTS

Resection of the pectoralis minor muscle is not difficult and does not lead to any substantial functional disability.[13] The operation may be performed by an anterior incision directly over the insertion of the pectoralis minor muscle or in the axilla. We prefer the axillary incision. Here a 5–8 cm incision is made in the axilla just above the hairline. This allows exposure of the axillary artery, as well as the pectoralis minor muscle. The pectoralis minor muscle may be fused with the pectoralis major muscle. However, with blunt dissection, the tendinous insertion at the coracoid can be identified and encircled with a finger. Here the muscle is resected with electrocautery. The nerves of the pectoralis major muscle pass through the pectoralis minor muscle and may be injured during dissection. Therefore, it is important to be as close to the coracoid as possible to prevent any functional pectoralis muscle disability. Furthermore, in a report by Sanders, patients with Langer's arch may be identified and the compression released simultaneously.[9]

The reported results of pectoralis minor muscle release are few. There are small case series of PMS associated with venous claudication and axillary vein thrombosis. Sanders and Rao reported axillary obstruction produced by the pectoralis minor muscle in six patients.[9] All patients experienced good to excellent relief of symptoms, without complication. Nakada reported a single patient with venous claudication with venographic evidence of muscle compression before and after muscle resection.[6] The patient also had an excellent result. In the original report by Lord and Stone, five patients underwent surgery with four having good relief.[10] The fifth patient was felt to have costoclavicular syndrome with more of a neurogenic component than venous obstruction.

Pectoralis minor muscle tenotomy is also useful in treating patients with neurogenic TOS symptoms. In 2010, Sanders and Rao reported one hundred consecutive operations for PMS alone or accompanied by neurogenic TOS.[8] The report includes a heterogeneous group of patients with both neurogenic PMS alone or patients with neurogenic TOS alone or in combination with neurogenic PMS.

The patients with neurogenic PMS alone were more often employed and had a much greater success rate than those who were unemployed and had the neurogenic thoracic outlet combination. The success rate at one to three years of follow up in the group with neurogenic PMS alone was 90%. However, in the combined group it was only 35%. Failure rate was 29% overall, 8% in the pectoralis muscle group and 46% in patients with both diseases. Interestingly, among patients who had both symptoms of neurogenic PMS and neurogenic TOS, 35% experienced improvement.

The complications associated with this procedure included wound infections (3%), temporary paresthesia in the thumb and index fingers (2%) and numbness and paresthesias on the underside of the arm (15%). Three patients experienced tenderness over the pectoralis minor muscles postoperatively, which responded to steroid injections. Interestingly, in patients who present with both neurogenic TOS and neurogenic PMS symptoms there was a 35% rate of success with pectoralis minor muscle release alone. This finding suggests that pectoralis minor muscle release should be performed initially as it is a minor procedure and thoracic outlet decompression postponed until failure of this operation. In addition, the pectoralis minor muscle tenotomy is useful in patients with recurrent neurogenic TOS. The use of this operation was first described by Ambrad-Chalela and colleagues.[5] In a group of sixty-five patients with recurrent symptoms, thirteen pectoralis minor tendon resections were performed with excellent results. However, most of these patients had combinations of other thoracic outlet procedures including resection of an intact first rib, residual first rib resection and repeat neurolysis.

COMMENT

Thoracic outlet syndrome is a complex group of diseases that occur in a single anatomic region. Due to lack of specificity of the diagnosis the results of surgery are often confusing and conflicting. Historically, the diagnosis was related to a specific etiology: the cervical rib syndrome, scalene anticus syndrome, costoclavicular space syndrome and hyperabduction syndrome. Because of the lumping of all symptoms in to one diagnosis the results have been varied and disappointing. The reemergence of the pectoralis minor muscle and subcoracoid space as an important location for neurovascular compression has added new specificity to this problem. Today with many patients sitting for many hours at desks performing data entry, shortening of the pectoralis minor muscle and its tendon occur. This results in atypical posture with depression of the clavicle resulting in rounding of the shoulders and closure of the costoclavicular space. As a result the shortening of the pectoralis minor muscle will produce hyperabduction and obstruction at the location of the pectoralis minor muscle tendon. Tenderness over the anterior chest wall and pectoralis minor muscle is usually solicited during physical examination. Patients with PMS alone have fewer symptoms in the cervical region with more in the chest and axilla. However, patients may have both conditions. Pectoralis minor muscle tenotomy is a simple procedure with few complications and gratifying outcomes. Patients who are good candidates for this procedure are those who improve with the pectoralis minor muscle block. The success rate is high, the disability and operative morbidity low. However, because of the coexisting neurogenic thoracic outlet in the costoclavicular space additional surgery may be required. Some authors have advocated scalenectomy along with pectoralis minor tendon release, while others have included a first rib resection as part of this procedure.

The pectoralis minor muscle and its tendon are assuming a greater role in the pathogenesis of neurogenic and venous TOS. Accurate identification of the process may be made on physical examination, with pectoralis minor nerve block, CTA venography/angiography or ultrasound. The obstruction or occlusion of these structures may be seen with the patient in a functional position. Surgical treatment with pectoralis minor muscle release can lead to excellent outcomes.

REFERENCES

1. Murphy JB. IV. A Case of Cervical Rib with Symptoms resembling Subclavian Aneurism. *Ann Surg*. Mar 1905;41(3):399–406.
2. Kirgis H, Reed A. Significant Anatomic Relations in the Syndrome of the Scalene Muscles. *Ann Surg*. June 1928 1948;127(6):1182–1201.
3. Falconer M, Weddell G. Costo-clavicular compression of the subclavian artery and vein: relation to the scalenus anticus syndrome. *Lancet*. 1943;2:539.
4. Wright I. The Neurovascular Syndrome Produced by Hyperabduction of the Arms. *Am Heart J*. 1945;29:1.
5. Ambrad-Chalela E, Thomas GI, Johansen KH. Recurrent neurogenic thoracic outlet syndrome. *Am J Surg*. Apr 2004;187(4):505–510.
6. Nakada T, Knight RT, Mani RL. Intermittent venous claudication of the upper extremity: the pectoralis minor syndrome. *Ann Neurol*. Apr 1982;11(4):433–434.
7. Sanders RJ. Recurrent neurogenic thoracic outlet syndrome stressing the importance of pectoralis minor syndrome. *Vasc Endovascular Surg*. Jan;45(1):33–38.

8. Sanders RJ, Rao NM. The forgotten pectoralis minor syndrome: 100 operations for pectoralis minor syndrome alone or accompanied by neurogenic thoracic outlet syndrome. *Ann Vasc Surg.* Aug;24(6):701–708.

9. Sanders RJ, Rao NM. Pectoralis minor obstruction of the axillary vein: report of six patients. *J Vasc Surg.* Jun 2007;45(6):1206–1211.

10. Lord JW, Jr., Stone PW. Pectoralis minor tenotomy and anterior scalenotomy with special reference to the hyperabduction syndrome and effort thrombosis of the subclavian vein. *Circulation.* Apr 1956;13(4):537–542.

11. Durham JR, Yao JS, Pearce WH, et al. Arterial injuries in the thoracic outlet syndrome. *J Vasc Surg.* Jan 1995;21(1):57–69; discussion 70.

12. Sucher BM. Thoracic outlet syndrome-postural type: ultrasound imaging of pectoralis minor and brachial plexus abnormalities. *Pm R.* Jan;4(1):65–72.

13. Scevola S, Cowan J, Harrison DH. Does the removal of pectoralis minor impair the function of pectoralis major? *Plast Reconstr Surg.* Oct 2003;112(5):1266–1273.

46

Contemporary Management of Aberrant Right Subclavian Artery

Grant T. Fankhauser, MD, Samuel R. Money, MD, MBA, and William M. Stone, MD

INTRODUCTION

An aberrant right subclavian artery is the most common anatomic anomaly of the aortic arch, occurring in 0.5–2.5% of the population.[1] Symptoms can range from dysphagia to airway compromise with potential rupture from aneurysmal degeneration, though in most cases the anomaly is asymptomatic. Treatment options are evolving through the use of endovascular methods, but open surgical intervention still plays a considerable role.

EMBRYOLOGY

The great vessels originate from six pairs of branchial arches that undergo complex development in the embryo between the 4th and 8th weeks of gestation.[2] Of note, much of the understanding regarding the embryologic development of the vascular system stems from the work of E.D. Congdon on 31 embryos in the 1920s.[3] Under normal circumstances the right subclavian artery is formed from the right fourth branchial arch, the right dorsal aorta distal to the fourth branchial arch, and the seventh intersegmental artery.[4] This development relies upon the involution of the right dorsal aorta distal to the seventh intersegmental artery. This involution severs the connection of the developing right subclavian artery from what will become the descending aorta. This results in the origin of the right subclavian artery originating in the proximal aortic arch via the brachiocephalic (innominate) artery. (Figure 46-1)

In the case of an aberrant right subclavian artery, the involution of the dorsal aortic arch distal to the seventh intersegmental artery does not occur, thus the developing right subclavian, with involvement of the seventh intersegmental artery, remains connected to what will become the descending aorta.[5] Involution of the fourth branchial

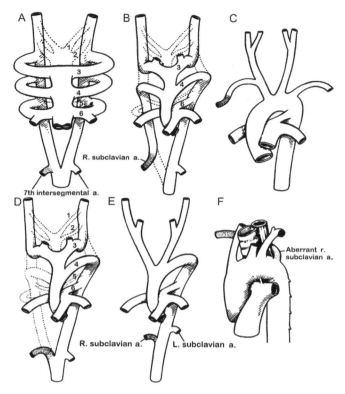

Figure 46-1. A–C: Normal development of the branchial arches with involution of the right aorta leading to the typical right subclavian artery anatomy. **D–F:** Failure of involution of the right distal aorta leading to aberrant right subclavian artery originating from the distal aortic arch.

arch separates the developing proximal arch from the aberrant right subclavian. This leads to an aortic arch with four branches (proximal to distal): right common carotid, left common carotid, left subclavian, and right subclavian.

ANATOMY

The development of symptoms from an aberrant right subclavian artery depend mostly on the course of the artery between the origin and the right upper extremity. In 80% of cases the artery courses posterior to the trachea and esophagus. In 15% of cases the artery courses between the trachea and esophagus, and in only 5% of cases does the artery course anterior to the trachea.[6]

Another factor contributing to the symptoms of an aberrant right subclavian can be the presence of an enlarged segment of the artery at its origin. This "infundibulum" was first described by Dr. Burckhard Kommerell in 1936 and retains his name: Kommerell's diverticulum.[7] This diverticulum occurs in up to 60% of patients and can cause mass effect or undergo aneurysmal degeneration.[8,9]

In patients with aberrant right subclavian arteries, the remainder of the aortic arch is usually normal although other abnormalities are possible. Other common abnormalities include origin of the left common carotid from the brachiocephalic ("bovine arch"), origin of the right inferior thyroid artery from the right carotid, aortic coarctation, and replaced right or left vertebral arteries.[8,10] The abnormal embryologic development that leads to an aberrant right subclavian artery also frequently leads to a non-recurrent right inferior laryngeal nerve.[11] This must be taken into account during surgery in the thorax or neck.

Cardiac anomalies are frequently encountered in patients with an aberrant right subclavian artery. Zapata et al. reviewed cardiac anomalies present in 117 patients out of 128 with aberrant right subclavian arteries.[10] Cyanotic defects were present in 62% of patients. The most common cardiac anomalies overall included truncus arteriosus (7%), double-outlet right ventricle (6%), aortic/mitral atresia (6%), and atrioventricular canal defects (5%). The incidence of associated cardiac anomalies was admittedly influenced by the study population, but this study stresses the importance of searching for other abnormalities before attempting intervention.

There is a strong association between trisomy 21 (Down syndrome) and aberrant right subclavian artery. Between 19–36% of prenatally diagnosed cases of trisomy 21 exhibit aberrant right subclavian artery.[12] This vascular malformation contributes to feeding difficulties in 10–20% of Down syndrome babies.[13]

SYMPTOMS

Most patients with aberrant right subclavian artery are asymptomatic but a significant number of patients will require intervention.[1,14] Symptoms, when they develop, depend on the presence of aneurysm and the relation of the artery to the trachea and/or esophagus. Symptoms can include dysphagia (*dysphagia lusoria*), airway compromise, aorto-esophageal fistula, or rupture.[15,16] Despite the presence of an aberrant vessel close to other structures since birth, symptoms may not appear until later in life. A proposed mechanism for this is progressive atherosclerosis of the vessel or decreased elasticity of the esophagus and surrounding tissues.[17] Another possible explanation may be progressive change in the vertebral column and thoracic skeleton with age- or hypertension-related vessel ectasia.[18]

DIAGNOSIS

The diagnosis of aberrant right subclavian artery is most commonly made with various imaging modalities. Additionally, the diagnosis has been described through upper gastrointestinal endoscopy. An extraluminal pulsatile mass may be identified during the examination. Lateral chest radiographs may show a posterior tracheal imprint but plain radiographs may miss the aberrant vessel if it does not impinge on the trachea or is not calcified.[19] Contrast esophagography can likewise reveal an extraluminal filling defect, suggesting the presence of an aberrant vessel. However, if there is not resultant esophageal compression this modality would not identify the aberrant subclavian artery.

Aortic angiography is the gold standard for delineating vascular anatomy. Angiography can reveal a Kommerell's diverticulum or other abnormalities of the arch. While angiography is excellent at visualizing the vasculature, it is less helpful in visualizing the relationship to the trachea and esophagus. For this reason, cross sectional imaging (computed tomography or magnetic resonance imaging) is the imaging modality of choice. It can show the course of the vessel, the presence of a Kommerell's diverticulum or atherosclerotic degeneration, and the relationship to the trachea and esophagus. Transesophageal echocardiography and endoscopic ultrasound can give similar information but are more invasive and provider-dependent. Ultrasonography has been used to visualize aberrant vasculature *in utero* and aid in the diagnosis of Down syndrome prenatally.[20]

TREATMENT OVERVIEW

The indication for intervention is dependent on the development of symptoms and/or aneurysmal degeneration. Asymptomatic aberrant right subclavian arteries without aneurysmal dilation generally do not require intervention. Such arteries may become symptomatic if they are in close proximity to the trachea or esophagus and aneurysmal changes develop or the vessel becomes sclerotic. Radiographic compression of the trachea or esophagus does not require treatment unless there is correlation with symptoms. Patients with Kommerell's diverticulum likewise do not warrant treatment unless aneurysmal degeneration occurs.

Intervention is warranted for the treatment of symptoms or if aneurysmal change develops in the aberrant vessel. Open surgical, totally endovascular, and hybrid (open and endovascular) options are available.

OPEN SURGERY

Open surgical intervention is aimed at alleviating symptoms from esophageal or tracheal compression or preventing rupture of an aneurysmal artery. Tracheal or esophageal compression by the aberrant subclavian artery usually requires division of the artery at its origin. This can be accomplished through a median sternotomy or left thoracotomy. The need for revascularization of the right subclavian depends on collateral flow. Collateral flow can be estimated by blood pressure in the right arm pre- and post-division of the subclavian artery or by back bleeding from the artery after division. Some have advocated mandatory revascularization given the likelihood of ischemia and the importance of the right vertebrobasilar system.[21] Although Robert Gross performed the first intervention for an aberrant subclavian artery, his procedure was ligation of the vessel at its orifice in a symptomatic child. Most adults when undergoing acute ligation of the subclavian artery develop ischemic symptoms and therefore ligation alone is not tolerated as in the pediatric population.[22] Revascularization can most easily be accomplished by right-sided carotid-subclavian transposition or bypass through a supraclavicular incision. A cross-over bypass from the left carotid, subclavian, or axillary arteries can also be used when the right carotid is inadequate.

Open surgical correction of an aneurysmal aberrant right subclavian artery is usually approached through a median sternotomy or left thoracotomy. The artery is divided at its origin and the aneurysmal section is excised. The necessity for and method of right subclavian revascularization proceeds as above. Aneurysmal dilation of the aortic arch involving the aberrant right subclavian artery may require arch replacement under hypothermic circulatory arrest.

HYBRID/ENDOVASCULAR OPTIONS

Several hybrid procedures utilizing endovascular techniques have been described in the treatment of aneurysmal aberrant right subclavian arteries. These techniques involve coverage of the orifice of the right subclavian artery and endovascular occlusion of the artery just proximal to the right vertebral.[23] An Amplatzer septal occluder (AGA Medical Corp, Golden Valley, MN) or Zenith iliac plug (Cook Inc, Bloomington, IN) are among the products that can also be used for endovascular occlusion after ostial coverage. Revascularization of the subclavian artery proceeds as described in the earlier section, most often through a supraclavicular incision. Totally endovascular management has been reported in the case of an aneurysmal subclavian treated with a PTFE-covered stent. Patency was maintained in the vessel and no additional revascularization was required.[24]

When aneurysmal dilation of an aberrant subclavian artery leads to dysphagia or airway symptoms, aneurysm exclusion may allow the aneurysm to shrink and symptoms to improve. Persistence of symptoms after aneurysm isolation may require open intervention with resection or decompression of the artery.

CONCLUSIONS

Aberrant right subclavian artery is the most common aortic arch anomaly. Most patients are asymptomatic, but may have concomitant anomalies. Dysphagia and aneurysmal degeneration are the most common indications requiring intervention. A thorough understanding of the anatomy is prerequisite to intervention while open, endovascular, and hybrid options are available.

REFERENCES

1. Stone WM, Ricotta JJ 2nd, Fowl RJ, et al. Contemporary management of aberrant right subclavian arteries. *Ann Vasc Surg.* 2011;25(4):508–14.
2. Congdon E. Transformation of the aortic-arc system during the development of the human embryo. *Contrib Embryol Carnegie Inst Wash.* 1922;14:65–10.
3. Myers PO, Fasel JHD, Kalangos A, et al. Arteria lusoria: Developmental anatomy, clinical, radiological and surgical aspects. *Annales de Cardiologie et d'Angeiologie.* 2010; 59:147–54.
4. *The Developing Human: Clinically Oriented Embryology.* 9th edition. By K. L. Moore. Philadelphia, London: W. B. Saunders. 2013
5. Edwards JE. Congenital malformations of the heart and great vessels. Section H. Malformations of the thoracic aorta. In: Gould SE, ed. *Pathology of the heart.* 2nd ed. Springfield (IL): Charles C. Thomas 1960. p. 391–462.
6. Harms J, Vogel T, Ennker J, et al. Diagnostic evaluation and surgical management of the aberrant right subclavian artery. *Bildgebung* 1994;61:299–303.
7. Kommerell BF. Verlagerung des oesophagus durch eine abnorm verlaufende arteria subclavia dextra (arteria lusoria). *Forstschr Geb Roetgenstr.* 1936;54:590–95.
8. Epstein DA, Debord JR. Abnormalities associated with aberrant right subclavian arteries – a case report. *Vasc Endovasc Surg.* 2002;36(4):297–303.
9. Salomonowitz E, Edwards JE, Hunter DW, et al. The three types of aortic diverticula. *Am J Roentgenol.* 1984;142(4):673–79.

10. Zapata H, Edwards JE, Titus JL. Aberrant right subclavian artery with left aortic arch: associated cardiac anomalies. *Pediatr Cardiol.* 1993;14(3):159–61.

11. Avisse C, Marcus C, Delattre JF, et al. Right non-recurrent inferior laryngeal nerve and arteria lusoria: the diagnostic and therapeutic implications of an anatomic anomaly. Review of 17 cases. *Surg Radiol Anat.* 1998;20:227–32.

12. Chaoui R, Heling K, Sarioglu N, et al. Aberrant right subclavian artery as a new cardiac sign in second- and third-trimester fetuses with Down syndrome. *Am J Obstet Gynaecol.* 2005;192: 257–63.

13. Bakker D, Berger R, Witsenburg M, et al. Vascular rings: A rare cause of common respiratory symptoms. *Acta Paediatr.* 1999;88:947–52.

14. Carrizo GJ, Marjani MA. Dysphagia lusoria caused by an aberrant right subclavian artery. *Tex Heart Inst J.* 2004;31:168–71.

15. Hardy JD. Aneurysm of aberrant right subclavian artery and Ondine's curse. *J Thorac Cardiovasc Surg.* 1989;97:319–20.

16. Guzzetta PC, Newman KD, Ceithaml E. Successful management of aberrant subclavian artery-esophageal fistula in an infant. *Ann Thorac Surg.* 1989;47:308–09.

17. Gross RE, Ware PF. The surgical significance of aortic arch anomalies. *Surg Gynecol.* 1946 (Oct);83:435–48.

18. Lunde R, Sanders E, Hoskam JA. Right aortic arch symptomatic in adulthood. *Neth J Med.* 2002; 60:212–15.

19. Hara M, Satake M, Itoh M, et al. Radiographic findings of aberrant right subclavian artery initially depicted on CT. *Radiat Med.* 2003;21:161–65.

20. Chaoui R, Heling KS, Sarioglu N, et al. Aberrant right subclavian artery as a new cardiac sign in second- and third-trimester fetuses with Down syndrome. *Am J Obstet Gynecol.* 2005;192:257–63.

21. Kieffer E, Bahnini A, Koskas F. Aberrant subclavian artery: Surgical treatment in thirty-three adult patients. *J Vasc Surg.* 1994;19:100–11.

22. Gross RE. Surgical treatment for dysphagia lusoria. *Ann Surg.* 1946;124:532–34.

23. Morris ME, Benjamin M, Gardner GP, et al. The use of the amplatzer plug to treat dysphagia lusoria caused by an aberrant right subclavian artery. *Ann Vasc Surg.* 2010; 24(3):416,e5–8.

24. Davidian M, Kee ST, Kato N, et al. Aneurysm of an aberrant right subclavian artery: Treatment with PTFE covered stentgraft. *J Vasc Surg.* 1998;28(2):335–39.

47

Neurogenic Thoracic Outlet Syndrome: Best Practice

Jason T. Lee, MD

Neurogenic thoracic outlet syndrome (TOS) is used to describe a wide variety of patient presentations, often encountered several months or even years after blunt trauma to the cervicobrachial region and presents both a diagnostic and treatment dilemma for practitioners. Upper extremity discomfort is noted by patients in posttraumatic situations, as well as work-related overuse injury and repetitive motion athletic injury. These patients are often referred with the request to "rule out thoracic outlet syndrome." First coined in 1956 by Peet et al, TOS can be categorized as vascular (arterial or venous) or neurogenic (nTOS).[1] While vascular-related TOS pathology is intuitively easier to understand and document due to more definitive imaging findings and symptoms, there remains significant controversy as to even the existence of nTOS.[2,3]

The anatomic issue in TOS occurs due to compression of the neurovascular bundle (the brachial plexus, subclavian artery, and subclavian vein) at the transition between the neck and axilla just above the first rib. Neurogenic TOS is much more common than vascular TOS, with most single-center series reporting ratios of twenty to one. Symptoms of nTOS referable to the upper extremity occur because of compression of the lower trunk of the brachial plexus due to a cervical rib or band and enlarged scalene muscles. Classically described or "true" nTOS with strict diagnostic criteria was outlined by Gilliatt et al in 1970,[4] but unfortunately, most reported series of nTOS to date rarely meet these criteria. Symptoms typically include arm discomfort, paresthesias of the inner surface of the hand and forearm, and weakness and atrophy of the thenar and intrinsic hand muscles of the affected side. Distinct anatomic and electrophysiologic findings include low compound muscle action potentials in the thenar and intrinsic muscles, abnormal sensory conduction of the ulnar nerve, prolonged F-wave latency of the ulnar nerve, and abnormal sensory conduction of the medial antebrachial cutaneous nerve.

Because these criteria are rarely documented in most patients referred for nTOS, Wilbourn introduced the phrase "disputed" or nonspecific nTOS (NnTOS),[3] which is not often referred to as such, and in fact, in most of the vascular surgery literature we use interchangeably the phrases nTOS and NnTOS. The controversy in the diagnostic workup for patients with suspected nTOS emanates from the fact that the presentation can be varied and overlaps with many other musculoskeletal issues of the upper extremities. Patients will typically have a history of a hyperextension neck injury such as whiplash from an automobile accident or a fall to the floor. Also very common is a work-related injury caused by repetitive movements.[5] Predisposing anatomic factors to nTOS include cervical ribs, anomalous first ribs, and congenitally narrowed scalene triangles. Another common presentation is athletes with repetitive upper limb movements including swimmers, divers, water polo players, rowers, baseball pitchers, and football quarterbacks.[6] Certainly, this very heterogeneous group of presenting patients will have a wide differential diagnosis, including and not limited to cubital and carpal tunnel syndromes, myofascial pain syndromes, and spinal stenosis.[7]

The evaluation when considering nTOS begins with a thorough history and physical examination, trying to elicit the exact nature of discomfort, paresthesias, and disability in the patient. An accurate physical examination documents whether certain nerves or nerve roots are involved. Roos and Adson tests as well as the simple straight-arm raise test are particularly helpful as the provocative positioning eliciting symptomatology or a change in the pulse is can be quite reproducible. The combination of any of the maneuvers that bring about symptoms or pulse dropouts are not very sensitive but can be quite specific in that not having any positive signs makes it unlikely that nTOS is the correct diagnosis.

Often overlooked and poorly documented in the literature is how these conditions disable people from activities of daily living. While we may ask and even write in the chart spontaneous comments about patients' limitations, the lack of a validated and objective measure makes follow-up and comparisons difficult. Some recent work uses standardized quality of life questionnaires, notably the QuickDASH (Disabilities of the Arm, Shoulder, and Hand) (QD) outcome measure, which generates a score that ranges from 0 to 100, with 100 indicating maximal disability, and that was initially developed and ultimately validated for upper extremity disorders and their surgical treatments.[8] The Johns Hopkins vascular group has applied this outcome measure to their large series of patients after thoracic outlet decompression of all types and found that the score correlates well with SF-36 surveys (which measure general health-related quality of life) and documents significant improvement after surgery.[9] We used a mini-QD score to document improvement in our series of 93 patients treated in the past decade.[10]

After the initial consultation, inventory of symptoms, accurate physical examination, and completion of the baseline QuickDASH survey, a multitude of radiographic tests can be ordered. Many patients in a referral practice have already had MRI or CT-Angiogram of the shoulder, since these patients are seen first to rule out musculoskeletal tears or neck pathology. Again, to reiterate the lack of sensitive radiographic findings for nTOS, the findings are often negative. Duplex imaging of the upper extremity is useful in assuring no venous component is present and is fairly sensitive and specific for arterial or venous involvement. We order for all nTOS patients a duplex using arterial digit plethysmography, which can document with provocative maneuvers the obliteration of waveforms suggestive of a narrowed thoracic outlet. This information can be useful when taken in the context of the entire diagnostic evaluation and has been found to be associated when present with improved outcome for surgery involving nTOS.[10]

The immediate treatment after initial consultation is always physical therapy. Conservative management is a safe and appropriate approach, and patients should be encouraged to exhaust all non-operative methods prior to undergoing surgery. In fact, Landry et al. described no significant difference at a mean of over 4 years after evaluation for nTOS in patients undergoing surgical treatment versus observational therapy.[11] The UCLA vascular surgery group who have taken an aggressive approach to surgical management has documented somewhat high long-term failure rates with surgery for nTOS, with only about one-half of patients after surgery who showed sustained improvement by 18 months postoperatively.[7] Subset analysis in these series and others have found poor predictors of long-term success to include worker's compensation cases,[12] duration of symptoms >2 years, and previous operations.

Given the unknown long-term issues with such an aggressive surgical approach, we believe a highly-selective algorithm is most useful for deciding on which patients can undergo operative management.[10] Our practice initially prescribes a two-three month trial of conservative management based on comprehensive physical therapy, preferably the TOS-specific algorithms described by Peter Edgelow.[13] Conservative measures also include relaxation/stretching exercises, biofeedback, muscle relaxants, analgesics, and anti-inflammatory medications. The Edgelow protocol focuses on breathing, relaxation, posture, and positioning to relieve stress on the narrowed thoracic outlet. Different protocols have been described that try to alleviate strain imparted to the neck region.

Upon returning for consultation after three months of conservative treatment, we then verify the patient has completed a satisfactory number of physical therapy visits. The number of visits to physical therapy often ranges from two visits total to two visits per week for the previous 12 weeks. We believe part of the success of surgical intervention relies upon postoperative physical therapy, and therefore commitment to the program preoperatively might indicate the patient's willingness to continue with physical therapy after surgery and maximize the likelihood of an improved outcome. At this three-month follow-up visit, the patient repeats the QuickDASH survey, and the next step in therapy is based on the change in score as well as the patient's subjective feelings. The Stanford protocol for deciding who should be offered surgery includes those that improve on their physical therapy regimen by a documented decrease in their QuickDASH disability score (Figure 47-1).

Based on our results, we therefore believe that those patients who show modest improvement with PT are the most likely to have some benefit from surgical decompression.[10] What is difficult to determine is the amount of time that PT should still be recommended until deciding when to operate. Most of the patients we eventually operated on from 2–4 months after initiation of PT had stagnated in their improvement, and continued to show disability (evidenced by relatively high QD scores still in 30s). The Edgelow protocol for TOS-specific PT relies on posture and breathing exercises that mimic surgical decompression. This concept is similar to the idea espoused by the UCLA group that pre-op response to Botox injection of the scalene muscle also predicts surgical success.[14] It is unlikely, though, we will have the perfect pre-op predictor of success for all patients, and again underlines the challenges of treating patients with nTOS.

Surgical approaches are varied in the literature, from transaxillary to paraclavicular to our preferred approach, the standard supraclavicular incision. Once through the platysma muscle, the clavicular head of the sternocleidomastoid muscle is transected.

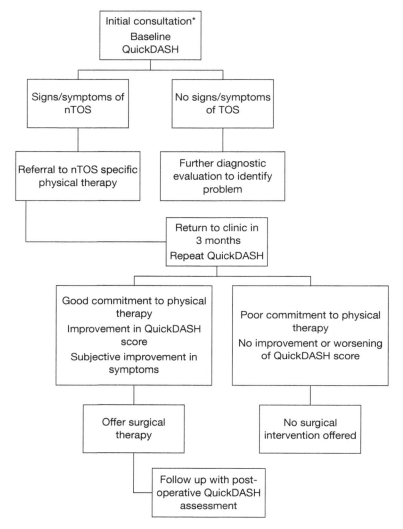

*Initial consultation includes history and physical exam, duplex ultrasound and occasionally other imaging studies such as MRI or CI. Duplex ultrasound is done with arterial plethysmography, which can document with provocative maneuvers the obliteration of waveforms suggestive of a narrowed thoracic outlet.

Figure 47-1. Stanford algorithm for workup and treatment of patients with suspected neurogenic thoracic outlet syndrome.

The anterior scalene fat pad is reflected superiorly, revealing the anterior scalene muscle and the phrenic nerve, which must be preserved and protected with a vessel loupe. The lymphatic ducts are carefully identified and suture ligated or cauterized with the aid of bipolar scissors. The anterior scalene muscle is released from the anterior surface of the first rib. The subclavian artery is identified, freed, and also encircled with a vessel loupe. This usually requires division of some side branches, including the thyrocervical trunk, to allow free mobilization of the artery. More laterally, the brachial plexus is identified. Many times, interdigitating fibers of the middle scalene weave their way through this area, and this contributes to the pathology. Sometimes, a cervical band pinches the brachial plexus. Most of the time, a prominent and flattened lateral part of the first rib is particularly compressing the brachial plexus. A clear silastic loupe is used to isolate and protect the brachial plexus, with the long thoracic nerve in the most lateral portion sometimes seen. The rib is cleaned from the posterior portion where the middle scalene fibers are taken down, and the rib is taken anteriorly, immediately below the subclavian and jugular vein confluence. A power saw with a mini-blade aids in the accurate transection of the rib, and the procedures is concluded after checking for pneumothorax or lymphatic leak after the rib is removed. This supraclavicular approach facilitates easy anatomic viewing of the structures in question and is cosmetically reasonable. Most operations take approximately 60 to 90 minutes, depending on the depth of the rib under the muscle and clavicle. The patient is observed on the postoperative floor overnight after a chest radiograph has been performed in the recovery room. Physical therapy, particularly range-of-motion exercises, is initiated immediately postoperatively, and the patient typically goes home the following day. Follow-up is in two to three weeks for a wound check and in six to eight weeks for a full symptom inventory and repeat QuickDASH questionnaire. Repeat visits are often made at six months and annually thereafter.

Improvement seen after surgery is best documented by objective measures of quality of life surveys, much like the miniQD score. In our experience, we have noted a significant trend towards improvement in overall upper extremity function in 90% of the patients up to one-year followup (Figure 47-2). These results from our highly-selective algorithm have given us confidence we can help certain patients with nTOS. Other studies have assessed long-term outcomes and attempted to determine predictors of success. Most have used subjective outcomes or non-validated tools [15-18] Reported negative predictors of surgical success for nTOS surgery have included poorly

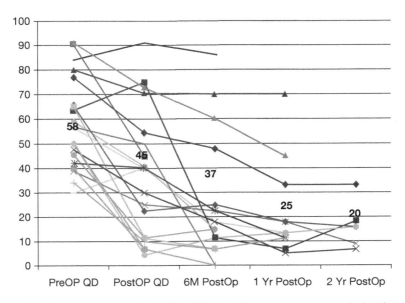

Figure 47-2. Individual improvement in QuickDASH (QD) disability scores among surgical patients (n = 21) in PERIOD 2 (100 indicates maximal disability) All patients (100%) reached 6-month follow-up with QD scoring, 12 (57.1%) had 12-month QD scores, and 6 (28.6%) reached 24-month QD scores. Mean # of post op surveys per patient was 2.8.

systematized neurological symptoms, extended resection of the first rib, severe post-operative complications, workers compensation cases, duration of symptoms >2 years and previous operations.[18–20] Axelrod et al. demonstrated an association between psychological and social factors (such as depression, marital status and education) on outcomes after operative decompression.[21] This may actually be another reason why our selective treatment algorithm may be effective in predicting outcomes, as the requirement of compliance with physical therapy and follow-up may select out patients with such comorbidities.

In summary, the diagnosis of nTOS is mainly clinical. Many other musculoskeletal and orthopedic conditions need to be ruled out, and patients need to understand that surgical outcomes currently are poorly reported without standardized guidelines. That said, surgery when performed by an experienced surgeon is safe and will rarely make symptoms worse. The holy grail of surgery for nTOS is selecting the patients who will have significant benefit. We have documented with up to two-year follow-up excellent results in up to 90% of operated patients a best-practice algorithm for surgical treatment of nTOS that includes the identification of appropriate findings on history and physical examination, demonstration of obliteration of waveforms on arterial duplex plethysmography that suggests the thoracic outlet is narrowed, a high baseline QuickDASH score, a sustained effort to undergo TOS-specific physical therapy for two to three months, and improvement after physical therapy documented subjectively and by improvement in the QuickDASH score. Continued improvement over the long-term and other groups adopting such algorithms to help decide which patients will benefit from operative decompression will be the necessary evidence required to allow patients and practitioners make the most informed decisions about treatment for neurogenic thoracic outlet syndrome.

REFERENCES

1. Peet RM, Henriksen JD, Anderson TP. Thoracic-outlet syndrome: evaluation of a therapeutic exercise program. *Mayo Clin Proc* 1956;31:281–287.
2. Roos DB. The thoracic outlet syndrome is underrated. *Arch Neurol.* 1990;47:327–328.
3. Wilbourn A. The thoracic outlet syndrome is overdiagnosed. *Arch Neurol.* 1990;47:328–330.
4. Gilliatt RW, Le Quesne PM, Logue V, et al. Wasting of the hand associated with a cervical rib or band. *J Neurol Neurosurg Psychiatry.* 1970;33:615–624.
5. Sanders RJ, Hammond SL, Rao NM. Thoracic outlet syndrome: a review. *Neurologist.* 2008;14:365–373.
6. Richardson AB. Thoracic outlet syndrome in aquatic athletes. *Clin Sports Med.* 1999;18:361–378.
7. Altobelli GG, Kudo T, Haas BT, et al. Thoracic outlet syndrome: Pattern of clinical success after operative decompression. *J Vasc Surg.* 2005;42:122–128.
8. Dorcas E. Beaton, James G. Wright, Jeffrey N. Katz and The Upper Extremity Collaborative Group. *J Bone Joint Surg.* 2005;87:1038–1046.
9. Chang DC, Rotellini-Coltvet LA, Mikherjee D, et al. Surgical treatment for thoracic outlet syndrome improves patient's quality of life. *J Vasc Surg.* 2009;49:630–637.
10. Chandra V, Olcott C, Lee JT. Early results of a highly selective algorithm for surgery on patients with neurogenic thoracic outlet syndrome. *J Vasc Surg.* 2011;54:1698–1705.
11. Landry GJ, Moneta GL, Taylor LM, et al. Long-term functional outcome of neurogenic thoracic outlet syndrome in surgically and conservatively treated patients. *J Vasc Surg.* 2001; 33:312–319.

12. Goff CD, Parent FN, Sato DT, et al. A comparison of surgery for neurogenic thoracic outlet syndrome between laborers and nonlaborers. *Am J Surg*. 1998;176:215–218.
13. Edgelow PI. Neurovascular consequences of cumulative trauma disorders affecting the thoracic outlet: A patient centered treatment approach. In: Donatelli, R (ed.) Physical Therapy of the Shoulder- 3rd ed. Churchill Livingston, New York, 1997.
14. Jordan SE, Ahn SS, Freischlag JA, et al. Selective botulinum chemodenervation of the scalene muscles for treatment of neurogenic thoracic outlet syndrome. *Ann Vasc Surg*. 2000; 14(4):365–369.
15. Sharp WJ, Nowak LR, Zamani T, et al. Long-term follow-up and patient satisfaction after surgery for thoracic outlet syndrome. *Ann Vasc Surg*. 2001;15(1):32–36.
16. Bhattacharya V, Hansrani M, Wyatt MG, et al. Outcome following surgery for thoracic outlet syndrome. *Eur J Vasc Endovasc Surg*. 2003;26(2):170–175.
17. Rochkind S, Shemesh M, Patish H, et al. Thoracic outlet syndrome: a multidisciplinary problem with a perspective for microsurgical management without rib resection. *Acta Neurochir*. Suppl 2007;100:145–147.
18. Degeorges R, Reynaud C, Becquemin J. Thoracic outlet syndrome surgery: long-term functional results. *Ann Vasc Surg*. 2004;18(5):558–565.
19. Goff CD, Parent FN, Sato DT, et al. A comparison of surgery for neurogenic thoracic outlet syndrome between laborers and nonlaborers. *Am J Surg*. 1998; 176(2):215–218.
20. Yavuzer S, Atinkaya C, Tokat O. Clinical predictors of surgical outcome in patients with thoracic outlet syndrome operated on via transaxillary approach. *Eur J Cardiothorac Surg*. 2004;25(2):173–178.
21. Axelrod DA, Proctor MC, Geisser ME, et al. Outcomes after surgery for thoracic outlet syndrome. *J Vasc Surg*. 2001;33(6):1220–1225.

48

Venous Thoracic Outlet Syndrome: Best Practice

Brandon W. Propper, MD and Julie A. Freischlag, MD

Thoracic outlet syndrome (TOS) is a term used to describe compression of one or more of the neurovascular structures as they exit a narrow aperture from the chest to the upper extremity. Classically, each syndrome presents following compression of one of three structures: subclavian artery (aTOS), subclavian vein (vTOS), or the brachial plexus (nTOS). Of the three, neurogenic is the most common, comprising more than 80% of cases. Venous compression accounts for 3% of TOS cases. This chapter will focus on the current management of vTOS.

Venous TOS is also known by three other names: Paget-Schroetter syndrome, axillo-subclavian vein thrombosis, or effort thrombosis. James Paget, a British surgeon, is credited with connecting venous thrombosis and arm swelling, while Leopold Von Schroetter linked the syndrome clinically to thrombosis of the axillary and subclavian veins. Peet initiated the term "Thoracic outlet syndrome" in 1956, in which he described exercise programs for treatment of compression syndromes. This is currently thought of as the first formal recommendation for physical therapy.[1] Ten years later, Roos published his experience with first rib resection via the transaxillary approach,[2] and this continues to be the procedure of choice for a large portion of the surgical community.

ANATOMY

The thoracic outlet can be thought of as a triangle with the apex of the triangle pointed toward the manubrium.[3] The first rib forms the lower border of the triangle and the clavicle marks the superior border. The medial connection, or the triangle apex, is the costoclavicular ligament (Figure 48-1). Exiting the triangle in the upper chest are the subclavian vein and artery and the brachial plexus. Moving anterior to posterior within the thoracic outlet the first structure encountered is the tendon of the subclavious muscle. This tendon inserts on the first rib and the muscle is attached to the inferior surface of the clavicle. Moving posterior, is the subclavian vein. Compression by the subclavious tendon can also be identified

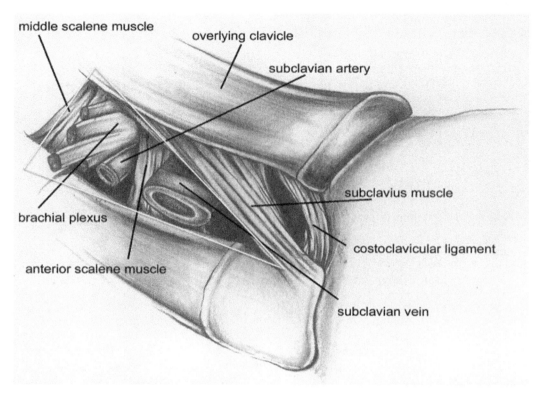

Figure 48-1. The thoracic outlet anatomy and thoracic outlet triangle.

when the angle between the fist rib and clavicle is acute. Separating the subclavian artery and vein is the anterior scalene muscle. The inferior portion of the muscle inserts on a small tubercle on the first rib and rises between the artery and vein into the neck. Identifying this structure is critical to performing surgical resection. Just posterior to the anterior scalene is the subclavian artery followed by the nerve roots of the brachial plexus. The superior nerve roots are formed from C4–C6, while C7–T1 roots are oriented inferiorly. The final structure encountered posterior lateral to the nerve root is the middle scalene muscle. The pleura is not part of the thoracic outlet, but worth noting as it is encountered posterior to the first rib. Understanding the relationship of these structures allows for safe surgical resection.

Special anatomic consideration is given to those with cervical ribs. Autopsy studies reveal that only 0.5% of the population has a cervical rib[4]; however, in population studies of TOS patients the incidence is higher. The rib can be fully developed or rudimentary. When present, subclavian artery is the structure most commonly affected, and only in rare occasions does a cervical rib cause true vTOS.

PRESENTATION AND PATHOPHYSIOLOGY

Venous compression typically presents in an otherwise healthy patients. The classic patient is young and involved in some sort of athletic endeavor or occupation that requires repetitive motion of the upper extremity. Examples include, swimming, baseball pitchers, weight lifting, and auto mechanics. Unlike arterial or neurogenic syndromes, vTOS presentation is acute and often dramatic. The patient notices swelling and color changes (rubor or cyanosis) of the upper extremity and medical attention is sought out early. The physician must be careful not to confuse the rubor with infection, as this can lead to a delay in treatment. If left untreated, arm swelling will usually resolve over a period of time as the body develops more substantial collateralization, but patients will not be able to perform physical activity without easy fatigue and swelling. Left untreated, venous hypertension and post thrombotic syndrome can ensue, although drastic changes such as phlegmasia are very uncommon with vTOS.

WORK UP AND TREATMENT

Given that presentation is acute, treatment should not be delayed. We recommend early treatment with intravenous heparin. During the initial lab draw a hypercoagulable work up should be initiated. It is worth noting that only 8% of patients with vTOS have a prothrombotic disorder, and extrinsic venous compression is far more common. In addition to lab work, initial testing should include chest radiographs to evaluate for a cervical rib and duplex ultrasonography. On duplex, evaluation should be conducted with the arm adducted, then repeated in abduction. When compression is present, "stressed" positioning (90 degree abduction) can help elucidate flow changes. Thus, full abduction will result in a decline in venous flow. Our practice uses absence of venous flow with abduction as diagnostic of venous compression.

Kunkel and Machleder published extensively on the safe use of thrombolysis as the initial treatment to a staged multidisciplinary approach ending in rib resection.[5–7] This has been widely accepted and modified by others.[8] Timing to surgical resection is highly varied among institutions. Previously, Machleder had advocated for a three-month delay in surgery to allow for intimal healing. This philosophy was widely adopted by many, although a subset of surgeons continued to practice urgent surgical intervention. Other more recent reports by have favored an "emergent" approach, utilizing thrombolysis and immediate surgery.[8,9] Most institutions have moved away from long delays prior to surgery. Our practice pattern has favored an individualized algorithm based on patient presentation. Largely patients fit into one of four treatment pathways that can be tailored for optimal treatment. Our multiple treatment algorithms are summarized below:[10]

The first group of patients included those with an acute thrombosis. These patients were treated with lysis initially and early transaxillary resection. All patients in the first group we discharged on low molecular weight heparin and had follow up venogram with venoplasty as needed at 2 weeks. Anticoagulation was continued until vein patency was achieved. Long-term follow up revealed that all of the veins were patent by 7 months.

The second group of patients included those with symptoms and a stenotic subclavian vein who were referred from outside institutions. This group had the initial event at varying times, but did not include acute presentation. The average time to presentation at our hospital was 22 weeks. These patients underwent rib resection with initiation of low molecular weight heparin followed by venogram at two weeks. Venoplasty was employed as needed and anticoagulation was continued until patency of the subclavian vein was present. At follow up venogram one third of the patients were open and anticoagulation was stopped. The other two thirds required venoplasty. Of those that required venoplasty, 92% were off anticoagulation with patent veins at three months.

The third group included those patients whom had intermittent occlusion but did not have thrombosis. These patients presented with life style limiting symptoms. Rib resection was accomplished and no anticoagulation was started unless duplex demonstrated stenosis or thrombosis. A quarter of these patients had residual symptoms or swelling post operatively and underwent venogram and venoplasty. This was successful and all patients were symptom free at follow up.

The final group included patients that presented with occluded subclavian veins months or years post initial event. This group was treated with transaxillary resection and venogram at two weeks. Anticoagulation was continued until vein patency was demonstrated by duplex. At six months 80% of group 4 had a patent subclavian vein. In our experience this multiple treatment algorithm has proved successful and 95% of our patients treated using this algorithm were patent and symptoms free at 10 month follow up.[10]

While establishing treatment algorithms has proved successful, the most important benchmark for vTOS is long term patency. Many groups has established multimonth follow up, but true long term follow up data was lacking. Using two week venography and repeated duplex remains the preferred method to evaluate the early response to rib resection and overall long term venous remodeling.

In our recent experience, 84 patients were identified over a six-year period.[11] The group consisted of 42 men and 42 women. The patient's clinical course was based on their initial presentation to our hospital and guided by the previously discussed algorithms. To gain additional information about long term patency, each patient underwent venography at two weeks. Venoplasty was used if a stenotic vein was encountered (Figure 48-2). Subsequently, each patient had venous duplex evaluation at 6 month intervals to assess for venous patency and the need for anticoagulation. Average follow up for the group was 22 months, which remains the longest follow up for a large group of vTOS patients undergoing transaxillary resection. A quarter of the patients had a patent vein on two week venography and follow up duplex showed continued patency long term. As such, patients that have a patent subclavian vein are not continued on anticoagulation.

The largest group of patients (55) had a stenotic subclavian vein on two week venography. Long term, 3 of the 55 patients had residual stenosis or clot, and only one patient had symptoms. Repeat imaging occurred at intervals of about six months and these three patients had additional dilation procedures that occurred at 27, 34, and

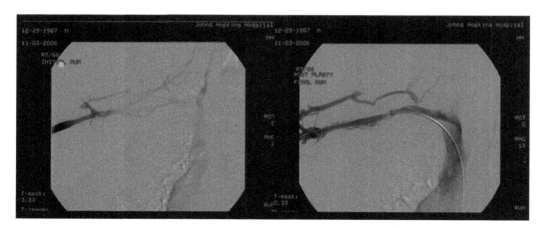

Figure 48-2. Stenotic subclavian vein and subclavian vein after venoplasty.

54 months post surgery. All were maintained on anticoagulation. Overall, 95% of those with a stenotic vein at two weeks were ultimately patent and off anticoagulation.[11]

Sixteen patients had a chronic occlusion at two weeks, and no intervention was performed. Anticoagulation was continued, and at six month follow-up 14(88%) recannalized.[11]

Since 2007 our practiced has matured and the treatment for acute presentation has been modified. Although widely accepted, our practice has moved away for pre-operative venography, venoplasty and thrombolysis. Our review has documented equivalent 16-month patency following rib resection in patients irrespective of early percutaneous intervention.[12] Given our referral base and wide array of patient presentation, we sought to compare those with pre-operative intervention to those with anticoagulation. A total of 45 patients undergoing pre-operative endovascular intervention were evaluated in addition to 65 patients whom were treated with just anticoagulation in the pre-operative period. At one year follow up both the intervention group (41/45) and anticoagulation group (59/65) had 91% venous patency with symptomatic improvement. Given that the anticoagulation group had equivalent one-year patency we prefer early transition to enoxaparin and avoidance of the potential complications and cost associated with thrombolysis.

One additional benefit to adopting this treatment paradigm has been shorter hospital stays and decreased cost. Earlier in the experience it was common for patient to spend three to four days in the hospital. While undergoing thrombolysis, patients were kept in the intensive care unit. With early transition to enoxaparin the current typical hospital stay is one night with planned surgical resection. We schedule surgery 2–4 weeks following initial discharge. This allows time for arm swelling to resolve, but does not create a large time interval between presentation and surgery. Patients prefer this approach as surgery can be scheduled at their convenience, without any adverse outcomes. As our experience continues to grow it continues to have change to maximize patient outcome. Our current treatment algorithm can be viewed in Figure 48-3.

Adolescent patients represent another group that requires specific forethought and consideration. As more children become involved in competitive athletics the strenuous workouts and repetitive motions elucidate those with venous compression. Specific sports of interest include swimming, baseball, softball, volleyball and weight lifting, as there is frequent repetitive motion and rigorous training. In this patient population, long term anticoagulation limits extracurricular activities and can be difficult for parents and adolescents to stay compliant.

We evaluated our experience from 2004–2010 to gain perspective on what can be expected in the younger patient.[13] This group includes 37 patients whom presented with a variety of TOS between ages 10–17. In this group, 17 patients had vTOS. All patients were evaluated and treated based on the Johns Hopkins clinical algorithm as previously discussed. In the adolescent group, two patients were patent at two-week venogram, 13 required dilation and two were chronically occluded. This group averaged 2.5 months of anticoagulation use. Of the two chronically occluded patients, one recannalized at 4 months and the other was diagnosed with Factor V Leyden deficiency and continued on lifelong anticoagulation.[13]

The important point for the adolescent patient is continued follow up and evaluation to eliminate long term anticoagulation use. In this group, two patients were identified to have contralateral asymptomatic venous compression and underwent elective transaxillary resection one year later to avoid future acute presentation.

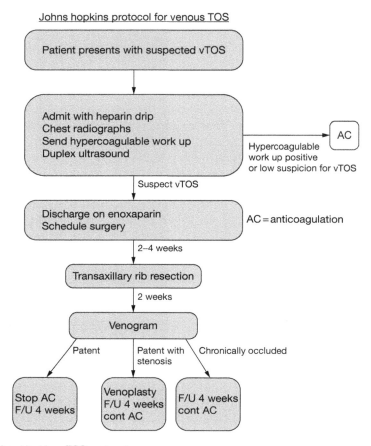

Figure 48-3. Johns Hopkins vTOS protocol.

Overall, adolescent patients respond very well to vTOS treatment and in most patients anticoagulation can be stopped early for return to normal activity.

SURGICAL APPROACH

The surgical approach for rib resection and scalenectomy is largely divided into two groups: trans-axillary resection and supraclavicular approach. For vTOS our practices favors the trans-axillary approach for all initial rib resections and only utilizes the supraclavicular approach for re-do surgery for vTOS.

Prior to the patient moving into the operating room, a conversation is held with anesthesia to ensure that all access is placed on the non-operative arm and that no long-term paralytics are used. Additionally, lighted retractors should be available for surgery. General anesthesia in used and the patient is placed in the lateral position with an axillary roll and beanbag for support. The operative field is prepped including the operative arm using a Machleder retractor (Figure 48-4). An incision is made at the inferior border of the hair baring line between the pectoralis major and latissimus dorsi. Dissection is carried down to the chest wall with care taken to stay above the axillary fat pad. Once the chest wall is encountered the Machleder retractor is raised and blunt dissection is used to identify the anterior scalene, subclavian vein and artery. Blunt dissection of the anterior scalene avoids vascular injury. Following, the first rib is dissected free using a periostial elevator (Figure 48-5). The anterior scalene is transected using multiple passes with a right angle clamp and scissors (Figure 48-5). Care is taken to transect the muscle superiorly, but careful identification of the subclavian artery is necessary as this represents a potential pitfall. With vTOS, the subclavious tendon should be identified and sharply cut from the first rib. This allows for additional freeing of the subclavian vein. At this point the first rib is ready for transection. The rib cutter is placed on the anterior portion of the rib first. Once cut, the rib tends to move superior to allow more visualization posterior. Additional posterior dissection with the periostial elevator is conducted to ensure the posterior curvature of the rib is free from muscle. The rib cutter can be inserted and the rib is cut just anterior to the nerve root. While it is tempting to make transect the rib posterior to the nerve root, this increases the likelihood of nerve injury. The rib specimen is removed. At this point additional rib posterior to the nerve root can be removed using rongeurs. This method allows for excellent visualization of the anterior and posterior rib segments and limits blind transection. In all cases, irrigation is placed into the wound and a valsalva maneuver if performed to evaluate for a pneumothorax. If present, a small chest tube is left in place between the 2nd and 3rd rib. The wound is closed in layers.

The supraclavicular resection can be performed with or without venotomy and venoplasty. The patient is positioned in the semi-Fowler position with the head facing away from the operative side. An incision is made 1–2 cm above the clavicle extending from external jugular vein to the sternocleidomastoid. The omohyoid muscle is divided and the underlying scalene fat pad is mobilized. Care should be taken to

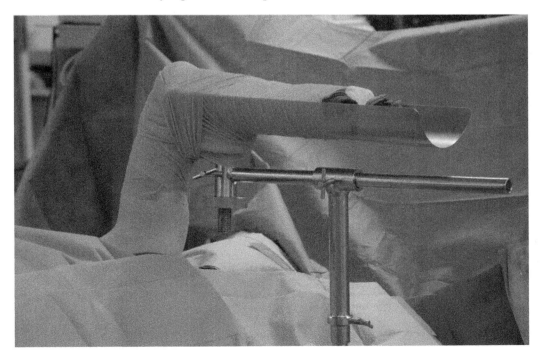

Figure 48-4. Operative photo of arm in the Machleder Retractor.

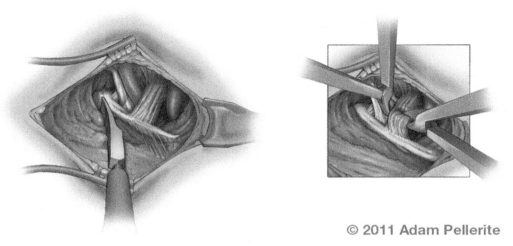

© 2011 Adam Pellerite

Figure 48-5. Removal of muscle off the first rib with periostial elevator and transection of the anterior scalene muscle.

avoid the phrenic nerve underlying the fat pad and anterior to the anterior scalene muscle. On the left hand side, the thoracic duct should be avoided or carefully ligated if in the operative field. The phrenic nerve should be mobilized and protected to expose the underlying anterior scalene. The muscle should be dissected free from the vascular attachments to the subclavian artery, vein and nerve roots. The anterior scalene is then divided close to the insertion on the first rib. At this point the middle scalene is dissected free off the first rib using a periostial elevator, with special attention to the long thoracic nerve to avoid injury. Once cleared of muscle, the first rib can be divided using bone cutters. Some groups favor full mobilization of the subclavian vein and venoplasty using saphenous vein. If this is to be employed the leg should be prepped at the beginning of the case.

In summary, vTOS can be treated with anticoagulation initially and followed by first rib resection and scalenectomy. Early thrombolysis is not necessary. Use of anticoagulation for 1–6 months following rib resection ensures vein patency. Postoperative venography is used at two weeks to evaluate vein patency, selectively dilate, and identify patients in which anticoagulation can be terminated. Children with vTOS can treated effectively.

REFERENCES

1. Peet RM, Hendricksen JD, Anderson TP, et al. Thoracic outlet syndrome: evaluation of the therapeutic exercise program. *Mayo Clin Proc.* 1956;31(28):281–87.
2. Roos DB. Transaxillary approach for first rib resection to relieve thoracic outlet compression syndrome. *Ann Surg.* 1966;163:354.
3. Machleder HI. *Vascular disorders of the upper extremity.* 3rd edition. Mt. Kisco, NY. Futura Press; 1999.
4. Roos DB. Congenital anomalies associated with thoracic outlet syndrome: anatomy, symptoms, diagnosis and treatment. *Am J Surg.* 1976;132:771–8.
5. Kunkel JM, Machleder HI. Treatment of Paget-Schroetter Syndrome. A staged, multidisciplinary approach. *Arch Surg.* 1989;124:1153–8.

6. Machleder HI. Evaluation of a new treatment strategy for Paget-Schroetter Syndrome: spontaneous thrombosis of the axillary subclavian vein. *J Vasc Surg*. 1993;17:305–17.

7. Kunkel JM, Machleder HI. Spontaneous subclavian vein thrombosis: a successful combined approach of local thrombolytic therapy followed by first rib resection. *Surgery*. 1989;106:114.

8. Urschel HC, Razzuk MA. Paget-Schroetter syndrome: what is the best management: *Ann Thorac Surg*. 2000;69:1663–9.

9. Molina EJ, Hunter DW, Dietz CA. Paget-Schroetter Syndrome treated with thrombolytics and immediate surgery. *J Vasc Surg*. 2007;45:328–34.

10. de León RA, Chang DC, Hassoun HT, et al. Multiple treatment algorithms for successful outcomes in venous thoracic outlet syndrome. *Surgery*. 2009 May;145(5):500–7. Epub 2009 Mar 21.

11. Chang KZ, Likes K, Demos J, et al. Routine venography following transaxillary first rib resection and scalenectomy (FRRS) for chronic subclavian vein thrombosis ensures excellent outcomes and vein patency. *Vasc Endovasc Surg*. 2012 Jan;46(1):15–20. Epub 2011 Dec 8.

12. Guzzo JL, Chang K, Demos J, et al. Preoperative thrombolysis and venoplasty affords no benefit in patency following first rib resection and scalenectomy for subacute and chronic subclavian vein thrombosis. *J Vasc Surg*. 2010 Sep;52(3):658–62.

13. Chang K, Graf E, Davis K, et al. Spectrum of thoracic outlet syndrome presentation in adolescents. *Arch Surg*. 2011 Dec;146(12):1383–7.

Index